Tumours of the Central Nervous System in Infancy and Childhood

Edited by

D. Voth P. Gutjahr C. Langmaid

With 136 Figures and 116 Tables

Springer-Verlag Berlin Heidelberg New York 1982

Professor Dr. med. DIETER VOTH, Neurochirurgische Klinik und Poliklinik, Klinikum der Johannes Gutenberg-Universität, Langenbeckstraße 1, D-6500 Mainz

Professor Dr. med. PETER GUTJAHR, Kinderklinik und Kinder-Poliklinik, Klinikum der Johannes Gutenberg-Universität, Langenbeckstraße 1, D-6500 Mainz

Mr. CHARLES LANGMAID, 174, Lake Road East, Roath Park, Cardiff CF2 5NR, South Glam. Wales, Great Britain

ISBN-13: 978-3-642-95415-3 e-ISBN-13: 978-3-642-95413-9
DOI: 10.1007/978-3-642-95413-9

Library of Congress Cataloging in Publication Data
Tumours of the central nervous system in infancy and childhood. Lectures given at a congress, held in Mainz, between 22 and 24 October 1981. 1. Tumours in children–Congresses. 2. Youth–Diseases–Congresses. I. Voth, D. (Dieter), 1935– . II. Gutjahr, P. (Peter), 1945– . III. Langmaid, C. (Charles), 1913– . [DNLM: 1. Brain neoplasms—In infancy and childhood. 2. Spinal cord neoplasms—In infancy and childhood. WL 358 T926] RC281.C4T857 1982 618.92'9928 82-10745

Preface

Tumours of the central nervous system in infancy and childhood show so many diverse pathomorphological characteristics and present so many diagnostic problems that a congress dealing specifically with the subject and thus bringing together a wide range of experts in the field seemed called for. The programme of the congress, held in Mainz between 22 and 24 October 1981, was designed to provide comprehensive coverage of diagnosis and the various therapeutic procedures, as well as of basic research in the field. The various lectures given are contained in this book, which thus reflects the complete spectrum of topics discussed.

The interest generated by the congress amply justified our decision to organize it. Representatives of various specialities, such as neuropathology, paediatrics, oncology, radiology, neurosurgery, paediatric surgery and neurology, and, last but not least, basic research, provided lively and interesting lectures which admittedly raised more problems than they solved. In addition to the actual papers presented, we attached considerable importance to the different opinions voiced during the congress, as reflected in the discussions included at the end of each chapter.

In organizing the congress we were supported by Prof. Dr. J. M. Schröder, Aachen, Prof. Dr. J. Kutzner, Mainz, and Dr. K. Kretzschmar, Mainz; we are very grateful for their help. Our thanks are also due to the publisher, who helped us to edit the congress reports in the form of a monograph. We are extremely hopeful that the book will present those interested with a concise account of "tumours of the central nervous system in infancy and childhood" and provide them with a summary of the present state of knowledge which will form a basis for further investigations.

Mainz – Cardiff THE EDITORS

Contents

Chapter 1 Basic Research and Special Pathology

Intracranial Tumours of Infancy and Childhood. By K. J. Zülch. With 1 Figure and 2 Tables 1

Remarks on the WHO Classification of Tumours of the Central Nervous System. By O. Stochdorph. With 2 Figures 17

Developmental Neuro-Oncogenesis in Experimental Animals. By P. Kleihues, S. Bamborschke, M. Kiessling, and O. Wiestler. With 4 Figures and 1 Table 19

Brain Tumours and Genetics. By J. Spranger. With 4 Figures and 4 Tables . 32

Interferon and Antitumour Effects. By H.-J. Röthig. With 1 Table 42

Rare Intracranial Tumours in Infancy and Childhood. By K. Jellinger and E. Machacek. With 3 Figures and 4 Tables 44

Intracranial and Spinal Tumours in Newborns and Infants. By H. Gerlach, W. Jänisch, and D. Schreiber. With 1 Figure and 4 Tables 53

The Usefulness of Immunocytological Demonstration of Glial Fibrillary Acidic Protein for Diagnostic Problems of Cerebral Tumours. By K. H. H. Merkel, M. Zimmer, W. Wahlen, and E. Schwarz. With 1 Figure and 1 Table 58

CNS Tumours in Infancy, Childhood, and Adolescence. By D. Schreiber, W. Jänisch, and H. Gerlach. With 1 Figure and 5 Tables 62

Congenital Intracranial Teratoma in a Newborn. By H. Klein and J. Klein. With 2 Figures 69

Discussion 72

Chapter 2 Clinical Presentation, Diagnosis, Follow-Up Studies

Clinical Presentation of Space-Occupying Lesions of the Central Nervous System. By G. Jacobi. With 2 Figures and 10 Tables 74

Cytology of Cerebrospinal Fluid in Children with Brain Tumours. By W. Dörffel. With 1 Figure and 2 Tables 85

Electrophysiological Diagnosis and Follow-Up Controls in Cases of Tumours of the Optic Chiasm. By D. Wenzel, D. Harms, U. Brandl, M. Klinger, and F. Albert. With 1 Figure and 2 Tables 90

Electroencephalograms in Long-Term Survivors of Primary Intracranial Tumours of Childhood. By E. Dieterich, B. Goebel, and P. Gutjahr. With 2 Tables 95

Early Auditory Evoked Potentials (EAEP) in Children with Neoplastic Lesions in the Brain Stem. By K. Maurer and M. Rochel. With 4 Figures and 1 Table 99

Conventional Investigations of CNS Tumours in Children. By C. R. Fitz. With 9 Figures and 1 Table 105

Computer Tomographic Diagnosis of CNS Tumours in Childhood. By E. Kazner and K. Kretzschmar. With 4 Figures 115

Radionuclide Imaging of Cerebral Tumours in Children. By K. Hahn. With 2 Figures and 3 Tables 122

Follow-Up Studies of Brain Tumours in Infants and Children. By K. Kretzschmar. With 5 Figures and 3 Tables 130

Computed Tomography and/or Ventriculography? By S. Wende, T. Kishikawa, N. Hüwel, E. Kazner, Th. Grumme, and W. R. Lanksch. With 1 Table 142

Ventriculography as a Diagnostic Procedure in CNS Tumours in Childhood: Its Indications and Interpretation. By H. Altenburg, M. Brandt, and H.-J. König. With 2 Figures 145

The Diffuse Brain Stem Astrocytoma in Childhood: Morphology, Course, and Prognosis. By H. P. Schmitt and W. Zeisner. With 1 Figure and 4 Tables 149

Astrocytoma with Extracranial Metastases. By R. Bubl, H. R. Hirt, H. Ohnacker, and A. Probst 165

Diktyoma (Medulloepithelioma). A Rare Neuro-Epithelial Tumour of the Eye. By G. Knoepfle, U. Bode, R. Hoischen, and H. J. Foedisch. With 2 Figures and 1 Table 169

Intracranial Teratoma of a Newborn. Computer Tomographic and Morphological Findings. By G. Ebhardt, H. Traupe, J. Könner, and L. Goerke. With 3 Figures 174

The Isolated Fourth Ventricle: Review of Current Concepts and Report on Three Cases in Children. By E. Mahlmann, D. Voth, and M. Schwarz. With 2 Figures 180

Follow-Up Findings with CT Scan and Ventriculography After Radiotherapy of Inoperable Midline Tumours in Childhood. By H.-J. König and H. Altenburg. With 1 Figure 186

Discussion 188

Chapter 3 Surgical Treatment

Evolutional, Developmental, and Clinical Aspects of Brain Stem Organisation. By P. Glees. With 9 Figures and 2 Tables 190

Standard Techniques and Microsurgical Procedures in the Removal of Supratentorial and Infratentorial Tumours. By D. Voth. With 9 Figures 199

Additional Operative Procedures (Shunt Systems, Leksell and Torkildsen Drainage). By M. Schwarz and D. Voth 214

The Significance of Continuous Recording of Intracranial Pressure in Children with Brain Tumours. By M. Brock and H.-J. Schmitz. With 2 Figures 218

Preoperative and Postoperative Intensive Care and Oedema Therapy. By J. Otte, P. Emmrich, and G. Meinig. With 1 Figure and 3 Tables . . . 222

Therapy of Peritumoural Brain Oedema. By G. Meinig. With 3 Figures and 1 Table 229

CT-Stereotactic Biopsy of Brain Tumours. By F. Mundinger. With 3 Figures and 3 Tables 234

Diagnostic Potential of Stereotactic Biopsy of Brain Tumours. A Report of 400 Cases. By M. Kiessling, J. Anagnostopoulos, G. Lombeck, and P. Kleihues. With 4 Figures and 5 Tables 247

Internal Shunt or Perioperative Pressure-Controlled Ventricular Fluid Drainage (C-VFD) in Children and Juveniles with Infratentorial Tumours. By K. E. Richard, R. Heller, and R. A. Frowein. With 2 Figures and 3 Tables 257

Indications and Experiences with the Ommaya-Reservoir for Treatment of CNS Neoplasms in Childhood. By K. Roosen, W. Havers, and J. Schaaf. With 3 Figures and 2 Tables 265

Indications for the Trans-Sphenoidal Approach to Craniopharyngioma Operations in Youth and Childhood. By E. Halves and N. Sörensen. With 2 Figures 270

Which Considerations Determine the Choice Between the Subfrontal and Trans-Sphenoidal Approach to Tumours of the Sellar Region in Youth and Childhood? By W. Ischebeck, S. Müller, and W. Braun 276

The Influence of Different Antihypertensive Drugs on Intracranial Pressure. By J. Hidding, C. Puchstein, and H. van Aken. With 2 Figures and 1 Table 278

Ventriculocisternostomy by the Method of Leksell – Indications, Technique, and Results. By D. Voth, K. Schürmann, and M. Schwarz. With 2 Figures 283

Discussion 289

Chapter 4 Radiotherapy

The Radiosensitivity of the Infant Brain. By W. Hinkelbein and M. Wannenmacher. With 4 Figures 291

Radiation Technique and the Planning of Treatment in Brain Tumours in Children. By J. Kutzner. With 3 Figures and 1 Table 301

Experiences with the Treatment of Cystic Craniopharyngiomas by Stereotactically Injected Radioisotopes. By V. Sturm, P. Georgi, H. Netzeband, K. E. Scheer, L. Strauss, W. Schlegel, H. Scharfenberg, H. Sinn, H. Gahbauer, and H. Penzholz. With 2 Figures 310

Radiosurgery in Intracranial Tumours and Arteriovenous Malformations in Children. By L. Steiner. With 3 Figures and 4 Tables 315

Radiation Therapy in the Treatment of the Astrocytomas and Midline Tumours of Childhood. By M. Herbst. With 1 Figure and 4 Tables 325

Radiotherapeutic Principles in the Combined Treatment of CNS Tumours in Children. By M. Bamberg and E. Scherer. With 1 Figure and 3 Tables . . 333

Postoperative Chemotherapy Prior to Radiotherapy in the Combined Treatment of Medulloblastoma, Ependymoma and Tumours of the Pineal Region: Early Results. By H. J. Habermalz, U. Stephani, H. Riehm, and F. Hanefeld. With 3 Figures and 4 Tables 338

Radiotherapy of Medulloblastoma: Radiation Technique, Results, and Complications. By E. A. Bleher, P. G. Poretti, and P. C. Veraguth. With 2 Figures 344

Report on the Medulloblastoma Study of the Society of Paediatric Oncology – Present Position. By M. Neidhardt 349

Data on the Biology of Medulloblastomas. By W. Müller, D. Afra, O. Wilcke, F. Slowik, R. Schröder, and M. Kordas. With 1 Figure and 5 Tables 350

Treatment of Meningeal Malignancy with Intrathecal ^{198}Au-Colloid and Methotrexate. The Example of Acute Lymphoblastic Leukaemia (ALL). By O. Metz. With 2 Figures and 2 Tables 354

Infratentorial Tumours – Treatment and Results in 109 Children. By P. Gutjahr, D. Voth, J. Heidfeld, B. Walther, J. Kutzner, and K. Kretzschmar. With 5 Figures 358

Discussion 365

Chapter 5 Chemotherapy, Late Effects, and After-Treatment

Cytostatic Monotherapy of Tumours of the Central Nervous System in Children. By B. Kornhuber. With 1 Table 367

Rationale of Combined Chemotherapy of Brain Tumours. By J. Hildebrand and D. Zegers de Beyl 374

Acute Toxicity of Chemotherapy of Tumours of the Central Nervous System in Children. By W. Havers. With 1 Table 378

Late Effects After Treatment of Brain Tumours in Childhood. By P. Gutjahr and B. Walther. With 3 Tables 383

Development After Treatment of Cerebellar Medulloblastoma in Childhood. By B. Walther and P. Gutjahr. With 1 Figure and 4 Tables 389

Spongioblastoma in Childhood. Remarks on Problems in Diagnosis and Treatment. By W. Entzian, L. Diaz, and H.-W. Schumacher. With 1 Figure and 3 Tables 399

Medulloblastoma. Relationship of Histologic Type to Survival. By H. Arnold, H. D. Franke, G. Langendorf, R. Olotu, and J. Grosch-Wörner. With 4 Figures 404

Ophthalmological Findings in Long-Term Survivors After Primary Brain Tumours in Childhood. By R. Rochels and Th. Neuhann. With 1 Table . . 410

Endocrinological Investigations in 68 Children with Brain Tumours. By W. Andler, K. Roosen, and H.-E. Clar. With 6 Tables 415

Supratentorial Tumours in Infants and Children. By S. Tiyaworabun, S. Kazkaz, N. Nicola, and M. Schirmer. With 3 Figures and 2 Tables . . . 420

Discussion 426

Final Comments and Summing-Up. By P. Gutjahr and D. Voth 427

Subject Index 433

List of Contributors

Afra, D., Dr. med., National Institute of Neurosurgery, Amerikai út 57, H-1145 Budapest

Aken, H. van, Dr. med., Klinik für Anästhesiologie und Intensivpflege, Universität Münster, Jungeblodtplatz 1, D-4400 Münster

Albert, F., Dr. med., Neurochirurgische Klinik der Universität Erlangen-Nürnberg, Schwabachanlage 6 (Kopfklinikum), D-8520 Erlangen

Altenburg, H., Dr. med., Neurochirurgische Klinik und Poliklinik der Westfälischen Wilhelms-Universität, Jungeblodtplatz 1, D-4400 Münster

Anagnostopoulos, J., Dr. med., Abteilung für Neuropathologie, Ludwig-Aschoff-Haus, Universität Freiburg, Albertstraße 19, D-7800 Freiburg

Andler, W., Dr. med., Kinderklinik, Universitäts-Klinikum der Gesamthochschule Essen, Hufelandstraße 55, D-4300 Essen

Arnold, H., Dr. med., Neurochirurgische Universitätsklinik Hamburg, Martinistraße 52, D-2000 Hamburg 20

Bamberg, M., PD Dr. med., Strahlenklinik am Klinikum der Gesamthochschule Essen, Hufelandstraße 55, D-4300 Essen

Bamborschke, S., Dr. med., Abteilung für Neuropathologie, Ludwig-Aschoff-Haus, Universität Freiburg, Albertstraße 19, D-7800 Freiburg

Bleher, E. A., Dr. med., Institut für Strahlentherapie, Inselspital Bern, CH-3007 Bern

Bode, U., Dr. med., Kinderklinik der Universität Bonn, Sigmund-Freud-Straße 35, D-5300 Bonn-Venusberg

Brandl, U., Dr. med., Kinderklinik der Universität Erlangen-Nürnberg, Krankenhausstraße 12, D-8520 Erlangen

Brandt, M., Dr. med., Neurochirurgische Klinik und Poliklinik der Westfälischen Wilhelms-Universität, Jungeblodtplatz 1, D-4400 Münster

Braun, W., Prof, Dr. med., Abteilung für Neurochirurgie, Krankenhaus Bethesda, Hainstraße 35, D-5600 Wuppertal 1

Brock, M., Prof. Dr. med., Abteilung für Neurochirurgie, Neurochirurgische/Neurologische Klinik und Poliklinik, Universitätsklinikum Steglitz, Freie Universität Berlin, Hindenburgdamm 30, D-1000 Berlin 45

Bubl, R., Dr. med., Kinderklinik, Universität Basel, Römergasse 8, CH-4005 Basel

Clar, H.-E., Prof. Dr. med., Neurochirurgische Universitätsklinik der Gesamthochschule Essen, Hufelandstraße 55, D-4300 Essen

Diaz, L., Dr. med., Neurochirurgische Universitätsklinik, Sigmund-Freud-Straße 25, D-5300 Bonn-Venusberg

Dieterich, E., PD Dr. med., Abteilung für Neuropädiatrie, Universitätskinderklinik, Schwanenweg, D-2300 Kiel

Dörffel, W., Dr. med., II. Kinderklinik, Städtische Klinik Berlin-Buch, Wiltbergstraße 50, DDR-1115 Berlin-Buch

Ebhardt, G., PD Dr. med., Max-Planck-Institut für Hirnforschung Köln-Merheim, Ostmerheimer Straße 200, D-5000 Köln 91

Emmrich, P., Prof. Dr. med., Kinderklinik der Universität Mainz, Langenbeckstraße 1, D-6500 Mainz

Entzian, W., Prof. Dr. med., Neurochirurgische Universitätsklinik, Sigmund-Freud-Straße 25, D-5300 Bonn-Venusberg

Fitz, C. R., Dr. med., Associate Professor of Radiology, Division of Special Procedures, Department of Radiology, Hospital for Sick Children, University of Toronto, 555 University Avenue, Toronto, Ontario, Canada

Foedisch, H. J., Prof. Dr. med., Institut für Kinderpathologie, Universität Bonn, D-5300 Bonn-Venusberg

Franke, H. D., Prof. Dr. med., Klinik für Strahlentherapie, Universitätskrankenhaus Eppendorf, Martinistraße 52, D-2000 Hamburg 20

Frowein, R. A., Prof. Dr. med., Neurochirurgische Universitätsklinik, Joseph-Stelzmann-Straße 9, D-5000 Köln 41

Gahbauer, H., Dr. med., Abteilung für Neuroradiologie, Universitätskliniken, Kirschnerstraße 1, D-6900 Heidelberg

Georgi, P., Prof. Dr. med., Nuklearmedizinische Abteilung, Deutsches Krebsforschungszentrum, Im Neuenheimer Feld 280, D-6900 Heidelberg

Gerlach, H., Dr. med., Institut für Pathologie, Martin-Luther-Universität Halle-Wittenberg, Leninallee 14, DDR-4020 Halle (Saale)

Glees, P., Prof. Dr. med. Dr. phil., Department of Anatomy, University of Cambridge, Downing Street, Cambridge CB 2 DY, Great Britain

Goebel, B., Kinderkrankenschwester, Universitätskinderklinik, Langenbeckstraße 1, D-6500 Mainz

Goerke, L., Dr. med., Max-Planck-Institut für Hirnforschung Köln-Merheim, Ostmerheimer Straße 200, D-5000 Köln 91

Grosch-Wörner, J., Dr. med., Abteilung für Pädiatrische Onkologie, Universitätskliniken Hamburg, Martinistraße 52, D-2000 Hamburg 20

Grumme, Th., Prof. Dr. med., Neurochirurgische Klinik im Klinikum Charlottenburg, Freie Universität Berlin, Spandauer Damm 130, D-1000 Berlin 19

Gutjahr, P., Prof. Dr. med., Kinderklinik und Kinder-Poliklinik, Klinikum der Johannes Gutenberg-Universität, Langenbeckstraße 1, D-6500 Mainz

Habermalz, H. J., Dr. med., Abteilung für Radiologie im Klinikum Charlottenburg, Freie Universität Berlin, Spandauer Damm 130, D-1000 Berlin 19

Hahn, K., Prof. Dr. med., Abteilung für Nuklearmedizin, Johannes Gutenberg-Universität Mainz, Langenbeckstraße 1, D-6500 Mainz

Halves, E., PD Dr. med., Neurochirurgische Klinik, Universität Würzburg, Josef-Schneider-Straße 11, D-8700 Würzburg

Hanefeld, F., Prof. Dr. med., Abteilung für Pädiatrische Neurologie im Klinikum Charlottenburg, Freie Universität Berlin, Spandauer Damm 130, D-1000 Berlin 19

Harms, D., Dr. med., Kinderklinik der Universität Erlangen-Nürnberg, Krankenhausstraße 12, D-8520 Erlangen

Havers, W., Dr. med., Kinderklinik im Universitätsklinikum der Gesamthochschule Essen, Hufelandstraße 55, D-4300 Essen

Heidfeld, J., cand. med., Kinderklinik der Johannes Gutenberg-Universität Mainz, Langenbeckstraße 1, D-6500 Mainz

Heller, R., cand. med., Neurochirurgische Klinik, Universität Köln, Joseph-Stelzmann-Straße 9, D-5000 Köln 41

Herbst, M., Dr. med., Abteilung für Radiotherapie, Universität Erlangen-Nürnberg, Krankenhausstraße 12, D-8520 Erlangen

Hidding, J., Dr. med., Neurochirurgische Klinik der Westfälischen Wilhelms-Universität, Jungeblodtplatz 1, D-4400 Münster

Hildebrand, J., Dr. med., Department of Neurology, Erasme Hospital, Free University of Brussels, Rue Héger-Bordet 1, B-1000 Brussels

Hinkelbein, W., Dr. med., Abteilung für Strahlentherapie, Universität Freiburg, Hugstetter Straße 55, D-7800 Freiburg

Hirt, H. R., Dr. med., Kinderklinik, Universität Basel, Römergasse 8, CH-4005 Basel

Hoischen, R., Dr. med., Abteilung für Mund- und Kiefer-Gesichtschirurgie, Universität Bonn, D-5300 Bonn-Venusberg

Hüwel, N., Dr. med., Abteilung für Neuroradiologie, Johannes Gutenberg-Universität Mainz, Langenbeckstraße 1, D-6500 Mainz

Ischebeck, W., Dr. med., Abteilung für Neurochirurgie, Krankenhaus Bethesda, Hainstraße 35, D-5600 Wuppertal

Jacobi, G., Prof. Dr. med., Abteilung für Pädiatrische Neurologie, Zentrum für Kinderheilkunde, Universität Frankfurt, Theodor-Stern-Kai 7, D-6000 Frankfurt 70

Jänisch, W., Prof. Dr. med., Institut für Pathologie, Rudolf-Virchow-Haus, Humboldt-Universität, DDR-1115 Berlin

Jellinger, K., Prof. Dr. med., L.-Boltmann-Institut für klinische Neurobiologie d. KRH Wien-Lainz, Wolkersbergenstraße 1, A-1130 Wien

Kazkaz, S., Dr. med., Neurochirurgische Klinik, Medizinische Einrichtungen der Universität Düsseldorf, Moorenstraße 5, D-4000 Düsseldorf

Kazner, E., Prof. Dr. med., Neurochirurgische Klinik im Klinikum Charlottenburg, Freie Universität Berlin, Spandauer Damm 130, D-1000 Berlin 19

Kiessling, M., Dr. med., Abteilung für Neuropathologie, Ludwig-Aschoff-Haus, Universität Freiburg, Albertstraße 19, D-7800 Freiburg

Kishikawa, T., Dr. med., Abteilung für Neuroradiologie, Johannes Gutenberg-Universität Mainz, Langenbeckstraße 1, D-6500 Mainz

Kleihues, P., Prof. Dr. med., Abteilung für Neuropathologie, Ludwig-Aschoff-Haus, Universität Freiburg, Albertstraße 19, D-7800 Freiburg

Klein, H., Dr. med., Institut für Klinische Neuropathologie des Zentral-Krankenhauses, Züricher Straße 40, D-2800 Bremen 44

Klein, J., Dr. med., Abteilung für Neurochirurgie des Zentral-Krankenhauses, Züricher Straße 40, D-2800 Bremen 44

Klinger, M., PD Dr. med., Neurochirurgische Klinik der Universität Erlangen-Nürnberg, Schwabachanlage 6 (Kopfklinikum), D-8520 Erlangen

Knoepfle, G., PD Dr. med., Abteilung für Kinderpathologie, Universität Bonn, D-5300 Bonn-Venusberg

König, H.-J., Dr. med., Neurochirurgische Klinik und Poliklinik der Westfälischen Wilhelms-Universität, Jungeblodtplatz 1, D-4400 Münster

Könner, J., Dr. med., Abteilung für Pathologie, Städtisches Krankenhaus Leverkusen, D-5090 Leverkusen-Schlebusch

Kordas, M., Dr. med., National Institute of Neurosurgery, Amerikai út 57, H-1145 Budapest

Kornhuber, B., Prof. Dr. med., Abteilung Hämatologie und Onkologie, Zentrum für Kinderheilkunde, Klinikum der Johann Wolfgang-Goethe-Universität, Theodor-Stern-Kai 7, D-6000 Frankfurt

Kretzschmar, K., PD Dr. med., Abteilung für Neuroradiologie, Johannes Gutenberg-Universität Mainz, Langenbeckstraße 1, D-6500 Mainz

Kutzner, J., Prof. Dr. med., Abteilung für Radiotherapie, Johannes Gutenberg-Universität Mainz, Langenbeckstraße 1, D-6500 Mainz

Langendorf, G., Dr. med., Klinik für Radiotherapie, Universitätskrankenhaus Hamburg, Martinistraße 52, D-2000 Hamburg 20

Langmaid, C., 174, Lake Road East, Roath Park, Cardiff CF2 5NR, South Glam. Wales, Great Britain

Lanksch, W. R., Dr. med., Neurochirurgische Klinik, Klinikum Großhadern, Ludwig-Maximilian-Universität München, Marchioninistraße 15, D-8000 München 70

Lombeck, G., Dr. med., Abteilung für Neuropathologie, Ludwig-Aschoff-Haus, Universität Freiburg, Albertstraße 19, D-7800 Freiburg

Machacek, E., Dr. med., L.-Boltmann-Institut für klinische Neurobiologie d. KRH Wien-Lainz, Wolkersbergenstraße 1, A-1130 Wien

Mahlmann, E., Dr. med., Neurochirurgische Klinik der Johannes Gutenberg-Universität Mainz, Langenbeckstraße 1, D-6500 Mainz

Maurer, K., PD Dr. med., Psychiatrische Klinik der Johannes Gutenberg-Universität Mainz, Langenbeckstraße 1, D-6500 Mainz

Meinig, G., Prof. Dr. med., Neurochirurgische Klinik der Johannes Gutenberg-Universität Mainz, Langenbeckstraße 1, D-6500 Mainz

Merkel, K. H. H., Dr. med., Institut für Pathologie der Universität des Saarlandes, D-6650 Homburg (Saar)

Metz, O., Dr. sc. med., Universitätskinderklinik, Carl-Zeiss-Stiftung, Kochstraße 2, DDR-6900 Jena

Müller, S., Dr. med., Abteilung für Neurochirurgie, Krankenhaus Bethesda, Hainstraße 35, D-5600 Wuppertal 1

Müller, W., Prof. Dr. med., Abteilung für Neuropathologie, Universität Köln, Joseph-Stelzmann-Straße 9, D-5000 Köln 41

Mundinger, F., Prof. Dr. med., Abteilung Stereotaxie und Neuronuklearmedizin, Neurochirurgische Universitätsklinik Freiburg, Hugstetter Straße 55, D-7800 Freiburg

Neidhardt, M., Prof. Dr. med., Kinderklinik des Krankenhauszweckverbandes, Stenglinstraße 47, D-8900 Augsburg

Netzeband, H., Dr. med., Neurochirurgische Universitätsklinik, Im Neuenheimer Feld 110, D-6900 Heidelberg

Neuhann, Th., PD Dr. med., Augenklinik der Johannes Gutenberg-Universität Mainz, Langenbeckstraße 1, D-6500 Mainz

Nicola, N., Dr. med., Neurochirurgische Klinik, Medizinische Einrichtungen der Universität Düsseldorf, Moorenstraße 5, D-4000 Düsseldorf

Ohnacker, H., Dr. med., Institut für Pathologie, Kantonsspital Basel, CH-4005 Basel

Olotu, R., Dr. med., Neurochirurgische Klinik, Universitätskrankenhaus Hamburg, Martinistraße 52, D-2000 Hamburg 20

Otte, J., Dr. med., Kinderklinik der Johannes Gutenberg-Universität Mainz, Langenbeckstraße 1, D-6500 Mainz

Penzholz, H., Prof. Dr. med., Neurochirurgische Abteilung des Chirurgischen Zentrums der Universität Heidelberg, Im Neuenheimer Feld 110, D-6900 Heidelberg

Poretti, P. G., Dr. med., Universitätsklinik für Radiotherapie, Inselspital Bern, CH-3007 Bern

Probst, A., Dr. med., Institut für Pathologie, Kantonsspital Basel, CH-4005 Basel

Puchstein, C., Dr. med., Klinik für Anästhesiologie und Intensivpflege der Westfälischen Wilhelms-Universität, Jungeblodtplatz 1, D-4400 Münster

Richard, K. E., PD Dr. med., Neurochirurgische Klinik, Universität Köln, Joseph-Stelzmann-Straße 9, D-5000 Köln 41

Riehm, H., Prof. Dr. med., Universitätskinderklinik, Kaiserin Auguste Viktoria Haus, Klinikum Charlottenburg, Freie Universität Berlin, Heubnerweg, D-1000 Berlin 19

Rochel, M., Dr. med., Kinderklinik der Johannes Gutenberg-Universität Mainz, Langenbeckstraße 1, D-6500 Mainz

Rochels, R., Dr. med., Augenklinik der Johannes Gutenberg-Universität Mainz, Langenbeckstraße 1, D-6500 Mainz

Röthig, H.-J., Dr. med., Behring-Werke AG, D-3550 Marburg (Lahn)

Roosen, K., PD Dr. med., Neurochirurgische Klinik im Universitäts-Klinikum der Gesamthochschule Essen, Hufelandstraße 55, D-4300 Essen

Schaaf, J., Dr. med., Neurochirurgische Klinik im Universitäts-Klinikum der Gesamthochschule Essen, Hufelandstraße 55, D-4300 Essen

Scharfenberg, H., Dipl.-Math., Nuklearmedizinisches Institut, Deutsches Krebsforschungszentrum, Im Neuenheimer Feld 280, D-6900 Heidelberg

Scheer, K. E., Prof. Dr. med., Nuklearmedizinisches Institut, Deutsches Krebsforschungszentrum, Im Neuenheimer Feld 280, 6900 Heidelberg

Scherer, E., Prof. Dr. med., Institut für Radiologie im Universitäts-Klinikum der Gesamthochschule Essen, Hufelandstraße 55, D-4300 Essen

Schirmer, M., PD Dr. med., Neurochirurgische Klinik, Medizinische Einrichtungen der Universität Düsseldorf, Moorenstraße 5, D-4000 Düsseldorf

Schlegel, W., Dr. med., Nuklearmedizinisches Institut, Deutsches Krebsforschungszentrum, Im Neuenheimer Feld 280, D-6900 Heidelberg

Schmitt, H. P., Prof. Dr. med., Institut für Neuropathologie, Universität Heidelberg, Im Neuenheimer Feld 220, D-6900 Heidelberg

Schmitz, H.-J., Dr. med., Abteilung für Neurochirurgie, Neurochirurgische/Neurologische Klinik und Poliklinik, Universitätsklinikum Steglitz, Freie Universität Berlin, Hindenburgdamm 30, D-1000 Berlin 45

Schreiber, D., Prof. Dr. med., Institut für Allgemeine Pathologie und Pathologische Anatomie, Medizinische Akademie, Nordhäuser Straße 74, DDR-5060 Erfurt

Schröder, R., Dr. med., Abteilung für Neuropathologie, Universität Köln, Joseph-Stelzmann-Straße 9, D-5000 Köln 41

Schürmann, K., Prof. Dr. Dr. h.c., Neurochirurgische Klinik, Johannes Gutenberg-Universität Mainz, Langenbeckstraße 1, D-6500 Mainz

Schumacher, H.-W., Dr. med., Neurochirurgische Universitätsklinik, Sigmund-Freud-Straße 25, D-5300 Bonn-Venusberg

Schwarz, E., Dr. med., Institut für Pathologie der Universität des Saarlandes, D-6650 Homburg (Saar)

Schwarz, M., Dr. med., Neurochirurgische Klinik, Johannes Gutenberg-Universität Mainz, Langenbeckstraße 1, D-6500 Mainz

Sinn, H., Dr. rer. nat., Nuklearmedizinisches Insitut, Deutsches Krebsforschungszentrum, Im Neuenheimer Feld 280, D-6900 Heidelberg

Slowik, F., Dr. med., National Institute of Neurosurgery, Amerikai ùt 57, H-1145 Budapest

Sörensen, N., PD Dr. med., Neurochirurgische Klinik, Universität Würzburg, Josef-Schneider-Straße 11, D-8700 Würzburg

Spranger, J., Prof. Dr. med., Kinderklinik, Johannes Gutenberg-Universität Mainz, Langenbeckstraße 1, D-6500 Mainz

Steiner, L., M. D., Ph. D., Associate Professor, Department of Neurosurgery, Karolinska Hospital, S-10401 Stockholm 60

Stephani, U., Dr. med., Universitätskinderklinik im Klinikum Charlottenburg, Freie Universität Berlin, Heubnerweg 6, D-1000 Berlin 19

Stochdorph, O., Prof. Dr. med., Institut für Neuropathologie, Universität München, Thalkirchner Straße 36, D-8000 München 2

Strauss, L., Dr. med., Nuklearmedizinisches Institut, Deutsches Krebsforschungszentrum, Im Neuenheimer Feld 280, 6900 Heidelberg

Sturm, V., Dr. med., Neurochirurgische Abteilung des Chirurgischen Zentrums der Universität Heidelberg, Im Neuenheimer Feld 110, D-6900 Heidelberg

Tiyaworabun, S., Dr. med., Neurochirurgische Klinik, Klinikum der Universität Düsseldorf, Moorenstraße 5, D-4000 Düsseldorf

Traupe, H., Dr. med., Max-Planck-Institut für Hirnforschung Köln-Merheim, Ostmerheimer Straße 200, D-5000 Köln 91

Veraguth, P. C., Prof. Dr. med., Universitätsklinik für Radiotherapie, Inselspital Bern, CH-3007 Bern

Voth, D., Prof. Dr. med., Neurochirurgische Klinik und Poliklinik, Klinikum der Johannes Gutenberg-Universität, Langenbeckstraße 1, D-6500 Mainz

Wahlen, W., Dr. med., Kinderklinik der Universität des Saarlandes, D-6650 Homburg (Saar)

Walther, B., Dr. med., Kinderklinik, Johannes Gutenberg-Universität Mainz, Langenbeckstraße 1, D-6500 Mainz

Wannenmacher, M., Prof. Dr. med., Abteilung für Strahlentherapie, Universität Freiburg, Hugstetter Straße 55, D-7800 Freiburg

Wende, S., Prof. Dr. med., Abteilung für Neuroradiologie, Johannes Gutenberg-Universität Mainz, Langenbeckstraße 1, D-6500 Mainz

Wenzel, D., Dr. med., Kinderklinik, Universität Erlangen-Nürnberg, Krankenhausstraße 12, D-8520 Erlangen

Wiestler, O., Dr. med., Abteilung für Neuropathologie, Ludwig-Aschoff-Haus, Universität Freiburg, Albertstraße 19, D-7800 Freiburg

Wilcke, O., Prof. Dr. med., Neurochirurgische Klinik, Universität Köln, Joseph-Stelzmann-Straße 9, D-5000 Köln 41

Zegers de Beyl, D., Dr. med., Department of Neurology, Erasme Hospital, Free University of Brussels, Rue Héger-Bordet 1, B-1000 Brussels

Zeisner, W., Dr. med., Abteilung für Neuropädiatrie, Universität Heidelberg, Im Neuenheimer Feld 150, D-6900 Heidelberg

Zimmer, M., Dr. med., Institut für Pathologie der Universität des Saarlandes, D-6650 Homburg (Saar)

Zülch, K. J., Prof. Dr. med., Max-Planck-Institut für Hirnforschung, Reference Centre of the WHO, Ostmerheimer Straße 200, D-5000 Köln-Merheim

Intracranial Tumours of Infancy and Childhood

K. J. ZÜLCH

The fact that in the last 50 years particular chapters or books have been published on this special subject could have two causes: (1) that diagnosis and treatment in this particular age group need special discussion and advice, or (2) that the pathology of tumours is different so that whereas some intracranial tumours occur in all ages, some other tumours develop preferentially or sometimes exclusively in infants and children [59].

Apparently O. T. Schultz [51] was one of the first to emphasize that the nature and distribution of neoplasms during this period varies greatly from those of adult life. Since "the peculiarities of intracranial tumours during infancy and childhood lacked precision", Bailey et al. [2] determined to accumulate and study the data of such a series and to condense them into a monograph. Other large contributions to our subject were made by Cuneo and Rand [13], Ingraham and Matson [23], and by the highly instructive monographs of Bushe and Glees [10] and Koos and Miller [29]; finally a volume on the pathology of tumours of the CNS in fetuses and infants by Jänisch et al. [24] has been published, to mention only a few of the pertinent contributions to the literature.

My own interest [54, 63, 64, 65, 66, 67, 69, 84] began with the classification and pathological description of some surprisingly large, mostly cystic, frequently calcified extraventricular tumours in that age group which Tönnis had observed. Here to our surprise the ependymomas turned out to form the majority of the cases [54]. Furthermore the whole series of young patients up to 20 years was classified.

The comparison of the 263 tumours we had observed in infancy and adolescence (Zülch [66]: Table 1) on the one hand and the cases in the middle and higher age groups on the other, actually proved again the above cited concept that the "spectrum of pathology in this age group was unusual".

Distribution of Age Groups

The first problem was to define the age group of infants and adolescence. Our basis was the particular pathology, yet, since biological phenomena like tumour growth are never sharply limited, it had to be decided whether the end of the 15th or 16th year had to be set as a limit or the end of the 20th year. The latter seemed appropriate to us.

If all the age incidence curves are plotted together, many of the lines crossed which showed the particular biological significance of the period at the end of childhood and of the adolescent years, e.g. around the twentieth year.

Other neurosurgeons such as Bailey himself, limited the "youth" at the age of 16, where the incidence of neoplasms typical of childhood fell off rapidly, as was evident from Cushing's graphs [14], but more clearly so in those of Ley and Walker [33] and Stern [53]. Yet at this age the incidence of those types characteristic of adult life had scarcely begun to make itself apparent.

At this age a crossing of frequency curves took place with the tumours of childhood being on the decline and the graphs of the typical tumours of "middle age" and "senescence" showing a rise.

I am aware of the fact that this limit stands in contrast to the ordinary limitation of admission to paediatric hospitals – usually the 14th year – and to most of the tumour series published in the literature. It is, however, in full agreement with the report of Foerster to the Society of British Neurosurgical Surgeons about the "101 tumours under the age of 20" (cited by Bailey et al. [2]).

Particular Spectrum of Pathology (Fig. 1, Tables 1, 2)

Which, then are the particular groups of tumours characteristic of this age group? According to the series in the literature including our own the prominent tumour groups are:

astrocytomas, pilocytic and others
medulloblastomas
craniopharyngiomas
ependymomas
pinealomas
choroid plexus papillomas and
various smaller groups

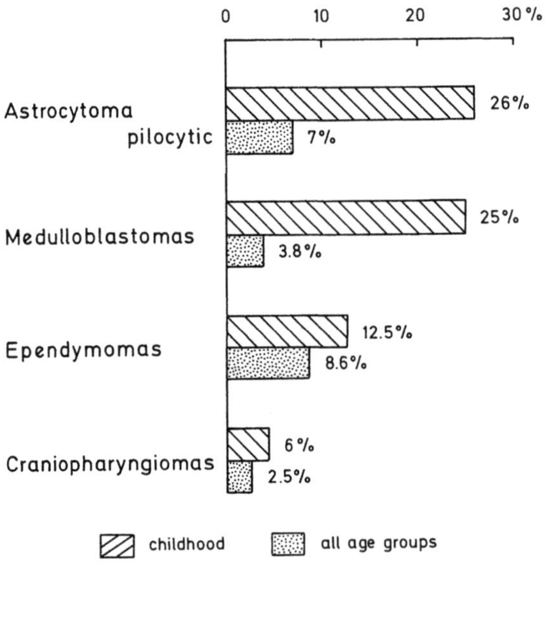

Fig. 1. Frequency of occurence (in percentages) of different types of brain tumours in childhood and all age groups. (After Behrend [5])

Table 1. Relative frequency of tumours in infancy and adolescence (percentage)

	Bailey and Cushing [3]: 154 cases	Zülch [65]: 263 cases	Cuneo and Rand [13]: 83 cases incl. Granulom.	Koos and Miller [29]: 700 cases
Astrocytomas (pilocytic and others)	36.5	29.3	31.3	21.7
Medulloblastomas	15.6	15.2	26.5	17.1
Craniopharyngiomas	13.6	6.0	10.8	8.2
Ependymomas	2.6 (!)	14.0	7.2	8.7
Pinealomas	2.6	2.3	3.6	1.6
Choroid plexus papillomas	0.6	1.9	3.6	1.6

Table 2. Relative frequency of intracranial tumours encountered in infants within the first year of life. (After Jänisch et al. [24])

Choroid plexus papillomas	19.5%	62.0%
Astrocytomas	12.9%	
Medulloblastomas	9.6%	
Ependymomas	6.4%	
Teratomas	13.6%	

A final proof that the profile of tumours in infancy and adolescence was unusual, was apparent from the age graphs of the various groups [25, 68, 72, 75, 78]. There were very well marked peaks for instance in the graph of the pilocytic astrocytomas around the 18th year, the medulloblastomas around the 12th year of age etc.

Classification

For a correct comparison of the series of various authors, the sometimes disturbing discrepancies in the terminology of classification has been a hindrance. However, a classification designed by a group of scientists of various schools and countries has now been worked out and accepted by all members of a group working for a pertinent division of the World Health Organization, Geneva. This group has now finished its work and it was published in 1979 [79, 80, 81, 82]. This should now make comparison of various series easy.

In the majority of tumour groups these experts agreed on definition in terminology. Only a few discrepancies remained unresolved.

One of the very great achievements was the unanimous agreement to replace the term "polar spongioblastoma" with pilocytic astrocytoma; furthermore the special biological properties of pilocytic astrocytomas were noted in contrast to the various other astrocytoma subgroups. Whether a particular "glial(?)" tumour was either classified as *giant cell glioblastoma* or *monstrocellular sarcoma* still remained under discussion and was left to the concept of the observer. *I have accepted and in future will use strictly this WHO nomenclature,* though a personal comment may be allowed.

In the tumours derived from the pineal parenchyma the former "well-known ("unisomorphous", "two-cell type") pinealoma" – so well known to the Europeans – is not included but is replaced by the term "germinoma". My personal concept is that a smaller group of *two- cell* true pinealomas actually exists. This is a tumour (a) derived from pineal parenchymal cells, (b) well defined by histochemical techniques, (c) and finally by metallic impregnations [41].

A last detail of terminology has to be emphasized from the many problems of semantics: in general pathology in the English-speaking world the ending "blastoma" is used in order to define a tumour with malignant tendencies. Ependymo-"blastoma" would then mean that this is an anaplastic form of an ependymoma. Bailey originally introduced this subgroup in his classification [3, 4] because of the similarity of the tumour cells with the so-called "ependymoblast" of embryology. It was later shown, particularly in the sub-group of ependymomas, that there were long fibrillary cells with long processes fixed to the vessel wall. These were similar to "ependymoblasts" and formed the particular pattern of the tumour, hence the name ependymoblastoma. However, the biological behaviour did not correspond to anaplasia or the other characteristics of malignancy. This has to be emphasized as the term "ependymoblastoma" [62] is still in use [43, 44, 62] in the field of experimental neuro-epithelial tumours.

Thus the meaning of the ending-"blastoma" was different in Bailey's concept from that used in general pathology, hence he abandoned it for this subgroup of the ependymomas. In using this classification we have been able to classify 9000 tumours (with a reclassification in 1974) as published in page 48 of the Atlas of Gross Neurosurgical Pathology [78].

To give a relevant summary in this part of our discussion, the following additional general statements about the tumours of infancy and adolescence seem appropriate: In childhood and adolescence the most common tumours of the cerebral hemispheres were ependymomas; other gliomas and ganglioneuromas occurred less often. Monstrocellular sarcomas were occasionally found and meningiomas were rare although they formed the largest single group in older patients. In the chiasmal region, craniopharyngiomas and pilocytic astrocytomas were common while pituitary adenomas were extremely rare. There was a complete absence of neurinomas. In the cerebellum, where the majority of all tumours occurred in younger subjects, medulloblastomas and pilocytic astrocytomas were the commonest types. Angioblastomas of the posterior fossa were uncommon. Teratomas and pinealomas occurred in this age group in the region of the quadrigeminal plate. Almost all pilocytic and other forms of astrocytoma of the aqueduct were found under the age of 20 years [63, 87]. Other tumours of childhood and adolescence were oligodendrogliomas of the thalamus and astrocytomas and pilocytic astrocytomas of the pons, and only very few pilocytic astrocytomas and ependymomas in the spinal cord (the spinal tumours are omitted here).

Sex Preferences

Interesting observations about certain sex preferences had already been made by Cushing [15, 16]. In malignant cerebellar medulloblastomas there was a higher incidence in males (2.3 : 1) and a preference for females in the pilocytic astrocytomas [7].

Age Preference

Furthermore, the above-mentioned age preference of certain tumours was evident in the series of all authors (see the graphs cited above). We may conclude then with the statement that in the intracranial tumours of childhood and adolescence there was a marked preponderance of typical tumour types in particular age groups (for instance medulloblastomas: 19.2% in children as against 7% of all age groups, and the pilocytic astrocytomas 25% as against 7% and a preference for the sexes [84]).

Preference in Location

A last particularity was the preference in site in the tumours [69, 76] of this age group. That craniopharyngiomas occurred only in the chiasmal region need not be discussed. Among the prominent gliomas of the cerebral hemispheres were the extraventricular large tumours, namely the ependymomas, as described by Tönnis and Zülch [54], which were one of the characteristics of this age, similar to the occurence in the basal medio-temporal region of the rare (and very benign) gangliocytomas [55].

The medulloblastomas are admittedly one of the two typical tumours of the cerebellar vermis and only a special variety – the final definition of which has not yet been clarified – namely the so-called "desmoplastic" type, is preferentially localized more frequently in the cerebellar hemispheres. Only the "desmoplastic" variety (classified as "cerebellar arachnoidal sarcoma" by the original describers Foerster and Gagel ([16], see also Rubinstein and Northfield [45]) occurs more frequently in the hemispheres. More details are contained in the relevant books [80].

We owe to Cuneo and Rand [13] an extensive monograph on the different forms observed in later childhood and adolescence. Here in their list of the 72 neoplasms the astrocytomas (14%), ependymomas (12.5%), sarcomas (15.6%), medulloblastomas (6.3%), neuroblastomas (7.8%) rank first. For further details see in Bailey et al. [2] and Koos and Miller [29].

Spinal tumours are certainly rare in childhood [40]; they never occur in the first year of life [24].

Morphology and Biology of the Tumour Groups Typical for Childhood and Adolescence

Histologically tumours of childhood can be traced to all three germ layers of the embryo. The stem cells of most tumours seemed to be identifiable as, for instance, the cells of the craniopharyngeal duct as the matrix of the craniopharyngiomas and the ependymal cells for the ependymomas. However, the pilocytic astrocytoma is definitely different in its derivation from other groups of astrocytic origin.

My own concept, supported by many morphological observations, is that they must be derived from the subependymal layer, because (1) their location is always in relation to the ventricular wall or central canal, (2) Rosenthal fibres [63, 67, 74] and "granular corpuscles" [67, 73] can be looked at as the "visiting-cards" of this tumour group. The undifferentiated cell type of the medulloblastoma is now still derived from highly "indifferent" cells like those of Schaper [49]. However, with discrepant concepts of Polak (1966 [39]: "neuroblastomas") or Gullotta (1967 [19]: "sarcomas") indicate attempts of derivation which, however, have not yet been accepted by other authorities.

Morphology and Biological Behavior

The following summaries may suffice to characterize the more common groups such as the pilocytic *astrocytomas* of infancy and adolescence, since they are sufficiently described elsewhere [67, 72, 75, 77, 78, 86]. They are the most benign and most common tumours of this age group with a certain preference for the female sex, occurring most frequently in the mid-cerebellar region, but not infrequently all around the neural axis as "midline" tumours: "pencil-like" gliomas of the spinal cord, pons, tectal region of the mesencephalon or aqueduct, hypothalamus, chiasm, optic fascicle and retina. They also occur (though not very frequently, but mainly in this age group) as extraventricular gliomas of childhood similar to the more common ependymomas; they frequently form large cysts, particularly in the cerebellar region, where tumour tissue may be then restricted to a mural nodule (similar to angioblastomas); they are rarely calcified. They are the most benign "glioma" although single cases with anaplasia are known [77, 78].

Medulloblastoma is a malignant tumour group [65] whose definite preponderance in the male sex is well-known; the occurrence of spontaneous metastases along the CSF pathways is remarkable: proximally into the region of the hypothalamus and ventricles, distally to the spinal cord, particularly to the cauda equina. Osseous metastases into the vertebral column and pelvis have been observed. The so-called "desmoplastic" variant is better delineated, harder, and preferentially occurs in higher age groups [45]. Its prognosis is better than that of the typical highly malignant medulloblastoma.

Craniopharyngioma. The typical tumour of the chiasmal region in the youth; preponderance in the male; its location may be intrasellar, suprasellar or even in rare cases within the third ventricle. Calcified and cystic, very benign.

Ependymoma. The typical site of most ependymomas is within the ventricles with preference for the lower end of the fourth ventricle; however, a well-defined group has an extraventricular location in the fronto-temporo-parietal region in youth and adolescence. The latter are large cystic frequently calcified tumours and supposed to have a less good prognosis than the intraventricular types of tumour. Ependymomas occur also as "pencil-like" tumours in the spinal cord and near the cauda equina but usually in higher age groups. Rarely they grow within the region of the aqueduct or the mesencephalon. Histologically different and also more common in older subjects is the ependymoma of the foramen of Monro.

Pineal Tumours. They are not uncommon in this age group, usually either as teratomas – and then easily removable by operation – or as "two-cell type" tumours (germinomas or pinealomas, see above) which are, however, infiltrating and spreading through the CSF. A very typical site is the "ectopic" pinealoma/germinoma in the infundibular region. Their biological prognosis as well as their derivation is still under discussion.

The fact that they are more frequently diffusely calcified, their growth is very slow and they are highly radiosensitive and finally their semibenign to – at most – semimalignant biological behavior and their histological particularities (see above) speak for the concept that one of the "two-cell/anisomorphous" subtypes has to be derived from the real pineal parenchyma and actually corresponds to the earlier commonly used term of "pinealoma", according to my personal interpretation [41].

Choroid Plexus Papilloma. They are always related to the special matrix tissue and most commonly situated in the temporal horn (often heavily calcified); however, they also occur more orally at the trigonum or in the third or fourth ventricle. In spite of their genuinely biological behaviour their "clinical" prognosis is not so good, since the artificial "transplantation" by the CSF at operation is not infrequent.

Grading and Prognosis

The introduction of stages of "malignancy" [42] or "grading" was introduced into neuropathology by Kernohan et al. [26], following the example of Broders [8].

The principle of "grading" [48] consisted in the estimating of the percentage of "dedifferentiated" cells in a carcinoma with up to 25% forming the grade I, up to 50% the grade II, up to 75% grade III and over this percentage the grade IV. Though it may have not been too difficult to define "dedifferentiated" cells in the field of "superficial" carcinomas (cervix, rectum etc.), this seems to be impossible in neuroepithelial tumours. We have no definition of a "dedifferentiated" ependymal or astrocytic cell.

The apparent exactness of such a procedure led to the acceptance of this "four grade scale of malignancy" in most parts of the English speaking world. Since the grades were grossly comparable with the terms "benign", "semibenign", "less malignant", or "highly malignant", the neurosurgeons were sufficiently informed about the prognosis by such an introduction of grades. However, grades have never been defined in *clinical* terms; that means in postoperative survival of months or years, which was the great advantage of the data given by Bailey and Cushing [3, 4: Table IV). To emphasize the procedure: the grading according to Kernohan was then an *interpretation of the morphological picture on* its cellular characteristics. This, however, lacked – primarily – any correlation to actual survival times apart from the gross correlation in the minds of the surgeons (they have talked of a tumour being

ningiomas, whereas the black soldiers had 19.47% of these tumours. This preponderance of meningiomas has also been observed – as stated above – in other epidemiological studies within the United States of America. However, other apparent preponderances will not be reported here after Schönberg's [50] discussion of the failures made in the procedural variations when collecting the data. Schönberg and Christine [50] believed that substantial numbers of any symptomatic tumours of the nervous system were missed, particularly in older individuals and that the age specific incidence patterns were largely dependent on the smaller proportion of patients with neoplasms coming later to autopsy. Therefore Kurland et al. [30] emphasized that the incidence rate of primary cerebral tumours is the same all over the world except for the meningiomas in negroes, and the pinealomas/germinomas in the yellow races. In conclusion: epidemiological studies (without known outer environmental factors) has not yet provided any stimulating concepts for pathogenesis.

Familial Occurrence

There is no general agreement about the deductions from the data, collected by Van der Wiel [61], who emphasized that there was a significantly higher occurrence of brain tumours amongst the relatives of brain tumour patients. This was energetically refuted by Koch in Germany [28], whose investigations about heredity are well known and fundamental.

Familial occurrence in one generation has been reported and we have seen it several times. Many cases of identical or non-identical twins are published in the literature and have been collected by Koch himself. The hereditary phacomatoses or hamartoblastomatoses need not be discussed here.

One has to emphasize here, however, that Kurland et al. [30], one of the best informed epidemiologists, is highly critical about most of the data that are available and he concludes that there is no geographic predilection of brain tumour growth apparent yet in man.

Environment. As an example of possible environmental influences the situation in Guam had been thoroughly investigated since cycasin is contained in the Cyca fruit and forms part of the nutrition of the inhabitants of this island. Yet, although this compound is carcinogenic in experimental animals it has induced no higher incidence and frequency of brain or other tumours in the population of Guam [52].

Meanwhile many environmental studies have been made around chemical factories suspected of inducing pollution (rubber and plastics factories etc.). Yet, indubitable increases of nervous neoplasia have not been observed.

Modern Methods of Identification of Cells

The use of ultrastructural methods brought the hope of getting more information on the cytogenesis or histogenesis of the tumour cells, on the rapidity of growth and on the processes of dedifferentiation and of malignancy. However, the yield of new data has not been very great in this regard. Facts that pilocytic astrocytomas had a high metabolic activity although they were so fibrillary in character, the ependymomas had their matrix cells probably not only in the ependymal but also in the subependymal glia, that choroid plexus papilloma cells corresponded to the normal epithelium, which underlined their benign nature, that pinealomas may be identified by their ultrastructure, and finally that gangliocytomas could be recognized because most of the tumour cells could be correlated to multipolar neuronal cells, was not really progress. Highly important, however, was the recognition of various kinds of fibrils, both glial or mesodermal [83].

In summarizing: the hope expressed by Bernhard in 1961 [6] that the problem of the transformation and the malignant behaviour of the cell could be clarified by ultrastructural studies has hardly been fulfilled yet.

Pathogenesis of Tumour Growth

Treatment in the field of intracranial tumours has remained almost conventional in the last 60 years. Operation followed by various, partly sophisticated, kinds of radiation have been the tools of the neurosurgical clinician, the only recent addition being cytostatic chemotherapy. However, life expectancy was not prolonged very much [22]. Immunology has not yet succeeded in changing the fate of the patient bearing an intracranial or intraspinal new growth.

What is the real cause of the lack of progress in the suppression of neoplastic growth, although diagnosis, surgical and anaesthetic techniques have made striking advances? Probably at this point of our discussion we have first to give a general survey of the present concepts of the production of tumours in the human as this may basically influence our approach to treatment.

Epidemiology. Is there an even distribution of the tumours known in our classification over the whole world, in the various regions, the various ethnic groups and environments? Epidemiology has provided a wealth of data and the attention of the reader should be directed to the relevant chapter written by R. Ch. Behrend in 1974 [5]. Yet, up to now only the following data seem able to stand up to systematic criticism: in the yellow races the pineal gland tumours are three to five times more common than in the other races. This is proved by large series of tumours in Japan [1, 47].

In the series of the Armed Forces Institute of Pathology [17] as in other circumscribed populations (Rochester/Minn., see Percy et al. [38]: The overall incidence appears stable ...) the Caucasians were represented with only 13.6% meningiomas, whereas the black soldiers had 19.47% of these tumours. This preponderance of meningiomas has also been observed – as stated above – in other epidemiological studies within the United States of America. However, other apparent preponderances will not be reported here after Schönberg's [50] discussion of the failures made in the procedural variations when collecting the data. Schönberg and Christine [50] believed that substantial numbers of any symptomatic tumours of the nervous system were missed, particularly in older individuals and that the age specific incidence patterns were largely dependent on the smaller proportion of patients with neoplasms coming later to autopsy. Therefore Kurland et al. [30] emphasized that the incidence rate of primary cerebral tumours is the same all over the world except for the meningiomas in negroes, and the pinealomas/germinomas in the yellow races. In conclusion: epidemiological studies (without known outer environmental factors) has not yet provided any stimulating concepts for pathogenesis.

Familial Occurrence

There is no general agreement about the deductions from the data, collected by Van der Wiel [61], who emphasized that there was a significantly higher occurrence of brain tumours amongst the relatives of brain tumour patients. This was energetically refuted by Koch in Germany [28], whose investigations about heredity are well known and fundamental.

Familial occurrence in one generation has been reported and we have seen it several times. Many cases of identical or non-identical twins are published in the literature and have been collected by Koch himself. The hereditary phacomatoses or hamartoblastomatoses need not be discussed here.

One has to emphasize here, however, that Kurland et al. [30], one of the best informed epidemiologists, is highly critical about most of the data that are available and he concludes that there is no geographic predilection of brain tumour growth apparent yet in man.

Environment. As an example of possible environmental influences the situation in Guam had been thoroughly investigated since cycasin is contained in the Cyca fruit and forms part of the nutrition of the inhabitants of this island. Yet, although this compound is carcinogenic in experimental animals it has induced no higher incidence and frequency of brain or other tumours in the population of Guam [52].

Meanwhile many environmental studies have been made around chemical factories suspected of inducing pollution (rubber and plastics factories etc.). Yet, indubitable increases of nervous neoplasia have not been observed.

Experimental Tumours and Carcinogens in the Chemical Environment

What about other carcinogens in the environment? They are not only promoted by modern industry and road traffic. Carcinogens however, are met with in nutrition and other environmental factors, in very low percentages. The formation of *N*-nitroso compounds in the stomach has been proved in rats, when given together with other chemical compounds which *per se* were not carcinogenic.

To summarize, we have not up to now found any reliable correlations between the findings in the experimental and the nitroso-urea tumours in particular (of which we have had extensive personal experience in our laboratory) and the genesis of brain tumours in man, although the resemblance has been very surprising, both microscopically and biologically in many of the forms we have induced. However, we are far away from a real understanding of the cancer problem. The wide range of tumours in the human, as described in the atlases of Cruveilhier [12] and Johannes von Müller [36] and in the publications of Virchow [56] and all their successors in the field of brain tumour pathology has not yet materially changed, since the increase of the pollution of our environment by modern industrialization.

Trauma

The human brain is well protected by its coverings. In the field of traumatic induction of tumour growth we still have only a few examples which appear to be beyond doubt. These were mainly meningiomas, but also very few glioblastomas. Altogether there may be between 20 and 40 cases in the whole world literature [71, 85] acknowledged or worth any discussion; even experimental studies have not shown that trauma has any influence [35].

Radiation

The influence of general terrestrial or cosmic radiation on the tissues of man before the atomic age has probably been below critical values as far as one knows. However, in regions with fall-out, an increase of cancer – generalized and also localized – is beyond any doubt. However, there is no hint to help our problem of tumour production in the CNS, an organ which is so well protected in its cavity.

The undoubted increase in the frequency of brain tumours in general is easily explained by the increasing average age of the human population in most parts of the world. It is now evident that most of the published divergences from this statement stem from methodological errors. That roentgen radiation can cause cancer in various parts of the body is well known since Roentgen's own experience. However, in our special field of intracranial tumours some fibrosarcomas of the dura have evidently been caused by radiation after operation, as we ourselves have published in 1952 [70]; see also Russell and Rubinstein [46], Wende [60], Waltz and Brownell [57].

Role of Viruses in the Causation of Neural Neoplasms

The possibility of a virological cause for brain tumours was emphasized early by Oberling and Guerin [37]. However, although it was their personal belief, they admitted that there was no proof. Yet, the reader is here directed to the excellent work of Laerum et al. [31] (Chapter IV in the UICC study 1978). A recent, very broad discussion by Ibelgaufts [21] still upholds this positive concept, but again without any definite proof.

It is my personal belief, that the only type of human CNS tumours possibly virologically induced could be the sarcomas, since they are the only neoplasms which have no preferences, either of age, of sex, or of location.

The whole field of experimental tumours which is so extremely interesting will not be discussed here, although we have spent much effort on both the morphological and biochemical aspects [9, 11, 27, 34, 58, and many other co-workers]. It will be covered in some of the following contributions.

Conclusions

At the end of this discussion we have to state, that our concept about the causation of neoplastic growth within and around the CNS is very diffuse. This is regrettable, because we cannot deduce any hints from these data which would provide a new approach to treatment.

Outlook

Still it may give us some hope, that a Reference Centre in Freiburg (under Kleihues) has commenced activity and that the installation of a General Cancer Register by the Federal Government is also being discussed. These may also initiate comprehensive studies on the genesis of brain tumours: epidemiology and experimental neuro-oncology are excellent tools, when concepts are in sight. Yet let us not forget those observations at the bedside which have provided decisive stimulation as to the direction which future research should take.

References

1. Araki, C., Matsumoto, S.: Statistical reevaluation of pinealoma and related tumours in Japan. J. Neurosurg. *30,* 146–149 (1969)
2. Bailey, P., Buchanan, D. N., Bucy, P. C.: Intracranial tumours of infancy and childhood. Chicago: University Chicago Press 1939
3. Bailey, P., Cushing, H.: Tumours of the glioma group. Philadelphia: Lippincott 1926
4. Bailey, P., Cushing, H.: Die Gewebsverschiedenheit der Gliome und ihre Bedeutung für die Prognose. Jena: Fischer 1930
5. Behrend, R. Ch.: Epidemiology of brain tumours. In: Vinken, P. J., Bruyn, G. W. (eds.): Handbook of clinical neurology, vol. 16/I, Tumours of the brain and skull. Amsterdam: North-Holland Publ. 1974, p. 56
6. Bernhard, W.: Elektronenmikroskopischer Beitrag zum Studium der Kanzerisierung und der malignen Zustände der Zelle. Verh. dtsch. Ges. Path. *45,* 8–37 (1961)
7. Borck, W. F., Zülch, K. J.: Über die Erkrankungshäufigkeit der Geschlechter an Hirngeschwülsten. Zbl. Neurochir. *11,* 333–350 (1951)
8. Broders, A. C.: Carcinoma: Grading and practical application. Arch. Path. Lab. Med. *2,,* 376–381 (1926)
9. Bücheler, J., Kleihues, P.: Excision of 0^6-methylguanine from DNA of various mouse tissue following a single injection of N-methyl-N-nitrosourea. Chem.-biol. Interact. *16,* 325–333 (1977)
10. Bushe, K.-A., Glees, P.: Chirurgie des Gehirns und Rückenmarks im Kindes- und Jugendalter. Stuttgart: Hippokrates 1968
11. Cooper, H. K., Bücheler, J., Kleihues, P.: DNA alkylation in mice with genetically difference susceptibility to 1.2-dimethylhydrazine-induced colon carcinogenesis. Cancer Res. *38,* 3063–3065 (1978)
12. Cruveilhier, J.: Anatomie pathologique du corps humain ou descriptions avec figures lithographées et coloriées des diverses altérations morbides dont le corps humain est susceptible. Paris: Baillière 1829
13. Cuneo, H. M., Rand, C. W.: Brain tumours of childhood. Springfield/Ill.: Thomas 1952
14. Cushing, H.: The intracranial tumors of preadolescence. Amer. J. Dis. Child *33,* 551–584 (1927)
15. Cushing, H.: Experiences with the cerebellar medulloblastomas. Acta path. microbiol. scand. *7,* 1–86 (1930)
16. Cushing, H.: Experiences with the cerebellar astrocytomas. Surg. Gynec. Obstet. *52,* 129 (1931)
17. Fan, K.-J., Kovi, J., Earle, K. M.: The ethnic distribution of primary central nervous system tumours: AFIP 1958 to 1970. J. Neuropath. exp. Neurol. *36,* 41–49 (1977)
18. Foerster, O., Gagel, O.: Das umschriebene Arachnoidalsarkom des Kleinhirns. Z. ges. Neurol. Psychiat. *164,* 565–580 (1939)
19. Gullotta, F.: Das sogenannte Medulloblastom. Monographien aus dem Gesamtgebiet der Neurologie und Psychiatrie, Heft 118. Berlin-Heidelberg-New York: Springer 1967
20. Hamperl, H.: Über die Gutartigkeit und die Bösartigkeit von Geschwülsten. Verh. dtsch. Ges. Path. *35,* 29–54 (1951)
21. Ibelgaufts, H.: Are human DNA tumour viruses involved in the pathogenesis of human neurogenic tumours? Editorial. Neurosurg. Rev. *5* (1982, in press)
22. Ilsen, H. W., Petrovici, J. N., Mennel, H. D., Zülch, K. J., Szymas, J.: Die Wirkung kombinierter Chemotherapie (Adriamycin/VM 26/CCNU) bei hirneigenen Tumoren des Erwachsenenalters und im Tierexperiment. Fortschr. Neurol. Psychiat. (in press)
23. Ingraham, R. D., Matson, D. D.: Neurosurgery of infancy and childhood. Springfield/Ill.: Thomas 1954
24. Jänisch, W., Schreiber, D., Gerlach, H.: Tumoren des Zentralnervensystems bei Feten und Säuglingen. Jena: Fischer 1980
25. Kautzky, R., Zülch, K. J., Wende, S., Tänzer, A.: Neuroradiology: A neuropathological approach. Berlin-Heidelberg-New York: Springer 1982 (in press)
26. Kernohan, J. W., Mabon, R. F., Svien, H. J., Adson, A. W.: A simplified classification of gliomas. Proc. Mayo Clin. *24,* 71–75 (1949)

27. Kleihues, P., Doejer, G., Swenberg, J. A., Hauenstein, E., Bücheler, J., Cooper, H. K.: DNA repair as regulatory factor in the organotropy of alkylation carcinogens. Arch. Toxicol., Suppl. *2,* 253–261 (1979)
28. Koch, G.: The genetics of cerebral tumours. Acta neurochir. (Wien), Suppl. X, 24–27 (1964)
29. Koos, W. Th., Miller, M. H.: Intracranial tumours of infants and children. Stuttgart: Thieme 1971
30. Kurland, L. T., Kurtzke, J. F., Goldberg, J. D.: Epidemiology of neurologic and sense organ disorders. Cambridge/Mass.: Harvard Univ. Press 1973
31. Laerum, O. D., Bigner, D. D., Rajewsky, M. F.: Biology of brain tumours. International Union Against Cancer, Geneva 1978
32. Lebert, H.: Über Krebs und die mit Krebs verwechselten Geschwülste im Gehirn und seinen Hüllen. Virch. Arch. path. Anat. *3,* 463–569 (1851)
33. Ley, A., Walker, A. E.: Statistical review of 230 consecutive cases of intracranial tumour. Folia neuropath. eston. *15/16,* 52–67 (1936)
34. Mennel, H. D.: Experimental tumours of the nervous system. Morphology and morphogenesis. Recent Results Cancer Res. *44,* 158–169 (1974)
35. Mennel, H. D., Sato, K., Zülch, K. J.: Traumatische Regeneration und Resorptivkarzinogenese am Zentralnervensystem. Acta neurochir. (Wien) *25,* 197–206 (1971)
36. Müller, J. von: Über den feineren Bau und die Formen der krankhaften Geschwülste. Berlin: Reimer 1938
37. Oberling, C., Guerin, M.: The role of viruses in the production of cancer. Adv. Cancer Res. *2,* 353–423 (1954)
38. Percy, A. K., Elveback, L. R., Okazaki, H., Kurland, L. T.: Neoplasms of the central nervous system: epidemiologic considerations. Neurology (Minneap.) *22,* 40–48 (1972)
39. Polak, M.: Blastomas del sistema nervioso central y periferico. Buenos Aires: Lopez Libreros 1966
40. Rand, W. R., Rand, C. W.: Intraspinal tumors of childhood. Springfield/Ill: Thomas 1960
41. Riverson, E. A., Zülch, K. J.: Pineal parenchymal tumours and germinomas (the problem of the so-called pinealomas). Editorial. Neurosurg. Rev. *2,* 3–11 (1979)
42. Rössle, R.: Stufen der Malignität. S.-B. dtsch. Akad. Wiss., Kl. med. Wiss., Berlin: Akademie-Verlag 1950
43. Rubin, R., Ames, R. P., Sutton, C. H., Zimmermann, H. M.: Virus like particles in murine ependymoblastoma. J. Neuropath. exp. Neurol. *28,* 371–387 (1969)
44. Rubin, R., Sutton, C. H., Zimmerman, H. M.: Experimental ependymoblastoma. J. Neuropath. exp. Neurol. *27,* 421–438 (1968)
45. Rubinstein, L. J., Northfield, D. W. C.: The medulloblastoma and the so called "arachnoid cerebellar sarcoma. Brain *87,* 379–412 (1964)
46. Russell, D. S., Rubinstein, L. S.: The pathology of tumours of the nervous system, 2nd ed. Arnold, London 1963
47. Sano, K.: Diagnoses and treatment of tumors in the pineal region. Acta neurochir. (Wien) *34,* 153–157 (1976)
48. Sayre, G. P.: The system of grading of gliomas. Acta neurochir. (Wien), Suppl. X, 98–106 (1964)
49. Schaper, A.: Die frühesten Differenzierungsvorgänge im ZNS. Arch. Entwickl.-Mech. Org. *5,* 81–130 (1897)
50. Schönberg, B. S., Christine, B. W.: Neoplasms of the brain and cranial meninges: a study of incidence, epidemiological trends and survival. Neurology (Minneap.) *20,* 399 (1970)
51. Schultz, O. T.: Tumors of infancy and childhood. In: Abts' pediatrics, vol. 8. Philadelphia: Saunders 1926, p. 641
52. Spatz, M., Laqueur, G. L.: Transplacental induction of tumors in Sprague-Dawley-rats with crude cycad material. J. nat. Cancer Inst. *38,* 233–245 (1967)
53. Stern, R. O.: Cerebral tumors in children. A pathologic report. Arch. Dis. Childh. *12,* 291–304 (1937)
54. Tönnis, W., Zülch, K. J.: Das Ependymom der Großhirnhemisphären im Jugendalter. Zbl. Neurochir. *2,*141–164 (1937)
55. Tönnis, W., Zülch, K. J.: Intrakranielle Ganglienzellgeschwülste (mit ausführlicher Beschreibung einer einheitlichen Gruppe im Großhirn). Zbl. Neurochir. *4,* 273–307 (1939)

56. Virchow, R.: Die krankhaften Geschwülste. Berlin: Hirschwald 1863/65
57. Waltz, T. A., Brownell, B.: Sarcoma: a possible late result of effective radiation therapy for pituitary adenoma. Report of two cases. J. Neurosurg. *24*, 901–907 (1966)
58. Wechsler, W.: Carcinogenic and teratogenic effects of ethylnitrosourea and methylnitrosourea during pregnancy in experimental rats. In: Tomatis, L., Mohr, U. (eds.), Transplacental carcinogenesis. Scientific Publ. No. 4, Internat. Agency for Research on Cancer, Lyon 1973, p. 127
59. Wechsler, W., Zülch, K. J.: Pathology of neurogenic tumours in childhood and adolescence. In: Bushe, K. A., Spoerri, O., Shaw, J. (eds.), Progress in paediatric neurosurgery. Stuttgart: Hippokrates 1974, p. 13
60. Wende, S.: Sarkom der Schädelkalotte nach Röntgentherapie. Fortschr. Röntgenstr. *96*, 278–282 (1962)
61. Van der Wiel, H. J.: Inheritance of glioma. Amsterdam: Elsevier Publ., 1960
62. Zimmerman, H. M., Netsky, M. G., Davidoff, L. M.: Atlas of tumors of the nervous system. Philadelphia: Lea & Febiger 1956
63. Zülch, K. J.: Zur Histopathologie der Großhirngliome in den ersten beiden Lebensjahrzehnten. Z. ges. Neurol. Psychiat. *158*, 369–374 (1937)
64. Zülch, K. J.: Die Hirngeschwülste des Jugendalters. Z. ges. Neurol. Psychiat. *161*, 183–188 (1938)
65. Zülch, K. J.: Das Medulloblastom vom pathologisch-anatomischen Standpunkt aus. Arch. Psychiat. Nervenkr. *112*, 343–367 (1940)
66. Zülch, K. J.: Hirngeschwülste im Jugendalter. Zbl. Neurochir. *5*, 238–274 (1940)
67. Zülch, K. J.: Über das "sog." Kleinhirnastrocytom. Virch. Arch. path. Anat. *307*, 222–252 (1940)
68. Zülch, K. J.: Die Hirngeschwülste in biologischer und morphologischer Darstellung. Leipzig: Barth 1951, 3. Aufl. 1958
69. Zülch, K. J.: Vorzugssitz, Erkrankungsalter und Geschlechtsbevorzugung bei Hirngeschwülsten als bisher ungeklärte Formen der Pathoklise. Dtsch. Z. Nervenheilk. *166*, 91–102 (1951)
70. Zülch, K. J.: Über die Pathologie und Biologie der Hirngeschwülste. Wien. med. Wschr. *102*, 711–715 (1952)
71. Zülch, K. J.: Hirngeschwülste als Schädigungsfolge. Ärztl. Forsch. *7*, 535–543 (1953)
72. Zülch, K. J.: Biologie und Pathologie der Hirngeschwülste. In: Olivecrona, H., Tönnis, W. (Hrsg.), Handbuch der Neurochirurgie, Bd. III. Berlin-Göttingen-Heidelberg: Springer 1956
73. Zülch, K. J.: Das Glioblastoma, morphologisch und biologisch gesehen. Acta neurochir. (Wien), Suppl. VI, 1–30 (1959)
74. Zülch, K. J.: La signification des fibres de Rosenthal. Colloque Internat. sur les malformations congenitales de l'encéphale, Paris 1961. Masson, Paris 1963, p. 61
75. Zülch, K. J.: Brain tumors, their biology and pathology, 2nd ed. New York: Springer-Publishing Comp. Inc. 1965
76. Zülch, K. J.: Einige Besonderheiten der Hirngeschwülste in Alter und Sitz sowie im Geschlecht der Tumorträger. Zbl. Chir. *90*, 890–898 (1965)
77. Zülch, K. J.: Atlas of the histology of brain tumours. Berlin-Heidelberg-New York: Springer 1971
78. Zülch, K. J.: Atlas of gross neurosurgical pathology, Berlin-Heidelberg-New York: Springer 1975
79. Zülch, K. J.: Principles of the new WHO classification of brain tumours. In: Frowein, R. A., Wilcke, O., Karimi-Nejad, A., Brock, M., Klinger, M.: Head injuries. Tumours of the cerebellar region. Advances in Neurosurg. 5. Berlin-Heidelberg-New York: Springer 1978, p. 279
80. Zülch, K. J. (in collaboration with pathologists in 14 countries): Histological typing of tumours of the central nervous system. International histological classification of tumours No. 21. World Health Organization, Geneva 1979
81. Zülch, K. J.: Principles of the new World Health Organization (WHO) classification of brain tumors. Neuroradiology *19*, 59–66 (1980)
82. Zülch, K. J.: Histological development of the classification of brain tumours and the new proposal of the World Health Organization (WHO). Neurosurg. Rev. *4*, 123–127 (1981)

83. Zülch, K. J.: Problems of the classification of tumours of the nervous system and the significance of electron microscopy (1981, in press).
84. Zülch, K. J., Borck, W. F.: Tafeln über die relative Häufigkeit der Hirngeschwülste in verschiedenen Altersklassen. Zbl. Neurochir. *12,* 93–97 (1952)
85. Zülch, K. J., Mennel, H. D.: Gehirntumor und Trauma. Hefte Unfallheilk., Heft *107,* 33–44 (1971)
86. Zülch, K. J., Mennel, H. D.: The biology of brain tumours. In: Vinken, P. J., Bruyn, B. W. (eds.), Handbook of clinical Neurology, vol. 16. Amsterdam: North-Holland Publ. Comp. 1974, p. 1
87. Zülch, K. J., Nachtway, W.: Pathologie und Klinik des Aquäduktverschlusses. Zbl. Neurochir. *18,* 80–106 (1958)
88. Zülch, K. J., Woolf, A. L.: Classification of brain tumours. Acta neurochir. (Wien), Suppl. X. Wien: Springer 1964

Remarks on the WHO Classification of Tumours of the Central Nervous System

O. STOCHDORPH

The 'Histological Classification of Tumours of the Central Nervous System' published by WHO has several remarkable shortcomings. Subdivision into chapters, e.g., does not follow a common principle. Closely related entities are separated from each other, and dissimilar entities are treated jointly.

The tumours traditionally designated glioblastomas are, according to the present state of knowledge, extremely anaplastic variants of astrocytomas, oligodendrogliomas, or ependymomas, or of glial cell tumours with indifferent cell forms (Fig. 1). Glioblastomas are not a separate tumour entity. This statement conforms to the opinion of Henschen [3] and to the experience of, e.g., Willis [5] or Ackerman and Rosai [1]. The latter authors even propose abolition of the term "glioblastoma" on the following grounds: "This term is unsatisfactory for several reasons. First, it implies an origin from (or at least a relationship with) the embryonal glioblast which probably does not exist. All the available evidence seems to indicate that this tumour is instead the result of progressive dedifferentiation in a neoplasm that originated in an adult cell. Second, it conveys the impression of a specific tumour type when it simply represents the undifferentiated form of all types of gliomas. Admittedly, the large majority of tumours called glioblastoma multiforme are of astrocytic origin, as demonstrated by special stains, tissue culture, and electron microscopy, but oligodendrogliomas and ependymomas may result in an identical microscopic appearance. Therefore it seems more logical simply to call these tumours undifferentiated gliomas." In any case, undifferentiated gliomas or glioblastomas are more closely related to glial cell tumours than nerve cell tumours. In spite of this, they are not listed together with glial cell tumours. They are, instead, combined with a mixed group of sundry embryonal tumours, among others with medulloblastomas, without any features of histogenesis, age distribution, or clinical behaviour being common to both groups.

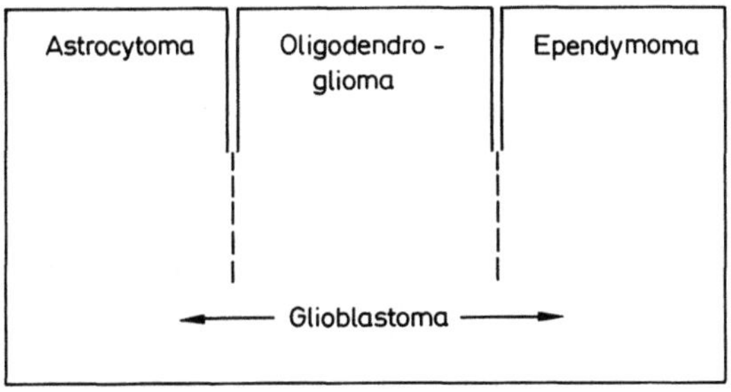

Fig. 1. Bi-dimensional system of glial tumours according to Henschen [3] with glial cell forms on one axis and degrees of anaplasia on the other

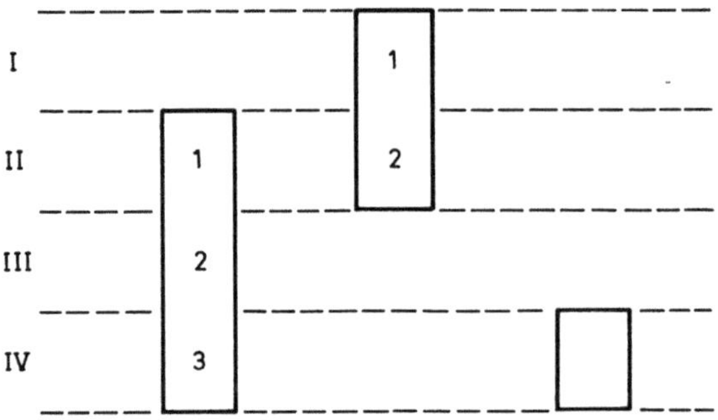

Fig. 2. Grades of anaplasia (*arabic numerals*) and degrees of prognostic value (*roman numerals*). From left to right: astrocytomas/glioblastomas – pilocytic cerebellar astrocytomas – medulloblastomas [3]

Combining ependymal tumours and tumours of the choroid plexus into one chapter is another aspect not justified by histology, as has already been pointed out by Rubinstein [4]. The ependyma arises through differentiation of neuroglia into a surface, and there is a smooth transition to the glial tissue beneath just as from a crust to the bread. In the choroid plexus, on the other hand, the total width of the hemisphere is transformed into a single epithelial layer. This layer is separated, just as any other epithelium, by a basal membrane from the underlying – leptomeningeal – tissue.

The WHO classification recognizes only glial cell forms commonly known around 1930. Modern concepts concerning the special histology of the so-called circumventricular organs and the existence of an additional glial cell form termed tanycyte, are not taken into account.

Even the designation as a classification of tumours of the central nervous system turns out to be a misnomer. Sheath cell tumours of peripheral nerves and/or roots, and tumours of the anterior pituitary are definitely not tumours of the central nervous system although they may be included in the category of intracranial tumours.

Perhaps the most important deficiency of the WHO classification arises from arbitrarily applying a different meaning to a term commonly used in tumour pathology, viz., to the term of grading. Grading was introduced by Broders [2] as a means of coding lesser or higher anaplasia among specimens of one single tumour type, in the original paper among lip carcinomas. The WHO classification denotes, instead, degrees of similarity in the clinical – and specifically in the prognostic – features of many different types of intracranial tumours as grades. This results in a sort of horizontal comparison as opposed to the vertical comparison of true grading (Fig. 2). Such an endeavour based upon clinical experience, is, of course, perfectly legitimate in its own field. However, those degrees should be denoted as degrees of "prognostic value" or by some similar formula. One should not, for this purpose, usurp the term of grading which has quite a different meaning in all other fields of tumour pathology.

References

1. Ackerman, L. V., Rosai, J.: Surgical Pathology, 5th ed., pp. 1248–1249. St. Louis: Mosby 1974
2. Broders, A. C.: Carcinoma: grading and practical application. Arch. Path. (Chic.) *2*, 376–381 (1926)
3. Henschen, F.: Tumoren des Zentralnervensystems und seiner Hüllen. In: Handbuch der spez. pathol. Anatomie, vol. XIII/3, pp. 413–1040. Berlin, Göttingen, Heidelberg: Springer 1955
4. Rubinstein, L. J.: Tumours of the Central Nervous System, p. 257. Atlas of Tumour Pathology, 2nd ser., fasc. 6. Armed Forces Institute of Pathology, Washington, D. C., 1972
5. Willis, R. A.: Pathology of Tumours. London: Butterworth & Co. 1948

Developmental Neuro-Oncogenesis in Experimental Animals*

P. KLEIHUES, S. BAMBORSCHKE, M. KIESSLING, and O. WIESTLER

Introduction

With the exception of some genetically determined neoplastic syndromes, the aetiology of human brain tumours is largely unknown. This is also true for CNS neoplasms in children. Their occurrence has been tentatively linked with prenatal exposure to environmental carcinogens but so far, no positive correlation has been established [35]. From observations both in humans and experimental animals it is known that the adverse effects of toxic compounds on fetal and postnatal development are not restricted to the causation of malformations. The first report on transplacental tumour induction in experimental animals was by Larsen in 1947 [28] who observed a high incidence of lung adenomas in the offspring of mice treated with urethane (ethyl carbamate) during the last three days of gestation. In 1964, Mohr and Althoff [31] reported an increased incidence of respiratory tract tumours in Syrian Golden hamsters after transplacental administration of diethylnitrosamine. At about the same time, the powerful perinatal neuro-oncogenic effect of ethylnitrosourea was discovered by Druckrey et al [5]. Since then, a great number of chemical carcinogens has been found to be similarly effective in a variety of experimental animals (Table 1). In 1971, Herbst et al. [17] and Greenwald et al. [11] reported the occurrence of vaginal adenocarcinoma in young women after maternal treatment with diethylstilboestrol (DES) but until now, DES has remained the only agent known to induce tumours transplacentally in humans.

In this article, some characteristic features of developmental neuro-oncogenesis in experimental animals are summarized. Several more extensive reviews on perinatal carcinogenesis in the nervous system and in other tissues have recently been published [27, 32, 41].

Developmental Neuro-Oncogenic Agents

More than 40 compounds are known to cause an increased risk of tumour in experimental animals if administered during fetal or early postnatal development [32, 41]. The principal site of tumour induction varies considerably in different species. In

* Supported by the Deutsche Forschungsgemeinschaft (SFB 31)

Table 1. Developmental neuro-oncogenesis in experimental animals[a]

Carcinogen	Species	Developmental stage at treatment (day)		Max. tumour incidence[b] (%)
Alkylnitrosoureas and related N-nitrosamides				
N-Methyl-*N*-nitrosourea	Rat	Prenatal	(21/22)	50
		Newborn		50
N-Ethyl-*N*-nitrosourea	Rat	Prenatal	(11–23)	100
		Postnatal	(1–30)	90
	Mouse	Prenatal	(19)	32
	Hamster	Prenatal	(11–15)	60
	Gerbil	Postnatal	(7/20)	43[b]
	Opossum	Postnatal		54[c]
	Rabbit	Prenatal	(8–10)	67
N-n-Propyl-*N*-nitrosourea	Rat	Prenatal	(19)	50
N-n-Butyl-*N*-nitrosourea	Rat	Prenatal	(22)	50
		Newborn		85
		Postnatal	(10)	95
N-Ethyl-*N*-nitrosobiuret	Rat	Prenatal	(15/22)	90
	Rat	Postnatal	(10)	100
N-Methyl-*N*-nitrosourethane	Rat	Prenatal	(18)	19[d]
Hydrazines, azo and azoxy compounds				
1,2-Diethylhydrazine	Rat	Prenatal	(15)	90
1-Methyl-2-benzylhydrazine	Rat	Prenatal	(15/21)	50[d]
Procarbazine	Rat	Prenatal	(22)	54
Azoethane	Rat	Prenatal	(15)	95
Azoxyethane	Rat	Prenatal	(15)	80
Azoxymethane	Rat	Prenatal	(22)	20[d]
Cycad meal	Rat	Prenatal		25
Dialkylaryltriazenes				
3,3-Dimethyl-1-phenyltriazene	Rat	Prenatal	(23)	42
3,3-Diethyl-1-phenyltriazene	Rat	Prenatal	(15)	92
3,3-Diethyl-1-pyridyltriazine	Rat	Prenatal	(15)	90
Alkylmethanesulphonates				
Methylmethanesulphonate	Rat	Prenatal	(15/21)	32
Ethylmethanesulphonate	Rat	Prenatal	(21)	16
Dialkylsulphates				
Dimethylsulphate	Rat	Prenatal	(15)	10
Diethylsulphate	Rat	Prenatal	(15)	10
Polycyclic aromatic hydrocarbons				
7,12-Dimethylbenz(a)-anthracene	Rat	Prenatal	(21)	75[d]
Miscellaneous				
Propane sultone	Rat	Prenatal	(15)	18

[a] For references see Kleihues [27]
[b] Neural crest-derived tumours (cutaneous melanomas)
[c] Tumours in the nervous system and various other tissues
[d] Tumours predominantly in the nervous system and kidney

rats, the most commonly induced neoplasms are malignant gliomas of the central nervous system (CNS), malignant neurinomas of the peripheral nervous system (PNS) and, less commonly, nephroblastomas. In contrast, mice show a general tendency to respond with an increased incidence of benign tumours of the respiratory tract (adenomas) and the liver (hepatomas). Among the different classes of chemical carcinogens, *N*-nitrosamides, aryldialkyltriazenes, hydrazine derivatives, and the polycyclic hydrocarbon 7,12-dimethylbenz(a)anthracene have to be classified as the most potent perinatal carcinogens. Their oncogenic effect on the developing nervous system of various species is summarized in Table 1.

Alkylnitrosoureas and Related *N*-Nitrosamides

Druckrey and his co-workers were the first to demonstrate that the neuro-oncogenic effect of these agents is greatly enhanced if the carcinogen is administered transplacentally. Prenatal administration of methylnitrosourea is limited by its strong cytotoxic effects but ethylnitrosourea, given to rats as a single intravenous dose of 40–80 mg/kg body weight on day 15 or 21 of gestation, induced malignant tumours of the nervous system in 98–100% of the offspring. The mean postnatal survival time ranged from approximately 180 to 210 days [12]. Administration of ethylnitrosourea to pregnant rats before day 12 of gestation did not produce tumours in the offspring. The developmental oncogenicity of ethylnitrosourea, when expressed as number of neurogenic tumours per animal or as Iball index, is highest during the last week of gestation and in newborn rats. During postnatal growth, the oncogenic effect gradually declines, with lower tumour incidence and increasing survival time.

In rats, the nervous system is the principal target organ, irrespective of the developmental stage at treatment. However, administration around birth or shortly thereafter will also induce some nephroblastomas. Stavrou and co-workers [39, 40] have shown that in rabbits there are distinct gestational periods for the induction of neural (day 8–10) and renal (day 18–31) neoplasms. In hamsters and mice, ethylnitrosourea induces a lower incidence of neural tumours and postnatal administration to Mongolian gerbils produced no tumours of the central or peripheral nervous system; however, 43% of the animals developed benign neural crest-derived cutaneous melanomas [22]. In Rhesus monkeys prenatal ethylnitrosourea was ineffective [43] but in Patas monkeys tumours were induced in different tissues, including the nervous system (J. M. Rice, personal communication).

The developmental carcinogenicity of ethylnitrosobiuret is largely identical with that of ethylnitrosourea, whereas the remainder of the *N*-nitrosamides (Table 1) are less effective, with the exception of butylnitrosourea, which is very potent when given postnatally. N-nitroso compounds are widely distributed in the environment, including food, and nitrosamines and nitrosamides can be formed non-enzymically in the body from their chemical precursors, i.e. amines and nitrites (for review see [30]). Ivankovic and Preussmann [13] showed that feeding of ethylurea and sodium nitrite to pregnant rats (day 13–23) induced neural tumours in more than 80% of the offspring. Similar experiments have been successfully carried out in hamsters and with sodium nitrite plus n-butylurea and related chemical precursors (for review see [30]). After systemic administration, ethylnitrosourea and related *N*-nitrosamides are rapidly distributed throughout the body, including placenta and fetuses. They easily cross the blood-brain barrier and there is no evidence for selective uptake in specific areas of the CNS [18]. Under physiological conditions, their breakdown proceeds spontaneously through base-catalysed hydrolysis yielding ethyl diazonium ion as the ultimate carcinogen. Decomposition in the intact animal occurs with a half-life of less than 10 minutes.

Hydrazines, Azo and Azoxy Compounds

1,2-Diethylhydrazine (DEH) is a very potent neuro-oncogenic agent when given transplacentally to rats [6]. Hydrazines require microsomal enzymes to be converted into their biologically active intermediates. The sequence of reactions causing the bioactivation of 1,2-diethylhydrazine is thought to start with two oxidation steps, giving rise to azoethane and azoxyethane. Both azoethane and azoxyethane are as effective as the parent carcinogen in the induction of neural tumours after prenatal administration [6]. Procarbazine (Natulan) is a derivative of methylbenzylhydrazine and widely used in the chemotherapy of human cancer, including brain tumours. It is itself a potent neuro-oncogenic agent when administered transplacentally to rats [14].

Dialkylaryltriazenes

The neuro-oncogenic effect of this class of carcinogens was first shown for 3,3-dimethyl-1-phenyltriazene (DMPT). After perinatal administration, the ethyl analogues of DMPT, 3,3-diethyl-1-pyridyltriazene and 3,3-diethyl-1-phenyltriazene are particularly effective [15]. Environmental or occupational exposure of humans is, to our present knowledge, negligible. Studies on the bioactivation of triazenes have focussed on DMPT. The initial step in the formation of an alkylating intermediate is the enzymic hydroxylation of one of the methyl groups which leads to the production of formaldehyde and 3-methyl-1-phenyltriazene (MPT). The latter has been postulated to be the proximate carcinogen of DMPT which, after hydrolytic fission, yields aniline and methyldiazonium hydroxide. As in the case of alkylnitrosoureas, this highly unstable product (or the released carbonium ion) is thought to methylate nucleophilic groups in cellular macromolecules. In vitro studies using microsomal fractions from various animal tissues [36] indicate that the nervous system, as the principal target tissue in the carcinogenicity of DMPT and related triazenes, is itself unable to metabolize DMPT. However, the half-life of MPT is sufficiently long ($\sim$ 20 seconds) to allow systemic distribution via the blood after its formation by hepatic microsomal enzymes. Furthermore, MPT is itself carcinogenic and methylates cellular DNA in the absence of drug-metabolising enzymes [29].

Owing to the inability of the CNS to metabolize dialkylaryltriazenes, the extent of DNA alkylation is considerably lower in the principal target organ (brain) than in liver and kidney. In fetuses no such differences exist, indicating that during prenatal development both liver and brain (and other tissues) are transplacentally methyl-

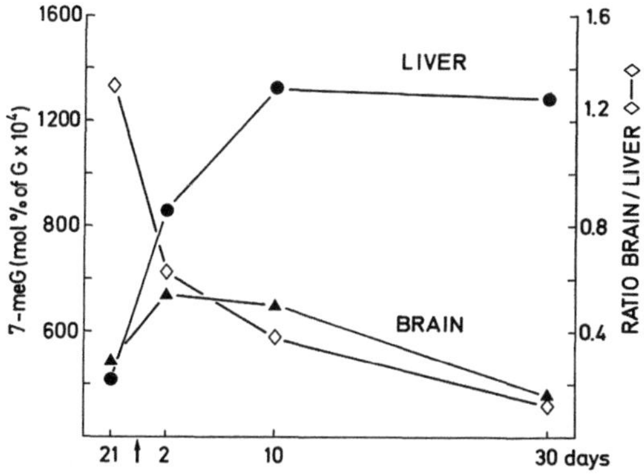

Fig. 1. Methylation by 3,3-(^{14}C)dimethyl-1-phenyltriazene of liver and brain DNA at various stages of development. The carcinogen was injected subcutaneously (100 mg/kg body weight) into pregnant (21st day of gestation) or into 2-, 10- and 30-day-old rats. Animals were killed 15 hours later and 7-methylguanine (7-meG) concentrations were determined in DNA isolated from the pooled organs of 3 (30-day-old) to 16 (fetuses) animals. The *arrow* indicates the time of birth. (Reprinted from Kleihues et al. [23])

ated by a proximate carcinogen produced in maternal organs (Fig. 1). After birth the rapid increase in the methylation of hepatic DNA reflects the maturation of the hepatic drug-metabolising enzyme system [23].

7,12-Dimethylbenz(a)anthracene (DMBA)

DMBA is the only polycyclic aromatic hydrocarbon known to exert a neuro-oncogenic effect after systemic administration. Intravenous injection in rats (25 mg/kg) on day 21 of gestation induced tumours of the nervous system (67% incidence) and the kidney (38% incidence) in the offspring [34]. After subcutaneous injection on day 20, Rice et al. [37] also found neural and renal tumours in the F_1 generation, in addition to tumours in various other organs. Both DMBA and one of its metabolites (7-hydroxymethyl-12-methylbenz(a)-anthracene) are embryotoxic and teratogenic [3].

Mechanism of Perinatal Tumour Induction: Reaction of Developmental Carcinogens with Cellular DNA

Chemical carcinogens or their electrophilic metabolites (ultimate carcinogens) react with various cell constituents, including nucleic acids and proteins. During the last decade evidence has accumulated that nuclear DNA is the relevant target molecule and that malignant transformation is initiated by a change in gene structure rather than in gene expression.

Monofunctional Alkylating Agents

Monofunctional aliphatic alkylating agents react at all available nucleophilic sites in DNA bases but the relative extent of reaction at these sites varies considerably and depends primarily on the reaction type of the respective alkylating agent. Comparative studies on the in vitro alkylation of DNA by various compounds have revealed that agents which react predominantly at ring nitrogen atoms in DNA bases are usually weak carcinogens (e.g. diazoalkanes, alkylmethanesulphonates), whereas agents which lead preferentially to O-alkylation (e.g. alkylnitrosoureas) usually exhibit a strong carcinogenic activity (for review see [2]).

In vitro studies using DNA polymerase and alkylated polydeoxyribonucleotides as templates have shown that mispairing during transcription is likely to result from substitution of O^6 of guanine, O^2 of cytosine and O^2 and O^4 of thymine, due to interference with hydrogen bonding between complementary DNA strands. If alkylation of DNA is a crucial event in the initiation of malignant transformation, one may expect that the extent of this reaction in different organs correlates with the location of tumours. However, no such correlation seems to exist for neuro-oncogenic agents. After systemic administration, alkylnitrosoureas are rapidly distributed throughout the animal, including the nervous system, and no accumulation occurs at sites of preferential tumour induction. Since enzymes do not affect their decomposition, levels of DNA alkylation by methylnitrosourea are similar in brain, liver, kidney intestines and other tissues [19]. Similarly, transplacental administration of ethylnitrosourea [9] and methylmethanesulphonate [20] did not show significant differences in DNA alkylation between target and non-target tissues. Prenatally, this is also true for 3,3-dimethyl-1-phenyltriazene (Fig. 1).

Numerous attempts have been made to correlate organ-specific tumour induction by chemical carcinogens with DNA repair capacities of the respective target tissues [2, 24, 38]. Promutagenic O-alkylated bases are, under physiological conditions, chemically stable but can be enzymically removed by a repair process, which has not yet been fully elucidated. Evidence for a differential repair capacity of various organs was first demonstrated for the neuro-oncogenic alkylnitrosoureas. O^6-Ethylguanine produced by a single injection of ethylnitrosourea into ten-day-old rats was found to be removed from DNA of the brain, which is the principal target

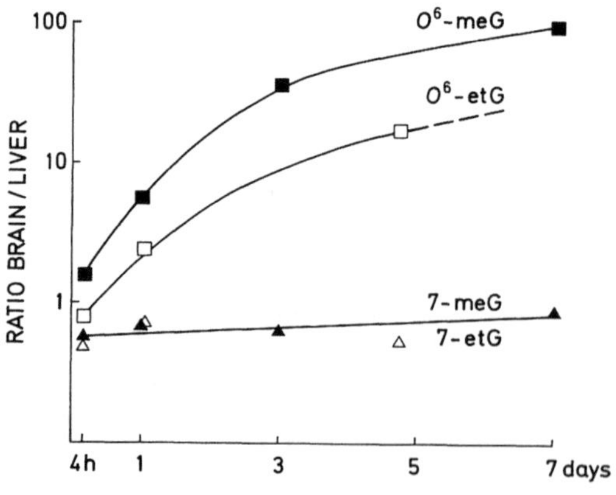

Fig. 2. Ratio of the brain and liver concentrations of O^6- and 7-alkylguanine after a single intraperitoneal injection of N-(^{3}H)-methyl-N-nitrosourea (10 mg/kg; *closed symbols)* or N-(^{14}C)-ethyl-N-nitrosourea (75 mg/kg; *open symbols)* in 10-day-old BD-IX rats. (Compiled from [10] and [23])

organ, at a much slower rate than from that of liver, a non-target organ in this animal [10]. Similarly, O^6-methylguanine produced by a single dose of methylnitrosourea to adult or ten-day-old rats [23, 24] persisted considerably longer in brain DNA than in that of other rat organs. Within one week after the administration of alkylnitrosoureas to ten-day-old rats, the amounts of O^6-alkylguanine present in cerebral DNA were about twenty times (ethylnitrosourea) and 90 times (methylnitrosourea) higher than in hepatic DNA (Fig. 2). This seemed to indicate that nervous-system specific carcinogenesis by aliphatic alkylating agents results from a deficient DNA repair capacity in the target tissues. However, comparative studies in mice showed a less consistent correlation [24].

In gerbils (Meriones unguiculatus) the repair capacity for O^6-methylguanine was even less than in rat brain, although this species is apparently not susceptible to the neuro-oncogenic effect of methylnitrosourea and related agents [25]. In conclusion, these data indicate that the formation and persistence of O^6-alkylguanine (and other O-alkylated bases) may constitute a necessary although not sufficient event for the initiation of organ-specific carcinogenesis by monofunctional alkylating agents.

7,12-Dimethylbenz(a)anthracene

According to the 'bay region hypothesis' of hydrocarbon activation [16] the carcinogenicity of benz(a)anthracene and its analogues should result from the formation of diol epoxides in the 1,2,3,4-positions of the molecule. Accordingly, 3,4-diol-1,2-epoxides would be expected to represent the ultimate carcinogens of DMBA and this view is supported by several reports on the mutagenicity of DMBA 3,4-dihydrodiols. In one experiment the reaction of ^{3}H-DMBA with DNA of maternal and fetal rat tissues was investigated [4]. After a single intravenous injection (15 mg/kg body weight) on day 21 of gestation, separation of enzymic DNA digests showed a chromatographic profile that was similar in all organs. Among the maternal organs the extent of adduct formation was highest in intestine, followed by liver, lung, spleen, kidney and brain. In intestinal DNA, adduct concentration was almost 15 times higher than in cerebral DNA. In fetal intestine and liver, concentrations were 34% and 16% lower than in the respective maternal organs. In contrast, the concentration of the major reaction product in fetal brain was 2.5 times higher than in maternal brain DNA.

In a further experiment ^{3}H-DMBA was directly injected into the amniotic fluid of 21-day-old rat fetuses [26]. Superimposed radiochromatographs of DNA hydrolysates from fetal brain after intravenous and intra-amniotic injection of ^{3}H-DMBA are shown in Fig. 3. In both conditions, the major product elutes at a similar position. However, the fraction of radioactivity present in the satellite peaks was considerably higher after intra-amniotic injection. This was also true for the incorporation of tritium into deoxyadenosine. Of all maternal organs investigated, only liver DNA contained measurable amounts of DMBA-DNA adducts (less than 10% of that in fetal DNA) after intra-amniotic injection. The observation that the chromatographic profile differs considerably depending on the route of administration suggests that bioactivation responsible for DMBA binding to fetal DNA may occur both in the fetus itself and in maternal organs. Autoradiographic

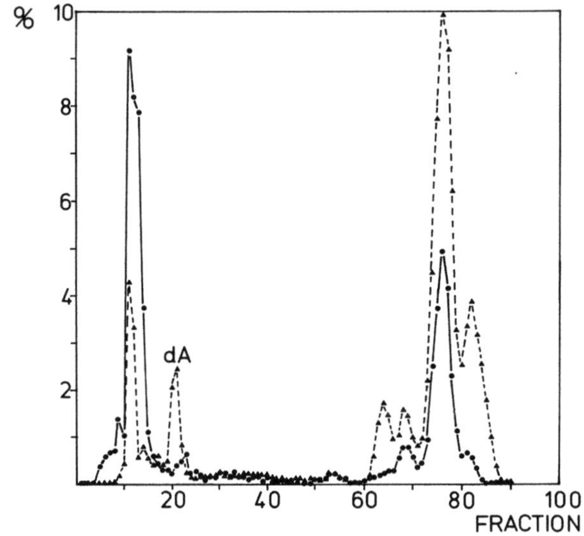

Fig. 3. Reaction of 7,12-dimethylbenz(a)anthracene (DMBA) with fetal rat brain DNA. ^3H-DMBA was administered intravenously to the pregnant female (15 mg/kg, *circles)* or directly into the amniotic fluid (4 µg/fetus, *triangles).* After 12 hours animals were killed. DNA was isolated, enzymically hydrolysed and separated on Sephadex LH-20 columns eluted with 20–100% aqueous methanol. Radioactivity of each fraction is expressed as percentage of the total radioactivity present. DMBA-DNA adducts elute between fractions 60 and 90; *dA,* deoxyadenosine. (From Kleihues et al. [27])

studies [27] indicate that DMBA crosses the placenta rather late. At 3.5 minutes after intravenous injection of ^{14}C-DMBA there is, in contrast to most maternal organs no detectable labelling of fetuses and even after 12 minutes they appear only moderately exposed. The possibility exists, therefore, that despite the capacity of fetuses to metabolize DMBA, proximate carcinogens produced by maternal organs may be included in the binding of DMBA to fetal DNA.

Comparative Aspects of Neuro-Oncogenesis During Development and in Adult Animals

The response to neuro-oncogenic agents of the developing nervous system differs considerably from that of adult animals. The most striking dissimilarities are summarized as follows.

Single Dose Compared with Chronic Carcinogen Administration

In adult animals, repeated administration of carcinogens is required to produce a high incidence of neurogenic tumours. In perinatal carcinogenesis, a single dose is sufficient to induce tumours of the nervous system in 90–100% of experimental animals.

Dose-Response Relationship and Induction Time

The neuro-oncogenic agents listed in Table 1 exert their adverse biological effects on fetuses at concentrations which produce little or no effects in the pregnant female. This is particularly true for ethylnitrosourea. When given transplacentally on day 15 of gestation, a dose of 3.2 mg/kg body weight (related to the pregnant female) is sufficient to induce a 50% incidence of malignant tumours of the nervous system in the offspring [12].

Even a dose of only 1 mg/kg, corresponding to 0.4% of the LD_{50} in adult rats, induces a tumour incidence of approximately 16%. In adult rats, ethylnitrosourea is also a potent carcinogen but the dose required for the induction of neural tumours in 50% of experimental animals is 160 mg/kg, i.e. approximately 50 times higher than that transplacentally. The exceptionally high susceptibility is also reflected by the short induction time. Administration of ethylnitrosourea to 30-day-old rats causes the development of nervous system tumours after a latency period approximately 2.5 times longer than following a similar dose on the first postnatal day.

Influence of the Developmental Stage on Incidence and Location of Tumours

Transplacental induction of neurogenic tumours in rats is possible only after day 11 of the gestation period. This is not due to a lack of penetration of carcinogens into fetal tissues since embryotoxic and teratogenic effects are known to occur after treatment during earlier stages of pregnancy. The susceptibility of the nervous system toward chemical carcinogens steadily increases after day 11 and reaches a maximum during the final period of intrauterine development. After the first month of postnatal growth the response to neuro-oncogenic agents approaches that of adult animals.

The biological basis of this phenomenon, which may also be present in other species, is not yet understood. In the rat, the nervous system is apparently the target tissue for any carcinogen which reaches the fetuses between 11 and 21 days of gestation. Administration of alkylnitrosoureas around birth produces, in addition, some nephroblastomas. In rabbits, on the other hand, exposure of fetuses to ethylnitrosourea during the early stages of gestation leads to the induction of neurogenic tumours, whereas in later stages the same carcinogen causes a selective induction of renal neoplasms. Considerable differences have been observed in the organ-specificity of carcinogens administered prenatally or after maturation.

1,2-Dimethylhydrazine (DMH) induces a low incidence of nervous system tumours perinatally; in adult rats it is a very powerful colon carcinogen. The ethyl analogue 1,2-diethyl-hydrazine is a very potent neuro-oncogenic agent when given prenatally; in adult rats, this compound induces a significant incidence of aesthesioneuroepitheliomas [7]. DMBA induces predominantly neurogenic and renal neoplasms transplacentally, in young female rats it causes a very high incidence of mammary tumours. These and other examples demonstrate that the susceptibility of various organs changes during development, and that carcinogenicity studies in adults do not allow any conclusions regarding the response of fetal tissues of the same species.

In adult animals, tumours are, with some exceptions, preferentially located in the brain. Perinatal administration leads to a higher proportion of tumours originating from the spinal cord and the peripheral nervous system. In BDIX rats, neurinomas of the trigeminal nerve occur most frequently after administration at the end of the gestation period [8] whereas neurinomas of spinal roots are more frequent after postnatal administration [33]. Similarly, the preferential location of CNS tumours varies with developmental stage and is, to some extent strain-dependant.

Carcinogenesis and Teratogenesis

The relationship between developmental carcinogenesis and teratogenesis has been widely discussed (for review see [21, 44]) and may be summarized in the statement that all developmental carcinogens are teratogenic, but only a few teratogens are carcinogenic. Depending on dose and developmental stage, alkyl-acylnitrosamides also cause a variety of teratogenic effects (for review see [44]). Dose-response relationships for the induction by ethylnitrosourea of neural tumours and malformations of the legs in rats on day 15 of gestation are shown in Fig. 4. These data show that the dose required to produce macroscopically detectable malformations was considerably lower than that needed for malignant transformation. The teratogenicity of perinatal carcinogens is based mainly on their cytotoxic effect on proliferating cells, e.g. the periventricular matrix cell layers of the brain. Since malignant transformation is also restricted to proliferating cell populations, a strong cytotoxic effect may reduce the target-cell population for tumourigenesis to such an extent that the tumour incidence in the offspring is greatly decreased. Methylating and ethylating carcinogens are similarly effective in adult rats. Transplacentally, however, ethylating agents are much more effective (Table 1). This has been shown for ethylnitrosourea compared with methylnitrosourea, 3,3-diethyl-1-phenyltriazene compared with 3,3-dimethyl-1-phenyltriazene and 1,2-diethylhydrazine compared with 1,2-dimethylhydrazine. This phenomenon can be explained by the relatively high toxicity of methylating agents, which react predominantly on nitrogen atoms in DNA bases. Ethylating carcinogens react more extensively on oxygen atoms and produce fewer cytotoxic effects, i.e. their balance between teratogenic and carcino-

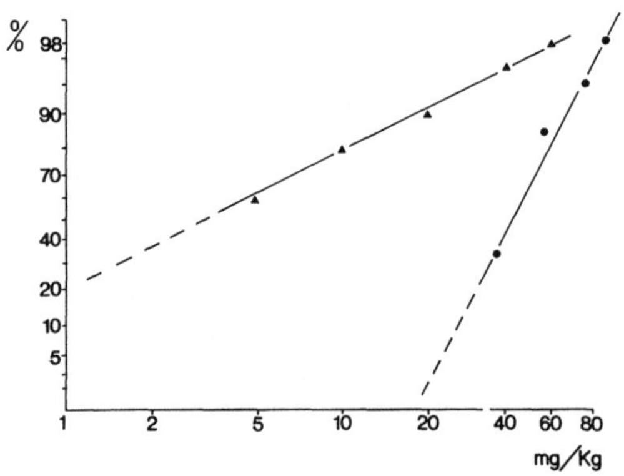

Fig. 4. Dose-response relationship for the carcinogenic (incidence of nervous system tumours, *triangles)* and teratogenic effects (hindleg and foreleg malformations, *circles)* or *N*-ethyl-*N*-nitrosourea in BD-IX rats. The carcinogen was administered as a single intravenous injection on day 15 of gestation. (Redrawn from figures published by Ivankovic and Druckrey [12])

genic effect is very much in favour of carcinogenicity (Fig. 4). Alexandrov and Napalkov [1] have elegantly demonstrated that pretreatment with methylnitrosourea significantly reduces the incidence of tumours produced by a subsequent dose of ethylnitrosourea. Pretreatment with X-rays is similarly effective [42].

References

1. Alexandrov V. A., Napalkov, N. P.: Experimental study of relationship between teratogenesis and carcinogenesis in the brain of the rat. Cancer Letters *1,* 345–350 (1976)
2. O'Connor P. J.: Interaction of chemical carcinogens with macromolecules. J. Cancer Res. Clin. Oncology *99,*167–186 (1981)
3. Currie A. R., Crawford A. M., Bird C. C.: The embryopathic and adrenocorticolytic effects of DMBA and its metabolites. In: Transplacental Carcinogenesis. IARC Scientific Publication No. 4, L. Tomatis, U. Mohr (eds.), pp. 149–153, International Agency for Research on Cancer, Lyon (1973)
4. Doerjer G., Diessner H., Buecheler J., Kleihues P.: Reaction of 7,12-dimethylbenz(a)anthracene with DNA of fetal and maternal rat tissues in vivo. Int. J. Cancer: *22,* 288–291 (1978)
5. Druckrey H., Ivankovic S., Preussmann R.: Teratogenic and carcinogenic effects in the offspring after single injection of ethylnitrosourea to pregnant rats. Nature *210,* 1378–1379 (1966)
6. Druckrey H., Ivankovic S., Preussmann R., Landschütz C., Stekar J., Brunner U., Schagen B.: Transplacental induction of neurogenic malignomas by 1,2-diethylhydrazine, azo- and azoxy-ethane in rats. Experientia *24,* 561–562 (1968)
7. Druckrey H.: Specific carcinogenic and teratogenic effects of 'indirect' alkylating methyl and ethyl compounds, and their dependency on stages of oncogenic developments. Xenobiotica *3,* 271–303 (1973)
8. Druckrey H.: Chemical structure and action in transplacental carcinogenesis and teratogenesis. In: Transplacental Carcinogenesis. IARC Scientific Publications No. 4, L. Tomatis, U. Mohr (eds.), pp. 45–58, International Agency for Research on Cancer, Lyon (1973)
9. Goth R., Rajewsky M. F.: Ethylation of nucleic acids by ethylnitrosurea-1-^{14}C in the fetal and adult rat. Cancer Res. *32,* 1501–1505 (1972)
10. Goth R., Rajewsky M. F.: Molecular and cellular mechanisms associated with pulse-carcinogenesis in the rat nervous system by ethylnitrosourea: Ethylation of nucleic acids and elimination rates of ethylated bases from the DNA of different tissues. Z. Krebsforsch. Klin. Onkol. *82,* 37–64 (1974)
11. Greenwald P., Barlow J. J., Nasca P. C., Burnett W. S. Vaginal cancer after maternal treatment with synthetic estrogens. New England J. Med. *285,* 390–392 (1971)
12. Ivankovic S., Druckrey H.: Transplacentare Erzeugung maligner Tumoren des Nervensystems. Z. Krebsforsch. Klin. Onkol. *71,* 320–360 (1968)
13. Ivankovic S, Preussmann R.: Transplazentare Erzeugung maligner Tumoren. Naturwissenschaften *57,* 460 (1970)
14. Ivankovic S.: Erzeugung von Malignomen bei Ratten nach transplazentarer Einwirkung von N-isopropyl-2-(methylhydrazino)-p-toluamid · HCl. Arzneimittel-Forschung *22,* 905–907 (1972)
15. Ivankovic S., Port R., Preussmann R.: Unterschiedliche carcinogene Wirkungen von 1-Phenyl- und 1-(Pyridyl-3)-3,3-diäthyl-triazen an BD-Ratten nach Gabe einer Einzeldosis am 1., 10. oder 30. Lebenstag. Z. Krebsforsch. *86,* 307–313 (1976)
16. Jerina D. M., Daly J. W.: Oxidation at carbon. In: Drug Metabolism, D. V. Parke and R. L. Smiths (eds.), pp. 13–32. London: Taylor and Francis Ltd. 1976
17. Herbst A. L., Ulfelder H., Poskanzer D. C.: Adenocarcinoma of the vagina. Association of maternal stilbestrol therapy with tumor appearance in young women. New England J. Med. *284,* 878–881 (1971)

18. Kleihues P., Patzschke K.: Verteilung von N-(^{14}C)Methyl-N-nitroso-harnstoff in der Ratte nach systemischer Applikation. Z. Krebsforsch. *75,* 193–200 (1971)
19. Kleihues P., Magee P. N.: Alkylation of rat brain nucleic acids by N-methyl-N-nitrosourea and methyl methanesulphonate. J. Neurochem. *20,* 595–606 (1973)
20. Kleihues P., Patzschke K., Margison G. P. Wegner L. A., Mende C.: Reaction of methyl methanesulphonate with nucleic acids of fetal and newborn rats in vivo. Z. Krebsforsch. *81,* 273–283 (1974)
21. Kleihues P., Lantos P. L., Magee P. N.: Chemical carcinogenesis in the nervous system. Int. Rev. Exp. Pathol. *15,* 153–232 (1976)
22. Kleihues P., Buecheler J., Riede U. N.: Selective induction of melanomas in gerbils (Meriones unguiculatus) following postnatal administration of N-ethyl-N-nitrosourea. J. Natl. Cancer Inst. *61,* 859–863 (1978)
23. Kleihues P., Cooper H. K., Buecheler J., Kolar G. F., Diessner H.: Mechanism of perinatal tumour induction by neuro-oncogenic alkylnitrosoureas and dialkylaryltriazenes. Natl. Cancer Inst. Monogr. *51,* 227–231 (1979)
24. Kleihues P., Doerjer G., Swenberg J. A., Hauenstein E., Buecheler J., Cooper H. K.: DNA repair as regulatory factor in the organotropy of alkylating carcinogens. Arch. Toxicol., Suppl. *2,* 253–261 (1979)
25. Kleihues P., Bamborschke S., Doerjer G.: Persistence of alkylated DNA bases in the Mongolian gerbil (Meriones unguiculatus) following a single dose of methylnitrosourea. Carcinogenesis *1,* 111–113 (1980)
26. Kleihues P., Doerjer G., Ehret M., Guzman J.: Reaction of Benzo(a)pyrene and 7,12-Dimethylbenz(a)-anthracene with DNA of various rat tissues in vivo. Arch. Toxicol., Suppl. *3,* 237–246 (1980)
27. Kleihues P.: Developmental Carcinogenicity. In: Developmental Toxicology. K. Snell (ed.), pp. 211–246. London: Croom Helm Ltd. 1982
28. Larsen C. D.: Pulmonary-tumor induction by transplacental exposure to urethane. J. Natl. Cancer Inst. *8,* 63–69 (1947)
29. Margison G. P., Likhachev A. J., Kolar G. F.: In vivo alkylation of foetal, maternal and normal rat tissue nucleic acids by 3-methyl-1-phenyltriazene. Chem.-Biol. Interactions *25,* 345–353 (1979)
30. Mirvish S. S.: Formation of N-nitroso compounds: Chemistry, kinetics, and in vivo occurrence. Toxicol. Appl Pharmacol. *31,* 325–351 (1975)
31. Mohr U., Althoff J.: Mögliche diaplacentar-carcinogene Wirkung von Diäthylnitrosamin beim Goldhamster. Naturwissenschaften *51,* 515 (1964)
32. Mohr U., Emura M., Richter-Reichhelm H.-B.: Transplacental carcinogenesis. Invest. Cell. Pathol. *3,* 209–229 (1980)
33. Naito M., Naito Y., Ito A.: Effect of age at treatment on the incidence and location of neurogenic tumors induced in Wistar rats by a single dose of N-Ethyl-N-nitrosourea. Gann *72,* 569–577 (1981)
34. Napalkov N. P., Alexandrov V. A.: Neutrotropic effect of 7,12-dimethylbenz(a)anthracene in transplacental carcinogenesis. J. Natl. Cancer Inst. *52,* 1365–1366 (1974)
35. Peters J. M. Preston-Martin S., Yu M. C.: Brain tumours in children and occupational exposure of parents. Science *213,* 235–237 (1981)
36. Preussmann R, von Hodenberg A.: Mechanism of carcinogenesis with l-aryl-3,3-dialkyltriazenes-II. In vitro-alkylation of guanosine, RNA and DNA with aryl-monoalkyltriazenes to form 7-alkylguanine. Biochemical Pharmacology *19,* 1505–1508 (1970)
37. Rice J. M., Joshi S. R., Shenefelt R. E., Wenk M. L.: Transplacental carcinogenic activity of 7,12-dimethylbenz(a)anthracene. In: Polynuclear Aromatic Hydrocarbons. Carcinogenesis, Vol. 3, P. W. Jones, R. I. Freudenthal (eds.), pp. 413–422. New York: Raven Press 1978
38. Singer B.: N-nitroso alkylating agents: Formation and persistence of alkyl derivatives in mammalian nucleic acids as contributing factors in carcinogenesis. J. Natl. Canc. Inst. *62,* 1329–1339 (1979)
39. Stavrou D., Hänichen T., Wriedt-Lübbe, I.: Oncogene Wirkung von Äthylnitrosoharnstoff beim Kaninchen während der pränatalen Periode. Z. Krebsforsch. Klin. Onkol. *84,* 207–215 (1975)

40. Stavrou D., Dahme E., Schröder B.: Transplacentare neuroonkogene Wirkung von Äthylnitrosoharnstoff beim Kaninchen während der frühen Graviditätsphase. Z. Krebsforsch. Klin. Onkol. *89,* 331–339 (1977)
41. Tomatis L.: Prenatal exposure to chemical carcinogens and its effects on subsequent generations. Natl. Cancer Inst. Monogr. *51,* 159–184 (1979)
42. Warkany J., Mandybur, T. I., Kalter H.: Oncogenic response of rats with X-ray-induced microcephaly to transplacental ethylnitrosourea. J. Natl. Cancer Inst. *56,* 59–64 (1976)
43. Warzok R., Schneider J., Thust R., Scholtze P., Potzsch H. D.: Transplacental tumour induction by N-ethyl-N-nitrosourea in different species. Zentralbl. Allg. Pathol. *121,* 54–60 (1970)
44. Wechsler W.: Carcinogenic and teratogenic effects of ethylnitrosourea and methylnitrosourea during pregnancy in experimental rats. In: Transplacental Carcinogenesis. IARC Scientific Publication No. 4, L. Tomatis, U. Mohr (eds.), pp. 127–142. Lyon: International Agency for Research on Cancer 1973

Brain Tumours and Genetics

J. Spranger

Only few central nervous system tumours are inherited. Though rare, they are proof that hereditary factors play a role in the causation and/or pathogenesis of at least some CNS tumours.

In the following sections I will briefly review evidence for genetic influences in CNS tumour formation. I will then proceed to discuss genetics and cancer in a more general way. How significant are genetic factors in carcinogenesis? What are the mechanisms and what is the relationship between genetic and epigenetic factors? Are there clinical observations which, as experiments of nature, give us some insight into the cellular, subcellular and molecular events leading to tumour formation?

CNS-Tumours and Heredity

Familial Aggregation of CNS-Tumours

CNS tumours occasionally aggregate within families. This is particularly true for gliomas and less common with meningiomas and medulloblastomas [12]. In general, the histological appearance and biological behaviour of the tumours is similar in family members. Though the familial aggregation of CNS tumours is of theoretical interest it is too rare to be of practical significance. Large statistics show that the risk of CNS tumours in relatives of an affected individual is small or negligible [12].

Genetic Disorders with CNS Tumours

There are at least seven genetic disorders in which CNS tumours occur regularly (Table 1). Four of them are so-called phakomatoses. The most common ones are neurofibromatosis and tuberous sclerosis.

Neurofibromatosis has an incidence of about 1 in 3000. It is inherited as an autosomal dominant disorder. It is highly variable in its manifestations and the diagnosis can only be made by the demonstration of café-au-lait spots and/or multiple fibromatous skin tumours. The diagnosis must be considered when a patient has more than five café-au-lait spots greater than 1.5 cm in diameter [10].

The most common tumours are acoustic neuromas, optic gliomas and meningiomas. Malignant degeneration has been reported in 3 to 15% of the cases [16]. Meningosarcomas occur more commonly in children than in adults [2].

Table 1. Inherited disorders with central nervous system tumours

Disorder	Genetics	Common CNS tumour
Neurofibromatosis	a.d.	(acoustic) Neurinoma (optic) Glioma Meningioma
Tuberous sclerosis	a.d.	Giant cell astrocytoma
v. Hippel-Lindau Syndrome	a.d.	Haemangioblastoma
Multiple naevoid basal cell carcinoma syndrome	a.d.	Medulloblastoma
Retinoblastoma	a.d.	Retinoblastoma
Multiple endocrine adenomatosis S. I	a.d.	Pituitary adenoma
Glioma-Polyposis-S.	a.r.	Glioblastoma multiforme Medulloblastoma

The pathogenesis is unknown. The clinical manifestations seem to be related to a defect of cellular growth regulation: cultured fibroblasts from patients with neurofibromatosis grow more slowly and stop growing at a lower population density than normal cells [26]. Humoral factors such as nerve growth factor may be involved [4]. These factors may even affect the embryo: children born with neurofibromatosis have a more severe disease when the mother is the affected parent than when the father is affected [17]. About 50% of all cases are caused by new mutations. It is not clear if the wide range of manifestations seen in neurofibromatosis is due to variability of expression of one and the same gene defect or if there is genetic heterogeneity with a central and a peripheral form of the disease. Families have been observed in which only the central nervous system was affected without peripheral involvement [5, 9].

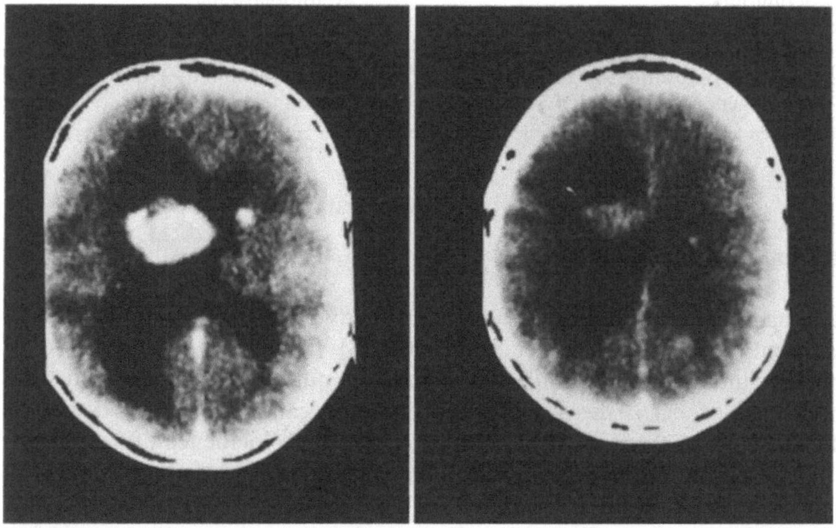

Fig. 1. Computerized cranial tomography of giant cell astrocytoma arising from tubera in tuberous sclerosis

Tuberous sclerosis occurs with a frequency of about 1 in 30.000. Its chief manifestations are epilepsy, mental deficiency and skin lesions. Epileptic seizures seem to occur in almost all and mental deficiency in about two thirds of the patients. The characteristic skin lesions – ash-leaf depigmented naevi – are probably already present at birth in most patients [7] and are an early clue to the diagnosis. Adenoma sebaceum develops later. The mass in the brain ("tuber") which gives it its name consists of gliomatous tissue with calcium deposits. They are easily detected by computerized tomography (Fig. 1) and can already be detected in infancy. From the tubers neoplasms may arise, mostly benign giant cell gliomas. Mixed embryonal tumours are found in the kidneys, rhabdomyomas in the myocardium, angiofibromas in the skin. The disorder is inherited as an autosomal dominant. About 85% of the cases are new mutations [17].

The Significance of Genetic Factors in Carcinogenesis

There are several lines of evidence to support the hypothesis that genetic factors play a major role in the aetiology and/or pathogenesis of neoplasms in general (Table 2).

Table 2. Lines of evidence for genetic influences in cancerogenesis

Evidence	Example
1) Familial aggregation of tumours	Familial adenocarcinomatosis
2) Neoplasias and genetic markers	Blood group A + stomach Ca
3) Hereditary tumours	Retinoblastoma
4) Genetic dysplasias with tumour disposition	Wiedemann-Beckwith syndrome
5) Neoplasias and single malformations	Aniridia + Wilms tumour
6) Neoplasias and chromosome aberrations	Retinoblastoma + 13q-
7) Neoplasias and genetic immunodeficiencies	Ataxia teleangiectatica

Familial Tumour Aggregation

The familial aggregation of brain tumours has already been cited. A similar association has been reported with other neoplasms [8]. Though the aggregation of tumour-bearing individuals in families is sometimes quite conspicuous it must be kept in mind that cancer is the second most common cause of death and that by statistical chance alone there must be families with a high incidence of neoplasms. The fact that certain tumours occur not only in various family members but also as multiple primary tumours in single individuals [8] supports the assumptions of a familial (genetic?) tumour predisposition. Twin studies have shown that genetic factors predispose to tumour type and location rather than to tumour frequency [24].

Neoplasms and Genetic Markers

A genetic marker is a protein or other phenotype determined by a single gene locus. Examples are the blood groups, the HLA system or the cerumen marker. By comparing the incidence of certain tumours in individuals with different genetic markers statistical associations have been found. For instance, cancer of the stomach and cancer of the salivary glands is more common in blood group A individuals [26]. Various HLA antigens have been found to be associated with neoplastic diseases though the statistical association is not as strong as, for instance, that between HLA B-27 and ankylosing spondylitis [21]. The statistical association of genetic markers and disease suggests that constitutional factors contribute to tumour formation.

Hereditary Single Tumours

There are at least 17 types of tumours which are inherited as single Mendelian traits [20] (Table 3). Fourteen are inherited as autosomal dominants and three as autosomal recessives. These tumours are proof that the mutation of single genes can induce and/or promote neoplastic growth at specific sites and tissues. The fact that some or all of these conditions can also arise on an apparently non-Mendelian basis suggests aetiological heterogeneity.

Table 3. Single tumours inherited as Mendelian traits (McKusick [17], adapted from Mulvihill [20])

Autosomal dominant	*Autosomal recessive*
Acoustic neuroma (10 100)	Juvenile fibromatosis (22 860)
Retinoblastoma (18 020)	Histiocytic reticulosis (24 640)
Paraganglioma (16 800)	Familial lipochrome histiocytosis (23 590)
Phaeochromocytoma (17 130)	
Multiple leiomata (15 080)	
Multiple lipomatosis (15 190)	
Familial polyposis coli (17 510)	
Gardner syndrome (17 510)	
Peutz-Jegher syndrome (17 520)	
Colorectal Ca	
Ovarian tumours (16 695)	
Multiple glomus tumour (13 800)	
Multiple trichoepithelioma (13 270)	
Squamous epithelioma (13 280)	

Genetic Dysplasias with Tumour Disposition

Dysplasias are inborn errors of tissue development, i.e. the result of dyshistogenesis [25]. Many of them are inherited as Mendelian traits and predispose to malignant degeneration. The 'genetic repertory of human neoplasia' lists 200 conditions with neoplastic tendencies [20]. Most of them are localized or generalized dysplasias. Examples are neurofibromatosis, the Wiedemann-Beckwith syndrome and enchondromatosis. The multiple tumour syndromes such as the multiple endocrine neoplasia syndromes or the Gardner syndrome also fall into this category.

Dominantly inherited dysplasias are mostly caused by defects of structural proteins, recessively inherited dysplasias by enzyme defects. Tumours are associated mainly with defects of structural proteins and with defective enzymes acting in nucleic acid metabolism. Enzyme defects affecting carbohydrate, lipid or amino-acid metabolism do not seem to lead to any increased tumour tendency (Fig. 2).

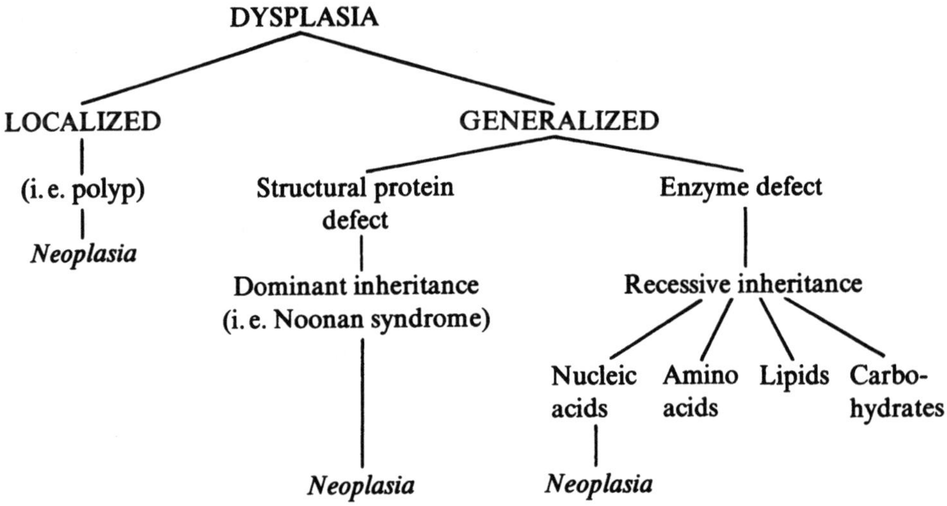

Fig. 2. Schema depicting the relationship between different types of dysplasias and their relation to neoplastic tendencies

Neoplasms and Single Malformations

Malformations are intrinsic errors of organ development [25]. Although it is frequently said that tumours occur commonly in association with malformations this statement must be qualified. Single errors of organ development such as heart defects, cleft lips, polydactyly are not associated with an increased risk of neoplasia. The exceptions such as aniridia or non-specific renal abnormalities in Wilms tumour patients are probably the result of prenatally occuring local dysplasias, and the relationship is identical to that outlined in Fig. 2. What is commonly called a 'malformation' is in reality a 'dysplasia'.

Neoplasms and Chromosomal Disorders

Tumour cells frequently show abnormalities of chromosome number and/or structure [23]. The best known example is the Ph^1 chromosome in myelogenous leukemia. Similar chromosome abnormalities can be produced by carcinogenic agents such as radiation or certain chemicals. They are probably secondary or correlated rather than causal phenomena reflecting a deep disturbance of mitogenic activity of the cell.

Table 4. Chromosomal instability syndromes and cancer

Condition (inheritance)	Major clinical manifestations	Complicating neoplasia	Major chromosomal changes
Bloom syndrome (a.r.)	Primordial dwarfism Characteristic face Sun sensitive telangiectatic facial erythema	Acute leukemia	Increased number of chromatic exchanges
Fanconi syndrome (a.r.)	Small stature Congenital heart defects Pancytopenia	Acute leukemia	Chromosomal breaks and gaps
Ataxia telangiectatica	Small stature Cerebellar ataxia Telangiectasias Decreased IgA levels	Cancer Lymphoma	Chromosomal breaks and rearrangements
Xeroderma pigmentosum (a.r.) (heterogenous)	Early photosensitivity Multiple skin lesions in sun exposed areas (including keratoses, keratocanthoma, angioma etc.)	Skin cancer	Chromosomal rearrangements

There are, however, a number of conditions in which chromosomal abnormalities antedate tumour development. Patients with Down's syndrome, for instance, have a higher than normal risk of developing leukemia suggesting that trisomy 21 predisposes to the formation (or lack of elimination?) of malignant bone marrow cells.

Of great interest in this respect are the so-called chromosome instability syndromes (Table 4). These disorders have in common a disposition to spontaneous chromosomal abnormalities, particularly breakage of chromosomes *in vitro,* and an increased tendency to develop malignancies.

Neoplasms and Hereditary Immunodeficiencies

The incidence of malignancy in patients with hereditary immunodeficiencies is estimated to be ten thousand times higher than in a comparable control population [9]. Most of the tumours involve the lymphoreticular system. The same tendency, although to a less marked degree, is observed in secondary immunodeficiencies such as those caused by immunosuppressive or cytotoxic drugs [15].

Genetic Mechanisms in Carcinogenesis

The clinical evidence cited above supports the principal role of genetic factors in carcinogenesis. But what are the mechanisms involved? Information regarding possible genetic mechanisms in carcinogenesis can be obtained at the tissue, cellular, nuclear and molecular level.

Tissue Level: Teratogenesis and Oncogenesis

Oncogenesis and teratogenesis are intimately related. Oncogens such as urethane, alcohol or irradiation are also teratogens [1, 3]. Both types of agent lead to abnormal tissue development (dysplasias) through dyshistogenesis.

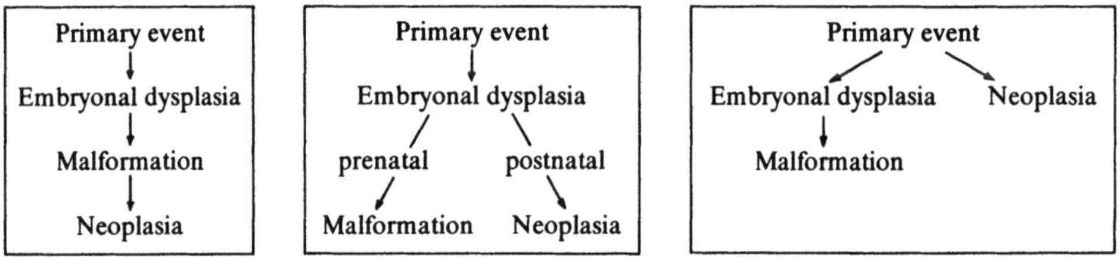

Fig. 3. Three models to explain dysplasias, malformations and the formal relationship between neoplasias

Most errors of morphogenesis recognizable postnatally with an increased tumour tendency are dysplasias such as polyps or osteogenesis imperfecta. Few are classified as malformations and they possibly arise from intrauterine dysplasias such as aniridia or renal abnormalities. There are three possibilities how dysplasia, malformation and neoplasia may formally be related (Fig. 3): A) The primary event such as a mutation or environmental agent causes an embryonal dysplasia which leads to a malformation. The tumour arises within this malformation. This concept is unlikely since malformations are almost never the morphologic basis of tumours. B) The primary event causes a mono- or polytopic dysplasia which prenatally may lead to a malformation and postnatally predisposes to tumour formation. In the case of the Wilms tumour – renal malformation association, malformation and tumour are contiguous. In the case of the aniridia-Wilms tumour association they are non-contiguous. The propensity of tumours to develop in dysplastic tissue such as a hamartoma or undescended testis is compatible with this concept. C) Embryonal dysplasia and postnatal neoplasia are independantly caused by the same primary agent. In this instance, dysplasia and neoplasia are not causally related but are independant manifestations of the same causal process. Whereas in B a tumour would always arise from dysplastic tissue this would not be the case in C.

Cellular Level: The Two-Hit Theory

Malignancy does not develop in all undescended testes and not all enchondromata become malignant. This observation is one of the reasons for formulating the so-called 'two-hit theory'. It claims that a cell is first brought to a pre-malignant state. A second event causes its malignant transformation (Fig. 4). Both events may be in-

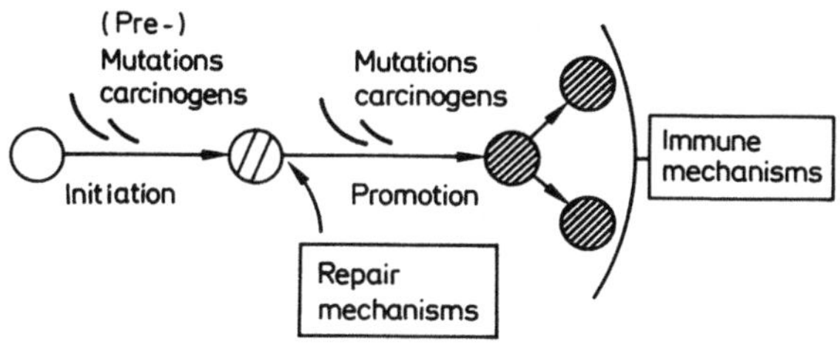

Fig. 4. Two-step theory of neoplastic transformation and defense mechanisms

dependant genetic mutations at different gene loci [16]. Or they may involve the same, labile gene which first undergoes a premutation and then a mutation [12, 13]. Both ideas are particularly suited to explain such partially hereditary tumours as retino-blastomas or chemodectomas.

On the other hand, one step may be caused by genetic and the other by epigenetic events or both may be caused by environmental agents.

Nuclear Level: Chromosomal Abnormalities

Chromosomes are DNA-histone complexes containing linear sequences of genetic information. The visibly recognizable chromosome changes in malignant cells and in cancer-prone states such as the Fanconi syndrome or Bloom syndrome show that carcinogenesis is deeply related to abnormalities of DNA structure and metabolism.

Molecular Level: Errors of DNA Metabolism and Immune Defense

Xeroderma pigmentosum is an experiment of nature which demonstrates the importance of nucleic acid metabolism in carcinogenesis. Patients with this disorder have freckles of different size and shape on sun-exposed skin, telangiectasia and white spots. In the skin, hundreds of tumours such as basal cell carcinomas, squamous cell carcinomas and melanomas can arise. The patients frequently die at an early age. There are at least five different mutations leading to xeroderma pigmentosum. They are caused by a number of defects in the repair mechanism of damaged DNA [2]. In the normal individual, spontaneously occurring or environmentally induced defects in the DNA chain are repaired through sequential mechanisms involving the incision and excision of damaged portions of DNA and their replacement through replicated normal patches of DNA. In xeroderma pigmentosum this repair process is disturbed. Though the defect seems to be directly related to carcinogenesis, it is probably not the primary, initiating or promoting event. It is rather a defect of a defense mechanism which corrects damage caused by unknown carcinogens (Fig. 4).

In the hereditary immunodeficiencies a second line of anti-cancer defense is damaged. Hereditary immunodeficiencies are caused by the faulty transcription of enzyme or structural proteins which are involved in the immune surveillance of, and in the immune response to tumour cells (Fig. 4). A defect in this recognition and elimination system leads to the uninhibited multiplication and spread of tumour cells.

Though xeroderma pigmentosum and the hereditary immunodeficiencies do not explain the primary events leading to malignant transformation of the cell they give an excellent insight into genetic mechanisms of metabolic control and immune defense which normally prevent the progression of a neoplastic process.

Summary. Central nervous system tumours are rarely familial and the genetic risk of recurrence is minimal except in a few genetically determined disorders with a high CNS tumour incidence such as neurofibromatosis, tuberous sclerosis, v. Hippel-Lindau disease and others. Tumour formation in general is, however, intimately related to genetic factors. The available evidence for the role of genetic factors in tumour formation is briefly reviewed. Disorders of DNA repair mechanisms and immunologic deficiencies have been shown to play a major role in neoplastic cell transformation The nosologic difference between malformations and dysplasias is stressed. Malformations are disorders of organ development and are only rarely associated with tumours. Dysplasias are disorders of tissue development and frequently predispose to tumour formation.

References

1. Bolande, R. P.: Childhood tumours and their relationship to birth defects. In (19), p. 43–76 (1977)
2. Cleaver, J. E.: Xeroderma pigmentosum. In: Stanbury J. B. et al. (ed.) The Metabolic Basis of Inherited Disease. New York, McGraw Hill, p. 1072 (1978)
3. Cohen, M. M.: Neoplasia and the fetal alcohol and hydantoin syndromes. Neurobehavioural Toxicol Teratol *3,* 161–172 (1981)
4. Crouse S. K., Berg, B. O.: Intracranial meningiomas in childhood and adolescence. Neurology *22,* 135–141 (1972)
5. Fabricant, R. N., Todar, G. J.: Increased serum levels of nerve growth factor in von Recklinghausen disease. Arch. Neurol *38,* 401–413 (1981)
6. Feiling, A., Ward, E.: A familial form of acoustic tumour. Brit. Med. J. *1,* 496–499 (1920)
7. Fitzpatrick, T. B., Szabo, G., Hori, Y, Simone, A. A., Reed, W. B., Greenberg, M. H.: White leaf-shaped macules. Arch. Dermat. *98,* 1–6 (1968)
8. Fraumeni, J. F.: Clinical patterns of familial cancer. In (19), p. 223–234 (1977)
9. Gatti, R. A., Good, R. A.: Occurrence of malignancy in immunodeficiency disorders. Cancer *28,* 89–98 (1971)
10. Gardner, W. J., Turner, O.: Bilateral acoustic neurofibromas: further clinical and pathologic data on hereditary deafness and v. Recklinghausen disease. Arch. Neurol. Psychiat. *44,* 76–99 (1940)
11. Haslam, R. H. A., Shulman, V.: Neurofibromatosis. In Bergsma, D. (ed.) Birth Defects Compendium. New York: Liss 1979
12. Herrmann, J.: Delayed mutation model: carotid body tumours and retinoblastoma. In (19), p. 417–438 (1977)
13. Herrmann, J., Elejalde, B. R.: Clinical Genetics and Pediatric Neoplasias. Pathogenetic and etiologic perspectives. Nat. Cancer Inst. Monogr. *51,* 7–18 (1979)
14. Horton, W. A.: Genetics of central nervous system tumours. Birth Defects Orig. Art. Series XII, *1,* 91–97 (1976)
15. Kirkpatrick, C. H.: Cancer and immunodeficiency diseases. Birth Defects Orig. Art. Series XII, 1 : 61–78 (1976)
16. Knudson, A. G.: Genetic end environmental interaction in the origin of human cancer. In (19), p. 391–400 (1977)

17. McKusick, V. A.: Mendelian Inheritance in Man, 5th ed. Baltimore, John Hopkins Univ. (1978)
18. Miller, M., Hall, J.: Possible maternal effect on severity of neurofibromatosis. Lancet *11*, 1071–1073 (1978)
19. Mulvihill, J. J., Miller, R. W., Fraumeni, J. F. (eds): Progress in Cancer Research and Therapy, Vol. 3. Genetics of Human Cancer, New York: Raven 1977
20. Mulvihill, J. J.: Genetic repertory of human neoplasia. In Mulvihill J. J. et al. (eds) Progress in Cancer research and therapy, vol. 3: Genetics of human cancer. Raven, New York, pp. 137–144
21. Murphy, G. P.: HLA and malignancy. Progr. Clin. Biol. Res., Vol. 16. New York, A. Liss 1977
22. Opitz, J. M., Herrmann, J.: Clinical genetics and cancer. In: Mulvihill J. J. et al. (eds) Progress in cancer research, vol. 3: Genetics of human cancer. Raven, New York, p. 465
23. Sandberg, A. A.: The Chromosomes in Human Cancer and Leukemia. New York, Amsterdam: Elsevier 1980
24. Spranger, J., V. Verschuer, O.: Untersuchungen zur Frage der Erblichkeit des Krebses. Nachuntersuchungen an der auslesefreien Zwillingsserie von v. Verschuer und Kober. Z. menschl. Vererb. Konstit. lehre *37*, 549–571 (1964)
25. Spranger, J., Benirschke, K., Hall, J. G., Lenz, W., Lowry, R. B., Opitz, J. M., Pinsky, L., Schwarzacher, H. G., Smith, D. W.: Errors of Morphogenesis. Concepts and terms. J. Pediat. (1982) in press
26. Vogel, F.: AB0 blood groups and disease. Am. J. Hum. Genet. *22*, 464–475 (1970)
27. Zelkowitz, M., Stambouly, J.: Short communication: neurofibromatosis fibroblasts: slow growth and abnormal morphology. Pediatr. Res. *15*, 290–293 (1981)

Interferon and Antitumour Effects

H.-J. Röthig

In 1957 Isaaks and Lindemann described the antiviral protection of cells by interferon [3].

A quarter of a century later our knowledge about interferon has widened enormously. Today we know more than 10 interferons.

Interferons are a group of highly active glycoproteins, synthesized and secreted by eukaryotic cells after stimulation (induction). The best known inducer is viral RNA. Interferons seem to have the features of intercellular transmitters.

The interferon produced depends on the cell stimulated and the inducer. The present nomenclature (Table 1) distinguishes three main groups. The investigations of interferon m-RNA's have shown that there are several subtypes within the HU IFN-α and HU IFN-β groups. The biological effects of these different polypeptides are not yet clear. Experiments showed a great variety of activity as regards growth inhibition. In combination, magnification and inhibition were observed.

The production of interferon is very expensive and the amounts are limited. The production of interferons by genetic engineering might solve these problems.

Now there is progress in the purification procedures. Older preparation had a purity of only 1 per cent whereas by using monoclonal antibody column techniques a purification up to 95 per cent is possible. Further preparations for clinical use should have a purity of 10–50%.

Antitumour effects of interferon were discovered when interferon was used for the treatment of animals infected with oncoviruses. Interferon therapy given over a long period was effective in preventing the development of leukemia and solid tumours. The action of interferon in these viral induced tumours was not astonishing because this could be explained by the antiviral activity. But in the next step interferon was tested in transplanted non-viral tumours and the treatment was also efficacious in these tumours, though not all animals could be cured from the tumours. The results were good and the animals could be cured if the tumour was small. If the tumour had grown to a big mass there was almost no effect. On the other hand animals bearing tumours which were not interferon sensitive also had an increased life span after interferon therapy, because of the immune stimulation in the host [2].

These encouraging experiments and the activity of K. Cantell who prepared leucocyte interferon in large amounts led to the first clinical investigations.

The results of Strander who treated patients with osteosarcomas are still under discussion as there was no control group in his study. In a study of advanced breast cancer leucocyte interferon showed effects like other chemotherapeutics and similar side reactions. Altogether there were 43 patients treated with no complete response

Table 1. Nomenclature of interferons

Human interferons	Type	Subtype	Molecular weight
Leucocyte interferon Lymphocyte interferon Lymphoblast interferon	HU IFN-α	HU IFN-α_{1-8}	15,000 – 20,000 165 amino acids
Fibroblast interferon	HU IFN-β	HU IFN-β_{1-2}	22,000 – 34,000 187 amino acids
Immune interferon	HU IFN-γ		40,000 – 60,000

and 12 partial responses. A few further studies with sufficient numbers of patients are not finished [1].

Interferon studies of brain tumours are rare. A group from Switzerland reported one complete clinical remission in four cases of astrocytoma. Several authors reported the intrathecal administration of fibroblast interferon in cases of meningeal leukaemia. The response to this treatment was good but all patients relapsed after several weeks.

In cell cultures a growth inhibiting effect of interferon could be seen for several brain tumours mainly for glioblastoma cells. But clinical experiences are still lacking in these cases.

In general the first clinical trials show results which could be expected from the animal data. Those who had hoped for wonders will now be disappointed [4].

Nevertheless there are so many facts about interferon's biological action that there is still hope for the future of interferon or interferon-like substances as antitumour agents.

References

1. Dunnick, J. K., Galasso, G. J.: Update on clinical trials with exogenous interferon. J. Infect. Dis. *142,* 293–299 (1980)
2. Gresser, J., Tovey, M. G.: Antitumour effects of interferon. Biochem. Biophys. Acta *516,* 231–247 (1978)
3. Isaacs, A., Lindenmann, J.: Virus interference. I. Interferon. Proc. R. Soc. London Ser. B *147,* 258–267 (1957)
4. Sikora, K.: Does interferon cure cancer? Brit. Med. J. *281,* 855–858 (1980)

Rare Intracranial Tumours in Infancy and Childhood

K. JELLINGER and E. MACHACEK

Intracranial tumours represent the second commonest malignancy in childhood with an incidence of 22–28 per million population under age 16 years [2, 11]. Although many studies have shown remarkable similarity in distribution of tumour types, their relation to age, sex, anatomical sites and prognosis are not constant, and considerable variation in the morphology and natural history of CNS tumours in infancy and childhood allow only limited comparison of statistical data. The purpose of this study is to demonstrate a number of rare neoplasms observed among 810 histologically verified intracranial tumours under the age of 16 years. They represent 10.8% of the Vienna Brain Tumour Registry between the years 1941 and 1980. Histological diagnosis followed the criteria of the WHO Classification [12].

The sex incidence – 58.5% males and 41.5% females –, the topographic pattern – 44.5% supratentorial, 52% infratentorial, and 3.5% supra- plus infratentorial or multiple –, and the preponderance of neuroepithelial tumours with a high incidence of astrocytomas, medulloblastomas, ependymomas, and malformative tumours (Table 1) agrees with the majority of the published series [2, 7, 9, 11]. Comparison of the relative prevalence of various types of neoplasm confirms the well known difference between children and adults (Table 2): gliomas, medulloblastomas, choroid plexus papillomas, craniopharyngiomas and other malformative tumours are frequent in children, while meningiomas, neurinomas, pituitary adenomas, and metastatic tumours are common in adults. Thirty-five cases or 4.3% of our total series of intracranial neoplasms were confirmed by biopsy and/or autopsy within the first year of life, the majority being congenital tumours [6] clinically presenting as progressive hydrocephalus or increased intracranial pressure (Table 3). In young infants, all types of tumours known in children and adults except for pituitary adenomas may occur, but there are considerable differences in their relative prevalence, choroid plexus papillomas, meningeal tumours and malformative tumours being more frequent under age one year. Comparison of our series of tumours in infancy with 575 cases collected from the literature [3] emphasizes the prevalence of neuroepithelial tumours with some differences in the relative incidence of gliomas, choroid plexus papillomas, and other neoplasms, our series showing only a small number of germ cell tumours and malformations (Table 4).

Among the nine intracranial tumours confirmed in the *neonatal period* (representing 25% of the tumours under age one year), there was a *primary malignant lymphoma* of the posterior fossa in a boy considered normal at birth who developed dizziness and respiratory disorders at 8 days and died in coma at the age of 16 days. A firm tumour 5×4×4 cm in diameter replaced parts of the cerebellum and lower brain stem. Histology revealed a circumscribed malignant lymphoma of high grade

Table 1. Intracranial neoplasms of childhood under 16 years (Vienna 1940 – 1980)

Histologic Diagnosis	Male	Fem.	Total	Supra tent.	Mid-line	S/I. T. multip.	Brain stem	Cere-bellum
1. *Neuroectodermal*								
Astrocytoma	67	49	116	63	6	5	42	–
Pilocyt. astrocytoma	101	75	176	12	38	–	4	122
Oligodendroglioma	9	4	13	12	–	–	–	1
Mixed oligo-astrocyt.	5	5	10	5	1	2	2	–
Ependymoma	46	32	78	38	–	2	34	4
Subependymoma	1	3	4	–	–	–	4	–
Ependymoblastoma	1	–	1	1	–	–	–	–
Plexus papilloma	5	4	9	6	–	–	3	–
Pineocytoma-blastoma	2	1	3	–	3	–	–	–
Gangliogliома	–	3	3	2	1	–	–	–
Neuroblastoma	3	4	7	4	2	–	–	1
Glioblastoma	15	10	25	13	2	1	7	2
Medulloblastoma	106	64	170	–	–	2	–	168
Medulloepithelioma	–	1	1	1	–	–	–	–
2. *Nerve sheath tumours*								
Neurinoma	2	1	3	1	–	2	–	–
Neurofibroma	3	–	3	3	–	–	–	–
3. *Meningeal tumours*								
Meningioma	9	3	12	8	2	1	1	–
Meningeal sarcoma	5	4	9	4	1	1	–	3
Fibroxanthoma	0	1	1	1	–	–	–	–
Fibroma	1	1	2	2	–	–	–	–
4. *Malignant lymphoma*	4	2	6	3	–	1	–	2
5. *Vascular tumours*								
Haemangioblastoma	4	5	9	–	–	–	–	9
Haemangiopericytoma	1	1	2	1	–	1	–	–
6. *Germ cell tumours*								
Germinoma, emb. carc.	4	4	8	–	8	–	–	–
Teratoma	4	2	6	–	6	–	–	–
7. *Other malf. tumours*								
Craniopharyngioma	29	21	50	–	50	–	–	–
Epidermoid, dermoid	8	9	17	10	3	–	–	4
Lipoma	3	2	5	1	1	–	3	–
Hypothal. hamartoma	2	–	2	–	2	–	–	–
8. *Pituitary adenoma*	5	4	9	–	9	–	–	–
9. *Regional tumours*								
Chordoma	1	–	1	–	1	–	–	–
Osteoma, fibr. dysplas.	3	5	8	7	–	–	–	1
Osteo-sarcoma	2	–	2	1	1	–	–	–
Rhabdomyosarcoma	1	1	2	1	–	1	–	–
Cylindroma	1	–	1	–	1	–	–	–
Histiocytosis X	6	5	11	10	1	–	–	–
10. *Metastatic tumours*	6	3	9	4	–	3	–	2
Leukemia, lymphomas	3	2	5	4	–	1	–	–
11. *Unclassified tumours*	2	2	4	2	–	1	–	1
Total	474	336	810	220[a]	139	24[a]	100	320[a]

[a] Several tumours

Table 2. Intracranial tumours in childhood and infancy (*n. e.* not examined)

Histological diagnosis	Age 0 – 16 years		Under age one year pers. series		Literature[a]	
	no	%	no	%	no	%
1. Neuroepithelial	451	55.7	16	45.6	308	53.6
Gliomas	428	(52.8)	11	(31.4)	176	(30.6)
Plexus papilloma	9	(1.1)	4	(11.4)	112	(19.5)
Pineal tumours	3	(0.4)	–		4	(0.7)
Nerve cell tumours	10	(1.3)	–		6	(1.1)
Medulloepithelioma	1	(0.1)	1	(2.9)	–	
1a. Medulloblastomas	170	21.1	5	14.3	55	9.6
2. Nerve sheath tumours	6	0.7	–		3	0.5
3. Meningeal tumours	24	3.0	5	14.3	38	6.6
Meningiomas	12	(1.5)	–		15	(2.6)
Mening. sarcomas	9	(1.1)	2	(5.7)	22	(3.8)
Fibromas	3	(0.4)	3	(8.6)	1	(0.2)
4. Malignant lymphomas	6	0.7	1	2.9	2	0.3
5. Vascular tumours	11	1.4	2	5.7	6	1.1
6. Germ cell tumours	14	1.7	1	2.9	78	13.5
7. Malformat. tumours	74	9.0	1	2.9	28	4.9
8. Pituitary adenomas	9	1.1	–		–	
9. Regional tumours	27	3.4	2	5.7	35	6.1
10. Metastatic tumours	14	1.7	2	5.7	n. e.	
11. Unclassified tumours	4	0.5	–		22	3.8
Total	810		35		575	

[a] Jänisch et al. [3]

malignancy, most probably an *immunoblastoma* ("reticulum cell sarcoma") arising from the leptomeninges of the posterior fossa, without other lymphatic malignancy elsewhere in the body. To the best of our knowledge, only one further case of congenital primary malignant lymphoma of the CNS has been reported in the posterior fossa [3], whereas medulloblastomas, cerebellar sarcomas or mixed glio-mesenchymal tumours of the cerebellum are rather common in early infancy [3]. They represented 14.3% of our infantile tumours, two of which were diagnosed in the neonatal period.

Among the rare types of *neuroepithelial* neoplasms showing clinical symptoms from birth or early infancy, there was a large cerebral *medulloepithelioma* in the right parietal region of a girl with congenital hydrocephalus, increasing head circumference and hemiparesis, who died in a decerebrate state at the age of nine months. Histologically, the tumour was composed of multilayered columnar bands with papillary structures, neural tubules and primitive medullary rosettes, and occasional primitive neuronal differentiation with neuroblastoma-like areas (Fig. 1 a,b). This rare tumour which is considered as the most primitive and multipotential prototype of neuroepithelial neoplasm recapitulates the features of the primitive medullary epithelium and divergent cellular maturation with the entire range of both neural and glial cells, occurs in about half of the 16 cases reported so far [8]. In

Table 3. Incidence and predominant age groups of brain tumours

Type of tumour	Average incidence (%)			
	Children[a]		All age groups[b]	
Neuroepithelial tumours	55 – 61	(55.7)[c]	35 – 51	(42.5)
Gliomas	50 – 55	(52.8)	35 – 51	(41.6)
Plexus papillomas	0 – 2.2	(1.3)	0.4 – 0.7	(0.5)
Pinealomas	0.8 – 3.4	(0.4)	0.4 – 1.0	(0.8)
Neuronal tumours	0.2 – 1.3	(1.2)	0.2 – 0.3	(0.2)
Medulloblastomas	14 – 22	(21.1)	0.5 – 4.3	(2.6)
Neurinomas	0.5 – 0.9	(0.7)	2.0 – 12	(6.9)
Meningiomas	1.4 – 3.0	(1.5)	13 – 18	(16.9)
Sarcomas + lymphomas	2.0 – 7.5	(2.2)	0.3 – 5.8	(2.7)
Angioblastomas	0.6 – 1.5	(1.3)	0 – 2.3	(1.6)
Germ cell tumours	1.0 – 6.4	(1.7)	0.4 – 3.4	(0.5)
Craniopharyngiomas	4.6 – 8.8	(4.8)	0 – 4.6	(2.5)
Other malform. tumours	2.2 – 2.8	(2.4)	0.4 – 4.4	(1.4)
Pituitary adenomas	0 – 1.5	(0.6)	4.7 – 18	(7.8)
Regional tumours	0 – 4.0	(3.4)	1.0 – 4.0	(1.5)
Metastatic tumours	0.4 – 0.6	(0.6)	4 – 24	(16.5)
Unclassified tumours	0.7 – 3.3	(2.2)	0 – 6	(2.0)

[a] See Jellinger and Seitelberger [5], Koos and Miller [7], Gjerris et al. [2], Schoenberg et al. [9], Yates et al. [11], pers. series (4800 cases)

[b] See Jellinger and Seitelberger [5], Jänisch et al. [4], Rubinstein and Herman [8], Arendt [1], Zülch [12], Zimmerman and others (40,000 cases)

[c] Numbers in brackets: Percentage of personal case series

a girl aged two years with a four month history of focal seizures and hemiparesis, a large, sharply demarcated, firm tumour showing massive invasion of the meninges was excised from the right parietal region. The child died after operation from respiratory arrest. Histology showed a poorly differentiated cerebral *neuroblastoma* with Homer-Wright rosettes (Fig. 2 a,b) areas of neuroblasts and dense connective tissue, but without differentiation to adult nerve cells or transition to ganglioneuroma as is occasionally seen in this rare tumour that is often apparent in infancy or early childhood [8]. No extracranial tumour was found, while the two *metastatic* malignancies under age one year were due to intracranial spread from adrenal sympathoblastomas in a stillborn and a seven-month-old girl.

Among the 11 *gliomas* occurring under age one year, there were six astrocytomas and five ependymomas. In addition to two cerebellar astrocytomas there was one congenital pilocytic *astrocytoma of the optic chiasm* removed from a boy aged eight months with amaurosis; optic gliomas are very rare in early infancy [3]. Among the three astrocytomas involving the cerebral hemispheres, one poorly differentiated tumour of the right frontal lobe was removed from a boy aged 21 days who died one day later [6], while autopsy on another boy aged eight months with a history of hemiparesis and increasing head circumference since the age of two months revealed an astrocytic *glioblastoma* replacing almost the whole right hemisphere. Glioblastoma, a common tumour in adults, is rather rare in children and accounts for 7–19% of all intracranial tumours in childhood [2, 9, 11], but only for 2–3.8%

Table 4. Intracranial neoplasms in infancy (under age one year) (*l. h.* large head; *ICP* increased intracranial pressure)

Sex	Age: Onset	Op.	Death	Histology	Location	Initial signs	Other symptoms
F	still-born			metastatic sympathoblast.	multiple	–	Adrenal tumor
M	prenat.	0	12 ds	teratoma	middle fossa	l. h.	increased ICP
M	5 ds	0	16 ds	lymphoma	post. fossa	l. h.	bulbar signs
F	birth	0	21 ds	osteoma/ lipoma	tentorium post. fossa	l. h. clefts	Dandy-Walker syndrome
F	birth	21 ds	22 ds	astro II	rt. hemisph.	l. h.	increased ICP
F	birth	2 mo	alive	xanthofibroma	occip. sinus	–	no increased ICP
F	birth	2 mo	?	haemangio-pericytoma	orbit-ant. fossa	amau-rosis	–
F	5 ds	0	3 mo	medulloblast. desmoblastic	cereb. vermis	fits	increased ICP
F	2 wk	2 mo	3 mo	medulloblast.	cereb. vermis	l. h.	hemiparesis
F	3 mo	0	5 mo	astro II	lft bas. ggl.	l. h.	hemiparesis
F	3 mo	0	6 mo	astro II	lat. ventric.	fits	tuberous scler.
F	6 mo	6 mo	7 mo	metastatic sympathoblast.	ant. fossa	l. h.	adrenal tumour
M	1 mo	7 mo	alive	fibroma	rgt occipit.	fits	no increased ICP
F	birth	0	8 mo	plex. papill.	rgt lat. vent.	l. h.	increased ICP
M	2 mo	8 mo	alive	astro I	opt. chiasm	amau-rosis	amaurosis
M	3 mo	0	8 mo	astro- III – IV	rgt pariet.	l. h.	hemiparesis
M	6 mo	0	8 mo	ependymoma	4th ventric.	vomit.	increased ICP
F	birth	0	9 mo	medullo-epithelioma	rgt pariet.	l. h.	hemiparesis
F	birth	9 mo	alive	ependymoma II	lft hemisph.	l. h.	increased ICP
F	8 mo	9 mo	alive	astro I	cerebellum	vomit.	ataxia, nystagm.
M	9 mo	9 mo	alive	fibroma	rgt frontal	fits	left VII paresis
M	7 mo	0	10 mo	medulloblast.	cereb. vermis	l. h.	ataxia, incr. ICP
F	9 mo	10 mo	12 mo	plex. papill.	rgt lat ventr.	l. h.	apathia, coma
M	birth	11 mo	alive	plex. papill.	lft lat. vent.	l. h.	increased ICP
M	8 mo	11 mo	22 mo	ependymoma II	4th ventr.	l. h.	increased ICP
F	3 mo	11 mo	15 mo	desmobl. medulloblast.	cerebellar hemisphere	l. h.	tremor, ataxia
F	10 mo	11 mo	28 mo	ependymoma II	4th ventric.	l. h.	tremor, ataxia
F	birth	12 mo	alive	epidermoid	occipital	tumour	occip. area
M	6 mo	12 mo	?	ependymoma II	4th ventric.	l. h.	increased ICP
M	6 mo	0	12 mo	rhabdomyo-sarcoma	middle fossa	fits	tumour pharynx
M	8 mo	0	12 mo	plex. papill.	temp. horn	l. h.	retard., vomit.
F	8 mo	12 mo	15 mo	desmobl. medulloblast.	mid. fossa vermis	fits	hemipares., coma
M	9 mo	0	12 mo	meningeal sarcoma	dienceph., cerebellum	l. h.	radiation, coma
M	10 mo	12 mo	?	sarcoma	lft temporal	fits	hemiparesis
M	11 mo	12 mo	12 mo	angioblastoma	cerebellum	fits	postop. death

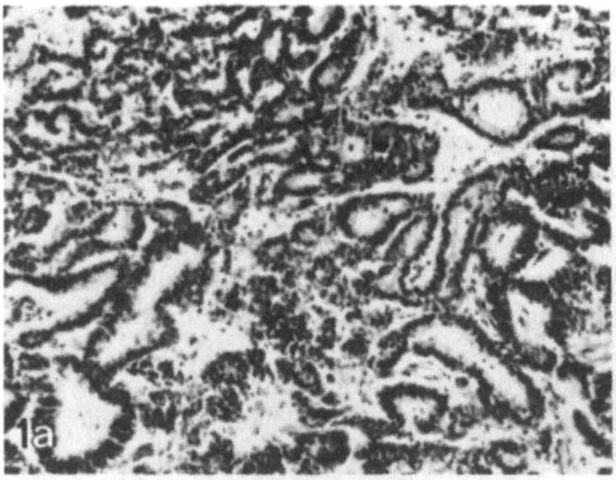

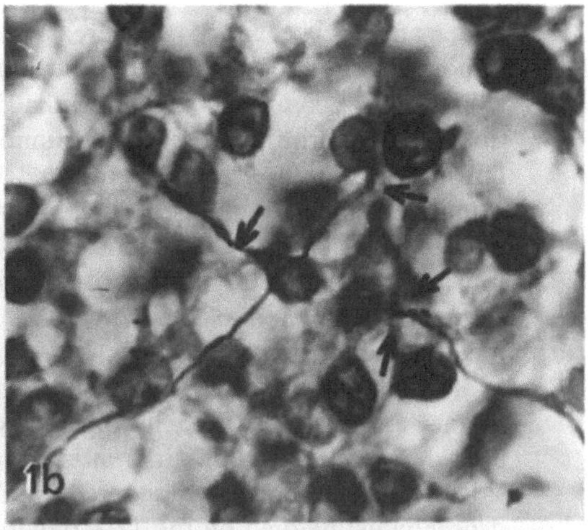

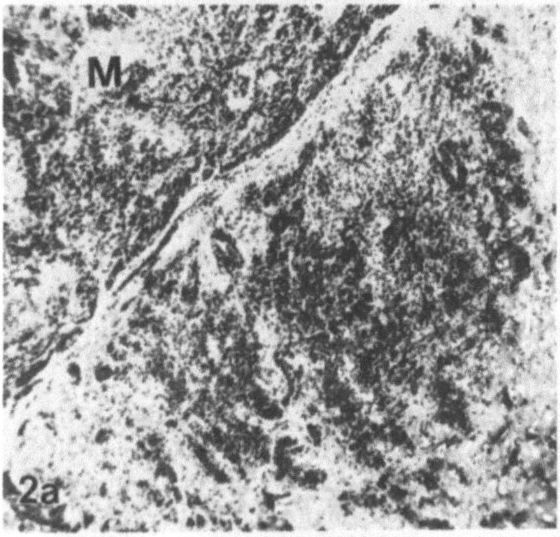

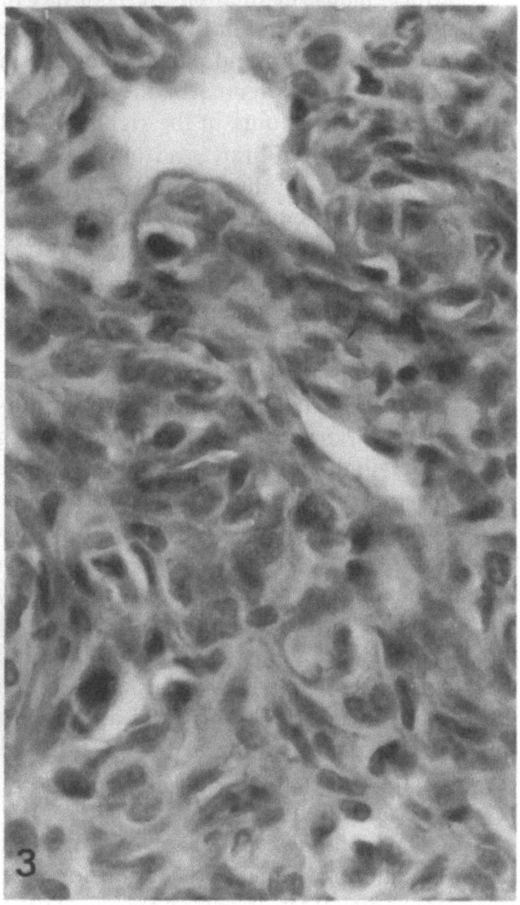

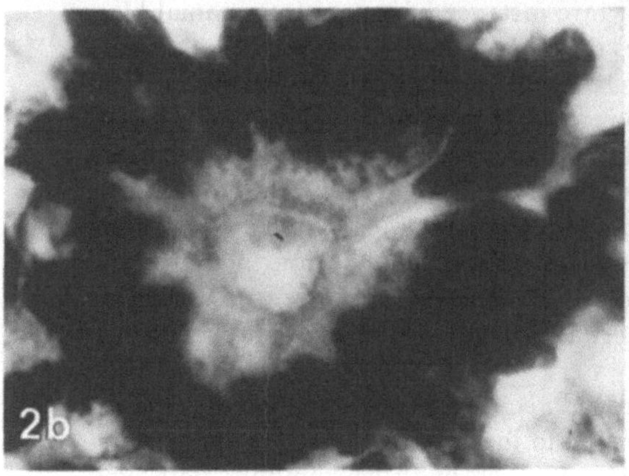

Fig. 1. **a** Cerebral medulloepithelioma with multilayered columnar bands and **b** local neuronal differentiation. **a** K. V., ×80, **b** Bodian, ×880

Fig. 2 a, b. Intracranial neuroblastoma invading the meninges (*M*) with Homer-Wright rosettes. **a** H.-E., ×40, **b** K. V., ×1480

Fig. 3. Recurrent meningeal haemangiopericytoma. H.-E., ×480

under age one year [3, 5]. Whereas ependymomas constitute 10 to 13% of brain tumours in childhood, being the fourth most common neoplasm at this age and 6 to 7 times more common than in adults [1], *ependymoblastoma* represents an exceptional type of primitive ependymal tumour in the cerebral hemispheres of young infants. This tumour, seen in a girl aged 16 months, is characterized by its high and primitive cellularity, the cell types often resembling spongioblasts but showing in places clear-cut ependymal rosettes with mitotic figures, some resembling the Flexner-Wintersteiner rosettes of retinoblastoma. Unlike the more differentiated form of ependymoma, focal invasion is frequent, and widespread cerebrospinal metastases may occur [8].

Among malformative tumours, *teratomas* are the second commonest tumours in infancy and the most frequent ones present at birth, most patients dying at or soon after delivery [3]. A large differentiated teratoma weighing 300 g was seen in the left side of the skull in a boy delivered by Caesarean section because of congenital hydrocephalus; he died on the 12th day [6]. Lipomas, being rather rare malformative tumours, occurred in five cases of our series: a girl aged 21 days with hypotelorism, bilateral cleft lip and palate, showed small lipomas in the cerebellar meninges, associated with osteoma of the tentorium, and Dandy-Walker malformation [6]. A cherry-sized lipoma in the right cerebello-pontine angle in association with pachygyria and Holt-Oran syndrome was seen in a mentally retarded boy who died at 19 months. Another lipoma of the cerebellum was combined with a desmoblastic medulloblastoma of the vermis and cerebellar micropolygyria, while a cherry-sized lipoma of the right pontine tegmentum in a mentally retarded boy aged eight years was associated with frontobasal epidermoid cyst and tentorial osteoma. The frequent combination of cerebral lipomas with other malformations is in favour of their hamartomatous nature.

Among *meningeal tumours,* we saw a congenital benign *xanthofibroma* arising near the occipital sinus of a two-month-old boy, while a large circumscribed *intracerebral fibroma* unrelated to the meninges was successfully removed from the frontal region of an 11-month-old boy who had suffered Jacksonian fits from the age of 9 months [7]. This fascicular fibroma is a rare instance of benign intracranial blastoma of mesenchymal origin with features different from meningiomas that are also rare in early infancy. A *meningeal sarcoma* with invasion of brain tissue in diencephalon and cerebellum was seen in a boy aged 12 months who developed signs of increased intracranial pressure at 9 months and after radiation therapy died in coma from focal radionecrosis of the hypothalamus. Other rare meningeal tumours of vascular origin were two instances of malignant haemangiopericytoma, one present since birth arising from the anterior fossa and retro-orbital region in a girl who underwent operation at two months, while the other was a recurrent lesion of the occipital region invading the brain in a girl aged eight years who underwent a second operation four years later (Fig. 3).

While *rhabdomyosarcomas* of the head and neck are frequent malignant tumours in childhood which in 35% develop extension to the meninges or CNS, primary intracranial RMS is extremely rare [10]. We observed two such tumours, both confirmed by electron microscopy in children: A large tumour attached to the lateral sphenoid and invading the temporal lobe was removed from a girl aged 12 who, after repeated operation, radiation and chemotherapy, died six years later with multiple metastatic tumours but without extracranial seeding. The other case was a 15-year-old girl from whom a right occipital mass was excised. Despite radiation, systemic and intrathecal chemotherapy, the girl developed a progressive neurological deficit with positive CSF cytology, and died five months after operation. Autopsy showed generalised cerebrospinal seeding. Histology of both highly cellular and pleomorphic tumours showed large ovoid and polygonal cells containing 12–15 nm myofilaments or disoriented myofibrils, suggesting *alveolar rhabdomyosarcoma,* a highly malignant tumour derived from multipotential mesenchymal tissue.

The reported examples of rare or atypical intracranial malignant lesions in infancy and childhood may demonstrate the difficulties and shortcomings in histological diagnosis and classification of CNS tumours in early life, where the criteria of the recent WHO classification [12] or other taxonomies cannot always be fully accepted for characterizing the biological behaviour and prognosis of some of these lesions.

Summary

Review of 810 histologically verified intracranial neoplasms between age 0 and 16 years observed over a 40-year period, showed a preponderance of neuroepithelial tumours and medulloblastomas. Among 35 cases (4.3%) confirmed within the first year of life, there were 45.6% neuroepithelial tumours, 14.3% medulloblastomas, 14.3% meningeal tumours (fibromas, sarcomas), 5.7% each of germ cell, malformative, vascular, other mesenchymal, and metastatic tumours (adrenal sympathoblastomas), but no pituitary adenomas, neurinomas and nerve cell tumours. Rare neoplasms occuring in the neonatal period included a primary malignant lymphoma of the posterior fossa, a large teratoma of the middle fossa, combination of tentorial osteoma and meningeal lipomas in Dandy-Walker syndrome, a dural xanthofibroma and malignant haemangiopericytoma of the anterior fossa (retro-orbital region) and two desmoblastic medulloblastomas. Other rare tumours included a medulloepithelioma and a poorly differentiated cerebral neuroblastoma of the cerebral hemispheres, a congenital pilocytic astrocytoma of the optic chiasm, cerebellar angioblastoma, and meningeal sarcoma, an intracerebral fibroma of the frontal region, a mixed medulloblastoma-lipoma of a microgyric cerebellum, a cerebral ependymoblastoma, and two primary intracranial rhabdomyosarcomas with cerebrospinal spread, both confirmed by electron microscopy. These rare tumours indicate the diagnostic difficulties of intracranial neoplasms in infancy and childhood.

References

1. Arendt, A.: Histologisch-diagnostischer Atlas der Geschwülste des Zentralnervensystems und seiner Anhangsgebilde. Jena: Fischer 1977
2. Gjerris, F., Harman, A., Kliken, L., Reske-Nielsn, E.: Incidence and long-term survival of children with intracranial tumours treated in Denmark 1935–1959. Brit. J. Cancer *38,* 442–451 (1978)

3. Jänisch, W., Schreiber, D., Gerlach, H.: Tumoren des Zentralnervensystems bei Feten und Säuglingen. Jena: Fischer 1980
4. Jänisch, W., Güthert, H., Schreiber, D.: Pathologie der Tumoren des Zentralnervensystems. Jena: Fischer 1976
5. Jellinger, K., Seitelberger, F.: Zur Neuropathologie der Hirngeschwülste im Kindesalter. Wien. med. Wschr. *120,* 855–861 (1970)
6. Jellinger, K., Sunder-Plassman, M.: Connatal intracranial tumours. Neuropaediat. *4,* 46–63 (1973)
7. Koos, W. T., Miller, M. H.: Intracranial tumours in infants and children. Stuttgart: G. Thieme 1971
8. Rubinstein, L. J., Herman, M. M.: Recent advances in human neuro-oncology. In: W. T. Smith, J. B. Cavanagh (Eds.) Recent Advances in Neuropathology, Vol. 1, Edinburgh-London-New York: Churchill-Livingstone, 1978, 179–223
9. Schoenberg, B. S., Schoenberg, D. G., Christine, B. W., Gomez, M. R.: The epidemiology of primary intracranial neoplasms of childhood. Mayo Clin. Proc. *51,* 52–56 (1976)
10. Yagishita, S., Itoh, Y., Chiba, Y, Fujino, H.: Primary rhabdomyosarcoma of the cerebrum. Acta neuropath. (Berl.) *45,*111–115 (1979)
11. Yates, A. J., Becker, L. E., Sachs, L. A.: Brain tumours in childhood. Child's Brain *5,* 31–39 (1979)
12. Zülch, K. J.: Histological types of tumours of the central nervous system. Histological Classification of Tumours, Vol. 21. Geneva: WHO 1979

Intracranial and Spinal Tumours in Newborns and Infants

H. GERLACH, W. JÄNISCH, and D. SCHREIBER

Tumours of the nervous system, especially those of the CNS, are the most common malignancy in early childhood [5]. A monographic review of primary CNS tumours histologically verified during the first year of life was given recently by Jänisch et al. [3]. Of these tumours 23.4% show a close time relationship to the perinatal period [2]. The purpose of the present study is to analyse these cases from some different points of view.

Materials and Methods

A total of 742 cases of microscopically verified CNS tumours with symptoms during the first year of life or after was collected. Fifty-six of them are our own cases or were made accessible to us by the courtesy of colleagues. The others were taken from reports in the literature since 1900 (for their origin, see [1, 2, 3]; for further cases, see [4, 6]). All available information regarding the case histories, the clinical and pathological findings were coded on punch cards and processed by a sorter. The following groups emerged: 1) Cases with histopathological confirmation at operation and/or autopsy during the first year of life. 2) Cases with onset of tumour symptoms during the first year of life but with histopathological confirmation during later life.

Results and Discussion

The most common tumour types are presented in Table 1. Many of them are regarded as congenital ones. Unfortunately, these terms were used with a different meaning by different authors [2]. It might be more preferable to classify these neoplasms as "tumours of the perinatal period", which comprises the time from the beginning of the 29th week of pregnancy until the first week after birth. By using this definition our study contains 173 CNS tumours which are time-related to the perinatal period. These tumours were divided into subgroups according to the following characteristics (1) neoplasms in stillbirths, (2) neoplasms with histological verification in the first week of life, and (3) neoplasms with symptoms since the first week of life and histological investigation performed later on.

Table 1. Survey on 742 histologically confirmed CNS tumours in infancy (group A = cases histologically verified during the first year of life; group B = cases with onset of tumour symptoms during the first year of life but with later confirmation)

Tumour types	Group A (589 cases)		Group B (153 cases)	
	n	%	n	%
Choroid plexus papillomas	113	19.2	8	5.2
Teratomas	80	13.6	2	1.3
Astrocytomas/spongioblastomas	76	12.9	59	38.6
Medulloblastomas	57	9.7	14	9.2
Ependymomas	39	6.6	11	7.2
Gliomas, not specified	30	5.1	3	2.0
Glioblastomas	23	3.9	4	2.6
Others	171	29.0	52	34.0

CNS Tumours in Stillbirths (Table 2)

Table 2 shows the types of CNS tumours in stillbirths and their sex distribution. To this group belong only intracranial, but no spinal tumours. In all cases the head was enlarged. This enlargement was due to the tumour mass or to the tumour-related hydrocephalus. Teratomas predominate strikingly among these 36 tumours (58.3%). They rank in the second position among CNS tumours histologically verified during the first year of life (Table 1, group A) and 65.9% of them are time-related to the perinatal period. The teratomas of this subgroup are mostly very large (largest diameter 20 cm, greatest weight 790 g). For that reason, in most cases the presence of the obstetrician was necessary for delivery (forceps, caesarian section, puncture, perforation, cranioclasia). In the cases of severe complications, therefore, reports on the location of the teratomas were incomplete. Four teratomas were sited at the base of the skull, two of them reached the left orbit. Other sites were the floor of the third ventricle, the right optic nerve and the right choroid plexus. In two cases episphenoides existed which grew into the cranial cavity and into the pharynx as well as into the mouth. In one report a brain tumour with two fetal parasites within was described (fetus in feto).

Histological investigation revealed mostly tridermomas with different degrees of maturation. Only one teratoma biphyllicum without entodermal structures has been

Table 2. Types and sex ratio in intracranial CNS tumours in stillbirths (36 cases)

Tumour types	Total		Females
	n	%	
Teratomas	21	58.3	10
Astrocytomas	6	16.7	3
Gliomas, not specified	4	11.1	1
Others	5	13.9	2

mentioned. In most of these teratomas the component with neural elements was very large. In this subgroup, beside the described teratomas, gliomas and other tumour types were found. Their number is too small for the evaluation of their morphological spectrum.

CNS Tumours with Histological Verification During the First Week of Life

Table 3 indicates intracranial neoplasms in stillbirths in comparison with the other subgroups mentioned. Thirty-eight tumours of the CNS were histologically verified during the first week of life. Teratomas predominate (11 cases = 28.9%). Their morphological pattern does not differ markedly from that in stillbirths. Large cysts very often exist. Nearly all teratomas are tridermomas. Two intracranial teratomas with epignathi were recorded and one of them was without entodermal structures.

Histologically investigated spinal tumours of the first week of life are shown in Table 4. This table also contains the 59 spinal tumours (=7.95%) from the whole material. Four of them were microscopically confirmed during the first week of life and teratomas predominate.

CNS Tumours with Symptoms Since the First Week of Life with Histological Verification Made Later

Table 3 contains intracranial tumours of this subgroup. Teratomas predominate here, too, but their relative frequency decreases with increasing age. Reports on these teratomas contain more data on tumour location. Three teratomas were situated at the base of the skull, two in the third ventricle, two others occurred in the pineal region. Other sites were the right choroid plexus, midbrain and the aque-

Table 3. Spectrum of intracranial tumours of the perinatal period (149 cases)

Tumor types	Stillbirths (36)		Histological confirmation during the first week of life (38)		Symptoms since first week of life (75)	
	n	%	n	%	n	%
Teratomas	21	58.3	11	28.9	15	20.0
Astrocytomas	6	16.7	3	7.9	9	12.1
Gliomas, not specified	4	11.1	5	13.2	4	5.3
Craniopharyngiomas	1	2.8	1	2.6	6	8.0
Choroid plexus papillomas	1	2.8	4	10.5	11	14.7
Others	3	8.3	14	36.8	30	40.0

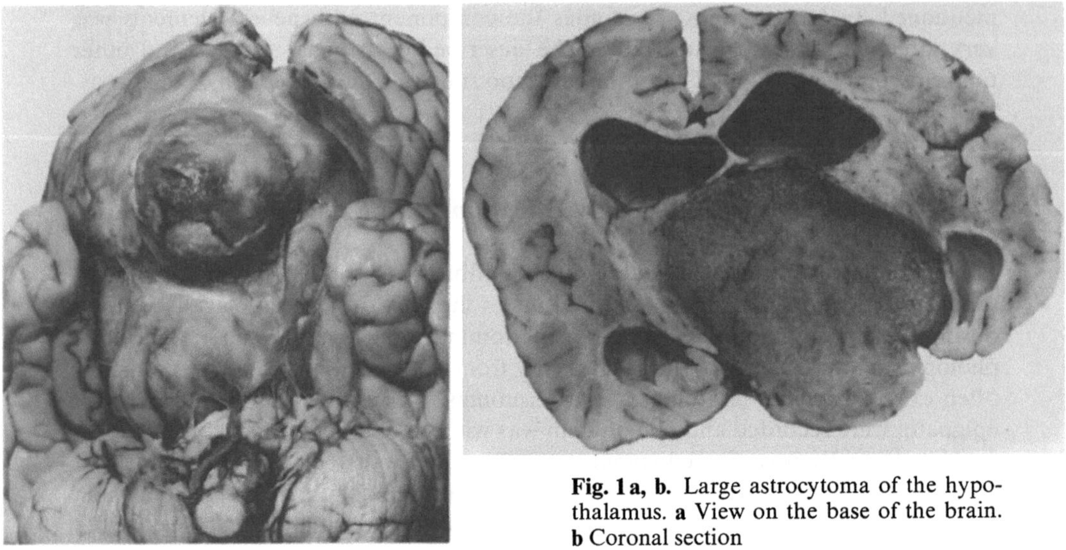

a b

Fig. 1 a, b. Large astrocytoma of the hypothalamus. **a** View on the base of the brain. **b** Coronal section

duct of Sylvius. The greatest tumour weight was 1850 g. The longest survival time in these teratomas was 15½ months. One extremely rare case was an intracranial teratoma which contained five fetuses; its survival time was 19 days. In this subgroup of CNS tumours, the number of papillomas of the choroid plexus was greater. These show the highest frequency among CNS tumours histologically verified during the first year of life [1, 3, 5].

It also seems necessary to draw attention to the astroglial tumours in this subgroup. Mostly, these are slowly growing neoplasms. One of our own cases (case 13, Fig. 1) is a typical example in this respect. The boy showed a paresis of the abducens nerve at birth. A craniotomy performed at the age of three years revealed an already inoperable brain tumour. The patient reached the age of 6 years and 8 months in spite of this tumour.

Most intracranial tumours which are time-related to the perinatal period affect midline structures. The high proportion of supratentorial tumours of this age group is mainly due to the situation of teratomas and choroid plexus papillomas.

Table 4. Types of spinal tumours of the perinatal period (59 cases)

Tumour types	Total (59)		Histological confirmation during the first week of life (4)	Symptoms since the first week of life (20)
	n	%		
Lipomas	18	30.5	–	8
Teratomas	13	22.0	2	5
Dermoids	6	10.2	1	3
Astrocytomas	6	10.2	1	–
Others	16	17.1	–	4

Lipomas predominate among histologically confirmed spinal tumours with symptoms since the first week of life (Table 4). Teratomas rank in the second position in this group. Of all spinal tumours with clinical manifestation in the first year of life 40.1% are time-related to the perinatal period.

Summary

A total of 173 CNS tumours related in time to the perinatal period is evaluated. These are 23.3% of all CNS tumours with clinical manifestation during the first year of life of our own cases and case reports in the literature. Among intracranial tumours teratomas predominate, their relative frequency decreases with increasing age. Of the spinal tumours 40.7% are time-related to the perinatal period, but without any predominance of special tumour types.

References

1. Gerlach, H.: Tumoren des Zentralnervensystems im frühen Kindesalter. Med. Dissertation (Promotion B), Halle 1979
2. Gerlach, H., Jänisch, W., Schreiber, D.: ZNS-Tumoren der Perinatalperiode. Zbl. allg. Path. path. Anat. Vol. *126* (1982) (in press)
3. Jänisch, W., Schreiber, D., Gerlach, H.: Tumoren des Zentralnervensystems bei Feten und Säuglingen. Häufigkeit, Pathogenese, Pathomorphologie, Krankheitsverläufe. Jena: VEB Gustav Fischer Verlag 1980
4. Nishimoto, A., Yagyu, Y.: A case of a brain tumour in a child manifested with emaciation and hypersecretion of plasma growth hormone (jap.). Shinkei Geko *6,* 121–129
5. Schreiber, D., Jänisch, W., Gerlach, H.: Tumoren des Zentralnervensystems im frühen Kindesalter. Dtsch. Gesundh.-Wes. *34,* 1577–1580 (1979)
6. Wexler, H. A., Poole, C. A., Fojaco, R. M.: The association of Wilm's tumour with second primary malignancies. Rev. Interam. Radiol. *1,* 15–18 (1976)

The Usefulness of Immunocytological Demonstration of Glial Fibrillary Acidic Protein for Diagnostic Problems of Cerebral Tumours

K. H. H. MERKEL, M. ZIMMER, W. WAHLEN, and E. SCHWARZ

Introduction

With the advent of the indirect immunoperoxidase procedure by Nakane und Pierce [13] and the peroxidase-antiperoxidase method by Sternberger et al. [14] we have methods at hand to demonstrate different antibodies in formalin fixed and paraffin embedded tissue.

An acidic protein (GFAP) was first localized in fibrous neuroglia [9]. Now, after purification, antibodies against this protein were raised [15]. Further studies localized GFAP in fibrillary astrocytes [1, 2]. A monospecific antiserum to GFAP was developed [10]. It proved to be very valuable in neuropathology for the diagnosis of tumours [3, 4, 5, 6, 7, 8, 10, 11, 17].

Materials and Methods

From our surgical files we collected 54 intracranial tumours in children under the age of 16 years. Sections of the paraffin embedded tissue were examined either with the indirect immunoperoxidase method or the PAP-method for the presence of GFAP. The PAP-method was carried out as follows:

Deparaffinize section in xylol. Block endogenous peroxidase in 0.75% hydrogen peroxide in methyl alcohol for 30 minutes. Rinse with tap water. Cover with normal swine serum (dilution 1 : 5 for 15 min). Incubate with rabbit-anti-GFAP antiserum for 2 hours. Dilution 1 : 128 to 1 : 512. Wash section in buffer solution for 15 min. Cover section with swine-antirabbit IgG for 30 minutes. Dilution 1 : 20. Wash in buffer for 15 minutes. Add rabbit PAP-complex for 30 minutes; dilution 1 : 50. Perform the 4-demethyl-aminoazobenzene (DAB)-reaction. Instead of using DAB one may use the chromogen carbazole.

We want to thank Dr. Eng from the Veterans Administration Hospital, Palo Alto, California, for the generous gift of the GFAP-antiserum. All other antisera were purchased from DAKO-Immunoglobulins, Copenhagen, Denmark. The DAB and carbazole were purchased from Sigma Chemicals, St. Louis, Missouri, U.S.A.

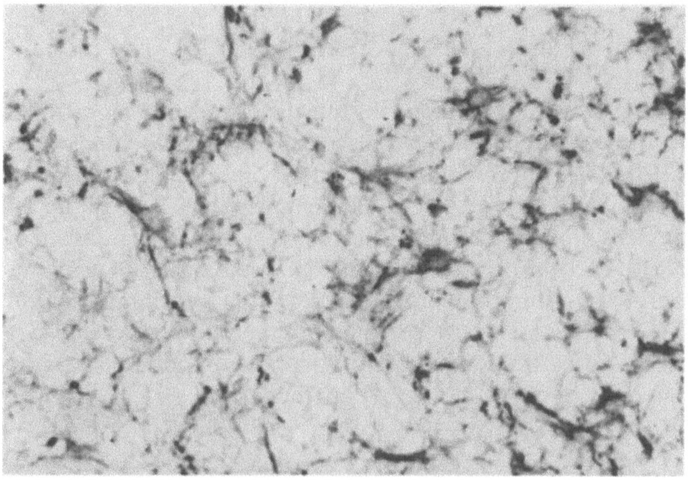

Fig. 1. GFAP in cells of astrocytoma. Peroxidase-anti-peroxidase. × 160

Table 1. Histological diagnosis and GFAP content of the examined glial and nonglial intracranial tumours

Tumor	Number of cases		GFAP +	GFAP –
Astrocytoma	5			
pilocytic		2	+	
anaplastic		2	+	
subependymal giant cell		1	+	
Glioblastoma multiforme	1		+	
Astroblastoma	1		+	
Medulloblastoma	26		10+	16–
Ependymoma	1		+ some cells	
Plexus papilloma	2			–
Subependymoma	1		+	
Oligodendroglioma	1			–
Mixed glioma	5			
astrocytoma/oligodendroglioma		4	+	
ganglioglioma		1	+	
Neurinoma	4			–
Haemangioblastoma	2			–
Meningeoma	1			–
Dural sarcoma	2			–
Craniopharyngioma	2			–
Total	54			

Results

Tumours of the astrocytic series of all different histological grades demonstrated GFAP in neoplastic cells. It was found in the cytoplasm surrounding the nucleus as well as in cell processes (Fig. 1). The brown or red reaction product was also found in bizarre cells of glioblastoma multiforme. We could demonstrate GFAP in the astrocytic component of mixed gliomas. Of interest certainly is the high number of medulloblastomas with scattered positive cells. Oligodendrogliomas, plexus papillomas, meningiomas, neurinomas, dural sarcomas, and craniopharyngiomas did not contain GFAP (Table 1). Reactive astrocytes surrounding the tumour were always heavily stained. The comparison of slides stained with both immunoperoxidase methods demonstrated superior results with the PAP-method.

Discussion

This study of paediatric intracranial neoplasms confirms other reports of tumours in adulthood in regard to the usefulness of the immunoenzymatic methods for the diagnostic evaluations of brain tumours [17, 4, 6, 7, 8, 10, 16]. By using the nuclear counterstain a much better evaluation of the tissue is possible compared to the immunofluorescence studies. With the PAP-method better results were obtained, since higher dilutions of the primary antiserum could be used. These methods are of great diagnostic value for differentiating meningeal sarcomas or certain neurinomas invading the brain. In our study we examined 26 medulloblastomas and found GFAP positive cells within the tumour masses in almost half of them. These cells were identified as part of the tumour by shape and location and not as remnants of the reactive astrocytes. This finding may be interpreted as a sign for differentiation in the astrocytic direction. Even though it is known that the GFAP concentration decreases in astrocytic tumours with the degree of differentiation [10, 16, 12], we could demonstrate tumour cells in glioblastoma multiforme and anaplastic astrocytomas that stained heavily for GFAP.

Summary

In a retrospective study we examined 54 intracranial tumours of children under the age of 16 years for the presence of glial fibrillary acidic protein (GFAP). We used the indirect immunoperoxidase method and the peroxidase-anti-peroxidase method. GFAP was present in astrocytes and tumour cells of the astrocytic lineage as well as in some cells of ependymomas. Of the 26 medulloblastomas ten showed scattered positive tumour cells. Oligodendrogliomas, choroid plexus papillomas, neurinomas, meningiomas, and craniopharyngiomas were negative. The PAP-method turned out to be more sensitive than the indirect immunoperoxidase method. Both are superior to the immunofluorescence method, since the slides can be stored without loss of the reaction product. The use of a nuclear counterstain greatly increases the information on the tissue. These methods turn out to be of great value in differentiating certain intracranial tumours and give hints regarding their histogenesis.

References

1. Bignami, A., Eng, L. F., Dahl, D., Uyeda, C. T.: Localization of the glial fibrillary acidic protein in astrocytes by immunofluorescence. Brain Res. *43,* 429–435 (1972)
2. Bignami, A., Dahl, D.: Astrocyte-specific protein and neuroglial differentiation. An immunofluorescent study with antibodies to the glial fibrillary acidic protein. J. Comp. Neurol. *153,* 27–38 (1974)
3. De Armond, S. J., Eng, L. F., Rubinstein, L. J.: The application of glial fibrillary acidic (GFA) protein immunohistochemistry in neurooncology. Path. Res. Pract. *168,* 374–394 (1980)
4. Deck, J. H., Eng, L. F. Bigbee, J., Woodcock, S. M.: The role of glial fibrillary acidic protein in the diagnosis of central nervous system tumours. Acta Neuropathol. (Berl.) *42,* 183–190 (1978)
5. Delpech, B., Delpech, A., Vidard, M. N., Girad, N., Tayot, J., Clement, J. C., Creissard, P.: Glial fibrillary acidic protein in tumours of the nervous system. Brit. J. Cancer *37,* 33–40 (1978)
6. Duffy, Ph. E., Graf, L., Rappaport, M. M.: Identification of glial fibrillary acidic protein by the immunoperoxidase method in human brain tumours. J. Neuropath. exp. Neurol. *4,* 645–651 (1977)
7. Duffy, Ph. E., Huang Yung-Yu, Rappaport, M. M., Graf, L.: Glial fibrillary acidic protein in giant cell tumours of brain and other gliomas. Acta Neuropath. (Berl.) *52,* 51–57 (1980)
8. Duffy, Ph. E., Graf, L., Huang Yung-Yu, Rappaport, M. M.: Glial fibrillary acidic protein in ependymomas and other brain tumours. J. Neurol. Sci. *40,* 133–146 (1979)
9. Eng, L. F., Vanderhaegen, J. J., Bignami, A. Gerste, B.: An acidic protein isolated from fibrous astrocytes. Brain Res. *28,* 351–354 (1971)
10. Eng, L. F., Rubinstein, L. J.: Contribution of immunohistochemistry to diagnostic problems of human cerebral tumours. J. Histochem. Cytochem. *26:* 513–522 (1978)
11. Goebel, H. H., Schlie, M., Spoerri, O., Eng, L. F.: Die immunhistologische Darstellung des Gliafaserproteins in der neuropathologischen Tumordiagnostik. Verh. dtsch. Ges. Path. *64,* 597 (1980)
12. Jacque, C. M., Kujas, M., Poreau, A., Raoul, M., Collier, P., Racadot, J., Baumann, N.: GFA and 5100 protein levels as an index for malignancy in human gliomas and neurinomas. J. Nat. Cancer Inst. *62,* 479–483 (1979)
13. Nakane, P. K., Pierce, G. B.: Enzyme-labelled antibodies: Preparation and application for the location of antigen. J. Histochem. Cytochem. *14,* 929–931 (1966)
14. Sternberger, L. A., Hardy, P. H., Cucutis, J. J., Meyer, H. G.: The unlabelled antibody enzyme method of immunocytochemistry. Preparation and properties of soluble antigen-antibody complex (horseradish peroxidase-antihorseradish peroxidase) and its use in identification of spirochetes. J. Histochem. Cytochem. *18,* 315–333 (1970)
15. Uyeda, C. T., Eng, L. F., Bignami, A.: Immunological study of the glial fibrillary acidic protein. Brain Res. *37,* 81–89 (1972)
16. Van der Meulen, J. D. H., Harthoff, H. J., Ebels, E. J.: Glial fibrillary acidic protein in human gliomas. Neuropath. appl. Neurobiol. *4,* 177–190 (1978)
17. Velasco, M., Dahl, D., Roessmann, U., Gambetti, P.: Immunohistochemical localization of glial fibrillary acidic protein in human glial neoplasms. Cancer *45,* 484–494 (1980)

CNS Tumours in Infancy, Childhood, and Adolescence

D. Schreiber, W. Jänisch, and H. Gerlach

Whereas CNS tumours of childhood and adolescence, are usually encountered in neurological and neurosurgical clinics as well as in related pathological institutes, the compilation of sufficient data on corresponding neoplasms in infancy has proved to be something of a problem. However, CNS tumours are not less common in infants than in later life [11]. They are of special interest because of

(1) their range as compared with neurogenic neoplasms in children, adolescents and adults,
(2) connections between CNS malformations and the origin of tumours,
(3) clinical peculiarities of tumour development at this age, and
(4) possible factors regarding tumour induction in the CNS.

Materials and Methods

To get sufficient information on CNS tumours in infancy we collected all the obtainable histopathologically verified tumours from the literature since 1900 (742 cases, Table 1). This material also includes 56 personal cases (for its origin see [4, 7]). The review of the European and American literature by Jellinger and Sunder-Plassmann [8] only comprised 335 histologically confirmed tumours up to one year of age. According to Jänisch et al. [7], Gerlach et al. [4] the 742 CNS neoplasms were divided into group A (cases with histological verification during the first year of life) and group B (cases with tumour symptoms since infancy but with histological confirmation in later life).

For comparison we added the autopsy reports on CNS tumours older than one year of age that were obtained at the Pathological Institute of the Medical Academy of Erfurt, GDR (1764 cases from 1953 up to 1980). Conclusions must be drawn cautiously because of the heterogeneity of the different tumour series. In spite of this, the CNS tumours in infants show several remarkable features as compared to neoplasms in later life.

Results and Discussion

Practically all CNS tumour types which are known in various age periods also occur in infancy. The only exception to this rule are pituitary adenomas because, to our

Table 1. Frequency of brain tumours at different age periods

Tumour types	Infancy (groups A + B)		1 < 20 years				≧ 20 years			
	n_0	%	n_1	%	n_2	%	n_1	%	n_2	%
Astrocytomas/ spongioblastomas	135	18.2	57	31.8	58	31.4	350	23.3	422	26.7
Choroid plexus papillomas	121	16.3	2	1.1	4	2.2	8	0.5	6	0.4
Teratomas	82	11.1	4	2.2	1	0.5	2	0.1	2	0.1
Medulloblastomas	71	9.6	41	22.9	37	20.0	16	1.1	10	0.6
Ependymomas	50	6.7	20	11.2	22	11.9	31	2.1	32	2.0
Glioblastomas	27	3.6	18	10.1	16	8.7	455	30.3	311	19.7
Meningiomas	18	2.4	1	0.6	–	–	325	21.6	371	23.5
Oligodendrogliomas	12	1.6	1	0.6	2	1.1	23	1.5	48	3.0
Others	226	30.5	35	19.6	45	24.3	292	19.4	377	23.9
Total	742	100.0	179	100.1	185	100.1	1502	99.9	1579	99.9

n_0 – according to Gerlach et al. [4]
n_1 – according to Jänisch et al. [7], Table 9
n_2 – autopsy material of the Pathological Institute of the Medical Academy of Erfurt (1953 – 1980)

knowledge, no reports exist in the literature up to date. Among the published cases of the first year of life astrocytomas, choroid plexus papillomas, and teratomas rank at the top (Table 1). The high frequency of choroid plexus papillomas and teratomas is especially remarkable since both tumour types are rare neoplasms in all other age groups as shown by the autopsy material of the Pathological Institute of the Medical Academy of Erfurt. These results are supported by other authors [1, 10]. Teratomas also comprise the greatest part of dysontogenetic neoplasms of the CNS which display signs of dysraphia in many cases. Table 2 shows the main types of dysraphia that have been observed in teratomas, epidermoids, dermoids, and lipomas. According to Tables 1 and 2, the dysraphia involved 14 out of 82 teratomas (17%). In the case of Pickens et al. [12] a cystic teratoma combined with agenesis of the cerebellar vermis extended from the posterior cranial fossa to the cauda equina. Besides teratomas with epignathi, rare inclusions of whole fetuses within the teratoma [2] are worth notice.

Morphologically, no striking differences exist in the naked-eye appearance and the histological structure between CNS tumours in infancy and adolescence or adulthood. Figure 1 shows a medulloblastoma involving the pons, medulla oblongata and leptomeninges in an eight-month-old female. In this case, metastases were found along the spinal cord. The neoplasm showed haemorrhages within the tumour tissue and subarachnoid space as is known from other samples of this age group [13].

Concerning the tumour site, however, differences occur between neoplasms in infancy and childhood. Among 606 reports with corresponding data 407 tumours of

Table 2. Survey on dysontogenetic CNS tumours in early life (groups A and B)

Tumour types	No. of cases	Main locations	Maximum tumour sizes	Main types of dysraphia	Age at histological verification	References according to Jänisch et al. [7]
Teratomas with dysrhaphia	10	intraspinal, especially lumbal; presacral; intracranial	whole spinal canal; 7×2 cm; 6 cm (diameter)	spina bifida aperta/occulta; encephalocele; agenesis of corpus callosum; cerebellar deformity	3 days up to 1 year	Table 38
Teratomas with epignathus	4	intracranial	10 cm (diameter)	persistent craniopharyngeal canal	birth	Table 37
Epidermoids and dermoids	10	intracranial (anterior and posterior cranial fossa); intraspinal, especially lumbosacral	larger than an apple	anencephaly; defects of os occipitale; dermal sinus	birth up to 28 months	Table 43
Lipomas	20	cerebello-pontine angle; cranial fossas; lateral ventricles; spinal cord; intraspinal, especially lumbosacral	whole spinal canal; plum-sized	defects of vertebral arc and os sacrum; hydromyelia; syringomyelia; dermal sinus	5 weeks up to 14 years	Table 44

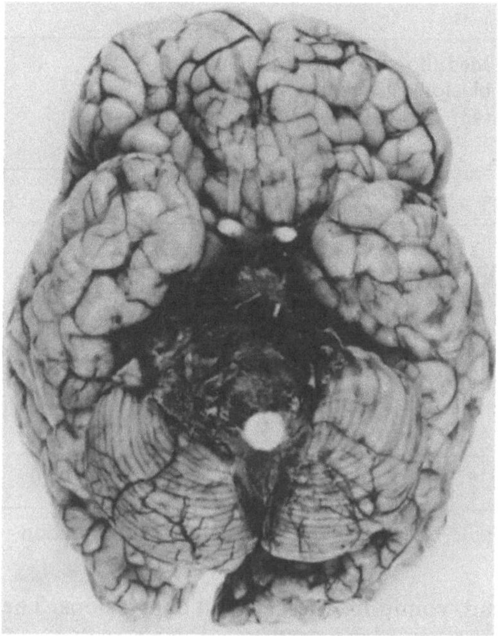

Fig. 1. Medulloblastoma of the pons involving the leptomeninx with haemorrhages (No. 1081/76). The tumour corresponds to case No. 20 of Jänisch et al. [7]

infancy (67%) were located supratentorially, 143 cases (24%) infratentorially, and 56 cases (9%) in both compartments. This ratio is remarkable since in children of all age groups up to 15 or 16 years an average of 59% of the intracranial neoplasms are situated in the infratentorial compartment [5].

Another peculiarity might exist regarding the sex distribution of medulloblastoma. Out of 62 medulloblastomas of groups A and B 34, corresponding to 54.8%, were registered in females. Contrary to this, among medulloblastomas of all age groups (2137 cases = 66% according to [5]) a striking predominance for the male sex was observed.

According to Table 3, a considerable proportion of neoplasms during the first year of life attained a large size. In group A about 27% and in group B 38% displayed diameters from 5 to 8 cm. The largest tumours were teratomas since 38 out of 63 cases (60%) measured more than 8 cm in diameter.

As mentioned recently [15], among brain tumours in early life the diencephalic syndrome or Russell's syndrome [14] plays an important role. It is clinically characterized by a striking emaciation despite good appetite, an alert appearance of the face, general hyperactivity and nystagmus. The typical location of a tumour causing this syndrome is the hypothalamus. Table 4 shows the tumour types in relation to the beginning of clinical symptoms during infancy. The predominating tumour types are astrocytomas including "spongioblastomas" and optic gliomas, respectively. Group B (41 cases) preponderates over group A (24 cases). This fact refers to the long duration of the disease in most of the reported cases.

Finally, the clinical symptoms of intracranial and intraspinal tumours in infancy subdivided into first and later signs are summarized in Table 5. Despite the large number of well-known symptoms there are only three main ones which deserve par-

Table 3. Size of brain tumours in infancy[a]

Diameter	Astro-cytomas (83)		Choroid plexus papillomas (79)		Tera-tomas (63)	Medullo-blastomas (43)		Ependy-momas (24)		Total			
	A	B	A	B	A	A	B	A	B	A	%	B	%
Up to2 cm	7	2	6	–	3	2	–	1	–	19	8.1	2	3.5
Up to 5 cm	10	6	29	2	4	13	2	5	1	61	26.1	11	19.0
Up to 8 cm	13	14	19	5	11	8	3	13	–	64	27.4	22	37.9
More than 8 cm	–	–	1	–	38	3	–	3	1	45	19.2	1	1.7
Large, not specified	12	19	17	–	7	9	3	–	–	45	19.2	22	37.9
Total	42	41	72	7	63	35	8	22	2	234	100.0	58	100.0

[a] The data of the tumour types differ from Table 1 because of incompleteness of information

ticular attention: enlargement of the head, vomiting, and cerebral convulsions. The enlargement of the head is due to the sutures of the skull being open at this age. This result corresponds to data of Table 3 concerning the tumour extension in early life.

The study of CNS tumours in infants offers opportunities for the careful analysis of pathogenesis. The maximum duration of tumour development can only amount to 21 months of the intrauterine and extrauterine life span. Within this time limit the stimulus for tumour induction must have acted. This comparatively short period should permit a tracing of the possible tumour producing agents. Today, informa-

Table 4. Time of first clinical symptoms in 65 brain tumour cases with diencephalic syndrome of emaciation (references see Gerlach [3])

Tumour types	1st trimester		2nd trimester		2nd half year		Total		
Groups	A	B	A	B	A	B	A +	B =	Σ
Astrocytomas/spongioblastomas	10	5	6	7	2	17	18	29	47
Optic gliomas	–	–	2	–	–	1	2	1	3
Gliomas, not specified	2	2	1	–	–	–	3	2	5
Ependymomas	–	1	1	–	–	2	1	3	4
Medulloblastoma	–	–	–	1	–	–	–	1	1
Oligodendroglioma	–	1	–	–	–	–	–	1	1
Glioblastoma	–	–	–	–	–	1	–	1	1
Neurofibroma	–	–	–	–	–	1	–	1	1
Ganglioglioma	–	–	–	–	–	1	–	1	1
Mixed glial-mesenchymal tumour	–	1	–	–	–	–	–	1	1
Total	12	10	10	8	2	23	24	41	65

Table 5. First and consecutive symptoms of intracranially and intraspinally localized tumours

Type of symptoms	First symptoms				Consecutive symptoms			
	Intracranial tumours (483)		Intraspinal tumours (56)		Intracranial tumours (483)		Intraspinal tumours (56)	
	n	%	n	%	n	%	n	%
Enlargement of head	148	30.6	4	7.1	186	38.5	2	3.6
Vomiting	112	23.2	–	–	132	27.3	–	–
Seizures	35	7.3	3	5.4	93	19.3	4	7.1
Paresis of extremities	9	1.9	15	26.8	57	11.8	13	23.2
Paresis of cranial nerves	17	3.5	–	–	113	23.4	3	5.4
Muscular hypotonia	1	0.2	5	8.9	62	12.8	8	14.3
Nystagmus	7	1.5	–	–	72	14.9	–	–
Other striking clinical symptoms	25	5.2	3	5.4	174	36.0	22	39.3
Non-characteristic clinical symptoms	129	26.7	10	17.9	332	68.7	14	25.0

tion about most of the glial, mesenchymal and mixed brain tumour types exists in experimental animals [6, 9]. This does not apply to dysontogenetic CNS tumours. A detailed analysis of glial tumours in infancy in the light of results obtained in experimental animals should help to clarify the possible aetiology of this tumour group.

Summary

742 CNS tumours of infancy are analyzed. The frequency of the tumour types, their site and size, as well as the relations between dysontogenetic tumours and dysraphia are summarized. Some peculiarities of neurogenic neoplasms in early life as against tumours in childhood and adolescence are mentioned. The diencephalic syndrome of emaciation deserves special attention. Possible relationships between neurogenic tumours in children and experimental animals should be noticed.

Note Added in Proof

Recently the two first cases of pituitary adenomas in infants were reported in the literature. An 8-month-old male with Cushing's disease (group A) showed a large inoperable adrenocortipin-producing pituitary tumour, measuring 12 × 8 × 5 cm, which had expanded in the sella turcica and the suprasellar region [16]. Another ACTH-secreting pituitary adenoma in an 18-month-old infant was described by Saeger et al. [17]; the symptomatology had started at the age of 9 months (group B).

References

1. Arendt, A.: Histologisch-diagnostischer Atlas der Geschwülste des Zentralnervensystems und seiner Anhangsgebilde. 2. Aufl. Jena: Fischer 1977
2. Fiedler, J., Röse, I.: Fetus in fetu im intrakraniellen Teratom eines Frühtotgeborenen. Zbl. allg. Path. path. Anat. *118*, 23–29 (1974)
3. Gerlach, H.: Tumoren des Zentralnervensystems im frühen Kindesalter. Med. Dissertation B. Halle/Saale 1979
4. Gerlach, H., Jänisch, W., Schreiber, D.: Intracranial and spinal tumours in newborns and infants. This Symposium, page 53
5. Jänisch, W., Güthert, H., Schreiber, D.: Pathologie der Tumoren des Zentralnervensystems. Jena: Fischer 1976
6. Jänisch, W., Schreiber, D.: Experimental tumours of the central nervous system. 1st Engl. edition by Bigner, D. D., Swenberg, J. A. Kalamazoo: Upjohn Co. 1977
7. Jänisch, W., Schreiber, D., Gerlach, H.: Tumoren des Zentralnervensystems bei Feten und Säuglingen. Jena: Fischer 1980
8. Jellinger, K., Sunder-Plassmann, M.: Connatal intracranial tumours. Neuropädiatrie *4*, 46–63 (1973)
9. Kleihues, P., Lantos, P. L., Magee, P. N.: Chemical carcinogenesis in the nervous system. Int. Rev. Exp. Path. *15*, 153–230 (1976)
10. Koos, W. T., Miller, M. H.: Intracranial tumours of infants and children. Stuttgart: Thieme 1971
11. Müller, J. H., Jänisch, W., Usbeck, W.: Geschwülste des Zentralnervensystems bei Kindern und Jugendlichen. Dtsch. Gesundh.-Wes. *26*, 643–646 (1971)
12. Pickens, J. M., Wilson, J., Myers, G. G., Grunnet, M. L.: Teratoma of the spinal cord. Arch. Path. *99*, 446–448 (1975)
13. Rothman, S. M., Nelson, J. S., DeVivo, D. C., Coxe, W. S.: Congenital astrocytoma presenting with intracerebral hematoma. J. Neurosurg. *51*, 237–239 (1979)
14. Russell, A.: A diencephalic syndrome of emaciation in infancy and childhood. Arch. Dis. Childh. *26*, 274–282 (1951)
15. Schreiber, D., Jänisch, W., Gerlach, H.: Tumours of the central nervous system during intrauterine life and in infancy. In: Brain tumours and chemical injuries to the central nervous system, ed. by Mossakowski, M. J. Warsaw: Polish Med. Publ. 1978, pp. 76–81
16. Miller, W. L., Townsend, J. J., Grumbach, M. M., Kaplan, S. L.: An infant with Cushings's disease due to an adrenocorticotropin-producing pituitary adenoma. J. Clin. Endocr. Metab. *48*, 1017–1025 (1979)
17. Saeger, W., Ruttmann, E., Lüdecke, D.: ACTH secreting pituitary adenoma in an infant of 18 months. Immunohistochemical, electron-microscopic, and in-vitro studies. Path. Res. Pract. *173*, 121–129 (1981)

Congenital Intracranial Teratoma in a Newborn

H. KLEIN and J. KLEIN

We give a summary of the clinical investigations and the operative findings, together with a clinical follow-up of a newborn with a congenital intracranial teratoma.

Case history: J. W., born 4. 2. 1981, a female infant, was the first child of healthy non-consanguineous parents. Delivery was effected by forceps without complication, birth weight 3550 g, body length 52 cm, head circumference 38 cm (macrocephaly). As her head rapidly increased in size in the postnatal period a cranial computerized tomography (CT) was done and was thought to show porencephaly. After admission to hospital (head size 44 cm) CT was repeated with intraventricular instillation of radiopaque contrast medium: a very large, lobulated tumour was found in the left lateral ventricle (Fig. 1). This tumour was surgically excised in two stages, 8 and 12 weeks after birth.

Histological diagnosis: teratoma.

Intraventricular bleeding (control CT) two days after the last operation required neurosurgical intervention but the postoperative course was uncomplicated. On discharge from hospital (9. 6. 1981) the child weighed 6860 g and the head circumference was 45.5 cm. A neurological examination six weeks later revealed some one-sided differences in motor function and retarded psychomotor development. Because of increase in the head circumference, 1.7 cm within one week, the infant was readmitted to hospital (19. 8. 1981). The fontanelle was bulging. A severe internal hydrocephalus was found in the CT and the intraventricular cerebrospinal fluid pressure measured 240 mm H_2O. An atrio-ventricular shunt (Hakim-Cordis, opening pressure 90–130 mm H_2O) was implanted without complications.

Histological findings: When the tumour sections were first examined the arrangement of nerve cells suggested the probable diagnosis of a gangliocytoma, but further examination of all the tumour tissue removed at the first operation (30–40 g) revealed glandular structures. The ependyma-like walls were surrounded by central nervous system tissue. Some papillary choroid plexus formations could be seen, so that it was finally possible to make the diagnosis of teratoma. The lobulated tumour excised at the second operation weighed 55 g. By the finding of cartilage, striated muscle and glandular structures suggestive of respiratory tract origin the diagnosis of an intracranial teratoma was confirmed (Fig. 2).

Discussion

Intracranial teratomata presenting at birth are rare. The incidence is estimated between 0.3–0.6% of all intracranial neoplasms. The rate increases to 2% if children under age 15 are considered.

In 1960 Greenhouse and Neuburger [2] published a review of a series of 25 cases gathered from the literature dating back to 1861. Following these authors the cases can be divided into three main groups with various characteristic clinical and patho-

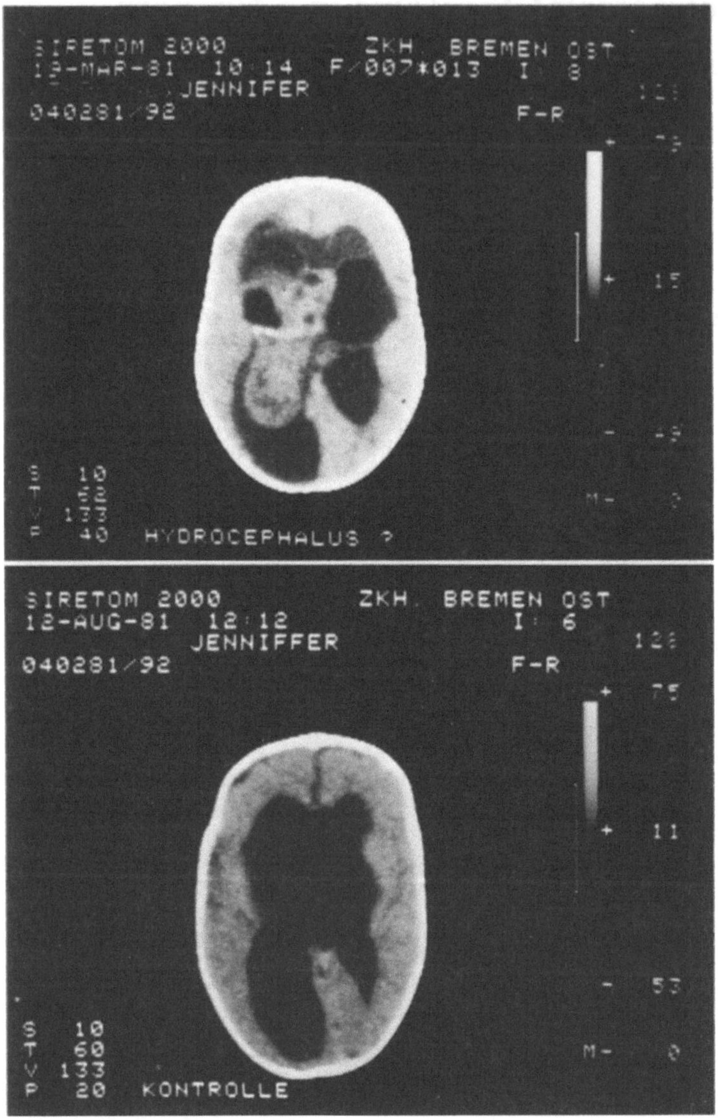

Fig. 1. CT after admission to hospital shows a large, lobulated tumour in the left lateral ventricle

logical features. The largest group comprises infants born dead with very big tumours, frequently completely replacing all cerebral tissue (see Vraa-Jensen [3]). The infants of the second group have an enlarged head as a result of the intracranial tumour, but they may survive delivery. The third group is made up of infants delivered normally with a head normal or nearly normal in size. In these an abrupt enlargement of the head occurs at periods varying from days to weeks after birth. The rapid growth of the tumours in the perinatal period may be related to the great-

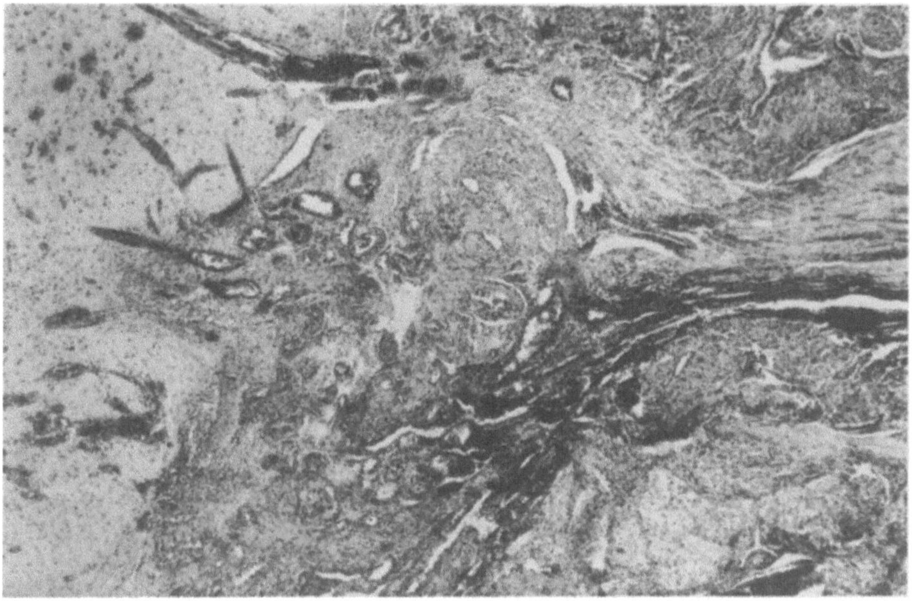

Fig. 2. The histological examination of the surgical specimen proves the diagnosis of a teratoma because of cartilages, transverse striated musculature and glandular structures

ly enhanced growth of the normal brain in this period of development [1]. This special growth effect may be transferred likewise to the central nervous tissue components of the intracranial teratoma. In our case these portions of the tumour by far exceeded those originating from the two other germinal layers. The commonest site of origin of these hamartomatous tumours is in the midline area, especially in the pineal and the pituitary. Some are situated in the lateral ventricle originating from the choroid plexus, as was evident in our case. An outstanding feature of these tumours is a tendency to obstruct the cerebrospinal fluid pathways. A rapid increase in head circumference in the postnatal weeks is suspicious and a highly suggestive sign of obstructive hydrocephalus. This sign should be noticed as early as possible to give way to further investigations, especially CT and, thence to any necessary surgical intervention.

References

1. Brandt, J.: Kopfumfang und Gehirnentwicklung. Klin. Wochenschr. *59,* 995–1007 (1981)
2. Greenhouse, A. H., Neuburger, K. T.: Intracranial Teratoma of the Newborn Arch. Neurol. *3,* 718–724 (1960)
3. Vraa-Jensen, J.: Massive Congenital Intracranial Teratoma. Acta Neuropath. *30,* 271–276 (1974)

Discussion

K. J. Zülch (Cologne) pointed out that every nomenclature represents a compromise. Neuropathology has been considerably stimulated from the clinical side. This also applies to the grading of cerebral tumours. Particularly with the American neurosurgeons the use of grading has expanded enormously and this has proved worthwhile for the practical procedures. A large number of the American neurosurgeons have a clear concept of the biological significance of this grading and correlate it with the traditional ideas of tumour pathology. Difficulties exist here in the understanding of the term; among neurosurgeons grading represents in practice their clinical experience with particular tumours, whereas in tumour pathology likewise a grading is familiar, that is supported by morphological criteria. These two forms of tumour assessment are not always identical.

K. Schürmann (Mainz) emphasized the importance of grading for the neurosurgeon in deciding as to how radical an excision should be attempted and also how to plan the subsequent treatment by radiotherapy or chemotherapy. He enquired further if the sex preponderance of certain tumours could be explained and whether it might shed further light on the problems. He stated that when a glioma recurred its malignancy was often increased.

K. J. Zülch (Cologne) said that it was scarcely possible to make any prediction about whether a glioma which recurred reached a higher grade of malignancy or not. In many astrocytomas one finds areas which could be called anaplastic, and could if they grew further lead to anaplasia of the whole tumour.

The question about the sex preference of particular tumours is extremely important, but definitive information about this is not yet available.

Müller (Hamburg) pointed out the difficulties, when small fragments of tumour are removed during operation, of giving any definite opinion about the nature of the whole lesion.

K. Jellinger (Vienna): Apart from the classification of the tumour in the sense of grading, an exact description of the tumour is extremely important, as the grading is not necessarily valid for all types of tumour. Thus, there are anaplastic ependymomas of the cerebral hemispheres with a survival of twelve or more years. In very many other tumours, even such as meningiomas, it cannot be foreseen whether they will dedifferentiate and become anaplastic. This opinion was confirmed by *J. M. Schröder (Aachen).*

Bohl (Mainz) also stressed that there were two different principles of classification, firstly the classification according to clinical experience with different types of tumour, and secondly according to the concepts of morbid anatomy. The danger exists of confusing these two procedures. Even grading according to clinical ideas should not be regarded as conclusive, as the prognosis of certain tumours had actually been improved by the treatment.

O. Stochdorph (Munich) stressed that grading in general, and not only in cerebral pathology is of importance for the analysis and codifying of the histological findings. His objection was that this subdivision according to clinical criteria was designated as "grading", in terms of its prognostic value. This term has already been reserved for a system of classification based on histological analyses.

S. Wende (Mainz) asked whether the large amounts of money which are being invested in experimental tumour research were being sensibly expended. He had failed to detect any relevant information concerning human pathology and stated that at times, completely absurd claims were published, particularly in the lay press, regarding cancer-producing substances.

These remarks were strongly contradicted by *P. Kleihues (Freiburg).* He pointed out that over twenty chemical compounds are known today, which demonstrably and not merely presumably can cause tumours in man. He mentioned the investigations which had proved the connection between cigarette abuse and bronchial carcinoma. In his opinion experimental carcinoma research has yielded a large number of important results, which justify further efforts.

These remarks were approved of by *D. Schreiber (Erfurt)*. He pointed out that in general brain tumours behave just like other tumours. In about 80% of all other tumours exogenous factors apparently play a part, aetiologically. Further, it is well-known that the blood-brain barrier does not represent any definite barrier, as animal experiments have shown that even in the brain, tumours can be caused by the oral administration of carcinogens.

K. J. Zülch (Cologne) stated that the discussion should become a little less heated! The endeavours of experimental carcinoma research had been very great and it had also had numerous successes, but in spite of that many things remain completely unexplained. Zülch further stated that he expected an important stimulus from a carcinoma register. He did not regard as valid the counter-arguments in Europe with reference to the confidentiality of records. It was his opinion that really important stimuli would come earliest from the clinical field.

K. Schürmann (Mainz) asked for some ideas as to how oncogenic substances produce tumours and was answered by *P. Kleihues (Freiburg)* who formulated a basic principle. All neuro-oncogenic compounds are also teratogenic. Conversely, however, not all teratogenic compounds are necessarily neuro-oncogenic. It is also a principle that the dose of such substances which leads to malformations, is as a rule significantly higher than the dose which suffices to cause tumours. Even the smallest doses, which have no cytotoxic and no teratogenic effect and even cause no dysplasia, can act as carcinogens.

G. M. Zu Rhein (Madison, Wis.) as a representative of basic research, confirmed the great importance of experimental tumour research. She supported this with other examples from her own field and stated that in the virogenesis of particular tumours human pathogenic viruses were used to some extent. This is a very important aspect.

K. J. Zülch (Cologne) returned to the question posed by *Jellinger (Vienna)* as to whether there was such a thing as an ependymoblastoma. It has been emphasized clinically that the tumours which one calls ependymoblastomas were indeed as relatively benign as the ependymomas (lower grade of malignancy).

The term "blastoma" was used as a rule, for a malignant tumour and an oligodendroblastoma was thus an anaplastic oligodendroglioma. Zülch did not regard this as a suitable basis for expressing grades of malignancy. Jellinger (Vienna) agreed, and stated that in his opinion, the anaplastic ependymomas were not identical with those tumours erroneously described in the American literature as ependymoblastomas.

Bohl (Mainz) asked *Jellinger (Vienna)* and *Gerlach (Halle)* how many premature babies had been in the group of congenital tumours, and also what was the earliest fetal age at which he had observed a tumour.

Jellinger (Vienna) replied that he had found nine tumours in the new-born, including two premature infants, and one still-born with generalized dissemination of a sympathoblastoma of the adrenal, and also one child with a teratoma.

H. Gerlach (Halle) stated in his reply, that the term "congenital" was not always used in the same sense. Many authors understood by this, also those tumours which showed themselves clinically in infants. To the second question from Bohl he mentioned a case of Tamura, who found a 22-week fetus with an extremely large teratoma.

P. Kleihues (Freiburg) asked *K. H. H. Merkel (Homburg)* if the detection of glial fibrillary protein in about half of all medulloblastomas, allowed one to express an opinion, that two types of tumour were involved, with possible different prognostic significance.

K. H. H. Merkel (Homburg) replied that any views about the prognosis on the basis of his investigations were not possible at present.

Clinical Presentation of Space-Occupying Lesions of the Central Nervous System

G. Jacobi

The clinical data of 192 children suffering from intracranial space-occupying lesions are presented here. Subtentorial tumours were encountered more often than supratentorial ones (Table 1). There was a preponderance in boys with the exception only of brainstem gliomas. Somatic symptoms, neurological findings, and cranial nerve (CN) involvement are thoroughly discussed below.

General Somatic Signs and Symptoms (Tables 2, 3)

About one half of all brain tumours in children are located within or near the midline. For this reason obstruction of the CSF pathways is encountered early. These children present with headache, vomiting, and papilloedema. Vertigo is rarely reported by children, apart from when they suffer from brain tumours. Increased head size is found in the huge gliomas of the cerebral hemispheres and in lesions of the supratentorial midline. A stiff posture of head and neck indicates pain originating from the dura in posterior fossa lesions. It can be seen from Table 2 that general signs very rarely lead to adequate clinical investigations whatever the reason might be in the individual case.

Table 1. Site-age-sex in 192 children with intracranial tumours

Age	Supratentorial			Subtentorial		N
	I= Cerebral hemisphere	II= Ventricles lat. and third upper brain stem	III= Supra-sellar	IV= Lower brain stem	V= Cerebellum (vermis, hemisphere)-fourth ventr.	
< 1 year	5	2	1	–	2	10
2 – 5 years	12	11	6	11	32	72
6 – 18 years	21	18	13	18	40	110
	38	31	20	29	74	192
Sex	27♂ 11♀	17♂ 14♀	12♂ 8♀	9♂ 20♀	50♂ 24♀	115♂ 77♀

Table 2. General somatic signs

General signs	Site of the tumour					N
	I	II	III	IV	V	
Headache	15 (2)	12 (6)	9 (3)	9	52 (4)	97 (15)
Vomiting	9 (2)	4 (1)	7 (1)	10	57 (10)	87 (13)
Vomiting before breakfast	1	3	1	3	23	31
Vertigo	1	3 (1)	2	2	11 (2)	19 (3)
Increased head circumference	7 (3)	11 (2)	–	–	12	30 (5)
Stiff head posture	–	–	–	5	14	19
Weight decrease	4	3	1	–	8	16
Weight increase	–	–	2	–	1	3

15 (2) means: of 15 patients with headache this prompted clinical investigation in 2

Table 3. Somatic symptoms

Symptom	Site of the tumour					N
	I	II	III	IV	V	
Neck rigidity or retraction	7	13	6	2	23	51
Head-tilt	–	2	–	5	20	27
Head circumference > P97	7	11	2	–	15	35
Limited bulging of the head	3	1	–	–	1	5
Protrusion of the eyeballs	5	1	–	–	2	8
Low stature (< P3)	–	5	11	–	3	19
High stature (> P97)	–	3	2	–	2	7
Anorexia	–	4	6	–	7	17
Hypoplasia of the genitals (♂) Amenorrhoea (♀)	–	1	7	1	–	9
Diabetes insipidus pre-operatively	–	2	–	–	–	2
Diabetes insipidus postoperatively	–	2	5	–	–	7
Sec. hypothyroidism pre-operatively	–	–	7	–	–	7
Sec. insufficience of the adrenals pre-operatively	–	–	3	–	–	3

Somatic symptoms might be the presenting or even the only finding in a child with a brain tumour. Panhypopituitarism is well known in children with craniopharyngiomas, leading to growth retardation, hypothyroidism, and genital hypoplasia. It is less well known that there might be excessive growth before puberty in children with craniopharyngioma or gliomas of the tuber cinereum (two cases and one case respectively). Moreover, there is a syndrome imitating anorexia nervosa in children with primary or secondary involvement of the lower brain stem, mainly pontine gliomas ([12], personal observations). The diencephalic syndrome of emaciation in tumours of the anterior hypothalamus is well known [19]. It might be diagnosed in late infancy or early childhood.

General Neurological Signs and Symptoms (Tables 4, 5)

The most important signs of supratentorial tumours are: seizures (Table 9), hemiparesis, visual impairment, and changes in behaviour. Gait disturbance on the other hand is the prominent feature of posterior fossa tumours which leads to proper investigations. Defective vision is detected late in most children, for there is usually no pain and no complaints from the child's side. He or she fixates in a parafoveal manner, gets very closely to the visual targets, or presents with pendular ocular movements. The exact site of the lesion in this latter symptom is not quite clear: it may be in the optic chiasm, the dorsal hypothalamus or the pretectal area?

Table 4. Neurological signs

Neurological sign	Site of the tumour					N
	I	II	III	IV	V	
Visual impairment	6 (4)	2 (2)	8 (5)	2	5 (4)	23 (17)
Squint – double vision	4 (2)	2	–	11 (2)	17 (5)	34 (9)
Defective eye-movements	–	–	1	2 (1)	2 (1)	5 (2)
Impaired hearing	1	–	1 (1)	2 (1)	3	7 (2)
Gait disturbance	3	–	2 (1)	15 (13)	26 (15)	46 (29)
Hemiplegia/Hemiparesis	5 (1)	8 (6)	1 (1)	7 (3)	–	21 (11)
Changes in behaviour	14	2	6	3	14	39
Depressed level of consciousness	8 (1)	4 (1)	3 (1)	2	17 (6)	34 (9)

Table 5. General neurological symptoms [*Va* midline: vermis. IV. ventricle; *Vb* cerebellar hemisphere(s)]

Symptom	Site of the tumour						N
	I	II	III	IV	Va	Vb	
Hemiparesis – hemiplegia	19 (4post)	10 (1post)	–	11	3	1	44
Paraplegia – tetraparesis	4	2	–	2	6	1	15
Hemisensory deficit	4	3	–	3	1	–	11
Homonymous hemianopic deficit	6	2	–	–	1	1	10
Dysphasia	6	1	–	–	–	–	7
Dysarthria	2	3	–	8	2	3	18
Gait ataxia – truncal ataxia	3	6	1	15	23	20	68
Tremor (all kinds)	1	3	1	9	9	6	29
Hypotonia	–	–	–	–	17	4	21
Choreoathetosis-dystonic posturing	2	2	1	–	2	1	8
Dysmetria-positive pronator sign	3	11	1	12	44	22	93
Rigidity-cogwheel phenomenon	2	3	–	4	4	1	14
(Pseudo)Bulbar paralysis	–	1	–	11	2	2	16
Number of patients in each group	38	31	20	29	50	24	192

Ocular Findings and Other CNS Involvement (Tables 6, 7)

There is no papilloedema in nearly all primary brain-stem tumours nor signs of raised intracranial pressure. Some children with long standing cerebellar lesions do

Table 6. Ocular symptoms

Symptom	Site of the tumour						N
	I	II	III	IV	Va	Vb	
Normal ocular fundi	14	10	6	28	15	10	83
Papilloedema	16	15	9	1	35	14	90
Optic atrophy (Foster Kennedy-syndrome)	8 (3)	6 (1)	5	–	–	–	19 (4)
Impaired pupillary reaction	7	5	2	4	7	–	25
IIIrd CN palsy	2	1	–	7	3	2	15
IVth CN palsy	–	1	–	3	3	–	7
VIth CN palsy – unilateral	2	3	–	14	12	6	37
VIth CN palsy – bilateral	2	2	1	8	15	3	31
Gaze paresis: lateral	–	2	–	6	3	5	16
Gaze paresis: vertical	1	2	–	–	2	–	5
Number of patients in each group	38	31	20	29	50	24	192

Table 7. Other cranial nerve symptoms

C. N. involved		Site of the tumour						N
		I	II	III	IV	Va	Vb	
Vth:	Motor	–	1	–	3	2	–	6
	Sensory	–	3	–	7	4	1	15
	Corneal reflex ∅	–	–	–	14	3	3	20
VIIth:	Supranuclear	10	5	–	16	4	3	38
	Nuclear-peripheral	1	3	–	9	4	4	21
VIIIth:	Acusticus	1	1	–	5	2	3	12
	Staticus	–	–	–	1	3	3	7
IXth:		1	1	–	5	–	1	8
Xth:	(N. recurrens)	–	–	–	3	–	1	4
XIth:		–	–	–	–	–	3	3
XIIth:		–	–	–	10	1	1	12
Nystagmus:	Vertical	–	–	–	1	1	–	2
	Lateral	1	–	–	5	6	6	18
	Gaze paretic	1	1	2	6	10	2	22
	Rotatory	–	1	2	2	4	2	11
	Dissociated	–	–	–	2	4	1	7
Number of patients in each group		38	31	20	29	50	24	192

not get papilloedema either. Optic atrophy at the time the diagnosis is made means amblyopia or even amaurosis, mostly on one side, rarely bilaterally. Pallor of the optic discs observed months after the operative procedures have been done does not mean such profound visual impairment compared with this finding in supratentorial lesions. The finding of a sixth nerve palsy on one side or bilaterally is an ambiguous sign: If there is raised intracranial pressure the cranial nerve palsy might be due to this, but if the pressure is normal it might indicate a pontine glioma, especially if there are other cranial nerve signs. This applies even more to the third (external) and fourth nerve palsies. Paresis of the trigeminal, acoustic, or hypoglossal nerve are important for the diagnosis of brain-stem intrinsic lesions. However, a seventh nerve palsy is a non-specific sign: if there is additional paresis of other cranial nerves, if there are long tract signs (pyramidal symptoms, truncal or peripheral ataxia), and a normal intracranial pressure, the diagnosis of a brain-stem tumour is almost certain.

Primary and Secondary Brain Stem Involvement (Table 8)

To eliminate all non-specific signs all observations in the patients in group IV and V were compared with the operative findings and/or the post mortem reports. The decisive question was: was there involvement of the lower brain stem or not. For instance: peripheral (nuclear) seventh nerve palsy is a non-specific sign and was therefore eliminated from the table, as also was lateral, gaze paretic or rotatory nystagmus. An accessory nerve palsy nearly always means an extrinsic lesion of the medulla oblongata, but if on the other hand there are two or more signs found which are listed in Table 8 an intrinsic lesion of the brain-stem might be diagnosed straight away. Any contemplation of a complete tumour removal should be rejected and strictly refused according to the author's personal experience.

Table 8. Neurological symptoms, two or more of them indicating brain stem involvement in 55 patients: All 29 group IV, 26 of group Va and Vb

Impaired pupillary reactions/not unilat. internal ophthalmoplegia		11 (all)
V:	Motor	5 (all)
	Sensory (Sölder's lines present)	12 (all)
	Corneal reflex depressed or absent	19 (of 20)
VIII:	N. acusticus	9 (of 10)
IX:		6 (all)
X:	(N. recurrens)	3 (of 4)
XII:		11 (of 12)
Vertical gaze paresis		2 (all)
Vertical nystagmus		2 (all)
Dissociated nystagmus		6 (of 7)
Alternating C. N. palsies (III – XII)		4 (all)
Vomiting *without* signs of raised intracranial pressure for months or years		6

11 (of 12) means: 11 of 12 patients who had P. of the hypoglossal nerve had brain stem involvement. Brain stem involvement was demonstrated intraoperatively and/or at autopsy

Unilateral deafness in a child scarcely ever means acoustic neurinoma. If there are neighbourhood cranial nerve palsies this indicates a cerebellar tumour of a doubtful nature in the cerebello-pontine angle, such as a medulloblastoma, (arachnoid) sarcoma or osteogenic tumour.

The clinical assessment viz., intrinsic or extrinsic lesion of the brainstem is not a substitute for proper neuroradiological investigation, but it is a supplementary way to consider the situation.

Seizures and Sudden Loss of Consciousness (Table 9)

Convulsions – before the diagnosis is established – are of great importance in supratentorial tumours (31 of 69 patients in group I and II). In subtentorial lesions they are generally due to a genetic predisposition. Seizures in supratentorial gliomas might remain monosymptomatic, even for years (10 cases). Tumour-epilepsy in a child is oligosymptomatic at the beginning and the patient responds well to anticonvulsant treatment. The seizures then get refractory to the drugs, increase in number, get longer, and complicated. One might observe adverse movements, dysphasic symptoms, and Todd's paralysis in the later stages. Most of the tumours are huge, benign gliomas. Sudden loss of consciousness is encountered in some children, simulating drop attacks. It might be due to some alteration of the blood flow in the midbrain region. We have reported paroxysmal dystonic movements without any clouding of consciousness in long-standing tumours of the medulla and cerebellum. These bouts last for half to one hour and might be accompanied by excessive salivation. Cerebellar fits occurred in some long-standing cerebellar lesions with ob-

Table 9. Seizures and sudden loss of consciousness

Clinical presentation		Site of the tumour					N
		I	II	III	IV	V	
Grand mal seizure (status)		4 (3)	7 (2)	–	1 (1)	3 (1)	14 (7)
Focal seizures:	Jackson adverse hemiconvulsion	4 (4)	2 (2)	1 (1)	1 (1)	1 (1)	9 (9)
Other focal:	akinetic myoclonic multifocal	6 (5)	2	–	–	–	8 (5)
Complex partial		3	3	–	–	–	6
Sudden loss of consciousness		–	1	2	–	3	6
Paroxysmal extrapyramidal syndrome		–	–	–	2	1	3
Cerebellar fits according to H. Jackson		–	1	–	–	7	8

Result: 37 (= 19.3%) out of 192 children with intracranial tumours had one or more seizure(s) before diagnosis of tumour was established

structive hydrocephalus. The patients present with loss of consciousness, pupillary changes, hyperventilation or apnoea, and decorticate or decerebrate posturing. In two cases these fits were mistaken for grand mal seizures and treated with diphenylhydantoin.

Changes in Behaviour (Table 10)

These might be due to raised intracranial pressure. Disturbances of consciousness and drive should also be mentioned here. They are sometimes characterized by a quick change in performance: the child has just responded alertly and was well oriented, but then becomes sleepy. Selective mutism has been seen in pre-school children with brain stem involvement. The symptom often cleared when they were treated by operation and/or by radiotherapy. Long-standing tumours often present in smaller children as regression, in the school-aged as retardation, and in adolescents as a puberty crisis [4, 6, 8].

In some supratentorial lesions there are distinct psychopathological syndromes: the cocktail-party syndrome in lesions of the midline with obstructive hydrocephalus, Gerstmann's syndrome and dysphasias in lesions of the dominant parietal or fronto-parietal lobe. In two children with tumours of the posterior hypothalamus, subthalamus, and splenium of the corpus callosum a very distinctive picture was

Table 10. Psychopathological findings

Presentation	Site of the tumour					N
	I	II	III	IV	V	
Reluctant to play – fatigue – apathy	10	5	3	2	17	37
Somnolence – stupor – coma	5	2	1	1	8	17
Close to tears – fearful – depressed – withdrawn	4	–	1	3	4	12
Performance at school worse	2	2	2	–	5	11
Mutism	1	1	–	7	5	14
Temper tantrums – aggressive – agitated	6	1	1	–	–	8
Speaks, laughs, cries unrestrainedly	1	–	–	3	1	5
Dysphasia – Gerstmann's syndrome	7	1	–	–	–	8
Cocktail party syndrome	1	3	–	–	–	4
Visual hallucinations with disintegration of visual perception	–	2	–	–	–	2
Retardation: Motor	3	1	2	–	2	8
Mental	5	3	1	–	2	11
Regression	–	1	–	–	8	9
Number of patients in each group	38	31	20	29	74	192

observed: they were disoriented in time, had visual hallucinations, especially during the night, leaving them frightened. Their field of visual perception disintegrated into three broad discs, insofar as the children were able only to recognize and to orientate spatially within the middle slice. One of them had a teratoblastoma, the other a non-classified sarcoma.

Some Considerations About the Different Types of Tumour

Supratentorial astrocytomas most often present as tumour-epilepsy. They are calcified in about 25% [13, 15, 21, 22]. The time for recurrence sometimes equals the time of primary growth (=length of past history) [14], but in some children there might be a rapid expansion after the first subtotal operation (three personal observations).

Oligodendrogliomas are much rarer in children than in adults [18, 23]. They are found in the supratentorial space almost exclusively. Epileptic seizures, too, might be the leading and only sign of presentation, in one of our cases for six years. Calcifications are found very often within the tumour. Today, therefore, they might be detected earlier by CT. Oligodendrogliomas are variants of malignant gliomas [22]. Recurrences might show an increase in malignant features [10, 14]. Astrocytomas might harbour small islets of oligodendroglioma the so-called "mixed glioma" of Rubinstein [18].

Ependymomas are different from the biological point of view if they are located supratentorially or within the posterior fossa. The supratentorial ones are calcified in 50–60% [13, 22]. They are found almost exclusively in a paediatric population. They do not seed along the CSF pathways, but have the tendency for local recurrence [7, 13, 22, 23]. They are situated within or near the ventricles. Of the children in a larger series 10% have multiple sites [7]. Only 10% of the children and adolescents survive the five years' period without additional radiotherapy [1, 7, 9, 20].

In subtentorial ependymomas Kricheff et al. [11] propose a staging:

T1: tumour limited to the fourth ventricle.
T2: tumour extends into the cisterna magna
T3: tumour extends beyond the cisterna magna and/or into the cerebellopontine cistern(s)
T4: invasion of the cerebellum and the brainstem
M: distant metastases.

Most authors conclude that childhood ependymomas have a worse prognosis than those of adults. They therefore plead for additional radiotherapy [1, 5, 11, 13, 16, 20].

Glioblastomas are much rarer in children than in adults. In general terms, the prognosis is hopeless as in later life. But in children there is one exception: the giant cell type in which long survival times have been observed ([10], two of nine personal observations).

Medulloblastomas might have their primary site within the brainstem (6 of 43 personal observations). The incidence in boys is twice that in girls [12, 22, 23]. Age and sex influence prognosis. According to Chatty and Earle [3] the mean time of survival in male patients is 21, in female 31 months. In children less than 15 years it is 11 months, in adolescents 50 months. Müller et al. (see p. 350) had similar results: they found survival times in the 1–5 years group of 11 months, from 6–10 years of 15 months, 11–15 years: 24 months and in patients older than 16 years: 48 months. On the other hand, they found no statistical difference in the so-called desmoplastic and the classical type of Rubinstein and Northfield [17, 18] as did Chatty and Earle.

In 1969 Chang et al. [2] gave a staging system which to-day is still in use in prospective therapeutic studies:

T1: tumour less than 3cm in diameter, lying within the fourth ventricle, the vermis cerebelli or in one cerebellar hemisphere
T2: tumour more than 3 cm in diameter invading adjacent structures
T3: tumour invading two adjacent structures or completely filling the fourth ventricle thus producing obstructive hydrocephalus
T4: tumour spreading through the iter to involve the third ventricle or midbrain, or extending to the upper cervical cord.
M0: no evidence of gross subarachnoid or haematogenous metastasis
M1: tumour cells found in the CSF on microscopy
M2: gross nodular seedings in the cerebellar or cerebral subarachnoid space or within the lateral or third ventricles
M3: gross nodular seedings in the spinal subarachnoid space
M4: extraneural metastasis.

Stage T3 is still subdivided by these authors [2] in T3a without, and T3b with, macroscopic evidence of the tumour's adhesion to the floor of the fourth ventricle.

My own opinion on this staging system is that the question of size and CSF blocking does not play an important role. The question of brainstem involvement does, as well as the question of seedings along the CSF pathways. Three personal observations should be mentioned here:

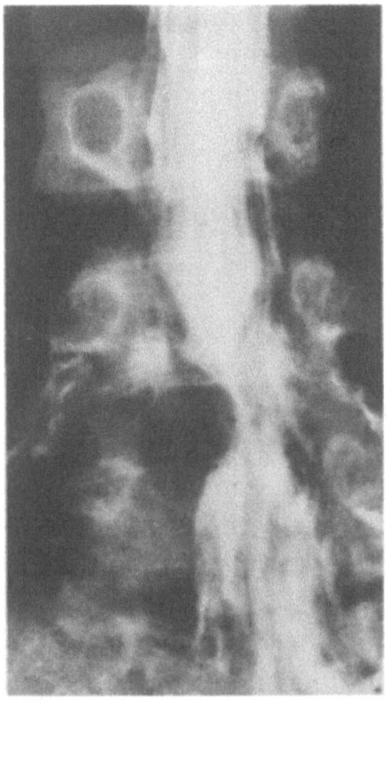

Fig. 1. Amipaque-myelogram of a boy, aged ten years and five months. He was operated on five months ago for a medulloblastoma of the cerebellar vermis. He presented with lumbar stiffness, flaccid paraparesis, and impaired bladder function. Intradural hold-up at L.1 was shown, tumour nodule at L 4/5, and infiltration of lumbo-sacral nerve-roots was demonstrated

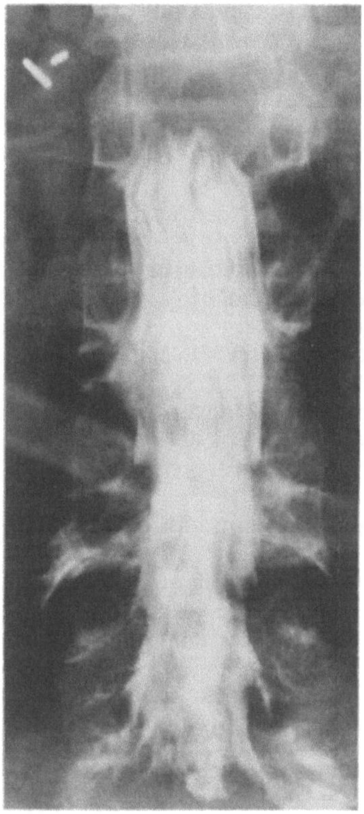

Fig. 2. Amipaque-myelogram of a boy, aged nine years and five months. He was operated on eight years ago for adrenal carcinoma on the right side (paravertebral clips). He presented with a mass lesion of the cerebellar vermis (medulloblastoma), and, at the same time, with transsection of the spinal cord. Intradural hold up at the L.2 level was shown. Note contrast filling defects of nearly bean-size below the lesion demonstrating the multiplicity of cerebrospinal fluid seedlings

1) In some cases (four in our own material) the lesion of the posterior fossa and the lumbar seedings presented at the very same time.
2) Carpet-like seeding on the floor of the lateral and third ventricles (three cases) might be detected late by CT but they are demonstrated earlier by ventriculography.
3) The spinal seedings are multiple and might spread along the nerve sheaths thus leading to extraneural metastases (Figs. 1, 2). We had spinal metastases in nine of our patients and extraneural tumour growth in two children without preceding shunts.

Summary

Clinical signs and symptoms of 192 children with brain tumours are given. Tumours might present with somatic, neurological or ophthalmological symptoms, seizure disorders and behavioural disturbance. Brain stem involvement might be diagnosed on clinical findings alone. This insight might give help in planning an operation and discussing it beforehand with the child's parents. The question of brain stem involvement also seems to be important in staging cerebellar medulloblastoma. Hope for final cure in this type of tumour is hampered by its biological behaviour: often it has already given rise to spinal seeding at the time of tumour detection producing much seeding along the neural axis. There are often recurrences after years.

References

1. Barone, B. M., Elvidge, A. R.: Ependymomas. A clinical survey. J. Neurosurg. *33*, 428–438 (1970)
2. Chang, C. H., Housepian, E. M., Herbert, C.: An operative staging system and a megavoltage radiotherapeutic technic for cerebellar medulloblastomas. Radiology *93*, 1351–1359 (1959)
3. Chatty, E. M., Earle, K. M.: Medulloblastoma. A report of 201 cases with emphasis on the relationship of histological variants to survival. Cancer *28*, 977–983 (1971)
4. Corboz, R.: Die Psychiatrie der Hirntumoren bei Kindern. Acta neurochir. suppl. *5*, 1–100 (1958)
5. Fokes, E. C., Earle, K. M.: Ependymomas: clinical and pathological aspects. J. Neurosurg. *30*, 585–594 (1969)
6. Gerlach, J., Jensen, H.-P., Koos, W., Kraus, H.: „Pädiatrische Neurochirurgie." Intrakranielle Geschwülste, 459–645 Stuttgart: Thieme 1967
7. Goutelle, A.: Les ependymomes intracraniens sus-tentoriels. Neurochirurgie (Paris) *23*, suppl. *1*, 53–66 (1977)
8. Hécaen, H., Ajuriaguerra, J. de: "Troubles mentaux au cours des tumeurs intracraniennes." Paris: Masson & Cie. 1956
9. Hoffmann, G. H., Thiry, S., Achslogh, J., Brihaye, J., Dereymaeker, A.: Etude statistique de 202 cas de tumeurs de la fosse postérieure de l'enfance. Neurochirurgie (Paris) *7*, 97–107 (1961)
10. Koos, W. T., Miller, M. H.: "Intracranial tumours of infants and children. Thieme, Stuttgart 1971
11. Kricheff, I. I., Becker, M., Schneck, S. A., Taveras, J. M.: Intracranial ependymomas: Factors influencing prognosis. J. Neurosurg. *21*, 7–14 (1964)
12. Maroon, J. C., Albright, L.: "Failure to thrive" due to pontine glioma. Arch. Neurol. *34*, 295–297 (1977)
13. Milhorat, T. H.: "Pediatric Neurosurgery". Chapter 8: Tumours of the Brain, Meninges, and Skull. 211–283. Philadelphia: Davis & Co. 1978
14. Müller, W., Afra, D., Schröder, R.: Supratentorial recurrences of gliomas. Morphological studies in relation to time intervals with oligodendrogliomas. Acta neurochir. *39*, 15–25 (1977)
15. Page, L. K., Lombroso, C. T., Matson, D. D.: Childhood epilepsy with late detection of cerebral glioma. J. Neurosurg. *31*, 253–261 (1969)
16. Pierluca, P.: Les ependymomes de la fosse cérébrale posterieure. Neurochirurgie (Paris) *23*, suppl. *1*, 111–148 (1977)
17. Rubinstein, L. J., Northfield, D. W. C.: Medulloblastoma and the so-called "arachnoidal cerebellar sarcoma". Brain *87*, 379–412 (1964)
18. Rubinstein, L. J.: "Tumours of the Central Nervous System." Atlas of Tumour Pathology, 2nd ser., fasc. *6*, Armed Forces Institute of Pathology, Washington, 1–17 (1972)
19. Russell, A.: A diencephalic syndrome of emaciation in infancy and childhood. Arch. Dis. Childh. *26*, 274 (1951)
20. Shuman, R. M., Alvord, E. C., Leech, R. W.: The biology of childhood ependymomas. Arch. Neurol. *32*, 731–739 (1975)
21. Tönnis, W., Borck, W. F.: Großhirntumoren des Kindesalters. Zentralbl. Neurochir. *13*, 72–98 (1953)
22. Walker, M. D.: Diagnosis and treatment of brain tumours. Pediatr. Clin. North Amer. *23*, 131–146 (1976)
23. Zülch, K. J.: "Atlas of Gross Neurosurgical Pathology." Berlin, Heidelberg, New York: Springer 1975

Cytology of Cerebrospinal Fluid in Children with Brain Tumours

W. Dörffel

There is still much controversy on the diagnostic value of cytologic examination of the cerebrospinal fluid [3]. Opinions differ greatly with regard to the value of tumour cell diagnosis in the CSF. In the first part of this paper the methods of cytologic examination of the cerebrospinal fluid in brain tumours and their effectiveness are discussed in the light of the literature as well as on the basis of our experience; the second part deals with our own results.

It is not my intention to describe the cell pictures characteristic of particular types of brain tumour – there is an excellent atlas of cerebrospinal fluid cytology – but to demonstrate the diagnostic relevance of identification of tumour cells in the CSF.

Table 1 presents some data about the *frequency of tumour cell identification* in children and adults with primary brain tumours. In cerebral metastases, particularly carcinoma metastases and haemoblastoses, the proportion of positive findings based on CSF cytologic examination is known to be increased. In benign CNS tumours it is rare for tumour cells to be detected in the CSF and their differentiation from cells found occasionally in the CSF of healthy children, as for instance choroidal or ependymal cells, is then extremely difficult.

The well-known cytological criteria of malignancy can be applied to malignant tumour cells in the CSF. Such tumour cells are characterized by anisocytosis and polymorphism as well as by an altered nuclear-cytoplasmic ratio usually in favour of the nucleus. There is an abnormal, irregular chromatic texture of the nucleus, often with hyperchromatism and with conspicuous nucleoli and the cytoplasm frequently stains dark blue. Typical cell clusters especially in glioblastoma multiforme, in medulloblastoma (Fig. 1 a) and in anaplastic ependymoma (Fig. 1 b) are helpful

Table 1. Tumour cells in the cerebrospinal fluid in primary brain tumours – data compiled from the literature

Authors	Number of patients	Identification of tumour cells	Suspicion of tumour cells	No tumour cells
Wieczorek [13]	119	17 (14%)		102 (86%)
Sayk and Olischer [9]	124	9 (7%)		115 (93%)
Den Hartog Jager [1]	142	22 (16%)	6 (4%)	114 (80%)
Stefanko and Kaluza [12]	144	17 (12%)		127 (88%)
Olischer [6]	208	20 (10%)		188 (90%)

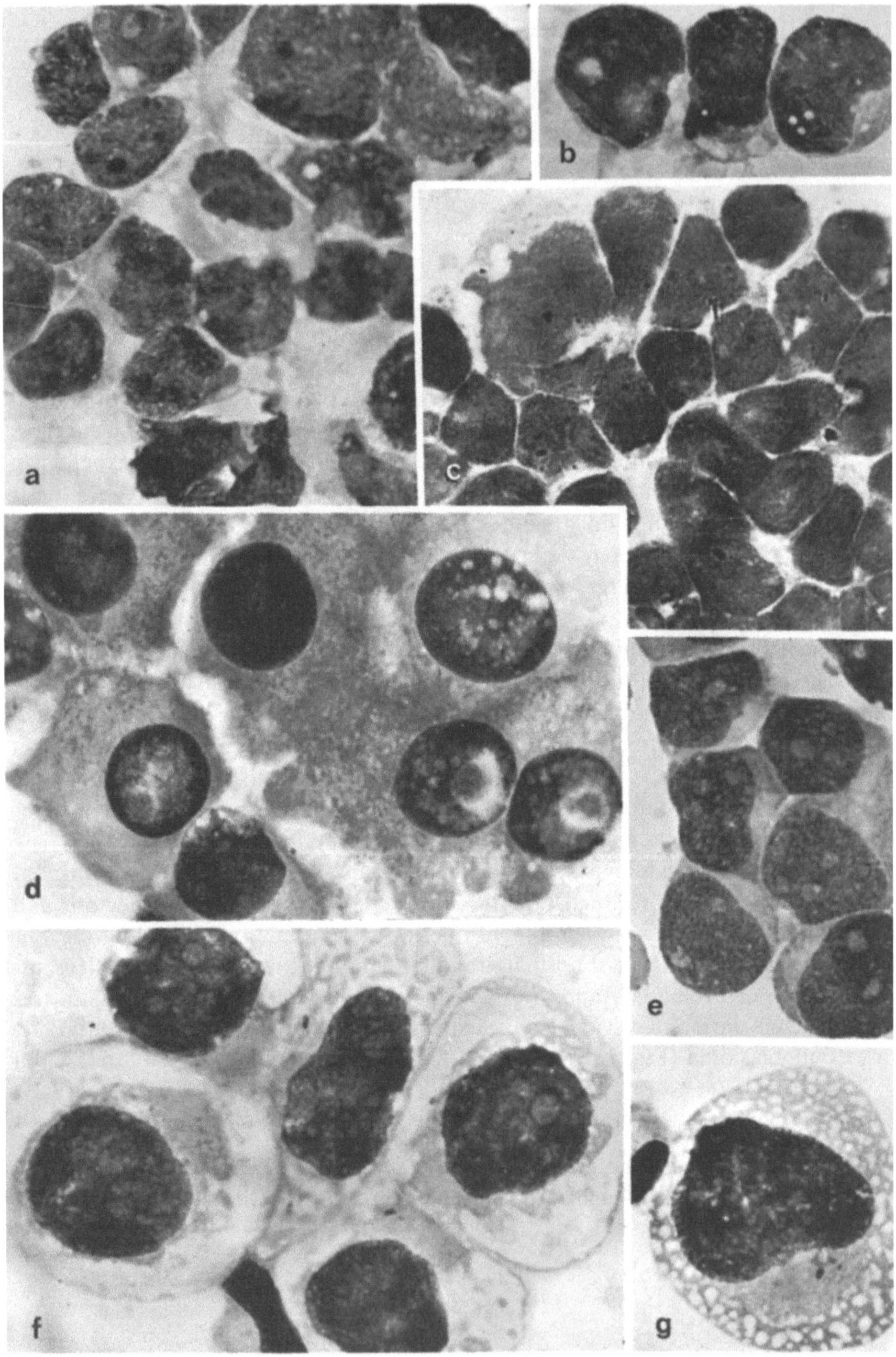

Fig. 1. Tumour cells in the CSF. **a** Cell clusters in medulloblastoma; **b** three tumour cells in anaplastic ependymoma; **c** tumour cell cluster in primary melanoma of the arachnoid; **d** cell cluster in reticulum-cell sarcoma; **e** tumour cell clusters in primary leptomeningeal sarcomatosis; **f, g** large tumour cells in anisomorphic pinealoma (germinoma)

in making the diagnosis. Mitoses occur in the CSF also in meningitides. They are increasingly but not always found when tumour cells are exfoliated into the cerebrospinal fluid.

The *rate of success of CSF cytologic examinations* in primary brain tumour depends upon the site and the histologic characteristics of the tumour. In tumours frequently exfoliating into the cerebrospinal fluid and tending to form so-called drip metastases in the spinal canal, tumour cells are quite often found in the CSF sample collected by lumbar puncture. However, even this correlation is only of statistical value, and there are, in fact, also false negative results, i.e. cases with diffuse leptomeningeal infiltration without evidence of tumour cells in the CSF. The fact that suboccipital and especially ventricular CSF samples contain tumour cells more often than lumbar CSF specimens do [5, 6], is true particularly with respect to cerebral tumours [4]. The success of the search for tumour cells is dependent upon the cerebrospinal fluid cell preparation rather than the way of collecting the CSF. Among the different methods of increasing cell concentration are the sedimentation techniques – we use the sedimentation chamber developed by Professor Sayk 25 years ago – and cytocentrifugation, have become widely used [2, 7].

A further development of the sedimentation chamber procedure, the absorption method developed by Sayk and Lehmitz [10] in which the CSF is absorbed in a cylinder made of porous ceramic material, is designed to ensure a higher number of cells and an even better quality of the cells settling on the slide.

In each case as many cell preparations as possible should be made from the same CSF. In some cases we obtained characteristic findings of tumour cells in one preparation only.

Panoptic staining after Pappenheim has proved to be the most suitable routine method. Additional staining methods – e.g. cresyl violet stain or fluorescent staining with acridine orange – may help support the diagnosis of "tumour cells in the CSF" in isolated cases. However, these stains are by no means pathognomonic of tumour cells. Moreover they yield negative results in many primary brain tumours, which renders their diagnostic value questionable. Last but not least, the training and experience of the examining physician may be of decisive importance in the cytologic assessment of the CSF in children with primary brain tumours. In the differential diagnosis of vague cerebral or spinal diseases CSF cytology by providing evidence of tumour cells may not only offer the key to the diagnosis but can also give valuable information about inflammatory lesions in the meninges or about bleeding in the subarachnoid space. In brain tumours with no evidence of tumour cells in the CSF there is quite often a meningeal irritative cell reaction with predominantly monocytic differentiation. Such irritations, however, also occur after puncture of the CSF spaces, after cerebral seizures, in the course of acute virus infections or in chronic inflammatory lesions. In such conditions atypical cells may also appear, which, judged by the above mentioned criteria of malignancy, may mislead an examining physician without sufficient knowledge of such disease patterns and thus result in a false positive assessment.

An accurate histologic diagnosis of tumour cells in the CSF is rarely possible but seems more likely in glioblastoma multiforme, in medulloblastoma and in cerebral metastases [11]. The cerebrospinal fluid offers characteristic cell pictures particularly in sarcomatous (Fig. 1 d, e) and leukaemic infiltration of the leptomeninges.

Table 2. Tumour cells in the cerebrospinal fluid of children with primary brain tumours (Municipal Hospital Berlin-Buch, June 1975 – July 1981)

Histology	Number of patients	Identification of tumour cells	Suspicion of tumour cells	No tumour cells
Medulloblastoma	19	11	1	7
Ependymoma	7	2	–	5
Astrocytoma	2	–	–	2
Spongioblastoma	1	–	–	1
Pinealoma (Germinoma)	2	–	1	1
Sarcoma	2	–	1	1
Melanoma of the arachnoid	1	1	–	–
Neuroblastoma	1	–	–	1
Choroid plexus papilloma	1	–	–	1
Sarcomatosis of the leptomeninges (autopsy result)	1	–	1	–
No histological evidence	5	–	1	4
Total	44	14 (32%)	5	23

Our Own Results

For several years in the neurosurgical clinic in Berlin-Buch[1] we have carried out cytologic examinations of the cerebrospinal fluid collected from children with tumours of the CNS or with vague cerebral disease patterns. Over the past six years we examined in this way CSF specimens taken from 42 children with primary brain tumours, most of them located infratentorially (Table 2). In 14 cases tumour cells were identified once or several times during check-ups in the sedimentation chamber preparation. A suspicion of tumour cells was raised in only five cases, and in 23 children no characteristic tumour cells appeared in the CSF. We were able to identify tumour cells most often in medulloblastomas, in 11 out of 19 cases with certainty, and only suspicion was raised in one case. In seven children with ependymoma tumour cell evidence was found in two cases, no evidence in three children with astrocytoma or spongioblastoma. Among another seven children with histological evidence of brain tumours tumour cells in the CSF were detected in one child with malignant melanoma originating from the arachnoid (Fig. 1c) and in two other cases one child with ectopic pinealoma (germinoma, Fig. 1f, g) and one child with reticulum-cell sarcoma (Fig. 1d) – a suspicion of tumour cells was raised. In six children with the clinically confirmed diagnosis of inoperable brain tumours two cases were highly suspicious of tumour cells, one of them with the histological diagnosis "leptomeningeal sarcomatosis" (Fig. 1e). Identification of tumour cells in the CSF

1 At this point I wish to thank Dr. Mateev in this clinic for her kind assistance

was of *clinical relevance* especially in two children in whom the cytological findings provided a clue for the diagnosis.

The first was a girl almost five years old, in whom an abacterial meningitis associated with Coxsackie virus type B 5 was diagnosed according to virologic and serologic examinations. Six months later, headache and vomiting occurred, followed by papilloedema. Pneumencephalography showed no filling of the ventricles. CSF examination now revealed 10% tumour cells. Subsequent ventriculography showed a space-occupying lesion involving the floor of the fossa rhomboidea. Histology showed the lesion to be a medulloblastoma.

The second child was a one and a half year-old boy, in whom Amipaque-ventriculography as well as pneumoencephalography did not demonstrate aqueduct obstruction, but showed a suprasellar space-occupying lesion the size of a cherry. By CSF examination, we suspected a highly malignant tumour such as a medulloblastoma, which was then confirmed by histology after operation.

We later saw two boys with germinoma and an ectopic anisomorphic pinealoma, respectively. With these tumour-types, Wiethölter and Oehmichen [14] question the diagnostic value of CSF examination, as they believe that the small lymphoid cells found in these patients cannot be regarded as tumour cells, but as immunologically stimulated T-cells. Apart from this cell-type, however, large pale "epithelial-like" tumour cells do occur in these patients with the "two-cell pinealoma" [8, 14]. Thus, in one of our patients, we found not only a lymphocytic pleocytosis, but also giant, malignant cells, which we believe to be true pinealoma cells.

References

1. Den Hartog Jager, W. A.: Cytopathology of the cerebrospinal fluid examined with the sedimentation technique after Sayk J. Neurol. Sci. *2,* 155–177 (1969)
2. Ducos, R., Donoso, J., Weickhardt, U., Vietti, T. J.: Sedimentation versus cytocentrifugation in the cytologic study of craniospinal fluid. Cancer *43,* 1479–1482 (1979)
3. Habeck, D., Perick, F.: Zum Stand der Liquordiagnostik in der Bundesrepublik Deutschland. Med. Welt *28,* 1070–1072 (1977)
4. Jänisch, W., Güthert, H., Schreiber, D.: Pathologie der Tumoren des Zentralnervensystems. Jena: VEB Verlag Gustav Fischer, 1976
5. Kölmel, H. W.: Atlas of cerebrospinal fluid cells. Berlin-Heidelberg-New York: Springer Verlag 1976
6. Olischer, R. M.: Zur Tumorzelldiagnostik im Liquor cerebrospinalis. Dt. Gesundh.-Wesen *32,* 601–605 (1977)
7. Olischer, R. M., Lehmitz, R., Zele, J.: Zur Zellanreicherung und ihren Ergebnissen in der Zytodiagnostik des Liquor cerebrospinalis. Dt. Gesundh.-Wesen *36,* 1027–1030 (1981)
8. Riverson, E., Brunngraber, C. V., Zülch, K. J.: Beitrag zur Frage der „ektopischen" Pinealome. Zentralblatt für Neurochirurgie *34,* 31–40 (1973)
9. Sayk, J., Olischer, R. M.: Fortschritte der Liquorzytologie bei der Diagnostik bösartiger Hirngeschwülste. III. Mitteilung. Psychiat. Neurol. med. Psychol. (Lpz) *19,* 88–99 (1967)
10. Sayk, J., Lehmitz, R.: Die Sorptionskammer. Eine neue Methode der spontanen Zellsedimentation. Dt. Gesundh.-Wesen *34,* 2561–2565 (1979)
11. Schmidt, R. M.: Atlas der Liquorzytologie. Leipzig: Johann Ambrosius Barth 1978
12. Stefanko, S., Kaluza, J.: La cytologie du liquide cephalo-rachidien dans les tumeurs du systeme nerveux. Schweiz. Arch. Neurol. Psychiat. *110,* 249–259 (1972)
13. Wieczorek, V.: Erfahrungen mit der Tumorzelldiagnostik im Liquor cerebrospinalis bei primären und metastatischen Hirngeschwülsten. Dtsch. Z. Nervenkh. *186,* 410–432 (1964)
14. Wiethölter, H., Oehmichen, M.: Liquor-zytologische Fehldiagnose bei anisomorphem Pinealom (Germinom). Nervenarzt *49,* 726–729 (1978)

Electrophysiological Diagnosis and Follow-Up Controls in Cases of Tumours of the Optic Chiasm

D. Wenzel, D. Harms, U. Brandl, M. Klinger, and F. Albert

Introduction

Visual disturbances are often the first signs of a space-occupying lesion in the chiasmatic region apart from the clinical signs of acutely raised intracranial pressure. Since on the one hand subjective data on visual field defects or loss of vision are usually lacking in children and since on the other hand, visual evoked potentials (VEPs) are assuming increasing importance in the topological diagnosis of lesions of the afferent visual tracts [2, 3], we have performed extended electrophysiological diagnosis in children with tumours of the optic chiasm. Besides pattern evoked potentials with chess-board reversal, we recorded flash evoked potentials in 12 children and compared the results of these findings with conventional EEGs. These electrophysiological results were compared with the ophthalmological findings depending on the location of the lesion. In 9 children we were able to compare the pre- and postoperative neurophysiological findings.

Patients and Method

Altogether 23 children ranging in age from 8 months to 22.4 years with space-occupying lesions near the optic chiasm as confirmed by operation and histology underwent ophthalmological and electrophysiological investigation. According to their location, the tumours were subdivided into one group (a: n = 16) with suprasellar extension and direct anatomical relationship to the anterior optic pathway (craniopharyngioma: 10, optic gliomas: 3, leiomyoma: 1, germinoma: 1, spongioblastoma: 1) and a group (b: n=7) with extension distant to the chiasm (intrasellar tumours: pituitary adenoma 2; located in the diencephalon: ependymoma 2, astrocytoma 2, spongioblastoma 1). The EEG recording in the children was performed with the 10–20 electrode system using silver-silver chloride electrodes over O_1-A_1, O_2-A_2 and O_z-A_1 with a conventional EEG apparatus. The averaging of these 1-second EEG sections which were timed to the light impulse, was carried out with a PDP-11 computer following artefact control and using our own programs.

Visual stimulation was performed separately for each eye using a chessboard pattern reversal stimulation with a constant light intensity (58 cd/m^2) via a television with a 20 angle field size. The pattern size of the individual square is variable from 12 minutes of arc to about 6 degrees visual angle. In 12 children stroboscopic light stimulation (3500 cd/m^2) was performed in addition to this pattern stimulation. Of the various EEGs carried out in the children, only the EEG recorded at the time of the VEP study was used for the comparison of electrophysiological results.

The VEPs were evaluted interindividually according to the latency time of the first large negative (N80) and the first large positive (P120) peak, as well as the amplitude (A) and the total wave configuration of the early and middle VEP components (up to 250 msec) for each eye separately following pattern stimulation as well as stroboscopic flash stimulation. Only the evoked potentials were compared in the pre- and postoperative electrophysiological follow-up studies. An immediate postoperative comparison of our EEG findings was not made because of the variability in the results caused by the operation.

Results and Discussion

The results of the ophthalmological and electrophysiological findings of the 23 children investigated are presented in Table 1 for both of the localization groups (a: suprasellar space-occupying lesion; b: lesion distant to the optic chiasm) together. In the group with suprasellar space-occupying lesions and anatomic relationships to the optic pathway (a) 14 of the 16 examined children demonstrated ophthalmological findings consisting of a more or less pronounced optic nerve atrophy and/or papilloedema as well as various visual field defects. Less common was a loss of vision. Reliable clinical data could be obtained only after the age of 5 years (8/23). In the group with lesions distant to the optic chiasm (b), only 1 of 7 children was found to have an incomplete bitemporal visual field defect. All other ophthalmological findings of this and the remaining 6 children were normal.

The electrophysiological studies revealed unspecific findings in the EEG in half of the cases (8/16) of group a, usually in the sense of a diffuse abnormality or abnormal rhythms of slow waves. Sometimes a focal slowing or hypersynchronous activity was also observed. Similar electroencephalographic findings were also detected in 5 of the 7 children in group b.

Table 1. Ophthalmological and electrophysiological findings in cases of chiasmatic lesion

	Suprasellar mass with direct contact and/or involvement of the optic system	Other tumors in proximity to the optic system
Ophthalmological signs	14/16	1/7
EEG	8/16	5/7
P-EP	16/16	7/7
Fl-EP	5/ 7	0/5

The visual evoked potential studies (VEPs) with pattern stimulation (P-EP) indicated one or more abnormal VEP parameters in 11 children such as prolonged latency time, intraindividual right/left eye amplitude differences or no response.

When the stroboscopic flash stimulation (Fl-EP) which is commonly used in paediatric studies is applied for the VEP investigation, then 5 of the 7 children with a suprasellar lesion and clinical signs of ophthalmological findings show pathological results in the sense of prolonged latencies and differences in amplitudes. However, 2 children with a clinically verified optic lesion manifesting as optic atrophy and a loss of vision as well as visual field defects were found to have normal flash VEPs. In the group with lesions distant to the optic chiasm (group b) all the flash evoked potentials (n = 5) were normal. However, pattern evoked potentials showed abnormalities in all these 5 children.

These results are therefore noteworthy for a number of reasons:

1. Pattern evoked potentials can be recorded in all children, even in infants.
2. Pattern evoked potentials revealed subclinical optic lesions in about one-third (8/23) of our cases.
3. Flash evoked potentials may be normal even in cases of clinically confirmed optic lesions.
4. Pattern evoked potentials are greatly superior to flash evoked potentials particularly in cases of slight disturbances in visual functions of the anterior visual pathway.
5. The EEG which provides other information about general brain function, reveals unspecific changes in about 60% of both groups (8/16; 5/7) independent of the localization of the space-occupying lesion.

In Table 2, the pre- and postoperative electrophysiological findings in 9 children are compared with the ophthalmological findings. For 6 of the 9 children, there was postoperative improvement of vision and/or a reduction in the visual field defect.

The same 6 children also showed an improvement in the pattern evoked potentials with decrease in latencies and an increase in amplitudes. On the other hand, an improvement was found in only 3 of the 8 children examined with flash evoked potentials. Clinical improvement and pattern evoked potentials correlated in all cases, while flash evoked potentials remained unchanged in 2 children with distinct clinical improvement.

A postoperative deterioration was found in 2 children as indicated by the pattern evoked potentials (P-EP), which manifested in a prolonged latency time and decreased amplitudes. In one of these children the clinical finding confirmed this de-

Table 2. Pre- and postoperative changes in the ophthalmological and electrophysiological findings

	Better	Worse	No change
Ophthalmological signs	6/9	1/9	2/9
P-EP	6/9	2/9	1/9
FI-EP	3/8	–	5/8
EEG	1/9	4/9	4/9

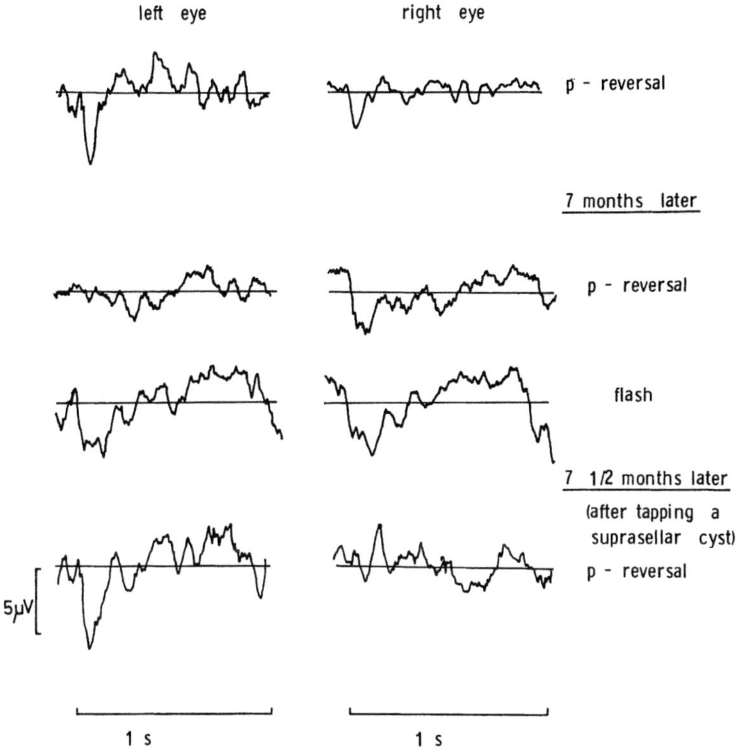

Fig. 1. VEP findings in cystic craniopharyngeoma. The first line shows pattern evoked potentials for left and right eye 6 months after subtotal removal of the tumour. The first positive component of the left eye (large downward deflection) is prolonged and on the right eye, there is a similar prolongation of latency of abnormally small amplitudes. The control 7 months later (second line) indicates a loss of pattern evoked potentials for the left eye and a more prolonged latency on the right. In line 3 the flash evoked potentials showed normal latencies for both eyes, although the computer tomogram revealed a left sided cyst recurrence. Following tapping of the cyst, the control pattern evoked potential 14 days later (line 4) showed results similar to line 1

terioration while the second child remained unchanged from a clinical viewpoint, while the computer tomogram revealed new tumour growth.

In 1 of 9 children there was no change in the pre- and postoperative P-EP finding, while flash stimulation revealed no change in 5 of 8 children (see Table 2).

These results indicate that pattern evoked potentials as a follow-up method correlate very well with clinical development for suprasellar lesions and that this method is superior to the clinical findings alone. This is particularly important in the group of young children since this age group cannot supply reliable clinical data as far as vision and field defects are concerned. The flash evoked potentials are much less sensitive to disturbances of visual function not only in the primary diagnostic study but also in the postoperative follow-up.

A comparison of the pre- and immediate postoperative EEG findings is not discussed, since the electroencephalogram shows rapidly changing findings due to the operation itself as well as due to the surgical procedures such as implantations.

A study of the EEG findings 6–12 months after operation revealed mostly unchanged recordings, in some cases with various unspecific abnormal findings. In 4 children the EEG findings deteriorated in that a focal change was now observed and hypersynchronous activity simultaneously occurred twice, while one child indicated an improvement with less focal changes. The EEG is no doubt important for postoperative follow-up studies, but it provides answers to questions other than possible tumour recurrence in the proximity of the chiasm.

In agreement with other authors [1–3], our results show that pattern evoked potentials are unusually accurate in the diagnosis of tumours of the anterior optic pathway. Beyond that we have shown that the information provided by pattern evoked potentials is better than that elicited by flash evoked potentials. This is true for clinically manifest optic nerve damage as well as in cases of slighter functional disturbances in vision, which is particularly important in practical early diagnosis.

Special advantages of this non-invasive and quite harmless method of pattern evoked potentials are apparent in all cases of lesions in the area of the anterior optic pathway particularly in small children, in the detection of subclinical losses of function as well as in postoperative controls of lesions in this area. Repeated postoperative follow-up studies are invaluable in recognizing early tumour recurrences in the case of suprasellar cystic craniopharyngiomas for example. This is illustrated in Fig. 1 where a tumour recurrence led to a new suppression of the pattern evoked potentials in one eye, which was reversible after tapping the cyst.

References

1. Celesia, C. G., Daly, R. F.: Visual electroencephalographic computer analysis (VECA). Neurology *27*, 637–641 (1977)
2. Desmedt, I. E. (Ed.): Visual evoked potentials in man: new developments. Oxford: Clarendon Press 1977
3. Halliday, A. M., Halliday, E., Kriss, A., McDonald, W. I., Muskin, J.: The pattern-evoked potential in compression of the anterior visual pathway. Brain *99*, 357–374 (1976)

Electroencephalograms in Long-Term Survivors of Primary Intracranial Tumours of Childhood

E. Dieterich, B. Goebel, and P. Gutjahr

Introduction

The value of EEG-recording in the diagnosis of intracranial tumours in children is well known [5]. However, there are only a few reports about EEG-findings and virtually no reports about the frequency of epilepsy in the long-term survivors of intracranial tumours in children [8].

EEG-findings in 29 children who are surviving free of recurrence three or more years after the diagnosis of a primary intracranial tumour are reported. The problem of the frequency of hypersynchronous activity and of epilepsy has been investigated and will be discussed.

Method and Patients

Twenty-nine children had EEG records $3\frac{1}{12}$–$17\frac{4}{12}$ years after the diagnosis of a primary intracranial tumour (there were 15 *posterior fossa tumours* and 14 *supratentorial tumours).*

The EEG-recording and interpretation was done according to the directions of the German EEG-society and the Workshop of Paediatric Electroencephalography [7]. In 9 of the 29 children the EEG could not be performed before treatment because the illness was so acute and needed immediate attention. The other 20 children in this series had an EEG before treatment.

Results

Among the long-term survivors, the EEG was normal in 13 of 15 children with *posterior fossa tumours* and in 7 of 14 who had *supratentorial tumours.* Two of the patients with former *posterior fossa* tumours had abnormal EEG tracings. One of them showed a diffuse slow delta activity; further investigations (computerized tomography) revealed a recurrence of the tumour. The other patient had primary generalized hypersynchronous activity (spikes and waves) and responded to photic stimu-

Table 1. EEG-findings before treatment and in the late stage of intracranial tumours (∅ = no record, – = normal finding, 1, 2, 3 = diverse degrees of diffuse slow activity, 4 = focal hypersynchronous activity, 5 = prim. general. hypersynchronous activity, 6 = photoconvulsive reaction, + = epilepsy, × = recurrence of tumour)

Tumour-location (No. of patient)	EEG before treatment	Survival (years)	EEG in late status
1 *supratentorial*	–	3.1	–
2 *supratentorial*	1	7.4	1, 4, 6, +
3 *supratentorial*	–	10.4	–
4 *supratentorial*	1	3.2	–
5 *supratentorial*	∅	9.2	4
6 *supratentorial*	∅	13.0	–
7 *supratentorial*	+	7.6	3, 4, +
8 *supratentorial*	1	4.4	–
9 *supratentorial*	2	7.6	–
10 *supratentorial*	1	17.4	–
11 *supratentorial*	∅	4.6	–
12 *supratentorial*	2	3.8	4
13 *supratentorial*	2,4	3.1	1, 4, +
14 *supratentorial*	∅	6.9	4
15 *posterior fossa*	–	7.3	–
16 *posterior fossa*	1	4.1	–
17 *posterior fossa*	1	5.9	–
18 *posterior fossa*	1	3.1	–
19 *posterior fossa*	1	4.1	3, ×
20 *posterior fossa*	∅	8.6	–
21 *posterior fossa*	1	6.1	–
22 *posterior fossa*	–	7.8	–
23 *posterior fossa*	–	7.2	–
24 *posterior fossa*	∅	11.9	–
25 *posterior fossa*	∅	12.3	–
26 *posterior fossa*	–	6.2	–
27 *posterior fossa*	∅	15.1	–
28 *posterior fossa*	∅	7.8	–
29 *posterior fossa*	1	8.0	5,6

Table 2. EEG-findings and frequency of epilepsy in the late stages after intracranial tumours

Finding n = 29	Infratentorial tumour n = 15	Supratentorial tumour n = 14
EEG		
normal	13	7
abnormal	2	7
Diffuse slow activity	1	2
Side-differences	0	5
Hypersynchronous activity		
sharp waves	0	6
spikes and waves	1	0
photoconvulsive reaction	1	1
Epilepsy	0	3

lation. These findings are genetically determined and have no connection with the former tumour and/or its treatment [4, 6].

During the investigations for this study, two other children had normal EEGs but had developed recurrences of their tumours.

In the group of patients with former *supratentorial tumours* the EEG was abnormal in 7 of 14 children (Tables 1, 2). In two children with a diffuse slow activity a recurrence of the tumour had still to be confirmed. Six other patients had developed hypersynchronous activity (sharp waves) and three of them had manifested focal epileptic convulsions with secondary generalized grand mal.

Discussion

Three or more years after the diagnosis of a primary intracranial tumour 20 out of 29 children showed normal EEG-findings. In all cases the tumour had been treated by operation (on the tumour itself, or a shunting operation); some of the patients had had radiation therapy and/or chemotherapy (systemic Vincristine and/or Cyclophosphamide and/or intrathecal Methotrexate).

All the EEGs which were abnormal before treatment had returned to normal in the long-term survivors. There were no abnormalities caused by chemotherapy and/or radiation therapy. This finding agrees well with our results in 188 children with different *extracranial neoplasms* treated with Vincristine or other cytostatics, who had no abnormal EEG related to the treatment of their long-term condition [1, 2].

It is further remarkable that two children with a normal EEG at the time of this investigation of long-term survivors had developed a recurrence of the tumour in the posterior fossa some time prior to the investigation. Thus, a normal EEG after treatment is not certain evidence of a good subsequent prognosis.

The abnormal EEGs in the group of patients after supratentorial tumours are primarily caused by the tumour itself and/or the operative treatment.

Epilepsy occurred in three cases. One child had been treated by a ventriculocisternal shunt and also radiation of the brain. In this case, the tumour itself and the treatment might be the cause of this event. In the second case, the epilepsy had appeared in the first year of life and long before any evidence of the tumour but it also persisted in the long-term. Early brain changes before the manifestation of the tumour may be the reason for epilepsy in this case. The third case with epilepsy in the late stages was a boy with an astrocytoma in one cerebral hemisphere; the tumour and/or the consequences of the operation may have caused epilepsy in this case.

Hypersynchronous activity was found in three other children, and so far they have not had any epileptic seizures. These EEG-tracings may be caused by the tumour itself or by operative treatment, because two of these three patients were treated without radiation or chemotherapy. This result agrees well with our findings in 40 other children with diverse neoplasms who had undergone irradiation of the brain two or more years earlier. In this group we found that abnormal EEG-tracings on account of radiation are apparently less frequent than morphological changes of the brain after radiation [3]; it is not necessary to assume that the latter always has an effect upon the function of the infantile brain (and vice versa).

In the late stages after primary supratentorial tumours the development of epilepsy is always a possibility. In 6 of 14 children a hypersynchronous focal activity was found, but only three of them developed a focal epilepsy. The other three children with focal hypersynchronous activity had not developed epilepsy up to $3\frac{8}{12}$, $6\frac{1}{12}$ and $9\frac{7}{12}$ years after diagnosis of their supratentorial tumour. Evidently the risk of developing epilepsy after supratentorial tumours in the late stages is not very high. Thus, "prophylactic" anti-epileptic treatment for all children with intracranial tumours does not seem to be indicated at all. In contrast to common opinions we do not know of any antiepileptic drug which has "prophylactic" effects at all. Besides, a great number of patients, in whom "prophylactic" anticonvulsant treatment is given, are certainly overtreated. Diphenylhydantoin for example is generally not able to prevent epileptic seizures in these patients.

References

1. Dieterich, E.: Zur Frage der Encephalotoxizität des Vincristin. Klin. Pädiat. *191*, 145–147 (1979)
2. Dieterich, E., Goebel, B., Gutjahr, P.: EEG-Befunde nach Vincristin-Behandlung. Mschr. Kinderheilk. *126*, 709–710 (1978)
3. Dieterich, E., Gutjahr, P.: EEG-Befunde im Spätstatus nach ZNS-Bestrahlung wegen maligner Neoplasien im Kindesalter. Strahlentherapie *155*, 549–552 (1979)
4. Doose, H., Gerken, H.: Photosensibilität. Genetische Grundlagen und klinische Korrelationen. Z. EEG-EMG **4,** 182–187 (1973)
5. Dumermuth, G.: EEG-Befunde bei Hirntumoren im Kindesalter. Arch. Psychiat. Nervenkr. *197*, 594–601 (1958)
6. Gerken, H., Doose, H.: On the genetics of EEG-anomalies in childhood (III. Spikes and waves). Neuropädiatr. *4*, 88–97 (1973)
7. Kruse, R., Scheffner, D., Weinmann, H.-M.: Ableitung und Beschreibung des kindlichen EEG. Richtlinien des Arbeitskreises für pädiatrische klinische Elektroencephalographie. Desitin-Werke, Carl Klinke Hamburg
8. Lipinski, C., Lorenz, H. M., Scheffner, D.: EEG-Veränderungen während der Therapie von Tumoren der hinteren Schädelgrube im Kindesalter. Z. EEG-EMG **6,** 188–194 (1975)

Early Auditory Evoked Potentials (EAEP) in Children with Neoplastic Lesions in the Brain Stem

K. MAURER and M. ROCHEL

Introduction

There are three groups of potentials evoked by an auditory stimulus: a very early series (early auditory evoked potentials – EAEP) in the initial 10 milliseconds (ms), a consistent middle latency sequence (8 to 40 ms) and the larger and longer latency "vertex-potentials" (50–300 ms) [6]. The shorter the latency of the waves the better the knowledge about their neural generators. The EAEP reflect the progressive activation of the auditory nerve and the brain stem auditory tracts and nuclei: cochlea and acoustic nerve (wave I), medulla oblongata (wave II), caudal pons (wave III), rostral pons (wave IV) and midbrain (wave V). EAEP are easily recorded from subjects of any age. Nearly all children are cooperative and tolerate wearing earphones and four EEG-electrodes glued on the scalp, and rest quietly during stimulation.

One of the most important physiological factors affecting latency and amplitude of EAEP is the age. Control values were therefore obtained in neurological and audiometric normal subjects ranging in age from a few days after birth to adulthood. Subjects were classified according to three age groups: newborn (birth–4 weeks), infants (4 weeks–3 years), children (3 years–adulthood). After establishing control values 17 children with infratentorial tumours were investigated. Abnormalities of each of the five components (waves I–V) were correlated with the location and extent of the neoplastic lesion.

Methods

Methods of recording have been published elsewhere [4]. Normal subjects and patients were examined in the supine position. Bipolar EEG-activity was recorded from the vertex (C_Z) and the mastoid ipsilateral to stimulation. The amplified and filtered signals (bandpass of the system: 300–3200 Hz) recorded in the first 20 ms poststimulus were summed with a signal averager (1024 sampling points). Electrically we used as stimulus a sine half wave with a duration of 250 μs; the acoustic result was a gaussian signal (tone-pip) with sharp rise and a duration of about 1 ms. The acoustic waveform corresponds to the gaussian elementary signal or "logon" [1]. The stimuli were presented monaurally by Beyer DT 48 earphones at a randomized rate of 10/s and an intensity of 60, 70 and 80 dBHL (decibels above the mean hearing threshold for normals). Masking white noise was presented to the contralateral ear. Normally two runs for each ear and for intensity were performed and only congruent components were accepted for evaluation. Since rarefaction and condensation stimuli produce different responses we evaluated the results of 1000 stimuli for each polarity separately. An automatic artefact rejector monitored the output of the amplifier continuously and averaging was not performed when the signal was contaminated with muscle activity and artefacts. All newborns and most of the infants slept during the entire session, none of the subjects were sedated. According to earlier reports [5] latencies were measured between the start of the tone-pip and the upward positive peak of each wave; the interpeak conduction times were determined between the different peaks. Amplitudes were measured from peaks to troughs. A latency delay or an amplitude reduction by more than 2.5 s.d. was considered to be significant. An otoscopy was done in all newborn and audiometry in cooperative children.

Results

Newborn, Infants, and Children

Since latencies and amplitudes correlate highly with maturation of peripheral and subcortical structures of the auditory pathway, it was important to determine normal values in newborn, infants and children. In 12 newborn it was possible to evoke waves I to V (Fig. 1, Table 1). With increasing age there is a shortening in latency and an increase in amplitude (Figs. 1, 2). The adult configuration of EAEP begins to emerge by 2–3 years of age. For children more than three years old, normal values of our control group described previously could be therefore be used [5].

Brain Stem Tumours

Seventeen patients with infratentorial neoplastic lesions were investigated. Seven children with medulloblastoma, five with cerebellar astrocytoma and five patients

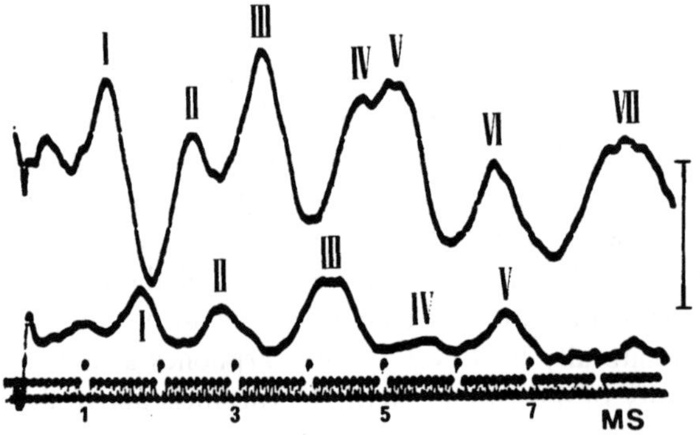

Fig. 1. EAEP, upper trace from adult, lower trace from a newborn subject. Calibration 200 nV

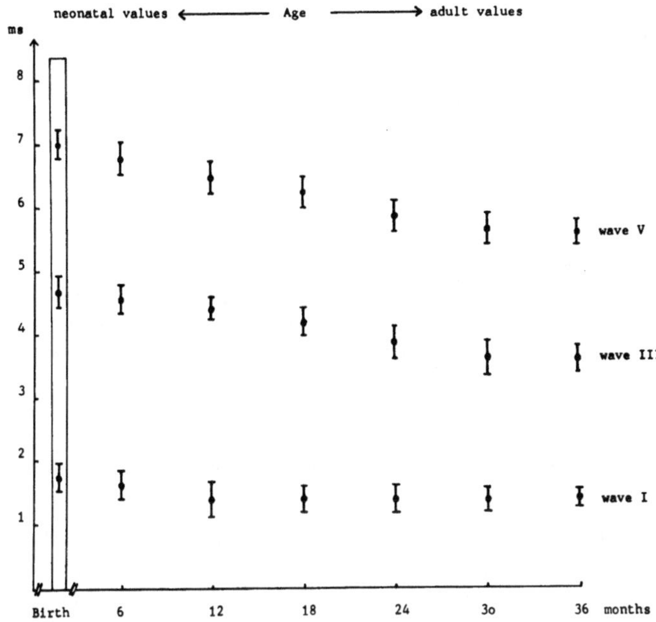

Fig. 2. Latencies of wave I, III and V, a function of age of subjects. Vertical bars enclose mean and standard deviation of 12 newborn, at least five infants in the period between six months and 30 months and of 50 adult subjects

Table 1. Latencies relative to stimulus onset and conduction times relative to waves I and II evoked by monaural stimulation at a level of 80 dBHL. I – II: peripheral conduction time (pct), II – V: central conduction time (cct). Amplitudes of EAEP (nV), monaural stimulation at a level of 80 dBHL

Relative to stimulus onset (ms)		
Wave	Mean	SD
I	1.85	0.26
II	2.95	0.22
III	4.65	0.28
IV	5.85	0.38
V	7.00	0.26
Relative to wave I and II (ms)		
I – II	1.1	0.25 pct
I – III	2.8	0.26
I – IV	4.0	0.28
I – V	5.15	0.21
II – V	4.05	0.22 cct
Wave	nV	SD
I	120	50
II	64	45
III	235	45
IV	75	30
V	160	55

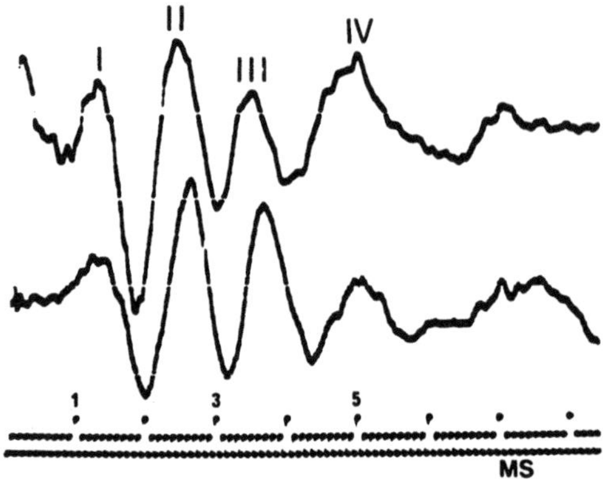

Fig. 3. EAEP in brain stem tumour, upper trace is from the left, and lower trace from the right ear. Amplitude of wave I (peak to trough: 230 nV)

with a tumour of the brain stem. Two cases will be described in more detail to demonstrate the topodiagnostic value of the EAEP.

Case 1: A 15-year-old girl complained of dysarthria, diplopia and a bilateral hearing loss. She had also noticed an unsteadiness in walking. Neurological examination revealed a horizontal eye movement paresis as symptom of a pontine lesion. The computerized axial tomography showed a tumourous mass in the pontine area. The EAEP indicated a ponto-mesencephalic lesion. On both sides waves I, II and III were normal, whereas wave IV was late and of reduced amplitude, wave V was not detectable (Fig. 3).

Case 2: A six-year-old girl with a brain stem glioma had several controls which confirmed the clinical deterioration (Fig. 4). The distal growth of the tumour could be correlated with gradual impairment of III and II so that finally only wave I and a spurious wave could be recorded.

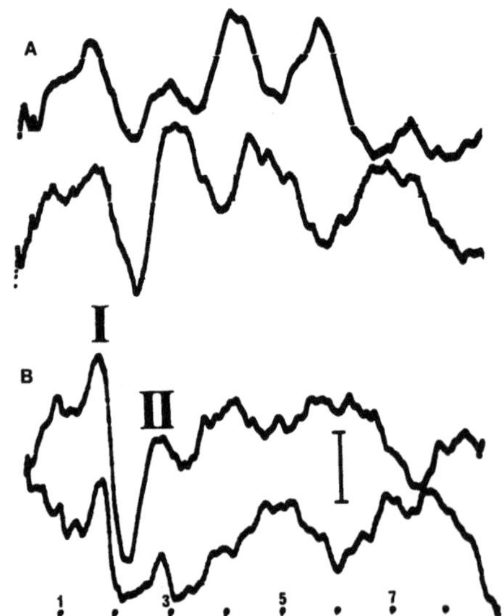

Fig. 4. Follow-up of EAEP in brain stem glioma. A: EAEP at date of admission to the hospital. B: EAEP six months later. Upper trace is from the left, and lower trace from the right ear. Calibration: 200 nV

Conclusions

Brain tumours are found in approximately two per cent of all necropsies. Common intracranial tumours in childhood are astrocytomas, medulloblastomas, craniopharyngiomas, brain stem tumours and ependymomas. Two-thirds of them are infratentorial. Common symptoms, caused by destruction of nuclear masses in the brain stem, are unilateral or bilateral paralysis of the fifth, sixth, seventh and tenth cranial nerves and paralysis of lateral gaze. An involvement of the cochlear nerve and auditory pathway nuclei is difficult to establish and patients seldom complain about it. Damage of the fibre pathways causes hemiplegia, hemianaesthesia or cerebellar disturbances. Increased intracranial pressure is a late sign. Often however, symptoms are mild and do not allow a localization of the lesion. Since the first description of EAEP in neurology [8, 9], reports have been published concerning mainly with maturational changes of the first five waves in normal children [3, 7]. There are, however, few reports about wave abnormalities due to a tumour in early childhood. In all newborn it was possible to evoke all waves of the EAEP. Besides absolute latencies interwave latencies were determined because they allow an evaluation of brain stem function even in the presence of a hearing disturbance. We considered the peripheral conduction time (pct), i.e. interwave latency between I and II, and the central conduction time (cct) i.e. interwave latency between II and V (brain stem transmission time). There are minor differences between the pct in newborns and adults, whereas the cct is significantly shorter in a mature auditory pathway. This confirms a nearly complete maturation of the inner ear at birth. It is probably within the external and middle ear, and more likely in the brain stem rather than in the cochlea itself, that the changes occur which would be responsible for improvement in brain stem transmission time. The knowledge about maturational changes of latencies and amplitudes is important since pathological conditions can produce similar wave alterations. Wave abnormalities of EAEP could be observed at each level of the auditory pathway between medulla and midbrain. Strictly unilateral changes prove the fact, that EAEP are generated from different levels of the auditory pathway of only one side. Waves I–V originate from the homolateral part of the brainstem, i.e. the side of the stimulated ear [4, 10]. It can be suggested, that bilateral abnormalities at the same level are produced by growth of a large tumour crossing the midline. It was possible to correlate wave abnormalities of waves II to V with well-defined neurological defects in the brain stem. We saw alterations of waves II and III in medullo-pontine tumours and alterations of waves IV and V in ponto-mesencephalic disorders. Besides the localisation by means of EAEP the side of tumour was confirmed in most cases by an axial computerized tomography.

As might be expected in tumours above the tentorium, waves I to V of the EAEP are normal. An exception is when there is increased intracranial pressure. If a midbrain syndrome is present, i.e. a compression of the inferior colliculi at the tentorium, wave V only is affected whereas impulse conduction remain normal from cochlea to the rostral pons (wave IV).

To summarize EAEP are a test which can be used to increase the level of diagnostic certainty in children with brain stem tumours. EAEP provide a method of searching for abnormalities in the medullary, pontine and mesencephalic part of the acoustic pathway.

References

1. Davis, H.: Principles of electric response audiometry. Ann. Otol. Rhinol. Laryngol. (Suppl.) *85,* 1–96 (1976)
2. Gutjahr, P.: Primäre Tumoren des Zentralnervensystems. In: Krebs bei Kindern und Jugendlichen (J. Oehme, P. Gutjahr, eds.) Köln-Lövenich: Deutscher Ärzte-Verlag (1981)
3. Hecox, K., Galambos, R.: Brainstem auditory evoked responses in human infants and adults. Arch. Otolaryngol. *99,* 30–33 (1974)
4. Maurer, K., Schäfer, E., Hopf, H. C., Leitner, H.: The location by early auditory evoked potentials (EAEP) of acoustic nerve and brain stem demyelination in multiple sclerosis. J. Neurol. *223,* 43–58 (1980a)
5. Maurer, K., Leitner, H., Schäfer, E.: Neurological applications of early auditory evoked potentials (EAEP) in acoustic nerve and brain stem disorders. Scand. Audiol. Suppl. *11,* 119–133 (1980b)
6. Picton, T. W., Hilliyard, S. A., Krausz, H. I., Galambos, R.: Human auditory evoked potentials. I.: Evaluation of components. Electroenceph. clin. Neurophysiol. *36,* 179–190 (1974)
7. Salamy, A., Mc Kean, C. M., Buda, F. B.: Maturational changes in auditory transmission as reflected in human brain stem potentials. Brain Res. *96,* 361–366 (1975)
8. Sohmer, H., Feinmesser, M., Szabo, G.: Sources of electroencephalographic responses as studied in patients with brain damage. Electroenceph. clin. Neurophysiol. *37,* 663–669 (1974)
9. Starr, A., Achor, L. J.: Auditory brain stem responses in neurological disease. Arch. Neurol. (Chic.) *32,* 761–768 (1975)
10. Thornton, A. R. D.: Interpretation of cochlear nerve and brain stem responses. In: Evoked Electrical Activity in the Auditory Nervous System (R. F. Nannton, C. Fernandez, eds.), New York: Academic Press 1978

Conventional Investigations of CNS Tumours in Children

C. R. Fitz

Introduction

In the era of CT, other examinations are often neglected in a determination to prove that the newest tool is always the best, rather than usually the best. There is a need to use other "conventional techniques" in some situations of central nervous system tumour diagnosis in children. These needs will vary with the facilities available, the expertise of the radiologist in various techniques, the needs of the surgeon, paediatrician, and chemotherapist, and the problems, age, and co-operation of the individual patient.

The physician's needs relate to the pathological and geographical accuracy required. The other factors are very inter-related. The newest bi-plane magnification angiogram equipment is of no use if the radiologist cannot catheterize the arteries of a 6 month old infant, or the anaesthetist is not skilled enough to anaesthetize the same child who is suspected of having a brain tumour.

In this discussion, I am assuming that CT is available and therefore, the further investigations needed are also dependant on the quality of the CT equipment in use at a particular hospital. Fewer conventional exams are usually required when a 3rd or 4th generation CT unit is used.

Patterns of Examination – Head

Figure 1 indicates the usual flow pattern of investigation at the author's hospital. After skull x-ray and CT, about 20% of children undergo angiography, 5% require contrast examination of the ventricle and/or subarachnoid space, and a small number of this 25% also get both examinations.

Skull X-Ray

This is a neglected exam. While it is now of limited value in adults, it still should be the first *routine* exam in children. The plasticity of the child's skull shows evidence of acute and chronic increased intracranial pressure, and may show local abnormalities. The sutures commonly will acutely split even at age 14. Abnormality or

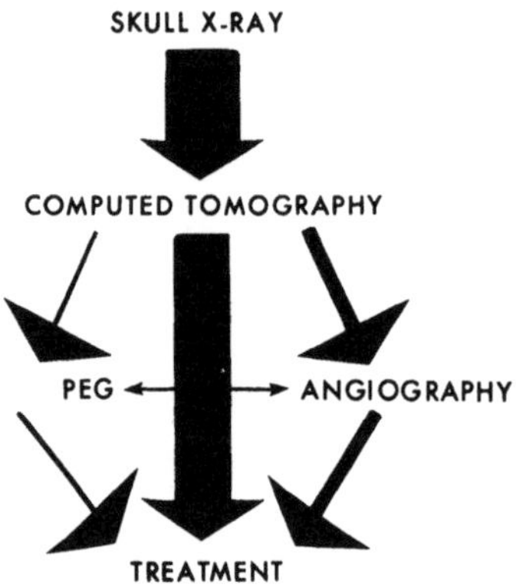

Fig. 1. Flow chart of tumour investigation at the Ho pital for Sick Children, Toronto

lack of it on skull X-ray is often an accurate guide as to the acuteness with whic other examinations should be done.

Conventional Tomography

Not listed in Fig. 1 is conventional tomography which by itself is considered usefi by the author only in one situation, that of examination of the optic canals in th axial position [3]. Conventional tomography still is the most accurate examinatio to see subtle canal enlargement or anterior clinoid erosions. Tomography as an ac junct to other examinations as angiography or pneumoencephalography (PEG) often quite helpful.

Radionuclide Brain Scan

This examination is not needed in the primary investigation of brain tumours, offe ing relatively poor specificity in spatial resolution in comparison with CT. For th investigation of metastases, there may well be some indication for radionuclic brain scanning, especially if an older CT unit is its companion. Radionuclide brai scanning has been reported to show metastases not seen on CT [4]. Positron emi sion tomography, with its ability to show physiological metabolic processes [1, 2] ha the potential for distinguishing different tumour types if they indeed have differei metabolisms.

CT Indications for Other Examinations

Angiography and contrast encephalography should be done following CT whe there is a need for them indicated by the CT. An outline of these conditions is liste in Table 1.

Table 1. CT indications for angiography and PEG

A. Location of tumour
   1. Adjacent to vessels
   2. Deep
   3. Superficial

B. Character of tumour
   1. Unusual shape
   2. Unusual pattern of enhancement
   3. Character odd for location

C. Normal or equivocal CT

D. Pathological diagnosis

Location

Here the need for further examinations is primarily dependant on the surgeon. If no operation is to be done, the exact relation of the tumour to vessels or other structures is of limited importance. If operation, even of a limited nature, will be done, this information is valuable and sometimes critical in the treatment of the child.

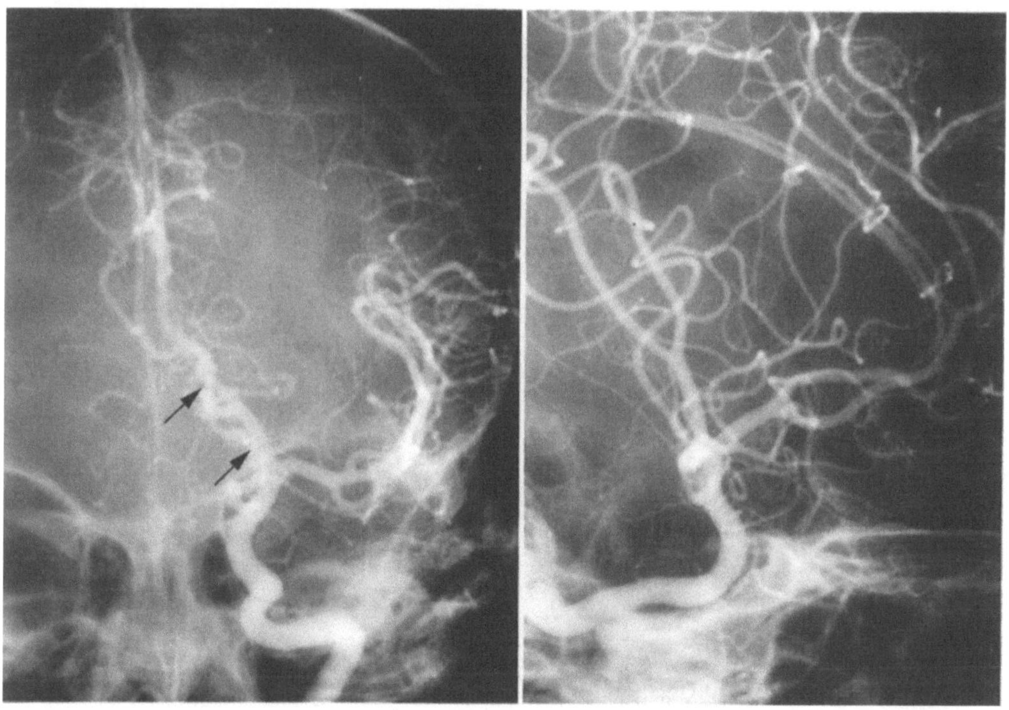

a b

Fig. 2a, b. Craniopharyngioma angiography. **a** AP arteriogram shows marked anterior cerebral artery elevation (*arrows*) by adherent tumour. **b** Lateral view shows a more subtle opening of the cartoid siphon from the tumour. Adjacent bone and cavernous sinus would totally mask this on CT

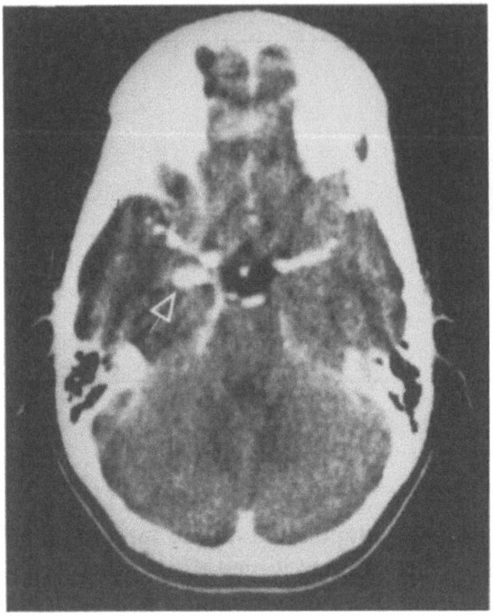

Fig. 3

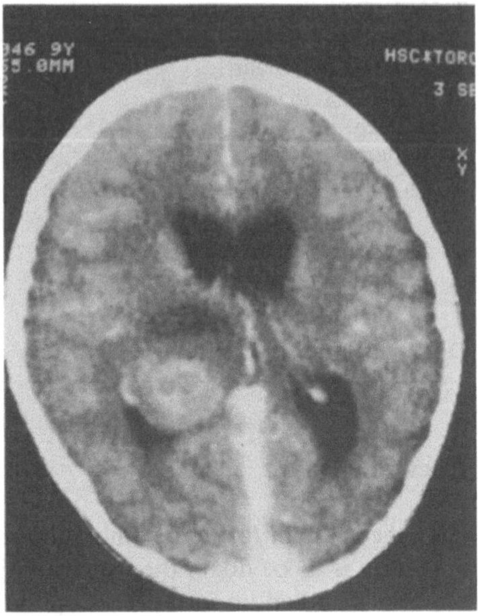

Fig. 4a

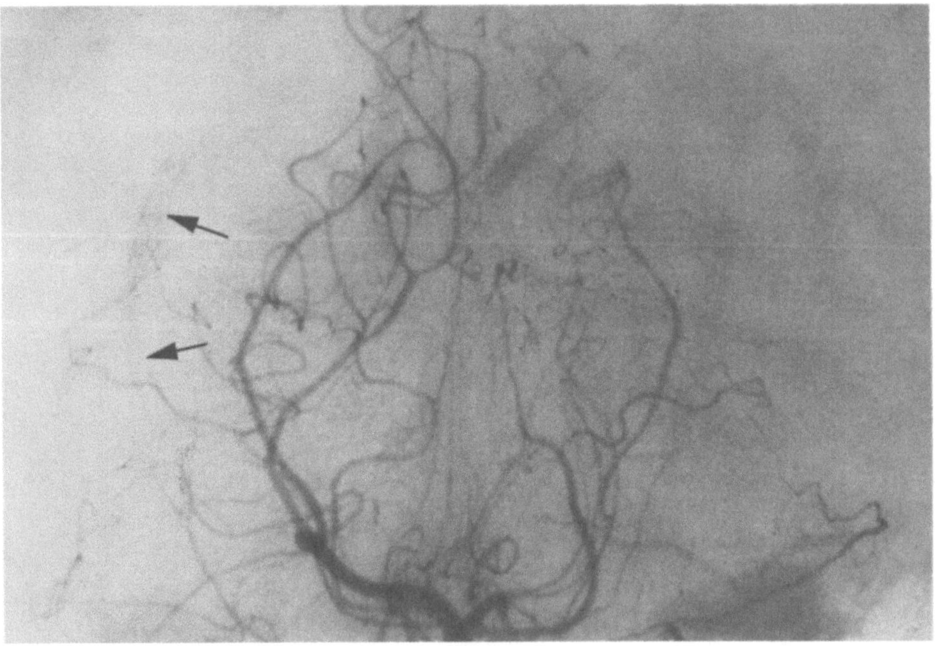

Fig. 4b

Fig. 3. CT of a child with seizures shows a calcified mass (*arrow*) resembling an aneurysm at the origin of the middle cerebral artery. Angiography showed no vascular abnormality

Fig. 4. Thalamic astrocytoma. **a** CT shows a large mass that could be interpreted as being intraventricular. **b** AP vertebral angiogram shows lateral displacement of the posterior lateral choroidal artery and choroid plexus (*arrows*), indicating that the tumour is medial to the ventricle and within the thalamus

Proximity to Vessels

By this is meant the situation where the location of the tumour on CT suggests major arteries or veins may be displaced and the knowledge of their location is critical to successful operation. In all cases angiography is the examination required. The most obvious example is that of a suprasellar tumour which is most often a craniopharyngioma in childhood. Here the location of major arteries is critical to the successful removal of the tumour (Fig. 2). Such displacements are not as well seen on CT, even with thin sections and reconstruction of images in coronal or sagittal planes.

One may uncommonly want to exclude a vascular lesion (Fig. 3), though the author has never found by any means an aneurysm or vascular malformation that was not clinically suspected.

Deep Location

This refers to tumours deep in the midline and periventricular regions. This indication may overlap with the previous category of proximity to vessels, as in a pineal tumour where location of the vein of Galen is of particular importance. It may be difficult to separate intraventricular from periventricular tumour by CT alone (Fig. 4a), but vascular displacement can accurately localize a mass (Fig. 4b), and cause a marked change in the operative approach to a tumour.

Deep tumours, especially those suspected of being intraventricular, may also be examined by ventriculography with air or water soluble contrast material such as metrizamide that is usually put into a ventricular shunt. As with CT, it can sometimes be difficult to differentiate a large tumour protruding into the ventricle from one arising from the ventricular surface.

Superficial Location

A mass that involves the cortex or calvarium should have angiography because meningeal tumours have a characteristic angiographic appearance. Knowledge of both major vessel displacement and external artery supply is again of surgical significance. Because superficial tumours in particular are likely to be meningeal, the possibility of making a pathological diagnosis is also important. Some meningeal tumours have a characteristic angiographic pattern (Fig. 5).

Character

To describe a tumour as having an unusual character on CT is subjective. Such description depends on the experience and skill of the radiologist. The author's criteria are those of an unusual shape, unusual pattern of intravenous contrast enhancement, and in general, an unusual appearance of a tumour compared to that usually seen in a common location such as the vermis.

Such a tumour is exemplified in Fig. 6, where a lobulated peripheral cerebellar tumour is seen. The location is typical of an astrocytoma, but the shape and contrast enhancement is not. Angiography suggested a medulloblastoma.

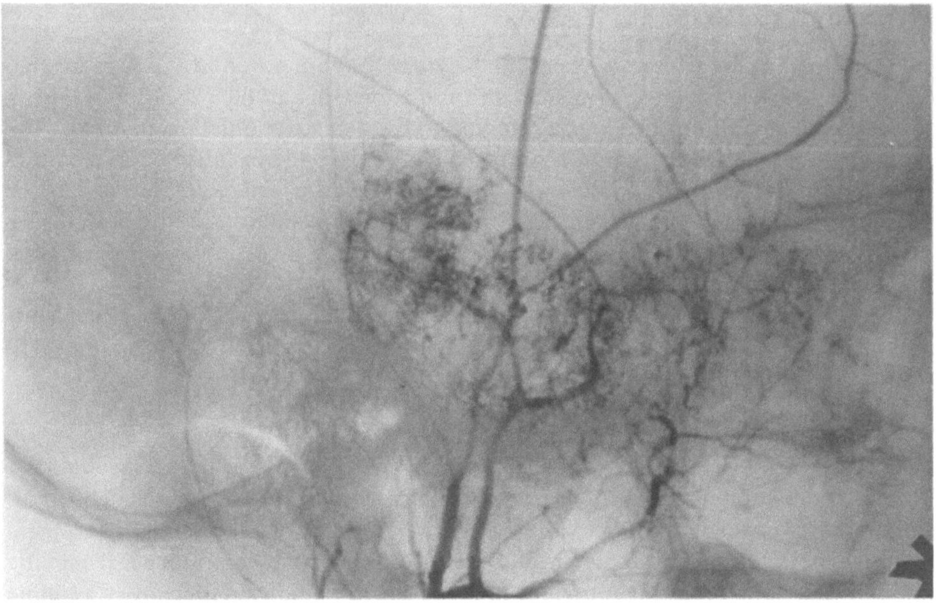

Fig. 5. Schwannoma. Lateral external carotid angiogram shows punctate tumour vascularity which persisted into the late venous phase. This is a typical finding in Schwannomas

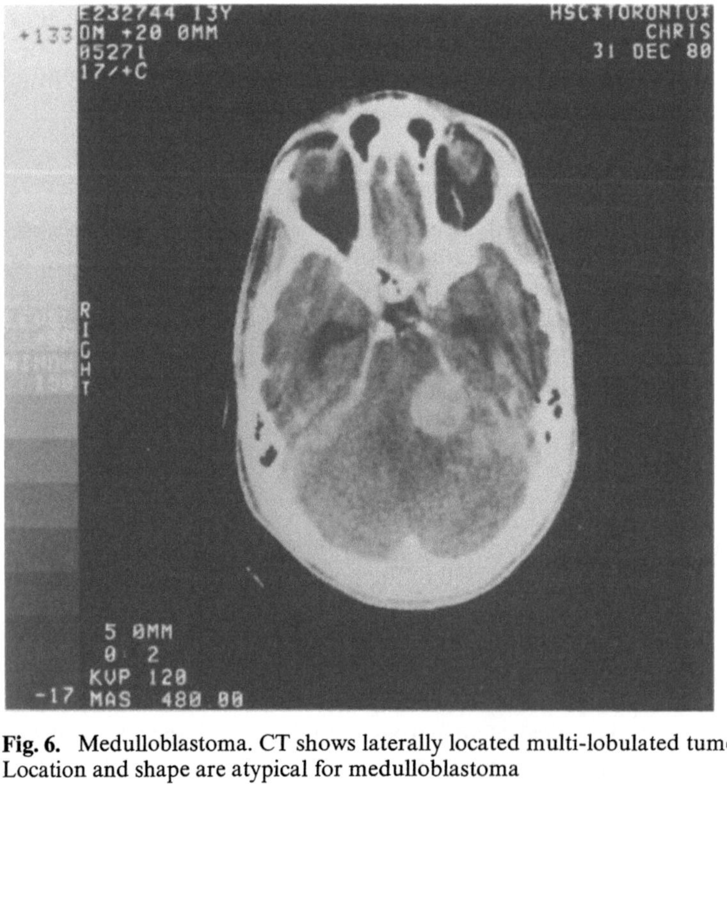

Fig. 6. Medulloblastoma. CT shows laterally located multi-lobulated tumour in a 13-year-old. Location and shape are atypical for medulloblastoma

Normal or Equivocal CT

This is very dependant on several factors. If there are strong clinical indications of a tumour with a normal CT, other investigations should be done. It is also quite dependant on the equipment and care with which examinations are done. Most of the problems arise in the area of the skull base; that is the brain stem, mid-brain, hypothalmus, and suprasellar regions. Both CT and other examinations must be done as skillfully as possible here.

A small brain stem tumour affecting only a short segment of the brain stem may still only be visible as a subtle stretching of the 4th ventricular floor on pneumoencephalography. A hamartoma of the tuber cinereum or intracranial extension of an optic nerve glioma may still be best seen on pneumoencephalography (Fig. 7). The region of the skull base remains a stronghold of investigation by contrast encepha-

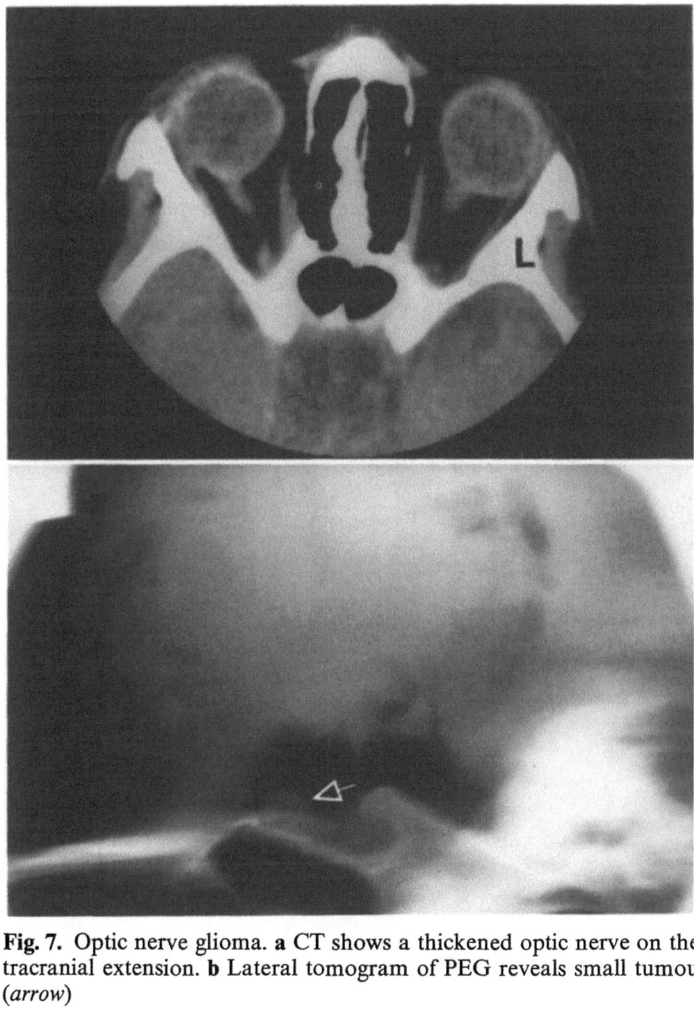

a

b

Fig. 7. Optic nerve glioma. **a** CT shows a thickened optic nerve on the left, but no definite intracranial extension. **b** Lateral tomogram of PEG reveals small tumour extension into chiasm (*arrow*)

lography, as the size of the tumours referred to cause a limited, if any, vascular displacement. The quality of CT equipment is of much importance in relationship to this indication. The author has found a reduction in the need for conventional examinations with the change from a 2nd to a 3rd generation scanner.

This brings up the matter of anaesthesia. The author believes that angiography and encephalography are best done under general anaesthesia. One may be tempted to spare a child an anaesthetic in favour of a repeat CT, but I am finding that the very thin 1–2 mm sections that can be done with newer CT units may also require an anaesthetized patient. Slight movement between CT slices will markedly degrade any multi-planar reconstruction, and such reconstruction is one of the chief benefits of thin section examination.

Pathological Diagnosis

The radiologist should strive for a pathological diagnosis to the degree that he is capable. This is especially true if no operative diagnosis will be attempted, though that is usually an unusual situation. If operation is done, the frozen section diagnosis may determine to what extent total tumour removal may be attempted. Frozen section diagnosis, like radiology, is sometimes both an art and a science, and radiological support or denial of an immediate pathological diagnosis is valuable.

Examples of the arteriographic patterns of meningeal tumours has already been mentioned. Suprasellar tumours may also be differentiated by angiography, as

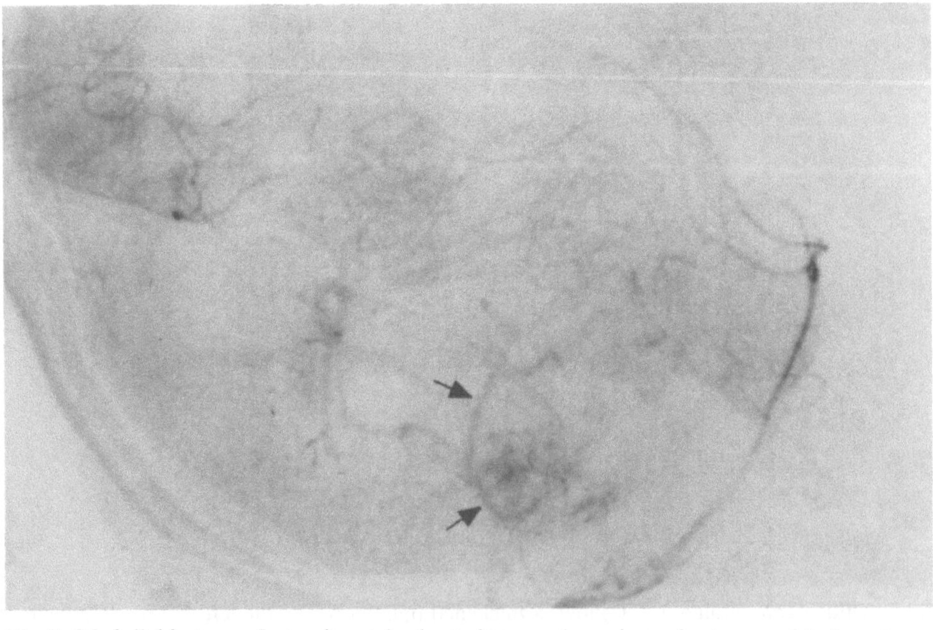

Fig. 8. Medulloblastoma. Lateral vertebral arteriogram shows irregular tumour blush and early draining vein (*arrows*) suggestive of medulloblastoma

craniopharyngiomas are avascular while malignant teratomas and adenomas are usually vascular.

In angiography, the picture of areas of vascular "blush" persisting into the venous phase, especially when combined with a paradoxical displacement of vessels, is very characteristic of medulloblastoma (Fig. 8).

The extent to which a pathological diagnosis can be made varies with the tumour type. On one hand the most information available is always the best. On the other hand, when there are no differentiating features by the radiological investigations done, this should be stated by the radiologist.

Surgical Roadmap

This is dependant on the needs of the surgeon. Some surgeons feel uncomfortable without an angiogram in nearly any operation, while others never want them. Both types of surgeons may have the same operative results, but it is the author's philosophy to try and give the surgeon more information if he strongly believes he needs it.

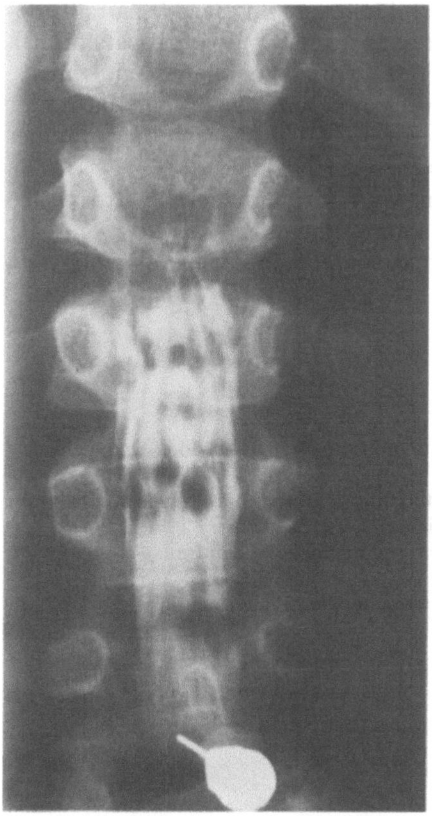

Fig. 9. Metastatic rhabdosarcoma. Metrizamide myelogram shows multiple metastatic nodules on the nerve roots and a complete block from intramedullary tumour at L1. CT revealed no further information

Examination of the Spinal Cord

Tumours of the spinal cord have more uniformity regardless of the radiological investigations done, and discussion of these will be brief. Even the best CT examination offers little definitive information regarding tumour pathology with either intrathecal or intravenous contrast material. Even tumour density and location of cyst is not reliably measurable on CT.

Myelography is needed for two reasons. It gives the surgeon or the radiotherapist a view of the spine that he is accustomed to for any operation or x-ray treatment, and myelography shortens any CT exam that might be necessary by showing the limits of the tumour. Myelography will show, fairly rapidly, the extent of most tumours (Fig. 9). Angiography has relatively little value in spinal cord lesions.

Conclusion

There is a continuing need for conventional radiographic examination in the diagnosis of central nervous system tumours in children, and this need is partially dependant on the amount of information required to treat an individual patient by a particular surgeon, oncologist, radiotherapist, or a combination of these individuals. The need for such exams has decreased since CT has become the primary means for tumour investigation, and may continue to decrease as CT further improves or other techniques such as nuclear magnetic resonance become available.

Developments of new contrast media, or new x-ray equipment may expand the usefulness of conventional techniques, and improvements in operative or other treatment forms may require the precision and complimentary investigation that combined radiographic techniques give.

References

1. Alavi, A., et al.: Mapping of functional activity in brain with F-Fluoro-Deoxyglucose. Seminars in Nuclear Medicine *11*, 24–31 (1981)
2. Wolf, A. P.: Special characteristics and potential for radiopharmaceuticals for positron emission tomography. Seminars in Nuclear Medicine *11*, 2–12 (1981)
3. Harwood-Nash, D. C.: Axial tomography of the optic canals in children. Radiology *96*, 367–374 (1970)
4. Raghavendra, B. N.: Computed tomography-nuclear medicine interface in the brain. Applied Radiology/NM pp. 141–144 (1978)

Computer Tomographic Diagnosis of CNS Tumours in Childhood

E. Kazner and K. Kretzschmar

The introduction of CT reduced the indications for conventional neuroradiological methods. Their diagnostic value is surpassed by CT.

Without any doubt CT leads to a simplification of the diagnostic procedures, and cerebral tumours can be demonstrated quite accurately.

Two hundred and sixty children, suffering from CNS tumours, were analysed by the university-clinics of Berlin, Mainz and Munich. In 94.6% of them the mass was shown by the first routine CT. Additional CT investigations allowed the tumour growth to be located in 4.6% of the cases. Therefore a single negative CT cannot definitely exclude a mass.

Two tumours (0.8%) could not be demonstrated either by CT or by other examinations. These tumours were verified at autopsy. A specification of the tumour type by CT is possible in about 90%. In other cases, especially in rare cerebral tumours, the classification can be predicted by CT-findings only in 50% of the children. However, this rate is still higher than results based on angiography or radionuclide brain scan.

On one hand the criteria for type diagnosis are based on the patient's history, his age and the site of the tumour. On the other hand the CT findings of the tumour, including the structure of the tissues, regressive changes and absorption values prior to and after injection of contrast medium, establish the pathological diagnosis.

In *cerebellar tumours* in childhood the main differential diagnosis is between medulloblastoma and pilocytic astrocytoma. One can distinguish both tumours quite precisely in 90% of the cases. In 5% of both types we found haemorrhages into the tumour tissue.

Medulloblastomas. In the majority of cases the routine scan shows a hyperdense mass. In about 20% a mixed density with hyperdense areas besides areas of primarily decreased density is apparent. Without injection of contrast medium 10% of medulloblastomas are isodense, and some necrotic tumours showed a reduced density (Fig. 1A). In general, non-necrotic parts of the tumour show a significant contrast enhancement. Also in tumours with necrotic areas the uptake of contrast medium in the solid parts of the tumour is significant for medulloblastomas. Preferably the tumour is located in the roof of the fourth ventricle and is growing in the middle of the vermis of the cerebellum. In general a primary hyperdense homogeneous tumour in the vermis of the cerebellum with contrast enhancement is considered to be a typical medulloblastoma.

The *desmoplastic medulloblastoma*, also known as arachnoid sarcoma, differs from the typical CT-appearance of a medulloblastoma. Its absorption values are similar, but it is situated laterally in the cerebellar hemispheres.

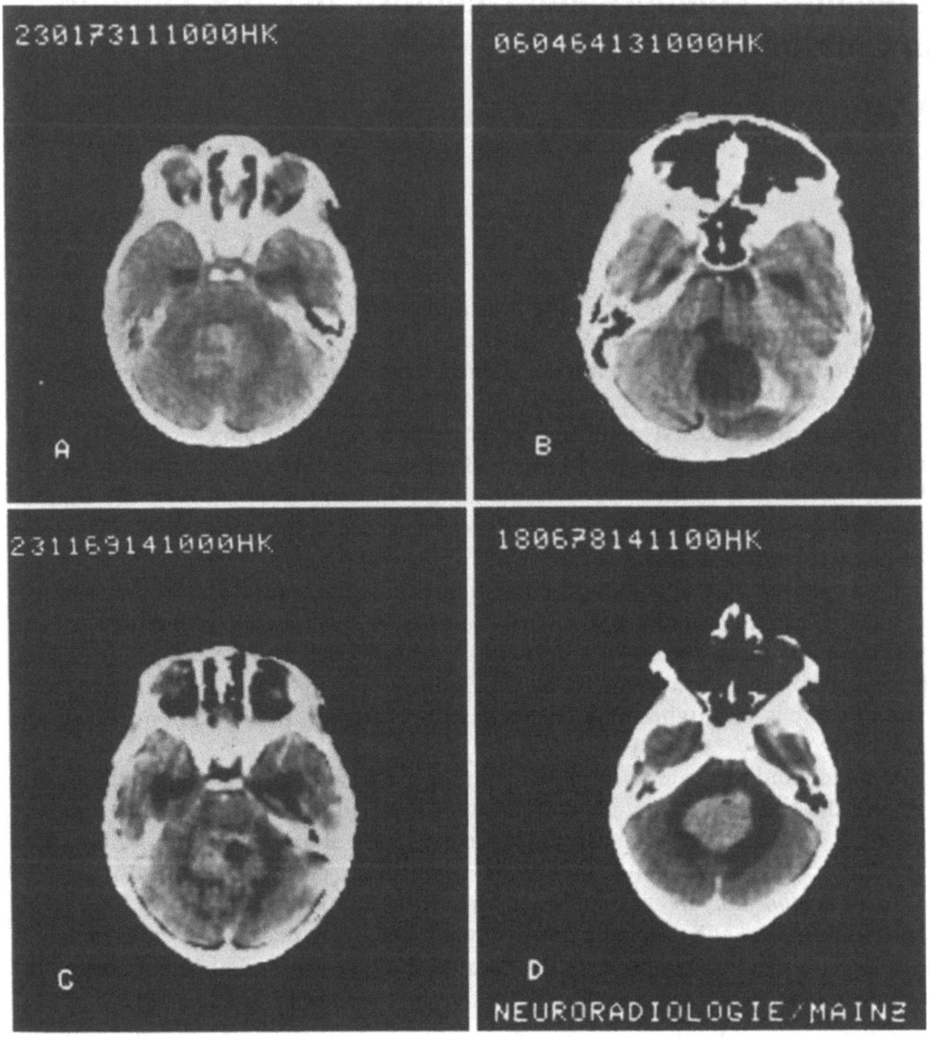

Fig. 1. A 7-year-old boy. Medulloblastoma. Contrast-CT. Hyperdense tumour in the roof of the fourth ventricle surrounded by perifocal oedema. **B** 14-year-old boy. Pilocytic astrocytoma (grade I). Contrast-CT. Cyst with marginally located solid tumourous nodules on the right side. **C** 10-year-old boy. Ependymoma (grade III). Contrast-CT. Mostly solid tumour with cystic and necrotic parts. **D** 3-year-old girl. Choroid plexus papilloma. Contrast-CT. Solid tumour of the fourth ventricle extending towards the rhomboid fossa

The differential diagnosis has to exclude the so-called *pseudotumour of the vermis.* In this case, the grey matter of the vermis is of a higher density than both cerebellar hemispheres, thus mimicking a hyperdense mass. Even a slight enhancement of the vermis is remarkable. However, there is no space-occupying effect. The fourth ventricle and the cistern of the superior vermis show a normal configuration.

Pilocytic Astrocytoma. Three different types can be distinguished. A big cyst dominates the CT appearance of the first type. A small nodular portion of the tumour can be found in the wall of the cyst, showing a distinct increase in density.

For the second type a nodular tumour with small cystic areas, even with ring-structures is specific. In the plain scan the solid areas are mostly hypodense, only a small number is isodense compared to the adjacent cerebellar tissue. After the injection of contrast medium there is a significant increase in density.

The third type consists of an area of reduced density without any cystic formation in the plain scan. Enhancement is also obvious here.

In all three types of pilocytic astrocytoma small spotty calcifications are to be seen in the nodular areas. The main site for pilocytic astrocytomas is in the cerebellar hemispheres, vermis and caudal brain stem (Fig. 1 B).

Ependymomas. In almost half of the ependymomas an increased density is already obvious early on. One third of these tumours demonstrates degenerative changes with small cystic areas and calcification. Generally ependymomas in the cerebellum show a less striking contrast enhancement compared to those situated in the cerebrum. The floor of the 4th ventricle is a typical site for the ependymomas. The flow of cerebrospinal fluid through the fourth ventricle is displaced dorso-laterally and shows a curved irregular outline around the tumour (Fig. 1 C).

In childhood the other tumours occurring in the cerebellar hemispheres can scarcely be classified by CT: fibrillary or gemistocytic astrocytomas, gangliocytomas or choroid plexus papillomas (Fig. 1 D).

Gliomas of the Pons. In the majority of cases the pons is affected by diffusely growing fibrillary astrocytomas, demonstrable in the CT as primary hypodense areas without any absorption of contrast (Fig. 2 A). In case of pilocytic or anaplastic astrocytomas a circular or nodular increase of density can be seen after contrast medium is injected (Fig. 2 B).

The growth of the tumour leads to an expansion and bulging of the pons. The fourth ventricle is displaced dorsally, the cisterns around the brain stem and pons are compressed.

The *supratentorial* masses are mostly located intra- or paraventricular near the midline.

Ependymomas, Ependymoblastomas. In childhood this type of tumour manifests a malignant character, and higher grades of malignancy are prevalent. CT is characterized by large cysts with a marginal tumour nodule, occasionally with calcification. In about 80% of the tumours a significant contrast enhancement in the solid part of the tumour is seen. The preferred localization is in the posterior part of the third ventricle or paraventricular in the temporal parietal or occipital lobe.

Pilocytic astrocytomas. In the plain scan this type of tumour is found isodense with occasional circular contrast enhancement. In contrast to the infratentorial pilocytic astrocytomas the division into 3 types of CT appearance as previously mentioned cannot be made. In general there is no typical formation of a large cyst with a small solid tumour nodule. Typically it grows in the basal ganglia close to the midbrain, in the medial temporal lobe or in the chiasm. The appearance of the mass is completed by areas of calcification and small cysts.

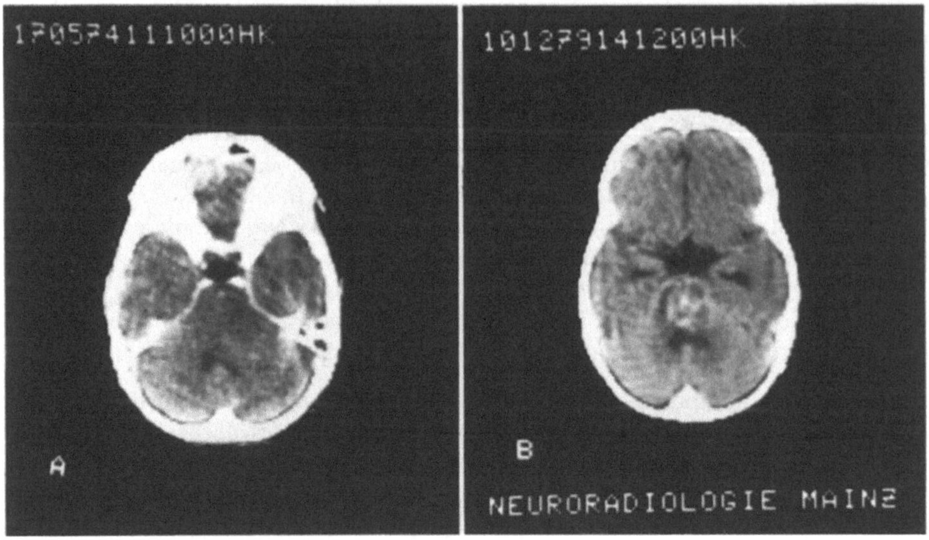

Fig. 2. A 7-year-old boy with a hypodense pontine tumour without any contrast enhancement. **B** 2-year-old boy. Contrast CT of a pontine glioma

The rarely occurring *hamartomas or gangliocytomas* can develop in the same site in the paramedian temporal lobe, but cannot be differentiated by CT from pilocytic astrocytomas.

As regards *ventricular tumours,* the plexus papillomas, subependymomas and subependymal giant cell astrocytomas are of clinical interest in childhood.

Plexus Papillomas. Plain scan demonstrates a solid, slightly hyperdense tumour with a shaggy surface. The richly vascularized mass shows a distinct homogeneous contrast enhancement. Calcification and rarely cysts, are seen. Their main location is in the fourth ventricle as already mentioned (Fig. 1 D).

In addition they may occur in the trigone of the lateral ventricles or they may originate from the choroid plexus of the third ventricle.

The diagnosis is based on the connection of the tumour with the choroid plexus and its intraventricular location.

Subependymomas. These tumours, situated in the lateral ventricle, appear as primary hypodense areas without contrast enhancement or as big cysts with a marginal enhancement zone.

Subependymal Giant Cell Astrocytomas. In the plain scan the tumour appears as isodense or slightly hyperdense, showing a homogeneous enhancement after contrast medium injection. Typically the mass grows on the floor of the anterior horn of the lateral ventricle, close to the foramen of Monro. Other ventricular locations are rare (Fig. 3 D).

The tumour process associated with tuberose sclerosis can be proved by calcification in the ventricular wall. The differentiation of intraventricular tumours has to take note of these types as well as the other subependymal tumours (Fig. 3 A) or astroblastomas (Fig. 3 B).

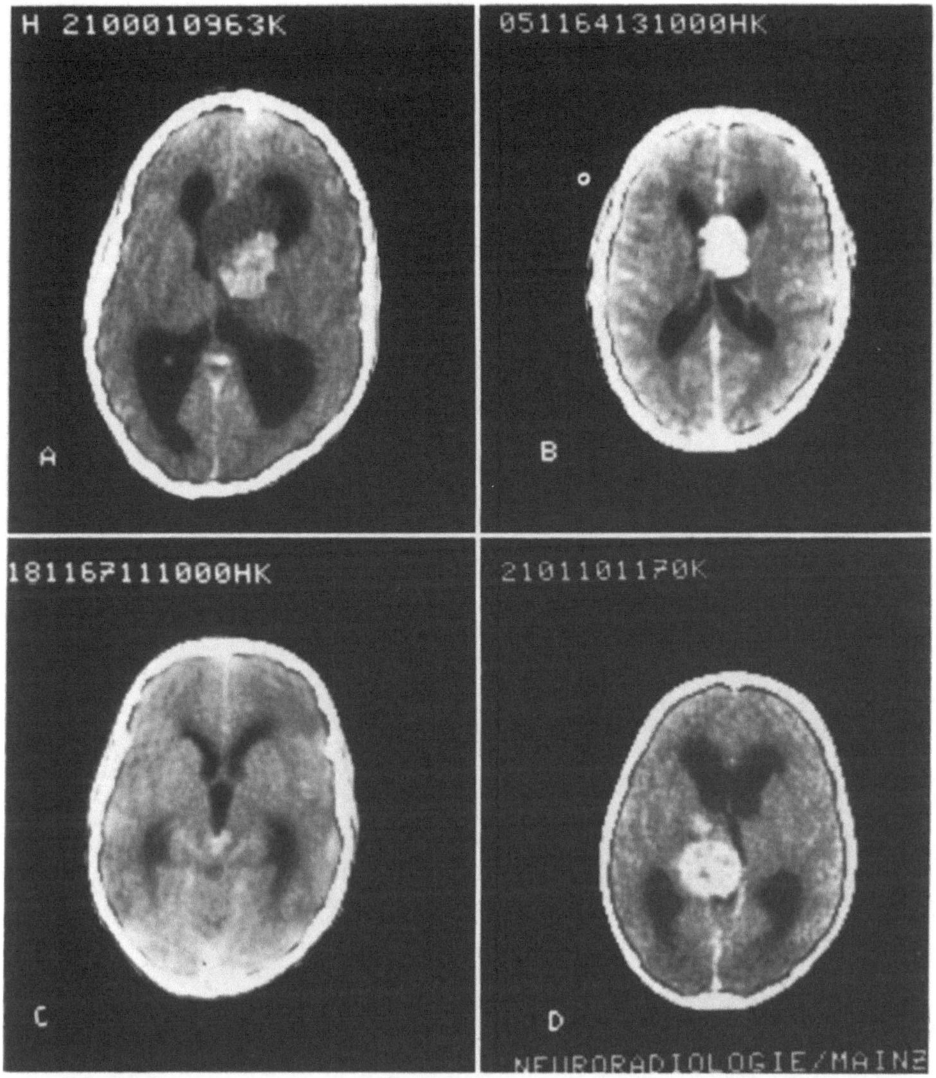

Fig. 3. **A** 14-year-old boy. Subependymal gemistocytic astrocytoma grade I–II. Contrast-CT. Partially solid, partially cystic tumour in the right lateral ventricle with occlusion of the foramina of Monro. **B** 15-year-old girl. Astrocytoma grade IV. Contrast-CT. Solid tumour in the right lateral ventricle. **C** 13-year-old boy with a small tumour in the pineal region (unknown histology). Contrast-CT. **D** 7-year-old boy. Subependymal giant cell astrocytoma grade III–IV. Contrast-CT. Unusual location in the left thalamus

Tumours of the posterior part of the third ventricle and the pineal region are mostly pinealomas (Fig. 3 C).

Pinealomas. The CT appearance of these very cellular tumours is characterized by a slightly increased density and an intensive uptake of contrast. In addition to the physiological pineal calcification there is calcification in the solid parts of the tumour in the majority of cases.

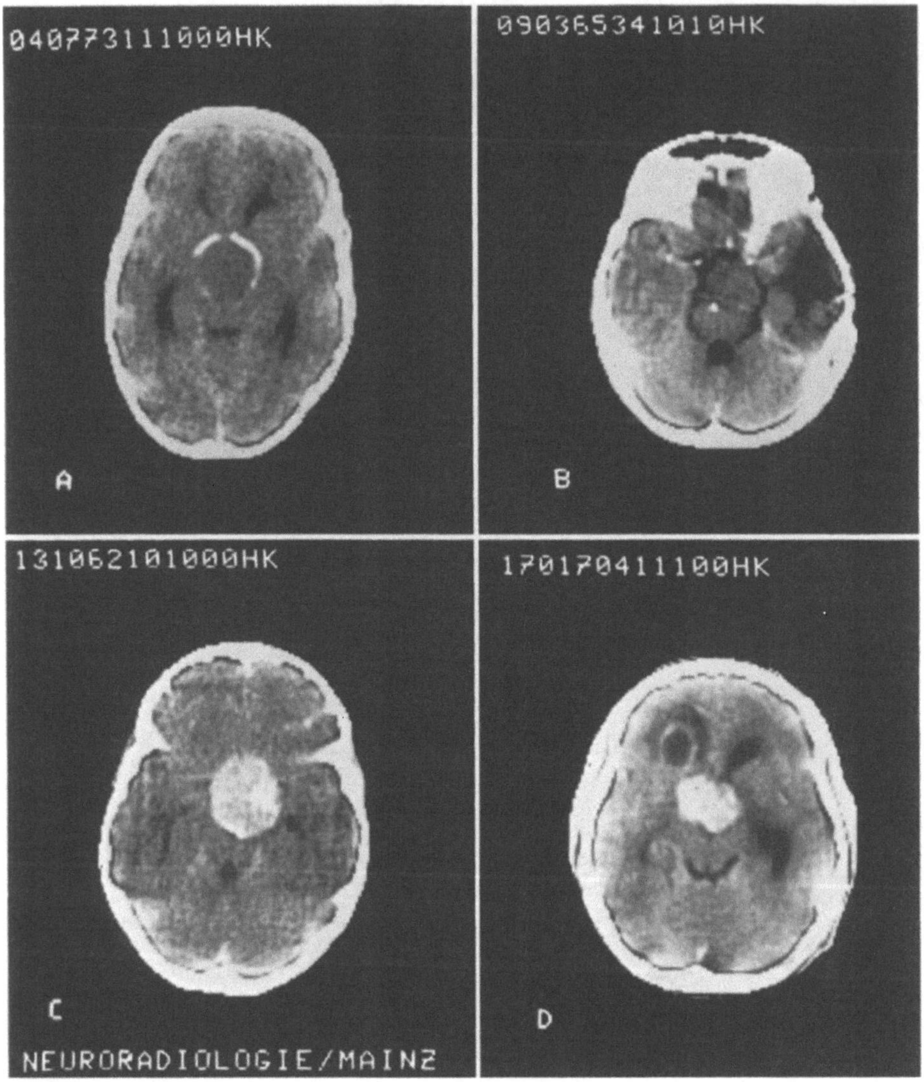

Fig. 4. A 7-year-old girl. Craniopharyngioma. Contrast-CT. Suprasellar tumour with scaphoid calcification and isodense content. **B** 14-year-old girl. Pilocytic astrocytoma grade I. Postoperative investigation (postoperative defect of the right temporal lobe). Isodense tumour originating from the hypothalamus and with a prepontine extension (contrast-CT). **C** 15-year-old boy. Endotheliomatous-psammomatous meningioma. Contrast-CT. Suprasellar tumour with central calcification. **D** 9-year-old boy. Teratoid with carcinomatous parts. Contrast-CT. Partly intraventricular tumour mostly solid

The tumours obstruct the outlet of the third ventricle and can cause obstruction of the aqueduct. All tumours of the pineal gland – whether they originate from the actual pineal tissue (pineocytomas) or from germinal cells (germinomas) – tend to disseminate in the CSF pathways. In a plain scan this formation of metastases can be proved by absence of the external CSF spaces and by a subarachnoidal contrast enhancement. The differential diagnosis of a mass in the posterior part of the third ventricle has to include ependymomas and congenital malformations, especially teratomas.

Germinomas in particular, the so-called ectopic pinealomas, can be found in the infundibulum of the pituitary gland. Other common tumours in the sellar region are craniopharyngiomas (Fig. 4A), pilocytic astrocytomas (Fig. 4B), meningiomas (Fig. 4C) and teratomas (Fig. 4D).

Craniopharyngiomas. In childhood they are the most important tumours of the sellar region. The craniopharyngioma is recognized by its variety of calcification, cysts and non-necrotic vital tumour areas of different density. The contrast uptake in solid, nodular parts is irregular or marginal. The characteristic intrasellar or suprasellar location simplifies the differential diagnosis.

In summary one can say that CNS tumours in infancy and childhood can almost without exception be classified in regard to their site, consistence and expansion and their space-occupying effect by the CT scan. In individual cases however, the diagnosis may be difficult to establish and sometimes is only possible by comparing with similar CT appearances in other tumours.

Concerning the uncertainties of the type specific tumour diagnosis, we expect to get some more details from angio-CT. However no significant results from this method are yet available.

Radionuclide Imaging of Cerebral Tumours in Children

K. HAHN

For many years radionuclide scanning has been the only noninvasive imaging procedure for studying children with suspected central nervous system tumours. Since the introduction of computerized axial tomography (CT) this procedure has proved to be the most effective noninvasive method for examining intracranial tumours in children. On the other hand, in recent years there has been important progress in nuclear medicine equipment by the development of high resolution gamma cameras and computerized data processing systems and the introduction of new ^{99m}Technetium labelled radiopharmaceuticals. This improvement of cerebral radionuclide studies has increased the accuracy and specificity of the results of radionuclide cerebral tumour imaging.

Radionuclide imaging visualizes vessels of the central nervous system in a normal brain as "hot" vascular channels whereas the brain is delineated as a "cold" area. Although the mechanism by which radiopharmaceuticals accumulate in cerebral tumours is not completely known, it is generally agreed that an alteration of blood-brain barrier is involved. Several changes that occur in brain lesions disrupt or alter this blood brain barrier permitting the localization or abnormal transport of radiopharmaceuticals, and these changes account for positive brain scans. Bakay [1] has listed several mechanisms that may account for the localization of tracer substances in brain tumours, many of which apply to other brain lesions as well.

1. Increased vascularity: This mechanism may be the only reason for detecting arteriovenous malformations, but many lesions have scarcely any increase in the numbers of vessels and yet strongly concentrate radioactive tracers.
2. Abnormal vascular permeability: The absence of vessels with a tight endothelial junction in most brain lesions is well demonstrated.
3. Pinocytosis: Healthy astrocytes inhibit pinocytosis in brain capillary cells. The absence of these cells in brain lesions may account for the accumulation of macromolecules such as labelled albumin.
4. Enlarged extracellular space and reactive oedema: Most brain tumours and many other lesions are associated with some oedema in surrounding brain tissue. The uptake of radiopharmaceuticals is often greater in this brain tissue than in the lesion itself.
5. Cellular metabolism: The metabolic activity in tumour cells may be greater than in normal brain tissue allowing transport of labelled tracers into the tumour along with metabolic substrates.

Positive uptake of a radiopharmaceutical in a given lesion cannot be explained by a single mechanism. It is most likely a combination of several processes, which would explain why brain lesions accumulate different kinds of molecules in different concentrations and why most lesions accumulate several molecules of widely varying size, ionic charge, and chemical characteristics.

Tumours, whose vessels still have nearly the same structure as normal cerebral vessels, such as very well-differentiated astrocytomas, grades I and II, do not accumulate radiopharmaceuticals and may result in negative brain scans. Meningiomas however, whose vessels are extremely pathological, accumulate the radioactive agents in a few minutes and show an abnormal scan.

With modern imaging techniques tumours of 1 cm or greater can usually be visualized. Smaller tumours are detected if associated haemorrhage or reactive oedema occurs. Tumours if they are located at the base of the brain or around vascular structures where interfering background activity is higher must be larger if they are to be shown.

Radionuclides Used in Brain Imaging

Of the many agents that have been used for brain scanning ^{99m}Technetium is the one most widely applied for static and dynamic imaging by virtue of its half-life of six hours, the emission of monoenergetic gamma rays of 140 keV energy and the low radiation absorbed dose. One of the main disadvantages of ^{99m}Tc-pertechnetate is that it localizes in the choroid plexus. Therefore ^{99m}Tc-labelled compounds that are excreted by the kidneys, such as DPTA, glucoheptonate, iron-ascorbate and citrate should be preferred. Clinical studies [6, 10–12], in which these compounds were compared with ^{99m}Tc-pertechnetate, showed in addition higher lesion:background ratios and therefore a better lesion detectability.

Dosage

The dosage of these ^{99m}Tc-complexes varies from one hospital to another. We prefer the dosage, which is used by D. L. Gilday, M. D. at the Hospital for Sick Children in Toronto, Canada, as set out in Fig. 1. The standard adult dose of 15–20 mCi is listed as 100% and the body weight in kilograms is plotted on the curve which results in a dose per body surface area.

Technique

For brain scanning in children a high resolution scintillation camera with a data processing system should be used. This equipment has enhanced the value of the brain scan by permitting direct assessment of cerebral vascularity. This added

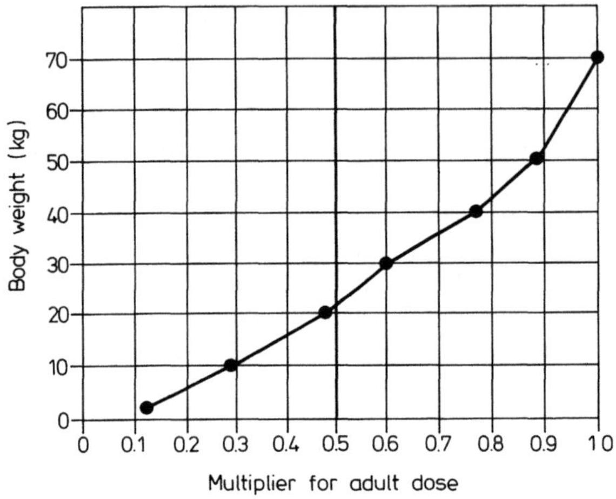

Fig. 1. Paediatric radiopharmaceutical doses per body surface area (by D. L. Gilday, M. D. Hospital for Sick Children, Toronto)

dimension is of special value in evaluating arteriovenous malformations that may not be evident in the static images, subdural and extradural haematomas, and cerebral death where internal carotid blood flow is markedly reduced. The dynamic flow study that means the study of the passage of the radioactive bolus through the brain, is usually performed in the anterior position, but may be also performed in the posterior, lateral, or vertex position for better definition if the site of the lesion can be located before starting the examination. Images are collected at 1 to 3 sec intervals by x-ray film, Polaroid film or by computer which allows the greatest flexibility of image presentation and analysis. During the arterial phase a five-pointed star pattern is formed by the two carotid arteries, the two middle cerebral arteries, and the combined anterior cerebral arteries. During the capillary phase a generalized distribution of activity is followed by a venous phase when the activity of the superior sagittal sinus prevails. The radionuclide angiogram should form an integral part of the brain scan since it increases the detection of pathological cerebral conditions by as much as 10 to 15%.

Whenever possible static brain images should be recorded immediately after the dynamic flow study in anterior, posterior, right and left lateral and vertex view.

The vertex view should be generally included because it is the best single view and is positive in 90% of lesions, having the advantage of being relatively uninfluenced by the unilateral, anterior, and posterior position of the lesion and being capable of detecting basilar brain lesions. These early scans show vascular details more prominently but frequently fail to delineate such lesions as haematomas and tumours. Delayed images 1 to 2 hours and occasional 2 to 4 hours after injection in five views are necessary, for it has been shown that delayed imaging will enhance detection of certain neoplasms, abscesses, infarctions, and abnormal dural fluid collections. This is presumably the result of an increase in accumulation of the radionuclide within the lesion simultaneously with a decrease in blood background.

By this technique the detection of those lesions of a highly vascular nature will be enhanced and also the superficial venous sinuses will be better delineated.

Tumours

Brain tumours seen in children differ both in type and distribution from those seen in adults, in whom most tumours are supratentorial and either meningiomas, glioblastomas, pituitary adenomas, or neurinomas. In contrast, two-thirds of tumours in children are infratentorial, and are either medulloblastomas, cystic astrocytomas, or ependymomas. In the one-third of tumours in children that lie above the tentorium, gliomas and craniopharyngiomas are most frequent.

In adults 85 to 90 percent of the patients with proven brain tumours have positive brain scans. Statistical analyses of large populations of patients imaged with ^{99m}Tc pertechnetate had a sensitivity of 81.5–83% for a proved neoplasm [13]. Maynard and Cowan reviewed the early literature on pertechnetate imaging and also compared their results with pertechnetate in 1,000 consecutive cases. They found a sensitivity of 75% for primary brain tumours and 90% for metastatic lesions [9].

Tanasescu et al. [14] reported about brain imaging with ^{99m}Tc-glucoheptonate in 859 patients. They found in patients with proved central nervous system tumours a sensitivity of 94%.

A review of the pediatric literature by Conway and Quinn [4] suggests that almost the same results are obtained in children (Tables 1, 2) but with the improved techniques of radionuclide cerebral angiography and emission tomography [2, 3] the results have improved considerably compared to this review. Tumours such as cerebellar astrocytoma, ependymoma, and glioblastoma multiforme virtually always had a positive scan. There were varying results in the literature in regard to medulloblastoma, but 11 of 12 in this series were positive. Well-differentiated cerebral astrocytomas were as difficult to diagnose in children as they are in adults.

Table 1. Positive brain scans in selected infratentorial brain tumours in children. (Review of literature, modified from Conway and Quinn [4])

Medulloblastoma	54	of	82	(66%)
Cerebellar astrocytoma	79	of	92	(86%)
Brain stem glioma	28	of	73	(38%)
Ependymoma	24	of	33	(73%)
Total	185	of	280	(66%)

Table 2. Positive brain scans in selected supratentorial brain tumours of children. (Review of literature, modified from Conway and Quinn [4])

Astrocytoma	47	of	56	(84%)
Glioblastoma multiforme	38	of	38	(100%)
Optic glioma	19	of	23	(83%)
Craniopharyngioma	12	of	30	(40%)
Total	116	of	147	(79%)

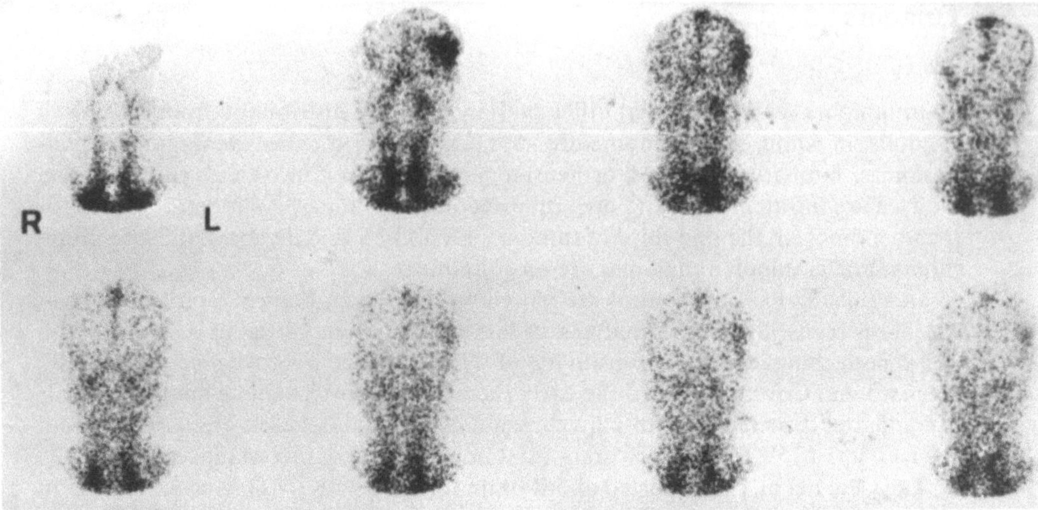

a

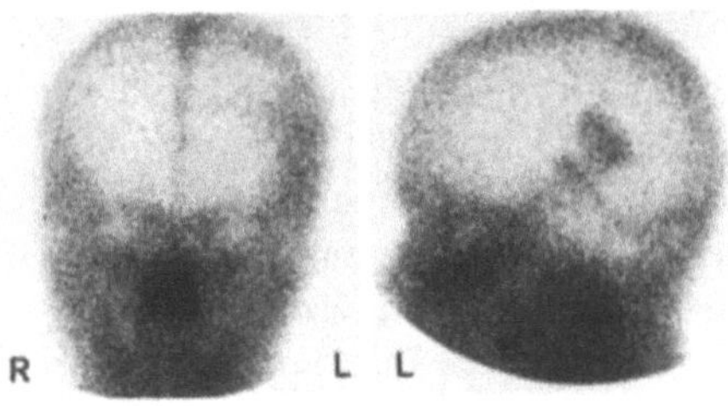

b

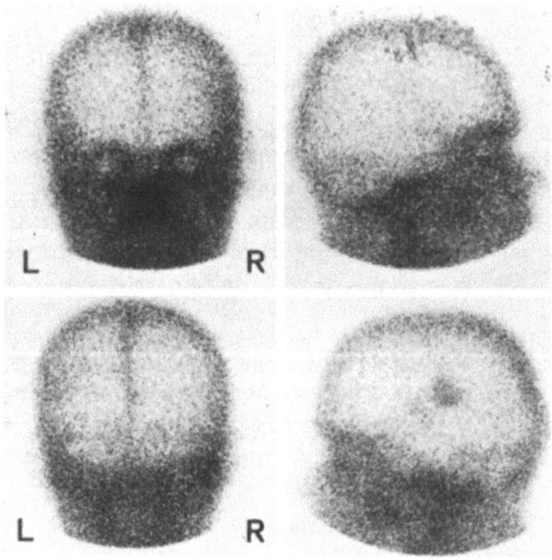

c

Fig. 2a–c. 14-years-old girl with arteriovenous malformation. **a** Radionuclide cerebral angiography showing early arterial increased activity in left hemisphere, which fades in the venous phase. **b** Early anterior and left static scan: large increased focal activity in left temporal region. **c** Anterior, right and left lateral and posterior view: well-demarcated increased radionuclide concentration left temporal but diminished compared to the early scans

Brain stem tumours were the most difficult brain tumours to diagnose by radionuclide techniques because the brain stem is a notoriously inaccessible site for routine brain imaging. The small size of the lesion, therefore, may be masked by the normal activity at the base of the brain. When results were positive it was usually because the tumour was very large. Craniopharyngioma, the commonest non-gliomatous intracranial tumour was also low on the list in percentage of positive studies. The radionuclide emission tomography may be of considerable help in delineating these tumours. The location of an abnormal radionuclide accumulation on the brain image was useful in predicting the histology of a lesion. For example, an intense radionuclide accumulation in a midline suprasellar lesion was more likely to be caused by optic glioma than craniopharyngioma. An intense peripheral radionuclide accumulation has been characteristic of meningeal sarcoma. Well-differentiated cerebral astrocytomas often accumulated minimal amounts of radioactivity within the lesion, whereas most glioblastoma multiforme lesions were indicated by an intense locus of radionuclide activity. In the posterior fossa, midline lesions probably represented medulloblastoma, whereas more deeply seated midline lesions were likely to be caused by brain stem glioma. Cerebellar hemisphere lesions were predominantly cerebellar astrocytomas.

Congenital Vascular Malformations

The two principal cerebral vascular malformations are aneurysms and arteriovenous shunts, called arteriovenous malformations (AVM). The incidence of these malformations constitutes about 2% of all symptomatic brain lesions. Reliable detection of congenital intracranial AVM's and aneurysms is important because the prognosis for these conditions has improved with advances in neurosurgery.

Aneurysms are not usually visualized by scanning unless they are exceptionally large. Congenital AVM's, on the other hand, are diagnosed with a very high degree of precision, especially by the radionuclide angiography in which they show an early activity that generally persists during the capillary phase (Fig. 2). The principal differentiating feature between AVM's and other vascular tumours, such as meningiomas, is that the latter become increasingly positive with time, while AVM's become less active in the venous phase. Gates et al. [5] evaluated nine children with AVM and a tenth with a cerebral aneurysm. These children underwent computer-processed dynamic scintigraphy with static scintigrams, transmission computed tomography (CT) with and without contrast injection, and radiopaque cerebral angiography. All ten lesions were detected by dynamic scintigraphy and with radiopaque angiography whereas two AVM's were missed on CT scans.

Radiation Dose

The estimated radiation exposure as a guideline for radionuclide cerebral imaging with ^{99m}Tc-pertechnetate and ^{99m}Tc-DTPA of children and newborns, described by Kaul and Roedler [7, 8], is shown in Table 3. As shown in this table, the radiation dose of the child caused by cerebral scintigraphy is low but it must be considered that there is not only a radiation exposure of the brain but also of the whole body and the ovaries and testes, due to the elimination of the radiopharmaceutical by the lower colon and the kidneys. The critical organ for ^{99m}Tc-pertechnetate is the lower large intestine, for ^{99m}Tc-labelled compounds, such as ^{99m}Tc-DTPA and ^{99m}Tc-glucoheptonate the kidneys and the bladder. A frequent emptying of the bladder will cause a substantial reduction of the gonadal radiation dose. As also shown in the table, it has to be considered that the radiation exposure will decrease slowly with the age of the children.

Table 3. Radiation dose caused by brain imaging of newborns and children. (Modified from Kaul and Roedler [7])

Organ to be investigated	Radiopharma-ceutical	Age (J)	Energy dose (mrd/μCi) in the		
			ovaries	testes	investigated or crit. organ
brain	^{99m}Tc-pertechnetate	0	0.22	0.10	1.9
		1	0.076	0.079	0.67 lower colon
		5	0.045	0.073	0.46
		10	0.032	0.066	0.33
		15	0.022	0.014	0.23
	^{99m}Tc DTPA	0	0.33	0.17	0.39
		1	0.11	0.13	0.15
		5	0.068	0.12	0.10
		10	0.049	0.11	0.068
		15	0.032	0.024	0.051

Indications for Radionuclide Imaging of the Brain in Children

1. In the evaluation of children with suspected intracranial mass lesions computerized cranial tomography (CT) is today generally the preferred initial diagnostic test. This is because it provides a more specific pathologic diagnosis and more anatomical detail than radionuclide imaging rather than a marked improvement in overall sensitivity. Perhaps in future the results of emission tomography will change this situation.
2. Radionuclide imaging should be first performed if CT is not practicable or if despite a persistent suspected mass lesion the CT is normal.
3. Radionuclide imaging should be done first in children with suspected congenital vascular malformations or cerebral vascular disease.

References

1. Bakay, L.: Basic aspects of brain tumour localization by radioactive substances: review of current concepts. J. Neurosurg. *27,* 239–245 (1967)
2. Biersack, H. J., Knopp, R., Wappenschmidt, J., Winkler, C.: "Single Photon" Emissions-Computertomographie des Hirns mit einer rotierenden Gammakamera – Ergebnisse bei 471 Patienten. Nuc. Compact *12,* 130–134 (1981)
3. Carril, J. M., MacDonald, A. F., Dendy, P. P. et al.: Cranial scintigraphy: value of adding emission computed tomographic sections to conventional pertechnetate images (512 cases) J. Nucl. Med. *20,* 1117–1123 (1979)
4. Conway, J. J., Quinn, J. L.: Brain imaging in pediatrics. In: James, A. E., Wagner H. N. Jr., Cooke, R. E. (eds.): Pediatric Nuclear Medicine, pp. 115–126, Philadelphia: W. B. Saunders 1974
5. Gates, G. F., Fishman, L. S., Segall, H. D.: Scintigraphic detection of congenital intracranial vascular malformations, J. Nucl. Med. *19,* 235–244 (1978)

6. Hör, G., el Helou, A.: Cerebrale Sequenz-Szintigraphie: Perfusionsdiagnostik in pädiatrischer Neurologie, Neurochirurgie und Perinatalogie, in: Hahn, K. (ed.): Pädiatrische Nuklearmedizin, pp. 3–11, Band 2, Mainz: Kirchheim 1980
7. Kaul, A., Roedler H. D., Hine, G. J.: Internal absorbed dose from administered radiopharmaceuticals. In: Medical radionuclide imaging, IAEA, Vienna 1977, Vol. II, p. 423
8. Kaul, A., Roedler, H. D.: Patients radiation exposition caused by radiopharmaceuticals. Nuc. Compact *9,* 22–28 (1978)
9. Maynard, C. D., Cowan, R. J.: Specific brain scan diagnosis. Curr. Probl. Radiol. *3,* 1–40 (1973)
10. Rollo, F. D., Cavalieri, R. R., Born, M. et al.: Comparative evaluation of ^{99m}TcGH, ^{99m}Tc O_4, and ^{99m}TcDTPA as brain imaging agents. Radiology *123,* 379–383 (1977)
11. Ryerson, T. W., Spies, S. M., Singh, N. B. et al.: A quantitative clinical comparison of three ^{99m}Technetium labeled brain imaging radiopharmaceuticals. Radiology *127,* 429–432 (1978)
12. Waxman, A. D., Tanasescu, D., Siemsen, J. K. et al.: Technetium-99m-glucoheptonate as a brain scanning agent: critical comparison with pertechnetate. J. Nucl. Med., *17,* 345–348 (1976)
13. Witcofski, R. L., Maynard, C. D., Roper, T. J.: A comparative analysis of the accuracy of the Tc-99m pertechnetate brain scan: followup of 1,000 patients. J. Nucl. Med. *8,*187–196 (1967)
14. Tanasescu, D., Wolfstein, R. S., Waxman, A. D.: Critical evaluation of ^{99m}Tc-glucoheptonate as a brain imaging agent. Radiology *130,* 421–423 (1979)

Follow-Up Studies of Brain Tumours in Infants

K. Kretzschmar

Introduction

The evaluation of curative measures in patients with cerebral tumours has been based upon clinical neurological findings, post-mortem examinations and survival-times [15, 20, 33, 34].

Of the neuroradiological investigations angiography and encephalography are less important in the control of treatment. The number of examinations is limited by the invasive nature of these procedures. Also a differentiation of postoperative changes, regression of tissue and tumour can only be made to a limited extent [4, 5, 24, 29]. However the diagnostic value of CT is also important for the planning of treatment, the assessment of treatment and for follow-up-studies of cerebral tumours [9, 12, 19, 32].

Method and Material

Our investigations are based on the progress of 84 children suffering from cerebral tumour. In these children CT-follow-up studies have been performed within the last six years. We had to have the CT-data of the initial findings at the end of treatment and the subsequent investigations.

Results

In Table 1 the histology of the tumours and the methods of treatment of the 84 children are summarized together with residual tumour detectable on CT.

On the basis of the report about total or incomplete removal, 73 operated cerebral blastomas are presented in Table 2.

The largest group is formed by 31 children suffering from an astrocytic tumour. Two thirds of them are pilocytic cerebellar astrocytomas, and the others include fibrillary, gemistocytic and protoplasmatic astrocytomas (grade II) of the cerebrum, two subependymal giant-cell astrocytomas and one astroblastoma (Table 3).

Table 1. Histology and treatment of 84 cerebral tumours in children (Cyt. = Cytostatics)

Treatment	N	Op.	Op. + ϟ	Op. + ϟ + Cyt.		Cyt.	CT with tum.	CT without tumour
Histology								
Astrocytoma	31	16	13	2	–	–	14	17
Glioblastoma	4	–	–	4	–	–	4	–
Pol. spongioblast.	1	–	–	1	–	–	1	–
Ependymoma	5	1	3	1	–	–	–	5
Medulloblastoma	15	–	–	15	–	–	7	8
Craniopharyngioma	11	2	9	–	–	–	9	2
Pituitary adenoma	2	–	2	–	–	–	2	–
Pineoblastoma	1	–	–	–	–	1	1	–
Haemangioblastoma	1	1	–	–	–	–	1	–
Dediff. sarcoma	3	–	–	3	–	–	1	2
Unknown histology								
Pons region	5	–	–	–	–	5	5	–
Sella region	3	–	–	–	3	–	2	1
Pineal region	2	–	–	–	–	2	1	1
	84	20	27	26	3	8	48	36

Table 2. Completeness of the operation and CT-findings in 73 tumours in children

Histology	N	Astro-cytoma	Glio-blast.	Pol. spongio.	Epen-dym.	Medul-lobl.	Cranio-phar.	Pit. adenoma	Sar-coma
Treatment									
Total extirpation	18	14	–	–	1	–	2	–	–
Total extirpation + ϟ	4	1	–	–	2	–	1	–	–
Total extirpation + ϟ + Cytostatics	10	1	–	–	–	7	–	–	2
CT with tumour	6	1	–	–	–	3	1	–	–
CT without tumour	26	15	–	–	3	4	2	–	2
Partial operation	2	2	–	–	–	–	–	–	–
Partial operation + ϟ	23	12	–	–	1	–	8	2	–
Partial operation + ϟ + Cytostatics	16	1	4	1	1	8	–	–	1
With tumour	33	13	3	1	–	4	8	2	1
Without tumour	8	2	–	–	2	4	–	–	–

Table 3. Treatment of the 31 astrocytomas (Cyt. = Cytostatics)

Treatment	N	Op.	Op. + ↯	Op. + ↯ + Cyt.	With tumour	Without tumour
Histology						
Pilocyt. astrocytoma	21	14	7	–	7	14
Astrocytoma (grade II)	7	1	4	2	5	2
Giant-cell astrocytoma	2	1	1	–	1	1
Astroblastoma	1	–	1	–	1	–
	31	16	13	2	14	17

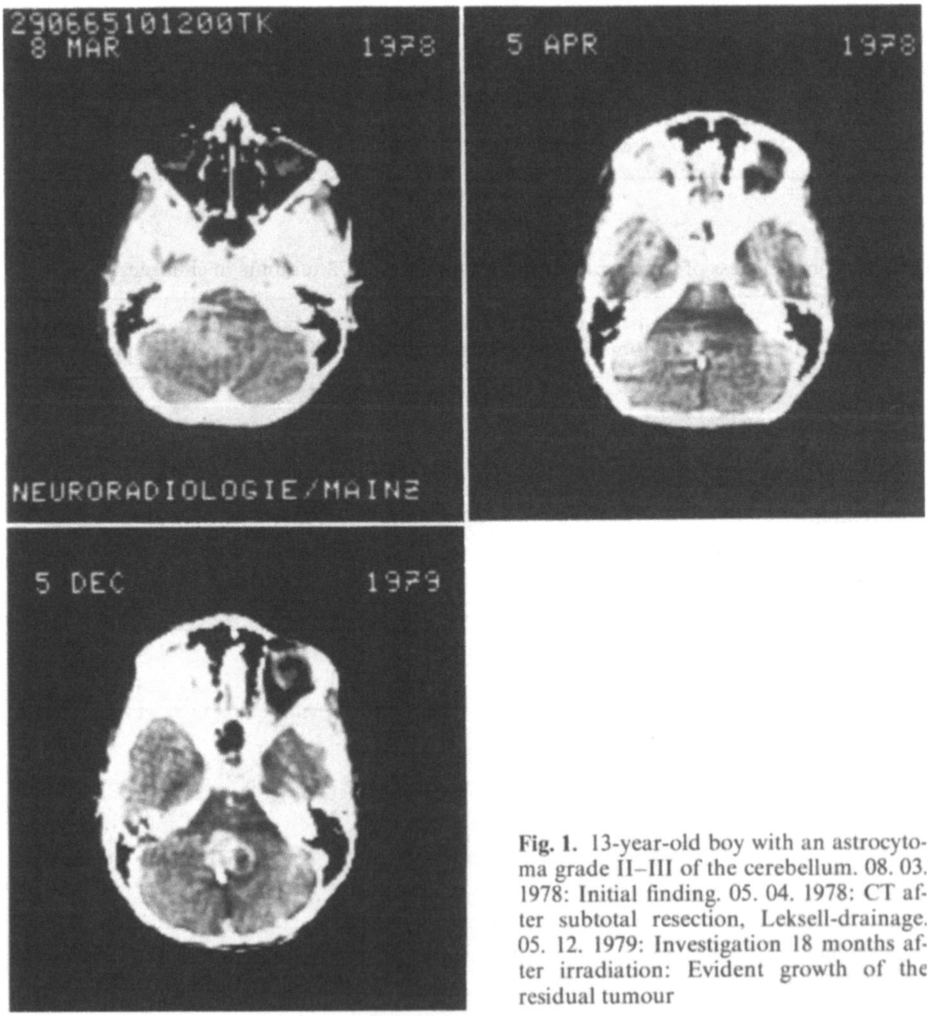

Fig. 1. 13-year-old boy with an astrocytoma grade II–III of the cerebellum. 08. 03. 1978: Initial finding. 05. 04. 1978: CT after subtotal resection, Leksell-drainage. 05. 12. 1979: Investigation 18 months after irradiation: Evident growth of the residual tumour

In 16 children operation alone was performed. Apart from a supratentorial protoplasmatic astrocytoma they have all been successful. In 15 cases irradiation and exceptionally cytostatics were given postoperatively. In two partially removed and post-irradiated astrocytomas no residual tumour can be demonstrated. The others show a diminution of a local tumour recurrence which has lasted six months. Since then a slow but continuous growth has been observed (Fig. 1).

Four patients suffered from *glioblastoma.* In one child the tumour developed in the temporo-parietal region eight years after the irradiation of a craniopharyngioma, which was given 60 Gy in opposing fields (Fig. 2). Al blastomas were removed subtotally and treated with radiation and cytostatics postoperatively. Already in the first year exacerbations of the tumour can be observed. Nevertheless one child still survives after two years under high doses of cytostatics.

The individual case of a *polar spongioblastoma* (grade IV) shows a rapid tumour growth after partial resection and combination therapy.

All the five children, whose *ependymoma* showed malignant areas remain without recurrence in a four years median control period on CT.

In the 15 patients with *medulloblastoma* just the combination of operation, radiotherapy and chemotherapy was used. In eight cases no recurrence can be seen, in two of these already for five years. Seven children showed extensive metastases along the cerebrospinal fluid pathways. In spite of this dissemination a survival of four years has been reached in two cases with the aid of additional courses of cytostatics (Fig. 3).

In the majority of the 11 children with a *craniopharyngioma* irradiation has been given as an adjunct to subtotal removal. Under CT-controls a diminution of the tumour can be seen. Cystic parts dry up, and solid portions get calcified. Also calciferous lumps can shrink. However, in the cases presented a residual part of the craniopharyngioma can still be proved for a median survival of about three years (Fig. 4).

A special case should be mentioned of a craniopharyngioma in a newborn with demonstrable intrasellar and suprasellar calcification two years later (Fig. 5).

In two chromophobe *pituitary adenomas* a slowly growing recurrence after an incomplete removal cannot be prevented, even with the aid of postoperative irradiation. In the present case of a *pineoblastoma, metastases into the CSF-spaces occur two years after irradiation and under cytostatic drugs.*

Although, according to the operation report, the haemangioblastoma was removed completely, CT follow-up studies show an enlargement of the operation cavity two years later. This finding might later be verified as a relapse.

Three children were affected with an *undifferentiated sarcoma.* In two cases no tumour was visible subsequent to postoperative irradiation and the administration of cytostatics.

Finally the material includes ten blastomas of *unknown histology.* In five *pontine tumours* first a slow and then a rapid growth is apparent on the computer-tomogram. Two of three tumours of the *sella region* show regressive changes after radiation treatment. The size of the tumour has not changed. A blastoma is melting progressively and disappearing. Four years of follow-up studies show no sign of recurrence in this child. The two tumours in the *pineal region* react differently to irradiation and chemotherapy. In one child the tumour has remained stationary for four years. In

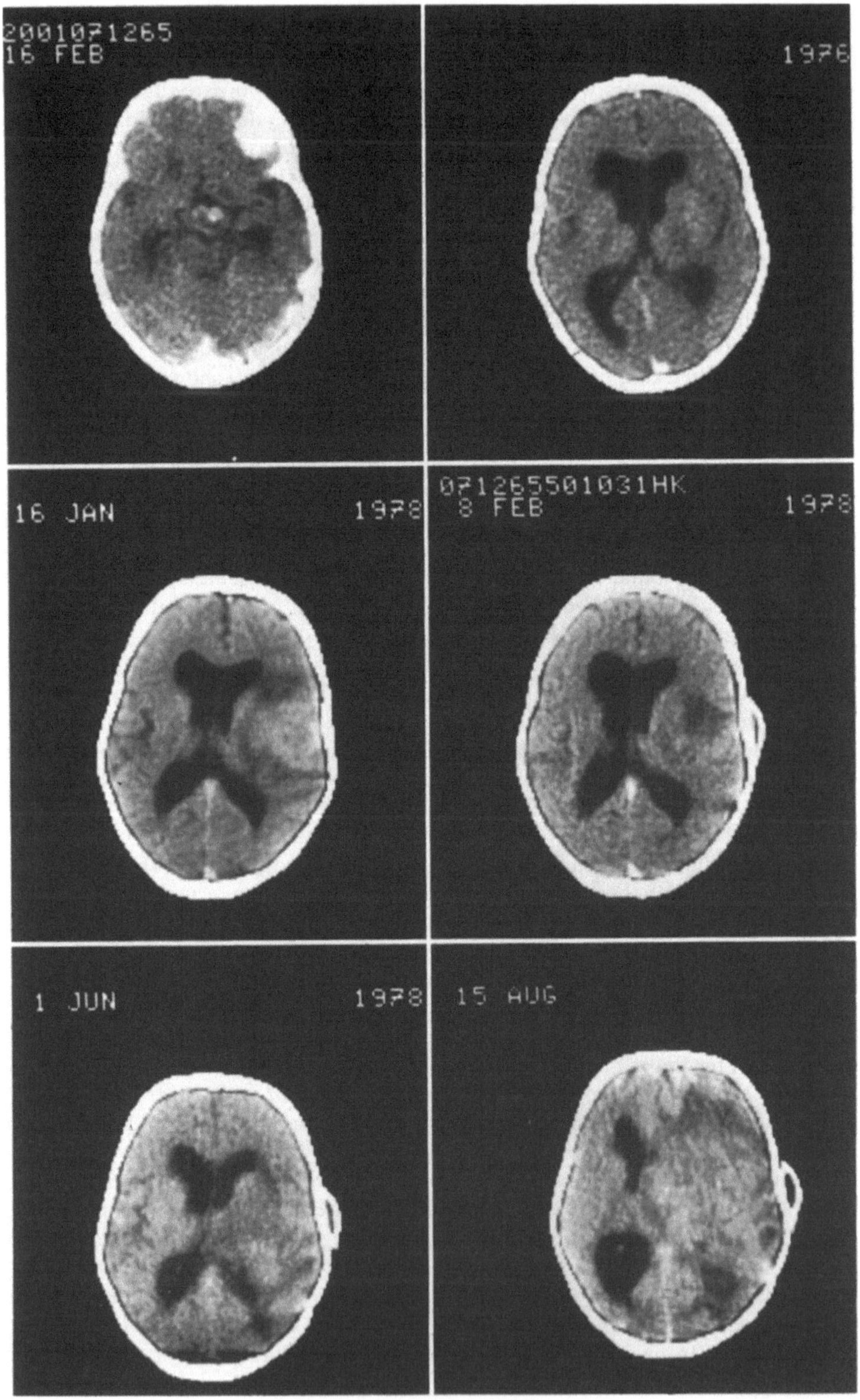

2001071265
16 FEB
1976
16 JAN
1978
071265501031HK
8 FEB
1978
1 JUN
1978
15 AUG

the other patient the blastoma and its metastases, already seen in the CT before the start of treatment, are receding completely. However, he has been observed for only ten months.

Discussion

All statistics about the therapeutic evaluation of cerebral tumours carry the risk, that there may be differences in the reaction of the host and of the biological behavior of the blastoma despite their showing the same histology [3, 34].

Gulotta [8] reports some doubts regarding the comparability and evidence of those studies. Certainly, the possibility of a biological maturation of the tumours remains unconsidered in older individuals. Therefore the stress has to be put more on the CT follow-up studies than on the discussion on lines of treatment.

In benign astrocytic tumours only a radical operation leads to a tumourless state. If there is any residue of the tumour demonstrable, its growth and a recurrence cannot be avoided, not even with the aid of a postoperative irradiation. The poor vascularization and rare mitosis determine the radioresistance of the gliomas, so that additional radiotherapeutic measures seem to be of dubious value [1, 33].

In *glioblastomas* no destruction of tumour can be obtained on the basis of conventional radiotherapy [18, 22, 23, 27]. By the additional administration of cytostatics the survival has been sufficiently prolonged [14, 31].

Our own follow-up studies however show an uninfluenced growth of the blastoma, despite postoperative radiotherapy and chemotherapy. Also the increase of a postoperatively residual portion of a polar spongioblastoma cannot be prevented at all. Zülch [36] reports about a polar spongioblastoma, which also grows rapidly in spite of radiotherapy. At the post-mortem examination no signs of any effect from the irradiation were provable in the tumour.

The CT-studies of children suffering from ependymoma do not show any failure. Not only in completely removed (N=3) but also in partially resected tumours no recurrence could be demonstrated in post-operative CT investigations.

The treatment of medulloblastomas by a combination of operation, radiotherapy and chemotherapy is now quite widely accepted. The value of chemotherapy is seen in a destruction of remaining tumour cells, in the avoidance of a local recurrence and invasion of CSF-spaces [2, 13, 30].

In the first results of this combined therapy a five years survival rate of 40% is reported (Seiler et al. 1978). The importance of additional therapeutic measures is also apparent in our own investigations. In seven children the medulloblastoma could be removed completely. In four of these children a recurrence has not ap-

Fig. 2. Subtotal resection of a craniopharyngioma in a 5-year-old girl (1970) after irradiation (60 Gy, opposing fields). 16. 02. 1976: The CT-investigation shows a remaining part of the craniopharyngioma and a dilatation of the ventricular system. The cerebral parenchyma is unremoveable. 16. 01. 1978: A glioblastoma occurs in the right temporoparietal lobe. 08. 02. 1978: Control after subtotally removal of the tumour, an Ommaya-Reservoir is implanted. 01. 06. 1978 and 15. 08. 1978: Investigations after irradiation and under the administration of cytostatics: The tumour is growing rapidly

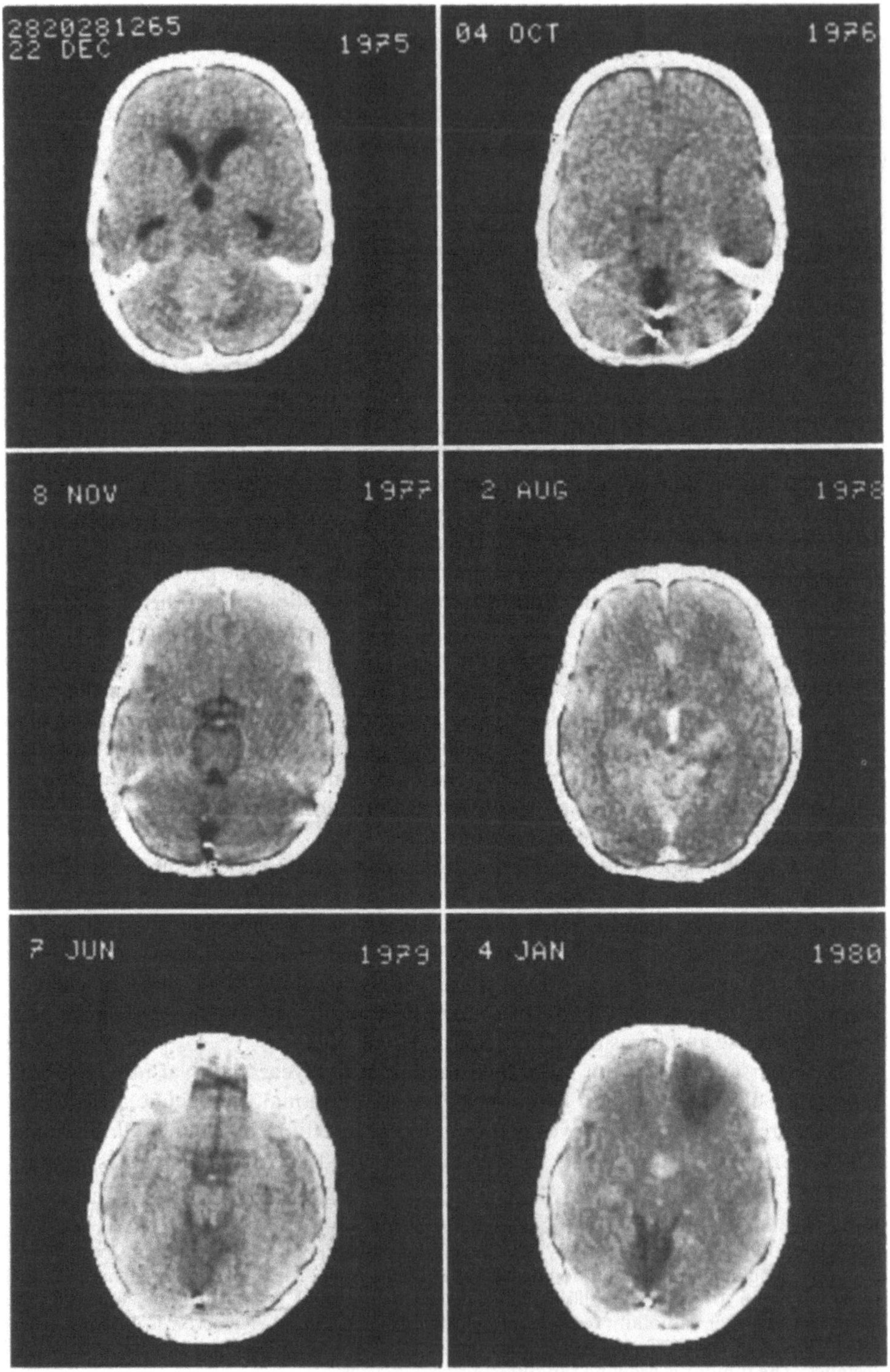
2820281265
22 DEC
1975
04 OCT
1976
8 NOV
1977
2 AUG
1978
7 JUN
1979
4 JAN
1980

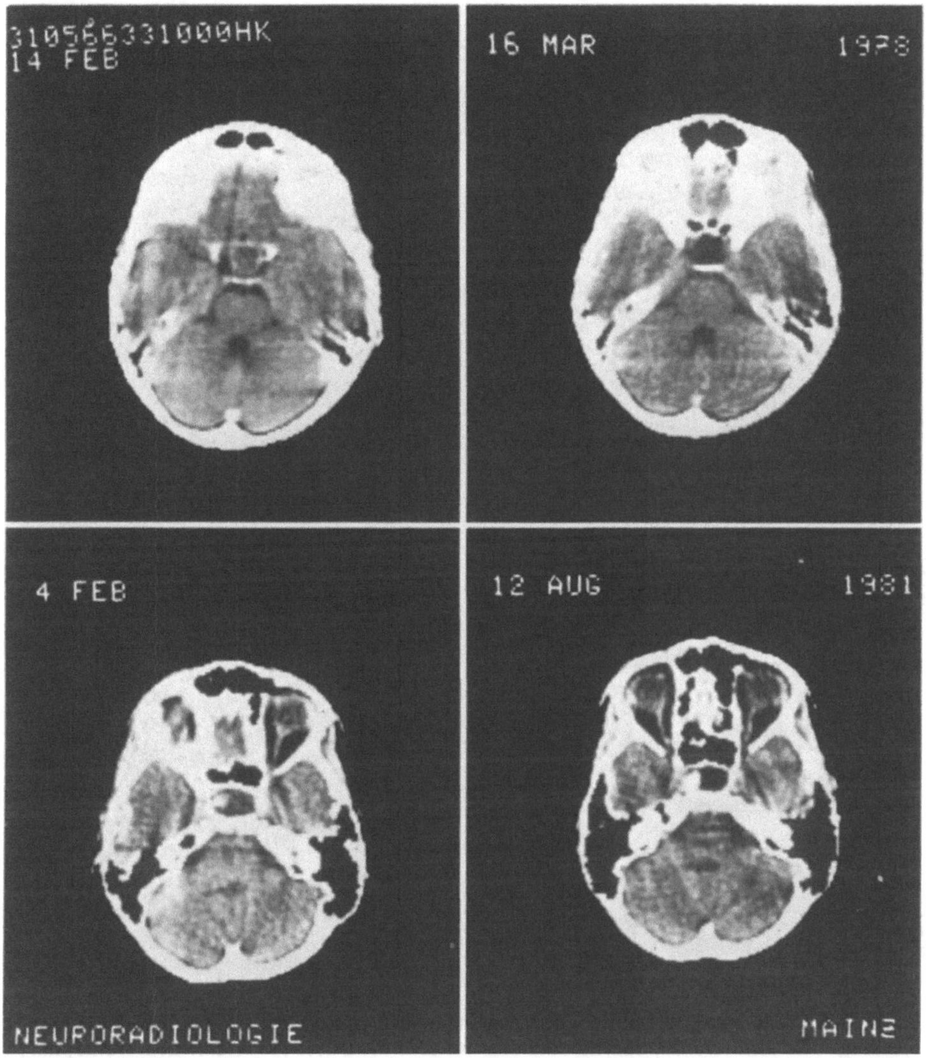

Fig. 4. 12 year-old boy with a craniopharyngioma. 14. 02. 1978: Solid, not calcified intrasellar tumour. 16. 03. 1978: Postoperative supervision (total removal): Empty sella. 04. 02. 1981: Beginning growth of the relapse, intrasellar on the left side. 12. 08. 1981: Enlargement of the intrasellar calcification. In the meantime a recurrence of the craniopharyngioma was verified by surgery

Fig. 3. 10-year-old boy with a medulloblastoma. 22. 12. 1975: Medulloblastoma with a size of 4 cm. 04. 10. 1976: Supervision after irradiation and under cytostatics: No pathological findings. No remaining tumour part. 08. 11. 1977: No tumour is provable. 02. 08. 1978: Disseminated CSF metastases. 07. 06. 1979: Repeated administration of cytostatics with subsequent regression of the dissemination. 04. 01. 1980: Recurrence of extensive metastases

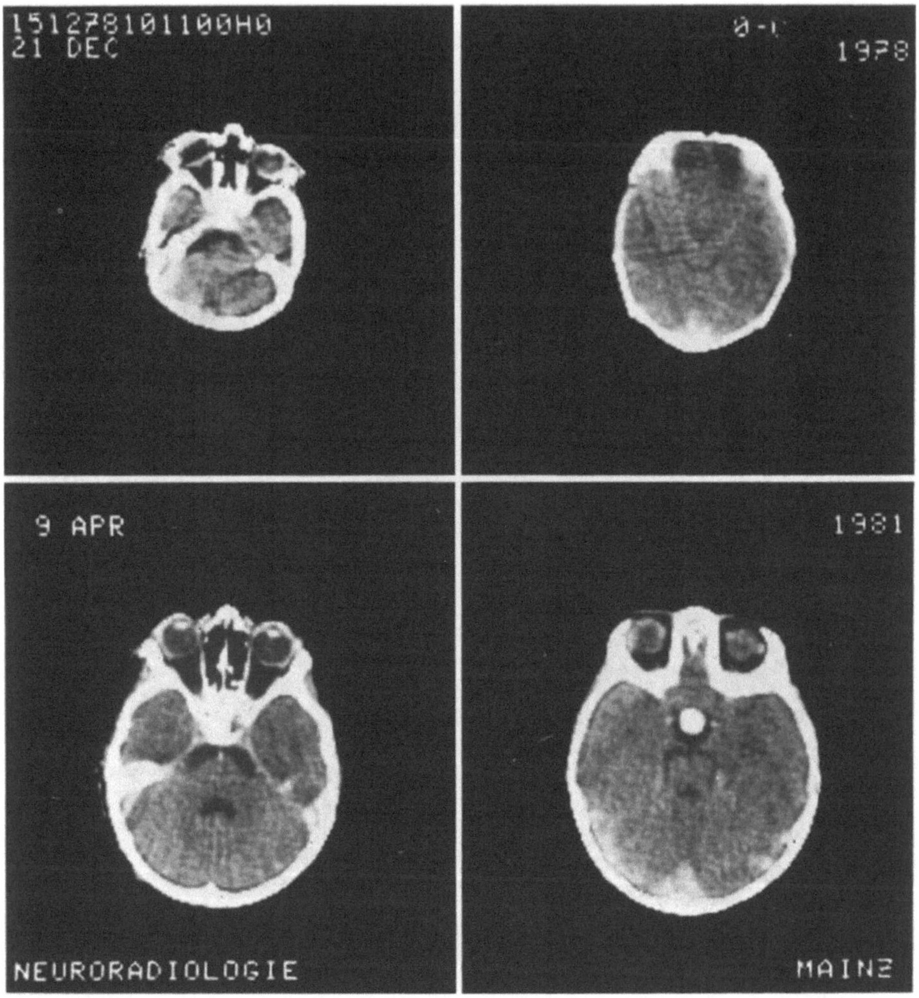

Fig. 5. 5-days-old male newborn with suspected birth injury. 21. 12. 1978: Subarachnoidal bleeding. The solid craniopharyngioma was missed. 09. 04. 1981: A calcified craniopharyngioma (operatively confirmed) is now obvious

peared within a three years mean time of supervision by CT. Two patients have survived five years.

Also in four out of eight partially removed medulloblastomas no relapse has occurred. Here, however, only CT-studies for a two years follow-up period are available. In conclusion a similar high percentage of children without any relapse occurs among the completely and the incompletely removed blastomas.

Radiotherapy of craniopharyngiomas should support the tendency of these tumours towards regressive changes. At the same time a dehydration of the cysts of the adamantinomatous tissue or of the epithelial cells can be observed [2, 10, 11, 21]. Of the 11 craniopharyngiomas only one child with a complete tumour removal has achieved a tumourless state. Postoperatively visible remnants of the blastomas indeed show increasing regressive changes, but six years after the initial treatment parts of the craniopharyngiomas can still be demonstrated.

The value of supplementary radiotherapy after a partial resection of a pituitary adenoma is not uniformly commended [3, 7, 16]. The CT follow-up studies presented here do not show any effect of the radiation on the growth of the adenoma.

On the other hand the undifferentiated forms of pinealomas belong to the most radiosensitive tumours [15, 17, 35, 36].

Despite this radiosensitivity the tendency of pinealomas to disseminate into the cerebrospinal fluid spaces determine the CT follow-up studies. Under the combination of irradiation and chemotherapy one child obtained a state of apparently complete remission.

A cure can be achieved by a complete removal of an angioblastoma [34]. Therefore any failure shown on the computer tomograph can only accounted for by a remnant of tumour left at the operation or by a second haemangioblastoma.

There are only case-reports available, concerning treatment of patients with a sarcoma [36]. Because of the different mesodermal origin of the tumours they are less amenable to comparison. After a complete removal two out of three tumours presented in follow-up controls remain without any relapse but a partially operated tumour is growing in spite of radiotherapy and chemotherapy.

According to Cocchi [6] one third of 20 patients with a histologically unclassified pons tumour survives three years after irradiation. In our cases all the five children died within one year. After radiotherapy and under cytostatics a short lasting regression of the volume of the tumours was observed by CT in only two cases.

In general we can say, that in benign tumours only a radical removal leads to freedom from tumour. If a remnant of the tumour can be seen postoperatively, a regression of the mass cannot be obtained, even with the aid of irradiation.

Concerning the recurrence-free interval children with a malignant blastoma do not show any interrelation with the completeness of removal. After incidental irradiation the remaining parts of the tumour show a diminution for six months. Afterwards the blastoma grows rapidly. If the operation is followed by a combination of radiotherapy and chemotherapy, on the average some regression of the tumour can be seen for one year. Independent of the site and malignancy of the recurrence any secondary treatment was unsuccessful. In two children CT-controls demonstrate regression of a tumour with unknown histology in the region of the sella and the pineal only after radiation and after radiotherapy and chemotherapy.

Finally the value of CT-investigations should be pointed out. One can obtain further informations and add the CT-appearances of tumour behavior to the therapeutic judgement of survival or the five-year survival rate. We have seen several children achieving a survival period of more than five years.

During this time, however, a slowly growing tumour can be verified on CT.

References

1. Arndt, J.:Indikationen und Grenzen der Strahlentherapie bösartiger Neubildungen. Stuttgart: Gustav Fischer-Verlag 1973
2. Bloom, H. J. G.: Combined modality therapy for intracranial tumours. Cancer *35*, 111–120 (1975)

3. Bouchard, J.: Radiation therapy of tumours and diseases of the nervous system. Philadelphia: Lea and Febinger 1966
4. Breit, A., Pfeiffer, J.: Mehrfache Angiographien während der Röntgenbestrahlung. Acta Radiol. *46,* 469–473 (1956)
5. Cocchi, U.: Radiotherapie des Glioblastoms. Zbl. Neurochir. *19,* 304–305 (1959)
6. Cocchi, U.: Die Bestrahlung von Hirntumoren. Strahlenforschung und Strahlenbehandlung, Band IV. Sonderbände Strahlentherapie *52,* 34–46 (1963)
7. Correa, J. N., Lampe, J.: The radiation treatment of pituitary adenomas. J. Neurosurg. *19,* 626–631 (1962)
8. Gulotta, F.: Bemerkungen zur Chemotherapie maligner Hirntumoren. Dt. Med. Wschr. *105,* 973–975 (1980)
9. Hyman, R. A., Loring, M. F., Liebeskind, A. L., Naidich, H. B., Stein, H. L.: Computed tomographic evaluation of therapeutically induced changes in primary and secondary brain tumours. Neuroradiology *14,* 213–218 (1978)
10. Kramer, S., Mc Kissock, W., Concannoni, J. P.: Craniopharyngiomas. Treatment by combined surgery and radiation therapy. J. Neurosurg. *18,* 217–226 (1961)
11. Kramer, S., Southard, M., Mansfield, C. M.: Radiotherapy in the management of craniopharyngiomas – further experiences and late results. Am. J. Roentgenol. *103,* 44–52 (1968)
12. Kretzschmar, K., Aulich, A., Schindler, E., Lange, S., Grumme, Th., Meese, W.: The diagnostic value of CT for radiotherapy of cerebral tumours. Neuroradiology *14,* 245–250 (1978)
13. Lampkin, B. C., Higgins, G. R., Hammond, D.: Absence of neurotoxity following massive intrathecal administration of Methotrexate. Cancer *20,* 1780–1781 (1967)
14. Levin, V. A., Crafts, D. C., Norman, D. M., Hoffer, P. B., Spire, J. P., Wilson, C. B.: Criteria for evaluating patients undergoing chemotherapy for malignant brain tumours. J. Neurosurg. *47,* 329–335 (1977)
15. Lindgren, M.: On tolerance of brain tissue and sensitivity of brain tumours to irradiation. Acta Radiol. Suppl. 170 (1958)
16. Löhr, H.-H., Vieten, H.: Die Strahlenbehandlung raumbeengender intrakranieller Prozesse. Handbuch der Neurochirurgie, Band 4. Eds.: H. Olivecrona, W. Tönnis. Berlin, Heidelberg, New York: Springer 1967
17. Mincer, F., Meltzer, J., Botstein, C.: Pinealoma. A report of twelve irradiated cases. Cancer *37,* 2713–2718 (1976)
18. Mundinger, F.: Erfahrungen mit der stereotaktischen interstitiellen Brachytherapie mit Ir 192-„Gamma-Med" bei infiltrierenden Hirntumoren. Fortschr. Röntgenstrahlen *110,* 259–261 (1969)
19. Norman, D., Enzmann, D. R., Levin, V. A., Wilson, C. B., Newton, T. H.: Computed tomography in the evaluation of malignant glioma before and after therapy. Radiology *121,* 85–88 (1976)
20. Pennybacker, J., Russell, D. S.: Necrosis of the brain due to radiation therapy; clinical and pathological observations. J. Neurol. Neurosurg. Psychiat. *11,* 183–198 (1948)
21. Petito, C. K., De Girolami, U., Earle, K. M.: Craniopharyngiomas. A clinical and pathological review. Cancer *37,* 1944–1952 (1976)
22. Salazar, O. M., Rubin, P., Mc Donald, J. V., Feldstein, M. L.: High dose radiation therapy in the treatment of glioblastoma multiforme: a preliminary report. Int. J. Radiat. Oncol. Biol. Phys. *1,* 717–727 (1976)
23. Schryver, A. De., Greitz, T., Forsby, N., Brun, A.: Localized shaped field radiotherapy of malignant glioblastoma multiforme. Int. J. Radiat. Oncol. Biol. Phys. *1,* 713–716 (1976)
24. Schwarz, G., Schreyer, H., Argyropoulos, G.: Radiology for detecting brain tumour recurrences. Acta Radiol. *17,* 193–199 (1976)
25. Seiler, R. W., Imbach, P., Vassella, F., Wagner, H. P.: Adjuvant chemotherapy with intraventricular methotrexate and CCNU after surgery and radiotherapy of medulloblastomas. Helv. paediat. Acta *33,* 235–239 (1978)
26. Sheline, G. E.: Radiation therapy of tumours of the central nervous system in childhood. Cancer *35,* 957–964 (1975)
27. Simpson, W. J., Platts, M. E.: Fractionation study in the treatment of glioblastoma multiforme. Int. J. Radiat. Oncol. Biol. Phys. *1,* 639–644 (1976)

28. Smith, N. J., El-Mahdi, A. M., Constable, W. C.: Results of irradiation of tumours in the region of the pineal body. Acta Radiol. Ther. Phys. Biol. *15,* 17–22 (1976)
29. Suzuki, J., Hori, S.: Evaluation of radiotherapy of tumours in the pineal region by ventriculographic studies with iodized oil. J. Neurosurg. *30,* 595–603 (1969)
30. Terheggen, H. G.: Die Therapie des Medulloblastoms und Ependymoms im Kindesalter. Dt. Med. Wschr. *102,* 899–901 (1977)
31. Weir, B., Band, P., Urtasun, R., Blain, G., Mc Lean, D., Wilson, F., Mielke, B., Grace, M.: Radiotherapy and CCNU in the treatment of highgrade supratentorial astrocytomas. J. Neurosurg. *45,* 129–134 (1976)
32. Zimmerman, R. A., Bilaniuk, L. T., Grundy, G., Littman, P.: Computed tomographic localization for radiotherapy of cerebral tumours. Radiology *119,* 230–231 (1976)
33. Zülch, K. J.: Biologie und Pathologie der Hirngeschwülste. In: Handbuch der Neurochirurgie, Band 3. Eds.: H. Olivecrona, W. Tönnis. Berlin, Göttingen, Heidelberg: Springer 1956
34. Zülch, K. J.: Über die Strahlensensibilität der Hirngeschwülste und die sogenannte Strahlenspätnekrose des Hirns. Dt. Med. Wschr. *85,* 293–298 (1960)
35. Zülch, K. J.: Morphologische Veränderungen an Geschwülsten nach Bestrahlung und Schädigungsmöglichkeit am normalen Hirn. Strahlenforschung und Strahlenbehandlung IV. Sonderbände Strahlentherapie *52,* 47–62 (1963)
36. Zülch, K. J.: Roentgen sensitivity of cerebral tumours and so-called late irradiation necrosis of the brain. Acta Radiol. Ther. *18,* 92–110 (1969)

Computed Tomography and/or Ventriculography?

S. Wende, T. Kishikawa, N. Hüwel, E. Kazner, Th. Grumme, and
W. R. Lanksch

In spite of the introduction of CT some clinics today are still using ventriculography with positive water-soluble contrast medium in order to diagnose space-occupying intracranial lesions.

In considering our own cases the following questions should be considered:

1) In which cases should a ventriculography be done in addition to CT?
2) What kind of positive evidence is provided by CT and ventriculography for the localization of a tumour and its differential diagnosis?

Our investigations have been done between 1975 and 1980, and in this time 134 patients had been studied (Mainz: 120 patients, Berlin: 10 patients, Munich: 4 patients). There were 93 children (up to 14 years old) and 41 adults. The number of patients is almost similar in all age groups, although a predominance of the 1st year of age (40 patients) is obvious.

Table 1 represents the different clinical syndromes leading to CT-investigations and ventriculography. The accuracy of localization and differential diagnosis is also indicated.

Referring to our own experiences and the results obtained ventriculography does not show any diagnostic advantage in cerebral tumours compared to CT. Also in the ventriculogram the tumour cannot be so clearly marked off and differentiated as is possible with CT. In fact just the opposite applies: With regard to the differential diagnosis computerized tomography is apparently superior to ventriculography. Also the question of operability of a tumour located in the region of the midline or in the posterior fossa cannot be answered better with the aid of ventriculography. Own investigations of the CT of patients who showed "inoperable" tumours in ventriculography proved that this diagnosis was not correct.

Certainly, some of the computed tomograms obtained by CT-scanners of the 1st and 2nd generation were hard to interpret, especially by the unexperienced, so that many neurosurgeons reverted to the familiar method of ventriculography. However, these problems which occurred at the beginning of the CT-era cannot be taken today as an indication for ventriculography, which anyway is an invasive method of investigation, occasions more stress for the patient, may show side-effects and can occasionally even lead to serious complications.

With the CT-scanners which are available today a tumour in the posterior fossa can be so clearly reproduced, that, in the majority of patients, the CT-scan is perfectly adequate for planning of a neurosurgical operation. Only in a few cases, especially in highly vascular lesions shown in the CT, is angiography necessary in addition to settle conclusively the differential diagnosis between tumour, angioma or aneurysm.

Undoubtedly in some cases the operability of a space-occupying lesion in the posterior fossa cannot be decided with certainty, either by CT or ventriculography. Therefore it is difficult to say before the operation, if a tumour in the fourth ventricle can be completely removed or not. Own experiences from the era of ventriculography are proving that sometimes a fourth ventricle tumour thought to be

Table 1

Tumour Nature and Site	n	CT		Ventriculography	
		Site +	Nature +	Site +	Nature +
Posterior Fossa Pilocytic astrocytoma Medulloblastoma Ependymoma Metastases Pontine tumour	32	32	22	24	–
Hemispheres Multiple abscesses Astrocytoma	3	3	3	1	–
Tumours of the Ventricle Thalamus Ependymoma	3	3	3	3	–
Tumours of the Midline Dermoid Craniopharyngioma Pinealoma	12	12	12	10	10
Tumours of the Cerebello-pontine Angle	5	5	5	3	–
Malformations Holoprosencephaly Encephalocoele Agenesis of corpus callosum Arnold Chiari Dandy-Walker	19	19	19	10	5
Nothing abnormal	3	–	–	–	–
Stenosis of the Aqueduct	32	32	–	28	–
Occlusion of the Aqueduct (Non-tumourous)					
Hydrocephalus (Non-tumourous)	18	18	–	18	–
Cysts	7	7	7	7	–
Third ventricle Posterior fossa Foramen of Monro					

inoperable could be removed completely, although ventriculography showed an "inoperable" tumour in the floor of the fourth ventricle. Finally, in every doubtful case the neurosurgeon is forced to explore the posterior fossa in order to clarify the situation by direct examination and possible biopsy. No method of investigation available so far is able to replace such an intervention, which may also lead to a definite histological diagnosis.

If hydrocephalus has already been diagnosed by computer tomography, it is still not possible when using the standard CT technique to decide whether the lesion present is a stenosis or a complete occlusion of the aqueduct. In such a case there is no doubt that ventriculography is superior to CT. At the same time it is necessary to consider whether a ventriculography is justifiable, because a shunt operation is indicated just as much in the case of an occlusion as with a stenosis. Also, if long-term pressure measurements are being made via an indwelling ventricular catheter with the aim of facilitating the choice of valve to be used, it is still not justifiable to inject positive contrast medium into the ventricles.

Because of the blockage of the cerebro-spinal flow many patients with posterior fossa tumours show an increase in the intracranial pressure, which can be recognized from the dilatation of the ventricles and a periventricular lucency in CT. In these cases many neurosurgeons think a release of pressure prior to the operation is necessary, and this can be done either as a temporary external drainage via a frontal burr-hole or a shunt system can be implanted. Very often this temporary and also long-lasting decompression is used to inject a positive contrast medium via an indwelling ventricular catheter in order to perform a ventriculography. However, when the diagnosis of a space-occupying lesion has been made by CT, it should not be verified once more by a further method of investigation. Ventriculography is not able to supply any additional useful information, with regard to the necessary neurosurgical intervention. It is just an increase of risk.

In former times a ventriculography was also done for the differential diagnosis of cystic lesions including congenital lesions and malformations, in order to verify the communication with the ventricles and/or the subarachnoid space. A CT after the intrathecal injection of a small amount of metrizamide is able to answer more exactly the question concerning the communication between cystic lesions and the cerebro-spinal fluid pathways. Here also a ventriculography is not necessary anyway.

To summarize we can say, that there is no longer any clear-cut indication for doing ventriculography in intracranial tumours and other space-occupying lesions. In some cases a CT-examination combined with metrizamide given intrathecally may be useful.

Ventriculography as a Diagnostic Procedure in CNS Tumours in Childhood: Its Indications and Interpretation

H. Altenburg, M. Brandt, and H.-J. König

Diagnostic procedures, treatment and follow-up in midline tumours of the brain have been changed by the CT scan [5].

Before the CT era tumours associated with raised intracranial pressure were usually detected by ventriculography. Nowadays the CT scan has to be compared with other neuroradiological methods, especially ventriculography with positive contrast medium [1, 3, 14].

CT is only one among a great variety of different diagnostic methods. Only a considered combination of procedures can give reliable results [11, 17, 19]. According to our experience ventriculography with water soluble contrast medium remains a valuable investigation [3, 9, 12, 14, 15]. Obstructive midline tumours which have already caused enlargement of the ventricles can be diagnosed and distinguished. Ventriculography may also be performed as an operative diagnostic procedure in cases where shunting or drainage of cerebrospinal fluid is necessary [2, 7, 15, 18] (Fig. 1).

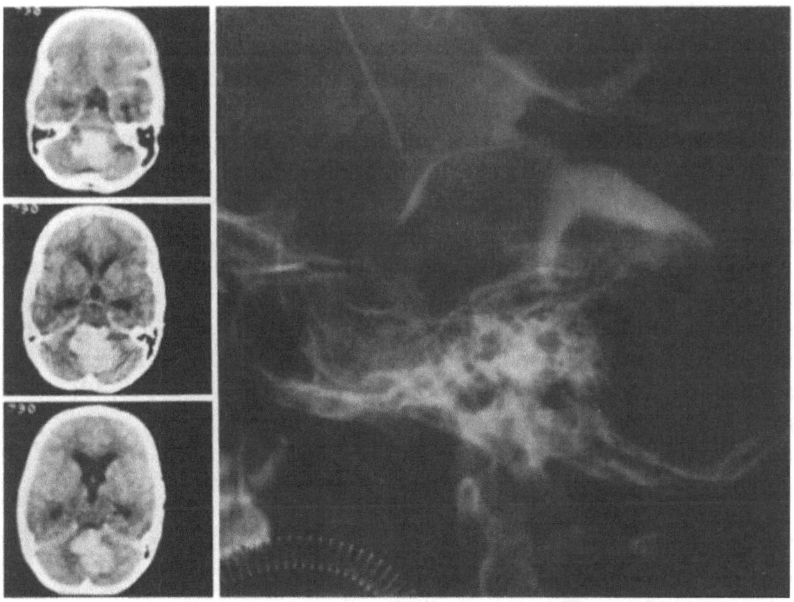

Fig. 1. CT and ventriculographic findings in posterior fossa tumour (medulloblastoma)

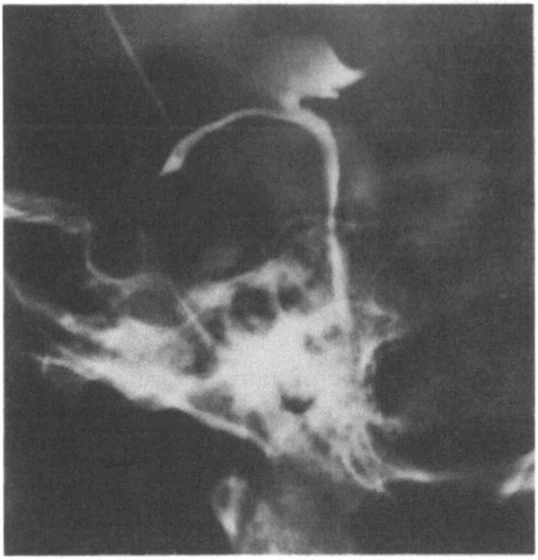

Fig. 2. Ventriculographic findings of a medial cerebellar tumour (lateral view): no tumour tissue on the bottom of the 4th ventricle

Even if a midline tumour can be detected by CT scan the surgeon may need more specific information for the planning and performance of the operation. Ventriculography gives more details about the exact location of space occupying midline tumours and their relation to surrounding brain structures [1, 3, 14, 18, 20] (Fig. 2).

If CT findings are negative or difficult to interpret ventriculography sometimes helps to complete the diagnostic procedure as well as it does in some cases of hydrocephalus [4, 6, 7, 10, 16, 17].

After chemotherapy or radiotherapy of midline tumours ventriculography can be useful to control the effect of treatment. It makes the diagnosis more reliable and answers the question as to whether the tumour can be operated upon or not.

Different neuroradiological methods should be performed in order to make a clear decision about the indications for operation, because in many cases an operation on a midline tumour carries with it a considerable risk for the patient.

In all cases the assault on the child must be recognised. Risky diagnostic procedure can only be performed, if good results can be expected. The evidence of the results of treatment after ventriculography should be undoubted [8, 12, 13, 19].

Some cases will show the value of positive contrast ventriculography.

1) With a midline tumour detected by CT scan one has to consider what kind of tumour it might be and obtain information about its operability.
2) Doubtful or negative CT findings.
3) Cause of hydrocephalus – this is of importance in deciding what particular neurosurgical procedure may be necessary (16).
4) Follow-up in cases with no effect from radiotherapy.
5) Decompression of cystic tumours during ventriculography.

Conclusion

Invasive diagnostic methods like positive ventriculography should be carefully performed after less invasive procedures have been done. Growing experience with CT scan means that the indications for ventriculography become progressively fewer. It should only be done in patients with raised CSF pressure. In cases of doubtful CT findings additional information may be necessary before undertaking surgical treatment [7].

If in spite of negative CT findings a tumour is suspected ventriculography should be performed, as well as in cases of hydrocephalus of unknown origin. In these cases it gives more information about which neurosurgical procedure is required.

References

1. Agnoli, , Eggert, H. R., Zierski, J., Seeger, W., Kirchhoff, D.: Diagnostische Möglichkeiten der positiven Ventrikulographie. Acta Neurochir. *31,* 227–243 (1975)
2. Albright, L., Reigel, D. H.: Management of hydrocephalus secondary to posterior fossa tumours. J. Neurosurgery *46,* 52–55 (1977)
3. Altenburg, H., Walter, W.: Die zentrale Ventrikulographie. Indikationen, Technik, Ergebnisse. In: Der Hirnstammtumor. Gund, A., Koos, W. (eds.), Stuttgart: Thieme 1982 (in prep.)
4. Belloni, G., Cardarelli, M., Di Rocco, S., Rossi, G. F.: Extra-axial subarachnoid cyst of posterior fossa: Clinical diagnostic studies. Acta Neurochir. *44,* 258 (1978)
5. Berger, P. E., Kirks, D. R., Gilday, D. L., Fitz, C. R., Harwood-Nash, D. C.: Computed tomography in infants and children: Intracranial neoplasms. Amer. J. Roentgenol. *127,* 129–137 (1976)
6. Bradac, G. B., Simon, R. S., Grumme, T., Schramm, J.: Limitations of computed tomography for diagnostic neuroradiology. Neuroradiology *13,* 243–247 (1977)
7. Camins, M. B., Schlesinger, E. B.: Treatment of tumours of the posterior part of the third ventricle and the pineal region: a long term follow-up. Acta Neurochir. *40,* 131–143 (1978)
8. Clar, H. E., Bock, W. J., Weichert, H. C.: Comparison of encephalotomograms and computerized tomograms in midline tumours in infants. Acta Neurochir. *50,* 91–101 (1979)
9. Cronqvist, S.: Ventriculography with Amipaque. Neuroradiology *12,* 25–32 (1976)
10. Davis, K. R., Taveras, J. M., Roberson, G. H., Ackerman, R. H.: Some limitations of computed tomography in the diagnosis of neurological diseases. Amer. J. Roentgenol. *127,* 111–116 (1976)
11. Davis, K. R., Poletti, C. E., Roberson, G. H., Tadmor, R., Kjellberg, R. N.: Complementary role of computed tomography and other neuroradiologic procedures. Surg. Neurol. *8,* 437–446 (1977)
12. Fitz, C. R., Harwood-Nash, D. C., Chuang, S., Resjo, I. M.: Metrizamide ventriculography and computed tomography in infants and children. Neuroradiology *16,* 6–9 (1978)
13. Helwig, H., Wooge, K.: Die Effektivität diagnostischer Maßnahmen in der klinischen Pädiatrie. Mschr. Kinderheilk. *126,* 583–587 (1978)
14. Kunze, St.: Ventrikulographie mit positiven Kontrastmitteln. In: Handbuch der medizinischen Radiologie XIV/2. Diethelm, L., Wende, S. (eds.). Berlin, Heidelberg, New York: Springer 1977
15. Leonardi, M., Cecetto, C., Fabris, G.: Corrales selective ventriculography in the study of posterior fossa pathology. J. Neurosurg. Sci. *21,* 65–70 (1977)
16. Palmieri, A., Menichelli, F., Paquini, U., Salvolini, U.: Role of computed tomography in the postoperative evaluation of infantile hydrocephalus. Neuroradiology *14,* 257–262 (1978)

17. Reisner, Th.: Möglichkeiten und Grenzen der kranialen Computertomographie. Wien. klin. Wschr. *89,* 541–547 (1977)
18. Thiebot, J., Launay, M., Merland, J. J., Fredy, D., Bories, J.: Mass lesions of the mesencephalon. J. Neuroradiology *5,* 83–90 (1978)
19. Winston, K. R.: Neurodiagnostic tests in children with brain tumours: Changing patterns of use and impact on cost. Pediatrics *61,* 847–852 (1978)
20. Yasuoka, S., Okazaki, H., Dambe, J. R., Mac Carty, C. S.: Foramen magnum tumours. Analysis of 57 cases of benign extramedullary tumours. J. Neurosurg. *49,* 828–838 (1978)

The Diffuse Brain Stem Astrocytoma in Childhood: Morphology, Course, and Prognosis

H. P. Schmitt and W. Zeisner

Introduction

Gliomas of the brain stem are widely regarded as a rather common and clinically unique neoplastic disease entity, although they are not actually unique with respect to their histological appearance. They occur mainly in childhood and adolescence (65–77 per cent, e.g. [16, 33]), but they are well known also in adults within a wide age range [e.g. 11, 14, 38].

Among twelve autopsy cases within the period given below we had only one woman aged 34, who had suddenly died from a massive pontine haemorrhage, and the glioma of the lower pontine region was only found by chance. Nevertheless she had had a 15 years history of sudden attacks of respiratory failure, excitement, postural hypotension, and other autonomic dysfunctions, but she had been regarded as a hypochondriac by various practitioners.

In large clinical series gliomas of the lower brain stem comprise about 15 per cent of all neuroepithelial tumours occurring in the posterior fossa [e.g. 5, 17]. They most often occur in or arise from the pons, although occasionally the midbrain and the medulla oblongata may also be the primary sites [1, 7, 9–11, 18].

Although not always primarily malignant, gliomas of the lower brain stem have, as a rule, a poor prognosis with only rather few exceptions, as will be shown later. This is due both to their unfavourable location and to their great tendency to undergo anaplastic transformation (e.g. 63 per cent [33]).

For a long time these tumours have attracted attention among both clinicians and pathologists [e.g. 36 to 31], and the number of cases reported in the literature amounts to at least 600 cases. This is still a comparatively small number if related to the total frequency of gliomatous tumours in infancy and childhood. The most complicated clinical problems such as clear diagnosis and indications for and mode of treatment as well as the assessment of the prognosis in the individual case, require much more experience with this group of gliomas.

Some people basically question the efficiency of any treatment in pontine astrocytomas of childhood and adopt a mood resignation. Progress regarding these problems can only be obtained by analysis of larger samples of clinical and pathological observations, which can only be achieved by pooling of the material from different medical centres and observers.

Hence, we do not only wish to comment on twenty cases with clinical and/or pathological data which have been observed in the Heidelberg Medical Centre in the years 1968 to 1981, but also on comparative data from the literature. We do this particularly with respect to the basic question, as to whether modern concepts of treatment, such as radiation and chemotherapy, have been able to improve significantly the poor prognosis of the primary brain stem tumours [e.g. 23], as compared to untreated cases or cases in former times, where treatment was either considered as impossible or was merely restricted to an attempt at a surgical approach. The latter, however, was most often limited to an operative exploration without any attempt to remove the tumour.

Personal Observations

Clinical Data. The main data of our cases can be derived from Tables 1 and 2. Eighteen of the 20 children had died within the period concerned. In 11 of them, a complete or partial autopsy (of the cranial cavity and of the spinal cord) could be performed. From one surgically treated child the exact anatomical situation was given by the surgical report, and microscopic slides were available from the files.

Ten children were male and ten female. The age at the onset of the first symptoms ranged from 2 to 13 years with an average of seven years. The mean age when death occurred was only about eight years, so that the average survival time (for the 18 victims) was only about one year. Their survival times ranged from one month to three years from the first onset of symptoms. Two children are still alive and are in fairly good condition. In one case the survival is already for nine years and in the other 13 years. So the survival time for the 20 children would average 22.5 months with a range from 1 to 156 months.

Hence, 90 per cent of the children died within three years, 85 per cent within two years and 65 per cent within one year from the onset of symptoms.

Treatment was omitted in only three children aged 5, 6 and 13 when they died. Their survival periods from the first symptoms to death were extremely short, i.e. 1, 2 and 3 months.

Seventeen children received treatment of various kinds, either radiation alone or combined with chemotherapy (see Tables 1 and 2). In some cases a ventricular shunt had to be inserted because of hydrocephalic complications, which, however, most often occurred at an advanced stage. In one child a surgical approach led to enucleation of a walnut-sized tumour of the pons, but there was an extension into the right cerebellar hemisphere. Despite additional repeated courses of radiation treatment with a high total dose (see Table 1, case 9) she expired 22 months after the first onset of symptoms.

The clinical symptoms varied somewhat depending on the site and spread of the tumour, but they were basically rather typical and in general coinciding with those outlined extensively in the literature (e.g. 11, 19, 25]). Strabismus and papilloedema were infrequent occurrences and increase of intracranial pressure, as a rule, occurred late, initiating the terminal phase. Headache, deviations of the head position, cranial nerve palsies, and hemiparesis (-plegia) or tetraplegia were most common.

Morphological data (Gross Appearance). In eleven of the twelve cases with either necropsy examination or surgical approach, the tumours seemed to have originated

Table 1. Brain stem tumours: clinical cases (without autopsy) (*VCR* Vincristine sulfate; *Cb* Cerebellum; *CCNU* 1-(2 chloroethyl)-3 cyclohexyl-1-nitrosourea)

Case	Name	Sex Month/Year of birth	Clinical diagnosis (location)	1st Symptoms		Death	Time of survival (months)	Therapy	
				Time	Age			Irradiation (dose)	Chemoth.
1)	Stephanie B.	Female 1/66	Pons glioma	4/76	10	4/77	12	5000 rads	VCR, CCNU
2)	Ralf D.	Male 8/67	Pons glioma	8/75	8	12/75	4	3560 rads (interrupted)	0
3)	Daniela H.	Female 7/65	Pons glioma	3/78	13	10/79	19	4800 rads	0
4)	Marion G.	Female 10/72	Pontomesencephalic glioma	10/75	3	6/76	8	4150 rads	0
5)	Alexandra V.	Female 6/73	Pons glioma	3/79	6	1/80	10	5000 rads	0
6)	Andreas W.	Male 7/66	Pons glioma	1968	2	–	156[a] (=13 years!)	4566 rads	0
7)	Roland D.	Male 8/67	Pons glioma	8/72	5	–	106[a] (= 9 years!)	5003 rads	0
8)	Hans-J. B.	Male 3/59	Pons glioma	6/72	13	6/75	3	5580 rads	0
9)	Tanja R.	Female 10/66	Pons → Cb glioma	3/70	4	1/72	22	7408 rads (following surgical removal of a walnut-sized pons tumour: astrocytoma grade II) (E.-No. 9698/70)	0

[a] Still living and in good condition

Table 2. Brain stem tumours: autopsy cases (*Bc* Basal cisterns; *Bg* basal ganglia; *Cb* cerebellum; *CSF* cerebrospinal fluid; *Dc* diencephalon; *Mb* midbrain; *Mo* medulla oblongata; *lv* lateral ventricle; *Spc* spinal canal; *VCR* vincristine sulfate; *CCNU* 1-(2 chloroethyl)-3 cyclohexyl-1-nitrosourea; *END* endoxane; *MTx* methotrexate)

Case	Autopsy no.	Sex Month/Year of birth	Tumour Location and spread	Histological diagnosis	1st Symptoms month/year	Death (age)	survival time (months)	Therapy	
								Irrad. (rads)	Chemoth.
1)	204/71	Male 7/65	*Pons* (right-sided maximum) ⇉ Cb, CSF, Infundibulum, olfactory bulb	Astrocytoma (IV) (glioblastoma)	12/70	2/71 (6)	2	0	0
2)	274/71	Female 5/66	*Pons* (right-sided maximum) ⇉ Cb, Mo	Astrocytoma (IV) (glioblastoma)	2/71	3/71 (5)	1	0	0
3)	86/74	Male 4/71	*Pons* → Cb	Astrocytoma (III) (with foci of primitive small cells like 437/79)	6/73	1/74 (3)	7	6500	MTx i. t.
4)	983/74	Male 5/66	*Pons* (maximum in the right Cb-pont. angle) ⇉ Cb, Mb, CSF (Spc, minor)	Astrocytoma (III – IV)[a]	9/73	9/74 (8)	12	4600	VCR, END, MTx
5)	1280/75	Female 6/69	*Pons* ⇉ Mo, CSF (Bc, Spc)	Astrocytoma (IV)	3/75	12/75 (7)	9	4010	0
6)	268/78	Male 6/72	*Pons* ⇉ Cb, Mb, Mo, (Bg)	Astrocytoma (III – IV)[a]	7/76	3/78 (6)	20	5000	0
7)	223/79	Female 10/73	*Pons* ⇉ Mb, Dc, lv (without CSF spread)	Astrocytoma (III – IV)[a]	1/78	3/79 (6)	14	4400	0

8)	437/79	Male 2/68	1) *Pons* → Mo 2) *Cerebellum*	1) astrocytoma (III) 2) Primitive undiff. "medulloblastoma"	12/78 (11)	5/79 (11)	6	5000	0
9)	610/79	Female 4/66	*Medulla oblongata* and *lower pons*	Astrocytoma (II – III)	4/79	7/79 (13)	3	0	0
10)	932/79	Male 9/66	*Pons* ⇉ Cb, Mo	Astrocytoma (III – IV)[a] (multiforme due to irradiation?)	12/78	10/79 (13)	10	5000	0
11)	124/80	Female 6/69	*Pons* ⇉ Mb, Dc, Cb, Mo	Astrocytoma (III)	10/77	2/80 (11)	28	5000	CCNU, VCR

[a] Clear decision could not be made due to therapy changes but grade III was at least estimated

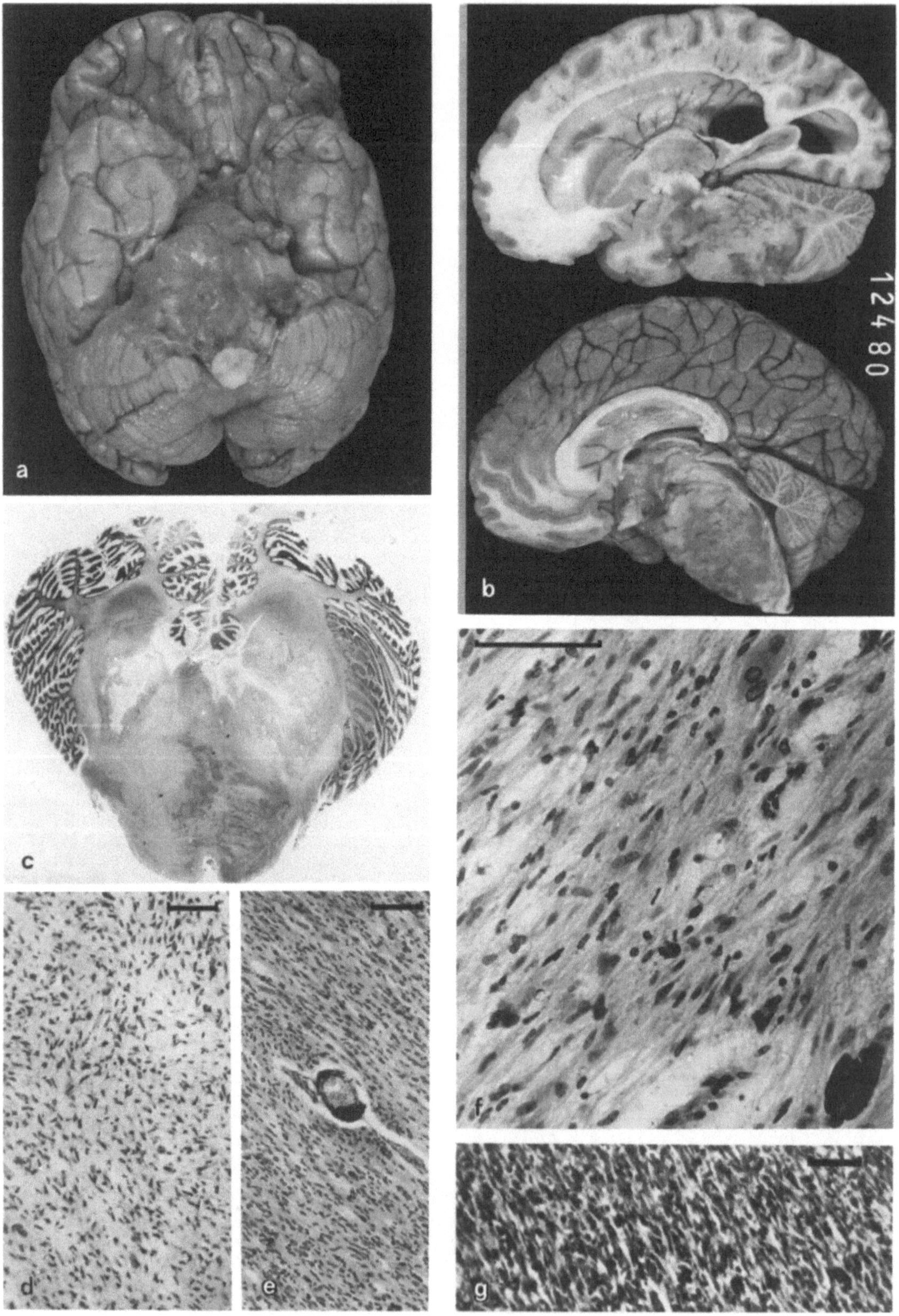
a
b
c
d
e
f
g

from the pons, but there was none which had remained confined to the pons. In one case it was difficult to determine clearly whether the tumour had arisen from the pons or from the medulla oblongata, both of which were partially involved. The clinical symptoms favoured an origin from the medulla. None of the tumours was sharply demarcated, all showing more or less extensive infiltration into the neighbouring structures such as the cerebellum, the midbrain, the diencephalon and the medulla. In two cases, there was clear evidence of spread throughout the CSF pathways (see Table 2 and Fig. 1).

Histological aspects: Almost none of the tumours showed a completely homogeneous picture. However, it was as a rule dominated by only one of the following microscopic characteristics: Most often areas with fusiform, spindle-shaped, piloid astrocytic elements, arranged according to the longitudinal fibre tracts (intrafascicular growth of Scherer [34]), alternating with areas characterized by stellate astrocytic cells. Fields composed of polymorphonuclear, often cytoplasm-rich cells with considerable variations of the ratio of nuclear size to cytoplasmic amount occurred somewhat less frequently. These cells were often consistent with the gemistocytic type of astrocytes. In one case (932/78) such areas dominated the picture, and suggested glioblastoma multiforme, but considerable effects of irradiation were obvious and complicated the assessment. More or less distinct palisading phenomena of the nuclei were often widely spread and sometimes the prevailing feature, not only in the most malignant tumours. Cystic mucoid replacement, calcification, vascular proliferation, and glial fibres, abundant in places, were further frequent features. Considerable haemorrhage occurred in some cases. The cellular density, although quite variable, was usually high. Mitotic figures were sometimes difficult to demonstrate, despite increased cellular density. In places they were numerous. Necroses were, as a rule, difficult to assess with respect to their significance for classification, because most of the patients had been given intensive radiation treatment. The same was true for the nuclear polymorphism. In two of the untreated cases, however, both were definitely primary features of the tumour. Previous radiation treatment was the main fact which made grading of the tumours most difficult in nearly all cases, particularly with respect to the differentiation between grade III and IV. Well-preserved neurons were not infrequently found in the midst even of highly cellular tumours.

Fig. 1 a–g. Pontine astrocytomas (data in Table 2). **a, b** Typical gross appearance of pontine astrocytoma: extension of the pons with nodular protrusions into the basal cisterns. Note the absence of the normal pontine striation due to destruction of the long fibre tracts in (**b**), and the infiltration of the cerebellum in the upper half of the picture (A.-No. 124/80). **c** Holoptic microscopic slide of a glioma mainly occupying the left half of the basis pontis and the tegmentum on both sides. Active infiltration into the cerebellum (A.-No. 268/78; staining according to Klüver-Barrera). **d–g** Histological appearance of different areas from the same brain stem glioma (A.- No. 437/79): medium cellular density of prevailingly small stellate astrocytic elements in (**d**); intrafascicular growth of pilocytic astrocytes with moderately increased cellular density in (**e**); higher magnification of a similar area in (**f**), displaying pilocytic astrocytes with increased nuclear polymorphism and a multinuclear giant cell at the top; highly cellular anaplastic region with proliferating strands of primitive glial cells in (**g**). (Black bars in **c–g** = 100 μm)

Seven tumours were at least considered to correspond to grade III (diffuse malignant astrocytoma), while three (two in the untreated cases) could definitely be judged as grade IV (glioblastoma). In only two cases was it very difficult to decide between grade II and grade III by histological means. In one of these cases, a non-treated child (610/79) with a course of only three months, the brain tissue was spoiled by an overlapping complete preterminal intravital circulatory necrosis, thus considerably complicating histological assessment. In the other case (Table 2, No. 9) too little material for a reliable conclusion as to the grade of the tumour, was found in the files. The specimens seemed to indicate grade II.

These problems, including the modifications due to therapy, generally remind us of the major hazards of grading tumours purely on histological grounds, which is in principle rejected by recognized authorities. In addition, the final stage at autopsy never allows a reliable conclusion as to the grade with which the tumour began. Its growth may have started long before the occurrence of the first symptoms with a slowly infiltrating but not destructive progress, thus corresponding to a grade I or II. The first clear symptoms and the following rapid course are probably often due to the occurrence of anaplastic transformation in such cases, as is well established in the literature [e.g. 12].

Hence, judgment should not particularly be related to the histological appearance but to the poor outcome in most of these brain stem gliomas, with a mortality rate of more than 80 per cent within two years from the first onset of symptoms.

In one very extraordinary case (437/79) with a survival time of only six months, a second tumour of entirely different microscopic appearance with the features of a desmoplastic medulloblastoma was found in the central part of the cerebellum, immediately adjacent to the diffuse astrocytoma of the pons, with transitional parts between both. This case has been [35] and will be further outlined elsewhere, more precisely with respect to its basic implications for developmental mechanisms in neuro-oncology. As the first clinical symptoms of the lesion pointed to the brainstem it is most likely that the already anaplastic astrocytoma of the pons was first, and it could be presumed that the second tumour had developed due to further anaplastic transformation, i. e. "dedifferentiation" of the malignant astrocytoma into a primitive tumour akin to a medulloblastoma. In another case (86/74) foci of similar primitive cells without reticulin formation were irregularly blended with the otherwise already malignant astrocytoma, which showed extensive palisading of long pilocytic cells as a prevailing feature.

All tumours showed an infiltrating mode of growth. The region adjoining the neighbouring normal tissue was never sharply demarcated. Only the primitive undifferentiated "mutants" in 437/79 and 86/74 showed a clear demarcation from the surrounding tissues.

Comparative Data from the Literature

From many more cases reported in the literature, a total of 485 (386) could be found with a fairly homogeneous documentation of relevant data for the present purpose. Nevertheless, as usual, establishing of the synopses given by Tables 3 and 4, was

Table 3a. Cases without modern therapy.[a] *AB* Astroblastoma; *AC* astrocytoma; *ACf* astrocytoma (fibrillary); *ACp* astrocytoma (protoplasmic); *E* ependymoma; *G* glioma; GC gangliocytoma; *GG* ganglioglioma; *GM* glioblastoma multiforme or malignum; *HB* haemangioblastoma; *MB* medulloblastoma; *MG* mixed glioma; *OG* oligodendroglioma; *SP* spongioblastoma polare

Author	No. of cases		Age		Time of survival (from 1st symptom)		Diagnosis	
	Male/Fem.		Mean (years)	Range (years)	Mean	Range (months)	Type	No.
1) Marburg	1		?		14	–	G	1
(van Rees) [23]	20		?		6[b]	1 – 60	G	20
2) Buckley [5]	10		~25	4 – 59	4	1 – 7	GM	10
	15			12 – 59	24	4 – 48	AC	4
							SP	3
							AB	1
							?	7
3) Hare and Wolf [15]	3	4	8	6 – 16	~16	2 – 60	GM	3
							SP	1
							ACf	3
4) Pilcher [29]	4	7	~12	3 – 35	~5	1 – 14	SP	11
5) Alpers and Watts [1]	1	3	~14	8 – 19	23	3 – 60	G	3
							AC	1
6) Alpers and Yaskin [2]	5	6	16	3 – 45	~3	1 – 14	G	1
							GM	4
							AC	6
7) Foerster et al. [8 – 11] (Bucy et al.) [6]	15	9	22	<3 – 63	25	1 – 171	AC	13
							GM	6
							SP	2
							GC, GG	2
							MB	1
8) Gagel [12]	–	1	–	9 –	–	78 –	AC	1
9) Renier and Gabreels	–	4	12	5 – 13	4	3 – 6	AC II	1
							AC III	3
10) White [38]	7	8	46	19 – 67	13	1 – 49	AC	7
							GM	2
							SP	1
							?	5
11) Lassman et al [21]	12		5	<3 – 13	4	1 – 8	AC	?
							SP	?
							GM	?
12) Panitch and Berg [28]	4	5	~9	0,5 – 20	~31	2 – 69	AC	5
							GM	2
							SP	1
							?	1
13) Bassoe and Apfelbach [3]	2	2	~19	6 – 38	~11	3 – 20	G	4
14) Cooper et al. [7]	9[d]	6[d]	26	2 – 58	~11[c]	1 – 26[c]	AC I	7
							AC III/IV	2
							E II	2
							OG	1
							?	4

Table 3a (continued)

Author	No. of cases		Age		Time of survival (from 1st symptom)		Diagnosis	
	Male/Fem.		Mean (years)	Range (years)	Mean	Range (months)	Type	No.
15) Mayer [26]	1	–	–	55 –	–	42 –	G (ACF)	1
16) Kaufmann [18]	6	6	22	5 – 48	29	1 – 228	GM	5
							ACf	2
							GIII	2
							ACp	1
							AB?	1
							MB	1
Total	176 57	 61	20 (5 – 55)	<3 – 67	19 (3 – 42)	1 – 228		

[a] Irradiation and/or chemotherapy
[b] Estimated from the author's data
[c] Time from the onset of symptoms to diagnosis; in six cases sudden death after admission to hospital; short survival times supposed for the rest (all autopsy cases)
[d] Tumours of the medulla oblongata

partly difficult, and in a few instances it could not be avoided that at least some values from the data originally supplied by the authors had to be estimated. This was only the case when reliable and reasonable calculations could be made which were in agreement with the author's general statements.

In Tables 3a and b special emphasis is put on the survival times and some further important data of the cases, separately for cases without modern therapy (irradiation and/or chemotherapy) and those which were given these treatments. Adult cases were not excluded from the surveys because it soon became clear from studies of the literature that their progress and prognosis did not in any way differ significantly from those in infancy and adolescence. The tables show that there was a wide range of survival times from 1 to 228 months with an average of 19 months in the untreated cases, and from 1 to 236 months, averaging 25 months in the treated ones. The difference between the means of only six months seemed to be significant in the "student's" t-test. However, on one hand one must bear in mind that in the statistics of Bray et al. (No. 2 in Table 3b) a mean for the group of eight cases could only be estimated as below 69 months from at most four precisely recorded survival times, which were 1 month, and 4, 6 and 13 years. Hence, the real average of this group must be considered to be far below 69 months, but in the calculation of the total average of table 3b, 69 months was taken as the mean. On the other hand, the data of all tables show that the frequency distributions of the survival times are markedly asymmetrical with an excessively leftsided peak. Application of the "student's" t-test to such distributions is hazardous because the present excessive left-sided asymmetry is probably far beyond what the t-test can "bear" with respect to deviations from the normal Gauss distribution.

Table 3b. Cases with modern therapy[a]

Author	No. of cases		Age		Time of survival (from 1st symptom)		Diagnosis	
	Male/Fem.		Mean (years)	Range (years)	Mean	Range (months)	Type	No.
1) Renier and Gabreels [31]	16	4	~7	2–15	20	4–120	AC III AC IV ?	2 9 9
2) Bray et al. [4]	24 8		~7	2–15	9 <69	? 1 –156	GM AC SP ?	5 3 2 22
3) Redmond [30]	23	19	~10[b]	3–53	20[b]	2 –>117	GM SP OG G ?	3 2 1 1 35
4) White [38]	13	16	40	17–57	32	1,5–120	GM AC III AC ?	9 2 5 13
5) Lassman et al. [21]	15		5	3–13	15	6 – 24	AC SP GM	? ? ?
6) Panitch and Berg [28]	17	14	~7	1–18	52	4 –236	AC SP GM MGIII ?	6 4 2 6 13
7) Golden et al. [13]	5 8		6.5 45	~1–11 30–56	~4 ~10	2.5– 8 1 – 26	{AC III {GM	5 8
8) Marsa et al. [24]	8	7	6	3–9	20	4 –116	AC III G III GM ?	2 1 5 7
9) Hara and Tachenchi [14]	13		29[b]	5–60	26	3 –178	AC GM	10 3
Total	210 77	 60	16 (5–44)	1–60	25	1 –236	class. ?	107 103

[a] Irradiation and/or chemotherapy
[b] Estimated from the author's data

The results of between 19 and 25 months of survival are in good agreement with our own survival average of about 23 months. If the two still living long term survivors were excluded, the average survival time would immediately fall to about 11 months.

Tables 4a and b summarize the long term survivors from both groups. It can be seen that the number of survivors of at least four years, or closely approximating 48

Table 4a. Longtime survivors[a] without modern therapy

Author	Total No. of cases	Survivors N	Survivors Time (months)	Survivors (percent)	Diagnosis[b] Type	Diagnosis[b] No.
1) Marburg [23] (van Rees)	20	1	60	5	G	1
2) Stroebe [36]	1	0	–	0	–	–
3) Bassoe and Apfelbach [3]	4	0	–	0	–	–
4) Mayer [26]	1	1[c]	>42	–	ACf	–
5) Buckley [5]	25	2	48, 48	8	AC	2
6) Hare and Wolf [15]	7	1	60	14.3	SP	1
7) Pilcher [29]	11	0	–	0	–	–
8) Alpers and Watts [1]	4	1	>61	25	G	1
9) Alpers and Yaskin [2]	11	0	–	–	–	–
10) Foerster et al. [8–11] (Bucy et al. [6])	24	3	>44[c], 80, 171	12.5	GG ACf	1 2
11) Gagel [12]	1	1	78	–	AC	1
12) Kaufmann [18]	12	1	228	8.3	ACf	1
13) Cooper et al. [7]	15	(probably) 0	–	–	–	–
14) White [38]	15	1	49	6.7	AC	1
15) Lassman et al. [21]	12	0	–	0	–	–
16) Panitch and Berg [28]	9	4	52, 64, 68, 69	44.4	AC ?	3 1
17) Golden et al. [13]	3	0	–	–	–	–
18) Renier and Gabreels [31]	4	0	–	–	–	–
Total	179	16	(average) *76* (>42 – 228)	8.9		

[a] From about 48 months on
[b] Histologically confirmed
[c] Probably longer because first symptoms probably earlier than deduced from the report

months, oscillates around an average of 9 to 10 per cent, as it is true for our own material. There are only two samples in table 4b (No. 3 & 5) with extraordinarily high percentages of long term survivors. Naturally, in more than half of these cases the diagnoses were not confirmed by histological examination, as is the rule among such cases for understandable reasons. However, considering this and the fact that these statistics are considerably higher than the rest without a significantly different mode of treatment, arouses suspicion that these samples included some strong bias. This could have been due not only to individuals, who did not really have gliomas, but also to some other reasons. It can be inferred from the literature that a number of different lesions may occur under the clinical picture of brain stem gliomas.

Table 4b. Longtime survivors[a] with modern therapy

Author	No. of cases (total)	Survivors N	Survivors Time (months)	Survivors (percent)	Diagnosis[b] Type	Diagnosis[b] No.
1) Bray et al. [4]	39	3	48, 72, 156	7.7	?	–
2) Redmond [30]	30	4	60, 62, 75, 117	13.3	?	–
3) White [38]	29	8	49, 72, 74, 78, 85, 86, 108, 120	27.6	AC ?	3 5
4) Lassman et al. [21]	15	0	–	0	–	–
5) Panitch and Berg [28]	31	9	58, 60, 83, 102, 151, 173, 222, 234, 236	29	AC SP ?	2 3 4
6) Lassiter et al. [20]	37	4	86, 103, 108, 159	10.8	?	4
7) Golden et al. [13]	10	0	–	0	–	–
8) Urtasun [37]	21	2	60, 60	9.5	?	–
9) Marsa et al. [24]	15	2	53, 116	13.3	?	–
10) Lee [22]	24	3	>60, >60 >120	12.5	?	–
11) Rosen et al. [32]	1	0	–	0	–	–
12) Milhorat [27]	10	2	>39 (48?) 132	20	ACf	2
13) Hara and Tachenchi [14]	24	2	55, 178	8.3	AC	2
14) Renier and Gabreels [31]	20	2	85, 120	10	?	2
Total	306	41	(average) *102* (>39 – 236)	13.4	AC(f) ?	9 29

(Without No. 3 & 5: Cases 246, survivors 24 = 9.8%; average s.-time 91 months)

[a] From about 48 months on

[b] Histologically confirmed

Nevertheless, even if these samples remain included in the calculations, the difference between 13.4% (41 cases) and 8.9% (16 cases) of long term survivors in both groups was not statistically significant in the χ^2-test with the contingency table ($\chi^2 = 2.17$, $P > 0.05$). However, if one considers the average survival times in the treated (102 months) and in the untreated (76 months) group, which could not be statistically tested because of difficulties arising from sampling of the data, it may at least be possible that modern concepts of therapy have somewhat increased the time of survival in those rather few individuals, although not their percentage.

Conclusions

The present data demonstrate that the situation of brain stem gliomas (mainly astrocytomas), whether in children or in adults, has changed but little since the pessimistic statement of Otto Marburg in 1926: "The prognosis *quoad vitam* is an absolutely unfavourable one in all cases".

Long term survivors occurred in the early reports as they do in the period of modern therapy. From our analysis it cannot be definitely proved that their survival has been significantly increased by the modern concepts of treatment. However, it remains at least possible that irradiation and/or chemotherapy have prolonged the times of survival in those individuals, who perhaps already have a "tendency" (whatever this may be) for a longer natural history of their tumours. In addition, the total statistics do not of course show whether the long term time survivors of former times and those of the period of modern treatment both survived for the same biological reasons. It cannot be excluded that in the individual case modern treatment has selected long term survivors, who would not have survived that long without treatment. Discussion of these problems would probably advance considerably if the attempt were made to confirm the diagnosis histologically in each case before treatment. This might well become possible by modern stereotactical procedures.

However, for the time being, one must conclude that the chance of attaining a significant success worthy of a human being with modern means of treatment is extremely slight. Hence, it must basically remain a matter of the personal ethical attitude of every single involved physician, whether he believes in this chance, or whether he sees the higher value for the patients in letting nature take its course without spoiling the predominantly short life-span; not only of the patients by a highly aggressive and exhausting treatment, but also for their relatives by the arousal of mostly unjustified hope – a basic problem of medicine, not only in the present context.

Summary

Twenty observations of gliomas of the lower brain stem in childhood (11 autopsy and nine clinical cases) from 1968 to 1981 are described. Ten were male and ten female. Their ages at the first onset of symptoms or when death occurred ranged from 2 to 13 years with an average of 7 years. Eighteen children had died within 36 months of the onset of the first symptoms; two were long term survivors, still living after a period of nine years in one case and 13 years in the other. The total survival time averaged 22.5 months; leaving out the long term survivors it is only 10.6 months. Seventeen children received treatment, either irradiation alone or in combination with chemotherapy. In one child a surgical approach was tried prior to irradiation. The three untreated children survived only 1, 2, and 3 months. In most of the cases the tumour had originated from the pons, but in none of the autopsy cases had it remained within this location. Most of the tumours in the autopsy cases and the single surgical case were at least malignant astrocytomas; only the latter was accorded grade II on the basis of only a small histological specimen from the files. Exact grading was greatly complicated in most of the cases by the changes due to radiation treatment.

In addition to the data of the personal observations a total number of 485 cases from the literature was evaluated mainly with respect to their survival times, separately for those which had and those which had not received modern therapy (i.e. irradiation and/or chemotherapy). No particular differences between the two groups could be detected, although it could not definitely be ruled out that modern treatment was mainly responsible for long survival times at least in individual cases. In addition, it might have prolonged the survival periods in the long term cases with treatment, as compared to those without. However, the lack of histological confirmation of the clinical diagnosis in many such cases leaves considerable uncertainty about the true nature of the lesions treated. Hence, it remains most doubtful, whether modern therapeutical approaches really significantly improved what is still essentially the very poor prognosis of the gliomas of the lower brain stem.

References

1. Alpers, B. J., Watts, J. C.: Mesencephalic gliomas. Arch. Neurol. Psychiat. *34,* 1250–1273 (1935)
2. Alpers, B. J., Yaskin, J. C.: Gliomas of the pons. Clinical and pathologic characteristics. Arch. Neurol. Psychiat. *41,* 435–459 (1939)
3. Bassoe, P., Apfelbach, C. W.: Glioma of the bulb and pons. Arch. Neurol. Psychiat. *14,* 396–408 (1925)
4. Bray, P. F., Carter, S., Taveras, J. M.: Brain stem tumours in children. Neurology (Minneap) *8,* 1–7 (1958)
5. Buckley, R. C.: Pontine gliomas; pathology study and classification of 25 cases. Arch. Path. *9,* 779–819 (1930)
6. Bucy, B., Foerster, O., Gagel, O., Mahoney, W.: Die Tumoren der Brücke; ein Fall von Astrozytom der Brücke. I. Mitteilung. Z. Neurol. Psychiat. *157,* 136–146 (1937)
7. Cooper, I. S., Kernohan, J. W., Craig, W. McK: Tumours of the medulla oblongata. Arch. Neurol. Psychiat. *67,* 269–282 (1952)
8. Foerster, O., Gagel, O.: Ein Fall von Gangliocytom der Oblongata. Z. Neurol. Psychiat. *141,* 797–823 (1932)
9. Foerster, O., Gagel, O.: Die Astrozytome der Oblongata, Brücke und des Mittelhirns. Z. Neurol. Psychiat. *166,* 497–528 (1939)
10. Foerster, O., Gagel, O.: Die encephalen Tumoren der Oblongata, Pons und des Mesencephalons. III. Mitteilung. Z. Neurol. Psychiat. *168,* 295–331 (1940)
11. Foerster, O., Gagel, O., Mahoney, W.: Die encephalen Tumoren des verlängerten Markes, der Brücke und des Mittelhirns. Arch. Psychiat. Nervenkrankh. *110,* 1–74 (1939)
12. Gagel, O.: Ein Pons – Oblongata – Astrocytom mit ungewöhnlichem Verlauf. Nervenarzt *14,* 343–347 (1941)
13. Golden, G. S., Ghatak, N. R., Hirano, A., French, J. H.: Malignant glioma of the brain stem; a clinicopathological analysis of 13 cases. J. Neurol. Neurosurg. Psychiat. *35,* 732–738 (1972)
14. Hara, M., Tachenchi, K.: A temporal study of survival of patients with pontine gliomas. J. Neurol. *216,* 189–196 (1977)
15. Hare, C. C., Wolf, A.: Intramedullary tumours of the brain stem. Arch. Neurol. Psychiat. *32,* 1230–1252 (1934)
16. Henschen, F.: Tumoren des Zentralnervensystems und seiner Hüllen. (p. 744) Gliome der Brücke. In: O. Lubarsch, F. Henke, R. Rössle (eds.) Handbuch der speziellen pathologischen Anatomie und Histologie, XII/3, Berlin-Göttingen-Heidelberg: Springer 1955
17. Jones, P. G., Campbell, P. E.: Intracranial and spinal tumours. In: Tumours of Infancy and Childhood, p. 231, Oxford: Blackwell 1976
18. Kaufmann, J.: Tumeurs pontines et bulbopontines. Schweiz Arch. Neurol. Psychiat. *64,* 197–252 (1949)

19. Koos, W. T., Miller, M. H.: Intracranial tumours in infants and children. Stuttgart: Thieme 1971
20. Lassiter, K. R. L., Alexander, E., Davis, C. H., Kelly, D. L.: Surgical treatment of brainstem gliomas. J. Neurosurg. *34,* 719–725 (1971)
21. Lassman, L. P., Lond, M. B., Arjona, V. E., Seville, L. M. S.: Pontine gliomas in childhood. Lancet *1,* 913–915 (1967)
22. Lee, F.: Radiation of infratentorial and supratentorial brainstem tumours. J. Neurosurg. *43,* 65–68 (1975)
23. Marburg, O.: Die Tumoren des Pons und der Medulla oblongata. In: G. Alexander, O. Marburg, H. Brunner (eds.) Handbuch der Neurologie des Ohres, Vol. III, p. 123–138, Berlin-Wien: Urban & Schwarzenberg 1926
24. Marsa, G. W., Probert, J. C., Rubinstein, L. J., Bagshaw, M. A.: Radiation therapy in the treatment of childhood astrocytic gliomas. Cancer *32,* 646–655 (1973)
25. Marsa, G. W., Goffinet, D. R., Rubinstein, L. J., Bagshaw, M. A.: Megavoltage irradiation in the treatment of gliomas of the brain and spinal cord. Cancer *36,* 1681–1689 (1975)
26. Mayer, C.: Blastom im Kleinhirnbrückenwinkel mit Entwicklungsstörungen im Bereich des Corpus pontobulbare ESSICK. J. Psychol. Neurol. *37,* 159–185 (1928)
27. Milhorat, T. H.: Pontine glioma (Letters). J. Amer. Med. Assoc. *232,* 595–596 (1975)
28. Panitch, H. C., Berg, B. O.: Brainstem tumours of childhood and adolescence. Amer. J. Dis. Child. *119,* 465–472 (1970)
29. Pilcher, C.: Spongioblastoma polare of pons. Clinicopathologic study of eleven cases. Arch. Neurol. Psychiat. *32,* 1210–1230 (1934)
30. Redmond, J. S.: The roentgentherapy of pontine gliomas. Amer. J., Roentgenol. *86,* 644–648 (1961)
31. Renier, W. O., Gabreels, F. J. M.: Evaluation of diagnosis and non-surgical therapy in 24 children with a pontine tumour. Neuropädiatrie *11,* 262–273 (1980)
32. Rosen, G., Ghavimi, F., Vanucci, R., Deck, M., Tan, Ch., Murphy, M. L.: Pontine glioma. High-dosage methotrexate and leucovorin rescue. J. Amer. Med. Assoc. *230,* 1149–1152 (1974)
33. Russell, D. S., Rubinstein, L. J.: Astrocytomas of the brain-stem. In: Pathology of Tumours of the Nervous System, p. 181–183, Baltimore: Williams & Wilkins, 4th Ed 1977
34. Scherer, H. J.: Structural development in gliomas. Amer. J. Cancer. *34,* 333–351 (1938)
35. Schmitt, H. P.: Brüsker Wechsel der phänotypischen Expression von Gliomen: Progression und Selektion in der Onkogenese. Annual Scientific Meeting of the Austrian Society of Neuropathology, May 7–8, Graz 1981. In: K. Jellinger, H. Gross (eds.) Current Topics in Neuropathology, Wien: Facultas (in press)
36. Stroebe, H.: Ueber Entstehung und Bau der Hirngliome. (p. 440) Glioma pontis. Beitr. path. Anat. *18,* 405–486 (1895)
37. Urtasun, R. C.: ^{60}Co radiation treatment of pontine gliomas. Radiology *104,* 385–387 (1972)
38. White, H. H.: Brainstem tumours occurring in adults. Neurology (Minneap.) *13,* 292–300 (1963)

Astrocytoma with Extracranial Metastases

R. BUBL, H. R. HIRT, H. OHNACKER, and A. PROBST

Extracranial metastases of primary brain tumours are rare. Smith et al. [22], examining 8,000 neuroectodermal tumours, found 35 cases of metastases outside the nervous system. Glioblastomas and astrocytomas formed the largest single group. A glance at the age distribution shows that the number of children affected is very small: In Pasquier's analysis [19] of 72 cases of metastasing glioblastoma, there were only 7 children under 16 years of age. Of these 7, 4 had undergone a shunt operation.

Case History

At the age of 6 years (1970), the patient became ill with postinfection encephalitis following measles, which resulted in a hemi-grand-mal seizure on the left side. The child recovered rapidly. The EEG showed initially a severe slowing on the right side which subsequently disappeared to a large extent. Two and a half years later, typical psychomotor seizures occurred. During the seizure-free period, a nonspecific focus was visible on the EEG in the right temporal region.

Neurological and psychiatric examination and radio-active scanning yielded no pathological findings. Anti-epileptic treatment was very difficult: The seizures persisted and behavioural disturbances became more frequent. Since the illness appeared to be progressive, the patient was readmitted to hospital four years later. In the x-rays of the cranium a pea-sized intracerebral calcification could be seen in the right temporo-basal region. The PEG showed enlargement and slight raising of the temporal horn. This finding was taken, in conjunction with the calcification, to indicate a dormant or very slowly developing hamartoma. The neurological status aroused no particular concern at this point. Only the CSF protein value showed a slight increase. Subsequently the frequency of the seizures diminished and there was an improvement in the behavioural disorders.

At a check-up six months later, however, bilateral papilloedema was found, with concentric contraction of the visual field. In the EEG an increase in the nonspecific disturbance in the right temporal region was found. On the CT an expanding lesion was visible in the right temporo-basal region. The carotid angiogram showed the middle cerebral artery pushed upwards and the anterior cerebral artery displaced to the left. These findings indicated a rapidly developing tumour in the anterior temporal region. At operation a tumour the size of a hen's egg was removed which at the base of the skull had invaded the dura mater and was only partially distinguishable from the normal brain-tissue. Histological examination revealed an anaplastic astrocytoma with marked desmoplastic reaction of the meninges. After operation, the tumour area was irradiated with LAC photons to a total dosage of 5,000 rad.

The child showed no further symptoms for over a year, after which there was a recurrence of frontal headache and impaired vision. The CT revealed compression of the suprasellar cistern and marked enhancement in the operation area. At operation, the suspected recurrence was confirmed. An intracerebral tumour was found in the right temporal lobe. A very hard portion of this was attached to the meninges, and had partially destroyed the bone. Histological examination again indicated an astrocytoma malignancy stage III.

$Iodine^{125}$ was now implanted stereotactically in the operated area. Three months later the patient suffered severe headaches, which were at first diagnosed as being caused by cerebral oedema, a local reaction to the beta emitters. Corticosteroids produced a good degree of improvement, but withdrawal resulted in recurrence of the headaches and impaired vision. The visual field showed an incongruous homonymous hemianopia. There was also slight spastic hemiparesis. The CT control showed an enhancing-positive lesion with perifocal oedema. This finding was interpreted as either a recurrence of the tumour or radiation necrosis with perifocal oedema. Diuretics (furosemide) and dexamethasone brought temporary relief from the headaches. However, the patient then began to experience neuralgic pain on the right side of the face. The CT now showed a definite recurrence of the tumour, with central necrosis. Since drugs had little effect on the facial pain, we hoped to relieve the child's suffering by operative obstruction of the affected trigeminal nerve. The pre-operative chest film showed hilar enlargement and several blurred rounded shadows.

Differential diagnoses considered were atypical pneumonia or pulmonary metastases. Tentative therapy with erythromycin produced no change in the pulmonary picture. It was therefore decided not to operate, and the patient was treated with analgesics. Ten months later, i.e. 2½ years after the first operation, the child died.

Neuropathological Findings

Autopsy revealed extensive recurrence of the tumour in the right temporal region. The tumour had destroyed the base of the middle cranial fossa and grown into the maxillary sinus and the right palatine vault. The gasserian ganglion, the lateral parts of the basal ganglion and the internal capsule were invaded. Considerable haemorrhage and necrosis were visible. The contiguous brain-tissue showed oedematous changes. Metastases were visible above all in the lungs and the cervical, hilar and periaortic lymph nodes. There were also metastases in the bone marrow and liver. The aortic arch, the jugular vein and the vena cava were surrounded by tumour masses.

Histology

The histological picture of the intracranial tumour and the metastases was similar. The tumour was characterized by its marked cellularity. The cells were extremely varied in size and form, with one or more nuclei, which were frequently hyperchromic. Many cells contained mitoses, some atypical. There was a marked desmoplastic reaction. No GFA protein was found in the tumour tissue.

Discussion

The case history of our patient extends over 10 years. It was initially characterized by focal seizures. A study of 72 children with a supratentorial tumour carried out by Jacobi showed that seizure was the first symptom in 10 cases [10, 15]. Two operations and repeated radiation treatment were followed by recurrence of the tumour. Histological examination of the operation and autopsy material, as well as that from the recurrent tumours and metastases gave identical findings. Because of the unusual course of the illness, the tumour was submitted to three reference centres:

Royal Manchester Children's Hospital
Armed Forces Institute of Pathology, Washington
Stanford University Medical Center (Calif.).

All three experts were unanimous that it was a primary intracranial tumour. Two pathologists confirmed the diagnosis of a metastasing astrocytoma. Professor Rubinstein assumed, in view of the invasion of the cranial fossa and lack of evidence of GFA protein, that it was a papillary meningioma. Pasquier [19] published details of a case of metastasing astrocytoma, where this reaction was evident only at isolated points in the tumour. The factors discovered by Perry [20] which favour metastasis all apply in the case of our patient:

1. Operation to remove recurrent tumour,
2. radiation treatment,
3. long period of survival.

The pattern of distribution of the organs affected by metastases also corresponds to data in the literature [13]. Glioblastomas and astrocytomas tend to metastase in the lungs and cervical lymph nodes.

The question whether a patient with metastases of a brain tumour should be subjected to chemotherapy is certainly not one which can be decided on the basis of purely medical criteria [14, 17]. We decided against it, in view of the long period of suffering the child had undergone and the extensive recurrence of the tumour.

References

1. Alvord, E. C.: Why do gliomas not metastasize? Arch. Neurol. *33*, 73–75 (1976)
2. Brander, W. L., Turner, D. R.: Extracranial metastases from a glioma in the absence of surgical intervention. J. Neurol. Neurosurg. Psychiat. *38*, 1133–1135 (1975)

3. Cappelaere, P., Glay, A., Adenis, L., Demaille, A., Laine, E.: Metastases of cerebral tumours outside of the cerebrospinal axis. Bull. Cancer (Paris) *72,* 235–254 (1972)
4. Dolman, C. L.: Lymph node metastasis as first manifestation of glioblastoma. J. Neurosurg. *41,* 607–609 (1974)
5. Duffner, P. K., Cohen, M. E.: Extraneural metastases in childhood brain tumours. Ann. Neurol. *10,* 261–265 (1981)
6. El-Gindi, S., Salama, M., El-Henawy, M., Farag, S.: Metastases of glioblastoma multiforme to cervical lymph nodes. J. Neurosurg. *38,* 631–634 (1973)
7. Glasauer, F. E., Yuan, R. H. P.: Intracranial tumours with extracranial metastases. J. Neurosurg. *20,* 474–493 (1963)
8. Hyman, R. A., Loring, M. F., Liebeskind, A. L., Naidich, J. B., Stein, H. L.: Computed tomographic evaluation of therapeutically induced changes in primary and secondary brain tumours. Neuroradiology *14,* 213–218 (1978)
9. Jackson, A. M., Graham, D. I.: Remote metastases from intracranial tumours. J. Clin. Pathol. *31,* 794–802 (1978)
10. Jacobi, G.: Die Bedeutung intrakranieller raumfordernder Prozesse für die Auslösung von Anfällen bei Kindern. 4. Jahrestagung des Arbeitskreises für Epilepsie, 1978
11. Jellinger, K., Schuster, H.: Extraneurale Metastasierung anaplastischer Gliome. Zbl. allg. Pathol. u. pathol. Anat. *121,* 526–534 (1977)
12. Komatsu, K., Hiratsuka, H., Takahashi, S., Kamisasa, A., Inaba, Y.: Widespread extracranial metastases of glioblastoma multiforme. Bull. Tokyo Med. Dent. Univ. *19,* 29, 49 (1972)
13. Kretschmer, H: Die extrakranielle Metastasierung intrakranieller Geschwülste. Zbl. Neurochir. *35,* 81–112 (1974)
14. Levin, V. A., Edwards, M. S., Wright, D. C., Seager, M. L., Schimberg, T. P., Townsend, J. J., Wilson, Ch. B.: Modified procarbazine, CCNU, and vincristine (PCV 3) combination chemotherapy in the treatment of malignant brain tumours. Cancer Treat. Rep. *64,* 237–241 (1980)
15. Mercuri, S., Russo, A., Palma, L.: Hemispheric supratentorial astrocytomas in children. J. Neurosurg. *55,* 170–173 (1981)
16. Montaut, J., Metaizeau, J. P., Gerbaux, A., Renard, M.: Les métastases extra-crâniennes des tumeurs primitives de l'encéphale. Neuro-Chirurgie *22,* 653–669 (1976)
17. Oster, M. W.: Combination chemotherapy for extracranial metastases of a primary malignant cerebral neoplasm. Cancer Treat. Rep. *63,* 1417–1418 (1979)
18. Pasquier, B., Pasquier, D., N'Golet, A., Panh, M. H., Couderc, P.: Le potentiel métastatique des tumeurs primitives du système nerveux central. Rev. Neurol. (Paris) *135,* 263–278 (1979)
19. Pasquier, B., Pasquier, D., N'Golet, A., Panh, M. H., Couderc, P.: Extraneural metastases of astrocytomas and glioblastomas. Cancer *45,* 112–125 (1980)
20. Perry, R. E.: Extracranial metastases in a case of intracranial ependymoma. Arch. Pathol. *64,* 337–341 (1957)
21. Slowik, F., Balogh, I.: Extracranial spreading of glioblastoma multiforme. Zbl. Neurochirurgie *41,* 17–68 (1980)
22. Smith, D. R., Hardman, J. M., Earle, K. M.: Metastasizing neuroectodermal tumours of the central nervous system. J. Neurosurg. *31,* 50–58 (1969)
23. Terheggen, H. G., Müller, W.: Extracerebrospinal metastases in glioblastoma. Europ. J. Pediat. *124,* 155–164 (1977)
24. Wakamatsu, T., Matsuo, T., Kawano, S., Teramoto, S., Matsumura, H.: Extracranial metastasis of intracranial tumour – review of literatures and report of a case. Acta Path. Jap. *22,* 155–169 (1972)

Diktyoma (Medulloepithelioma). A Rare Neuro-Epithelial Tumour of the Eye

G. Knoepfle, U. Bode, R. Hoischen, and H. J. Foedisch

Retinal medulloepithelioma is a very rare form of neoplasm generally occurring in infancy; it is congenital in most cases [1, 15]. About 100 cases have been described so far. Some time ago, we had the opportunity of diagnosing a growth of this kind in a 10-year-old girl.

Case History

E. F., born in 1971 (Medical Record # 18832/81, Paediatric Hospital, Bonn University).

Family Case History. Not contributory.

Anamnesis. The girl, who had not been seriously ill before, had had her left eyeball removed two and a half years earlier. As early as three months after enucleation, a preauricular node began to manifest itself. The node was not tender on pressure, but subsequently grew in size.

In the diagnosis submitted to us the node was described as a malignant tumour of the carcinoma type.

Condition on Admittance. A normally developed girl without nutritional or general deficiencies. The left temporal, malar, and submandibular regions were covered by an extremely prominent hard growth with a slightly nodular surface which had spread across the midline of the neck to the right-hand side. This growth had displaced the left external auditory meatus and led to an induration of the floor of the mouth (Fig. 1).

At the same time, a structurally identical tumour mass filled half of the left eye socket. Except for enlarged lymph nodes found on the left side, towards the nape of the neck, no more clinical or neurological symptoms were found.

Laboratory Findings. Leucocytosis of 12,400 cells; erythrocyte sedimentation rate (ESR) markedly increased; slightly reduced serum iron level.

Ophthalmologically, the right eyeball was found to be normal. The cerebrospinal fluid was also normal.

X-Ray Findings. Thorax scans in two planes were not contributory. Plain films and tomograms of the facial part of the skull showed the bone at the left angle of the mandible to be disintegrating, but scans of other segments of the skull, especially in the vicinity of the base, showed no indications of further bone lesions.

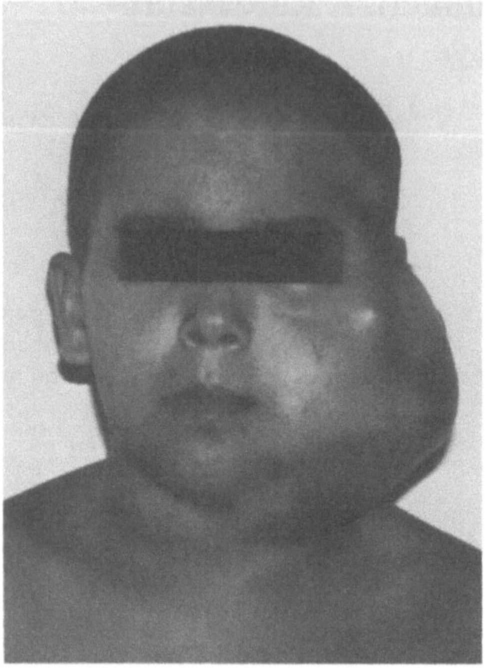

Fig. 1. A ten-year-old girl. Condition after removal of the left eyeball because of teratoid medulloepithelioma. Excessively large metastatic growth covering the left side of the face and jaw

Even by computer tomography we were unable to find anything pointing at an invasion of the interior of the skull by the tumour.

A biopsy sample (K 569/81) excised from the preauricular part of the growth was *classified pathologically and anatomically as a malignant teratoid medulloepithelioma.* Clinically, the growth was in a far-advanced stage of extension involving local infiltration and destruction of adjacent tissue as well as the formation of metastases in the left part of the face and neck.

Development. An attempt at therapy involving the infusion of high doses of methotrexate over a period of 42 hours, followed by the administration of cyclophosphamide and adriamycin, did not succeed in reducing the tumour. After a brief phase of stagnation, it continued to grow rapidly. As the neoplasm was very poorly supplied with blood vessels, it did not seem promising to instil cytostatic drugs intraarterially; we therefore decided to extirpate the tumour, to resect part of the lower mandible and malar bone, to dissect the left side of the neck, and to remove the right carotid triangle.

Four weeks after this operation, a new fast-growing tumour appeared in the scar tissue. This time, it was established by computer tomography that the tumour had in fact invaded the sphenoidal sinus and the ethmoidal cells on the left. Segments of the growth in the parietal and temporal regions had already begun to compress the ventricular system on the left and to displace the midline structures to the right.

Macroscopically, the operative specimen (K 1842/81) was moderately firm in consistency and uniformly greyish-white in colour. The primary tumour, which consisted of numerous nodules of various sizes, had already begun to erode a large

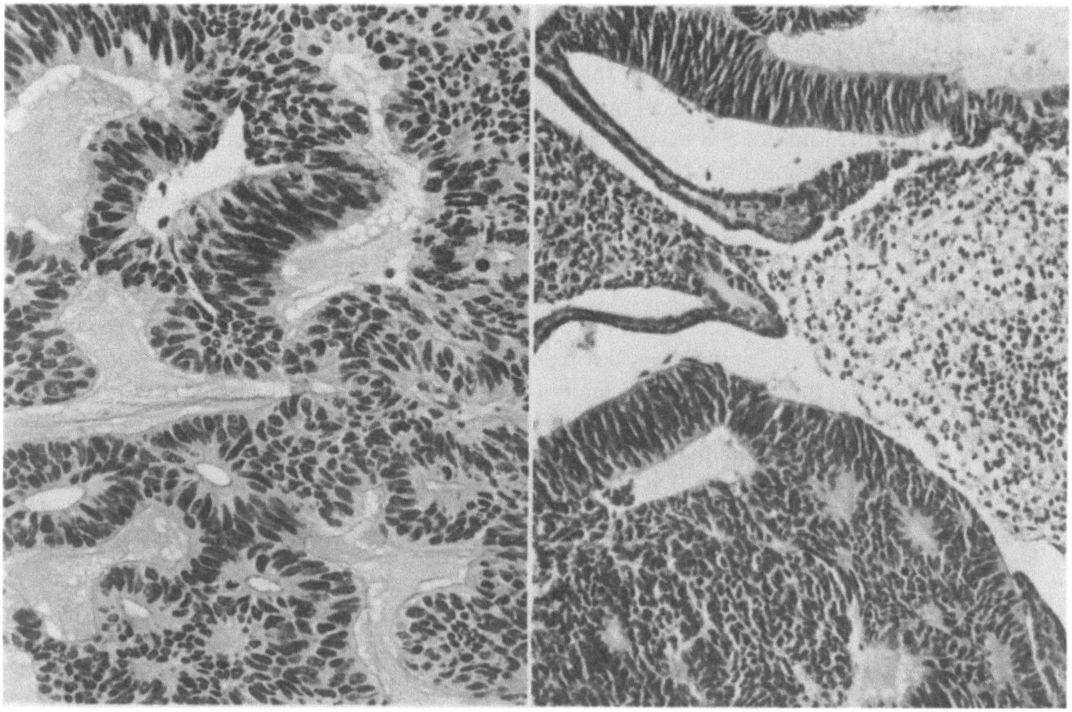

Fig. 2. a Photograph showing the typical histological structure of a malign medulloepithelioma of the eye, consisting of strings of epithelial cells, adeniform structures, rosettes, and areas of solid tissue. Sample # K 569/81. Haematoxylin and eosin, × 350. **b** Malignant teratoid medulloepithelioma (sample # K 1842/81). Combination of solid epithelial tissue and neuroglial differentiation (on the right). Haematoxylin and eosin, ×255

part of the angle of the mandible; the bone now showed holes up to 1 cm in diameter.

Histologically, the neoplasm was composed entirely of a multitude of different tissues. In a partially hyalinised stroma bed of low fibre density we found strings of epithelial cells of uneven height, trabecular and adeniform structures as in embryonal medulloepitheliomas, as well as small or slightly larger islands of solid matter which, while beginning to form rosettes in a few instances, were clearly malignant in view of the prevalence of both polymorphism and mitoses.

That the growth was teratoid was established by the presence of hyaline and often atypical cartilaginous islands as well as extensive neuroglial elements which in some cases even contained fully mature ganglion cells (Fig. 2).

Clinically, as we said before, this growth was a medulloepithelioma or diktyoma. Neoplasms of this type are characterized by the fact that they are essentially embryonal. On the one hand, the presence of pseudorosettes and genuine rosettes is somewhat reminiscent of retinoblastomas, while on the other hand there are also more sophisticated and differentiated structures like glands, papillae, and microcysts. The so-called *teratoid* variety of medulloepithelioma, which encompasses 30 to 40% of all cases as well as the case described in this paper, is characterized by the simultaneous presence of varying quantities of neuroglial structures, ganglion cells in all stages of maturity, and muscular as well as cartilaginous tissue [3, 4, 6, 15].

According to the histogenetic classification evolved by Zimmerman in 1971 which has since been adopted almost without change by the WHO Commission, medulloepithelioma of the eye is a neuroepithelial growth which manifests itself in the embryonic retina [14]. Most of these neoplasms develop in the unpigmented epithelium of the ciliary part of the retina. So far, only four cases have been described where the tumour was located either in the sensory retina or in the vicinity of the optic papilla [7, 13]. We distinguish between benign and malignant forms according to their biological behaviour [2, 11]. According to the criteria postulated by Andersen in 1962 [2], only one in four growths can be called malignant, while according to the criteria of malignancy evolved by Broughton and Zimmerman in 1971 [4], two out of three growths are malignant (Table 1). It is quite remarkable that only about 20% of all benign neoplasms are of the teratoid variety, whereas nearly half (45%) of the malignant growths feature heteroplastic histodifferentiation [7, 8].

Table 1. Malignancy criteria of embryonal medulloepitheliomas (Broughton and Zimmerman [4])

1) The presence of tissue elements composed of immature neuroblastic cells, with and without formation of rosettes.
2) A high rate of mitosis and/or marked pleomorphism.
3) Sarcomatous differentiation.
4) Growths invading the uvea, cornea, or sclera; the neoplasm may or may not spread into extraocular regions.

Unlike retinoblastomas, medulloepitheliomas are always solitary and unilateral, occurring with approximately the same frequency in both sexes. Another typical factor is that there is no heredity or genetic disposition. On an average, manifestation begins at an age of 3½ to 4 years; after the age of ten, it becomes extremely rare [4, 9, 12].

Among clinical symptoms, loss of vision and pain are most frequently named (70%), while the most frequent pathological phenomena found are a nodular growth in the anterior region of the eye, secondary glaucoma, and cataract [4, 5].

To begin with, the expansion of medulloepithelioma is primarily local, with the neoplasm spreading in most cases from the posterior into the anterior chamber of the eye; as a rule, this is a slow process. In nearly 40% of all cases, the tumour invaded the uvea, cornea, or sclera, and in about half of these cases extraocular growths were reported [1, 4, 10].

Prognosis is generally good in all cases where benign and even malignant growths have remained confined to intraocular expansion in the anterior sections of the eye. What affects clinical prognosis most unfavourably is the growth of an extraocular tumour which in most cases would be located in the retrobulbar tissue; in all such cases, the mortality rate is not less than 50%. As a rule, the death of the patient is caused by the spread of an intracranial growth. Instances of the tumour forming metastases either in the mediastinal lymphatic nodes or in the lungs via the lymphatic or vascular system are extremely rare, as are metastases in the parotid. Almost without exception, recurrence is confined to the period between 12 and 30 months after excision of the primary tumour; should the patient survive for more than five years without recurrence experience suggests that he is as good as cured [2, 4].

Adequate treatment of medulloepithelioma depends mainly on the degree to which the tumour has expanded; generally, it would consist in the removal of the affected eyeball. According to our admittedly limited experience it would seem that radiotherapy alone is not effective. We know of only one case where systemic chemotherapy in combination with irradiation was reported to be effective [4].

References

1. Andersen, S. RY.: Medullo-epitheliomas, diktyoma and malignant epithelioma of the ciliary body. A general review and a new case of diktyoma. Acta ophthal. (Kbh.) *26,* 313–330 (1948)
2. Andersen, S. RY.: Medulloepithelioma of the retina. In: Zimmerman, L. E. (Hrsg.): Tumours of the eye and Adnexa. Int. ophthal. Clinics *2,* 483–506 (1962)
3. Andersen, S. RY.: Tumours of the eye and its adnexa. Acta ophthal. (Kbh.) *54,* 1–16 (1976)
4. Broughton, W. L., Zimmerman, L. E.: A clinicopathologic study of 56 cases of intraocular medulloepitheliomas. Amer. J. Ophthal. *85,* 407–418 (1978)
5. Cardell, B. S., Starbuck, M. J.: Diktyoma. Brit. J. Ophthal. *43,* 217–224 (1959)
6. Carrillo, R., Streeten, B. W.: Malignant teratoid medulloepithelioma in an adult. Arch. Ophthalmol. *97,* 695–699 (1979)
7. Green, W., Iliff, W. J., Trotter, R. R.: Malignant teratoid medulloepithelioma of the optic nerve. Arch. Ophthalmol. *91,* 451–454 (1974)
8. Harry, J., Morgan, G.: Pathology of a unique type of teratoid medulloepithelioma. Brit. J. Ophthal. *79,* 321–329 (1975)
9. Jakobiec, F. A., Howard, G., Ellsworth, R. M., Rosen, M.: Electron microscopic diagnosis of medulloepithelioma. Amer. J. Ophthal. *79,* 321–329 (1975)
10. Klien, B. A.: Diktyoma retinae. Arch. Ophthalmol. *22,* 432–438 (1939)
11. Mullanex, J.: Primary malignant medulloepithelioma of the retinal stalk. Amer. J. Ophthal. *77,* 499–504 (1974)
12. Naumann, G. O. H.: Retinoblastom. In: Doerr, W., Seifert, G., Uehlinger, E. (Hrsg.) Pathologie des Auges. Bd. 12. Spezielle pathologische Anatomie, Springer, Berlin, Heidelberg, New York, 1980
13. Reese, A. B.: Medullo-epithelioma (Diktyoma) of the optic nerve. Amer. J. Ophthalmol. *44,* 4–6 (1957)
14. Zimmerman, L. E.: Verhoeff's "Terato-neuroma". A critical reappraisal in light of new observations and current concepts of embryonic tumours. The Fourth Frederick H. Verhoeff Lecture. Amer. J. Ophthalmol. *72,* 1039–1057 (1971)
15. Zimmerman, L. E., Font, R. L., Andersen, S. RY.: Rhabdomyosarcomatous differentiation in malignant intraocular medulloepitheliomas. Cancer *30,* 817–835 (1972)

Intracranial Teratoma of a Newborn. Computer Tomographic and Morphological Findings

G. Ebhardt, H. Traupe, J. Könner, and L. Goerke

Intracranial teratomas are a rare type of neoplastic malformation. Together with dermoids and epidermoids the frequency is about 1%. Teratomas by themselves account for approximately 0.3% [7]. Typical locations are the pineal or the sella turcica region. Rarely intracerebral teratomas can be found in the floor of the third ventricle or in both lateral ventricles [5]. If one considers only reports of those intracranial teratomas with parts of all three germ layers, reports with CT-scans are rare [1, 3, 7, 12]. The following study gives a report of an unusual intracerebral neoplastic malformation misdiagnosed by CT-scan.

Case Report

The parents and a 13-year-old brother are well. No familially inherited diseases are known. The mother used oral contraceptives for several years, which she stopped in 1979 when she wanted another child. Ovulatory cycles restarted spontaneously. Last menstrual period on June 16, 1980. Estimated date of delivery March 23, 1981. She took antiemetics only in the first period of pregnancy, but she did not receive any other drugs or radiation therapy.

Smear bleedings occurred in the 15th week of pregnancy. Treatment with bed-rest and tocolysis by a β-sympathomimetic given intravenously. During the 31st week of pregnancy ultrasonic results for the first time seemed to indicate macro-

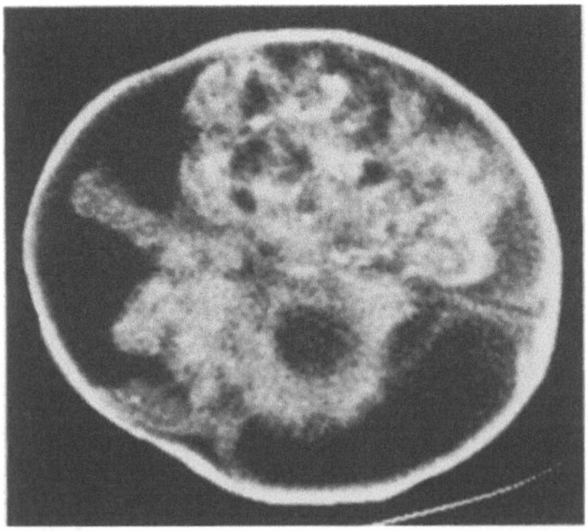

Fig. 1. Non-contrast CT-scan showing irregular tumour masses with various values of density. In the right parasagittal region there is a ring of large calciferous nodules joined by other calcifications within the region of the left hemisphere

cephaly. Further ultrasonic tests confirmed the pathological conditions. At the 35th week of gestation a premature male infant was delivered by caesarean section. The head circumference was 50 cm. The child was moaning and the skin was kept pink only by administration of oxygen. Tonus was reduced and a decrease in spontaneous motor activity was evident. Within three days the child became moribund and died. At the autopsy there were no indications of extracranial malformations.

On the first day of life a CT-scan was taken, with the following results: Base of the skull and cranium are deformed. The cranial cavity is filled by several nodular tumours of varying density. Besides extensive hypodense areas there are areas with strong increase of density already in the plain CT-scan (Fig. 1). With contrast medium these hypodense structures also show enhancement. Extensive liquid filled cavities are situated in the intracranial tissues frontally and occipitally. An exact identification of brain structures such as the hemispheres or the diencephalon is impossible, and it is therefore supposed there is a malformation of the brain. Cerebellum and medulla oblongata seem to be regular.

Autopsy Findings in the Head

Sutures widely separated and fontanelles bulging. Flattening of the middle and anterior cranial fossa. No malformation of the cranial skeleton. Dura tense and on opening it a large amount of blood-stained fluid drained away. Both cerebral

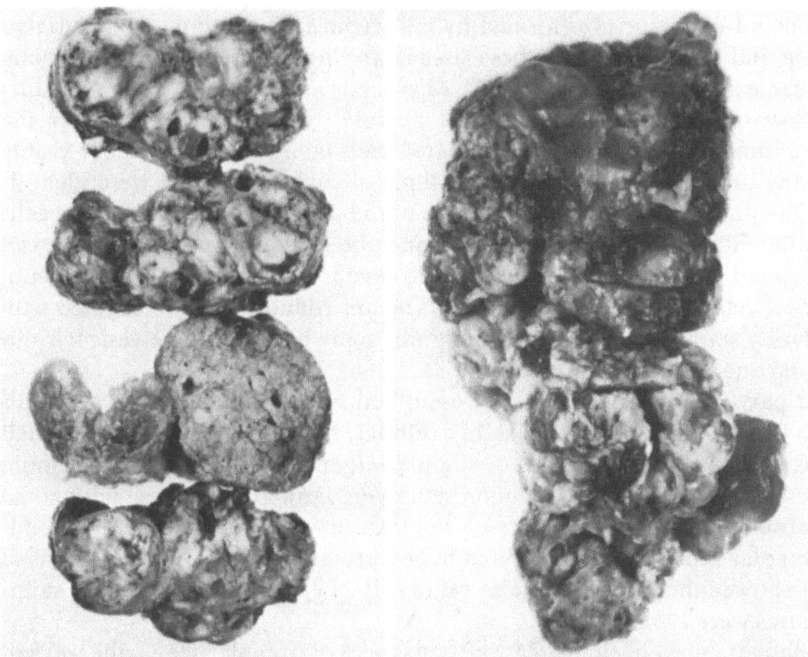

a b

Fig. 2. a The cut surface of the tumour: large solid fleshy areas. **b** Large tumour with a smooth surface and numerous nodular protrusions separated by areas of cartilage, numerous yellowish foci, haemorrhages and cystic spaces

hemispheres were formed regularly but the convolutions were flattened and the fissure of Sylvius had completely disappeared. The grey and white matter were greatly thinned with a maximum thickness of 4 millimetres. The corpus callosum was not identifiable. The diencephalon and the brain stem were disorganized and destroyed by the tumour and could not be identified. Both hemispheres completely enveloped huge nodular tumour masses. The tumour contributed approximately 500 g of the total brain weight of 910 g. During dissection the tumour separated into two larger and numerous smaller parts, some of these connected with brain tissue. In between the parts of the tumour large blood clots were found. The surface of the tumours was smooth with numerous tuberous protrusions (Fig. 2b). The cut surfaces of the tumours were spotted with large solid fleshy areas often separated by areas of bone and cartilage in between, while numerous yellowish foci, haemorrhages and cystic spaces were also to be found (Fig. 2a).

Microscopic Examination

The tumour showed parts of all three germinal layers which seemed to be in a state of senseless disorder and showed varying degrees of differentiation. Embryonic neuroepithelial structures were abundantly present. Also visible were islands of immature and mature partly ossified cartilage, areas of respiratory and digestive epithelium, gland-like structures formed by tall vacuolated columnar cells, striated muscle tissue and fatty tissue. All these tissues are interspersed with loose young connective tissue stroma and blood vessels. Microcysts and macrocysts were lined by flat cells. Foci of haemorrhage and small necroses were scattered all over the tumour. In addition islands of undifferentiated cells could be seen without visible relation to any organ. Neuroepithelial structures of complex pattern were identifiable within the tumour and in the brain tissue of the diencephalon. Most of the cells were less differentiated judging by the size and the shape of the nuclei. The cell bodies were small. The nucleocytoplasmic ratio favoured the nucleus. The nuclei of the majority of cells were polymorphous, that means round, oval or elongated with abundant darkly staining chromatin. Among this some cells had large vesicular nuclei containing one large nucleolus.

In some parts the cyto-architecture resembled a neuroblastoma or a medulloblastoma. The picture was that of highly cellular, homogeneous masses of small regular cells as large as lymphocytes or slightly larger. The nuclei were sometimes carrot-shaped, forming distinctive pseudorosettes (Fig. 3a). Only in these parts could mitoses be observed. Around blood vessels the texture was often composed of bundles of long bipolar spindle cells with ovoid hyperchromatic nuclei. Other portions of the tumours showed the architecture and cellularity of ependymomas. The most important features were rosettes.

Occasionally there were elongated clefts or spaces of irregular shape, the walls of which are covered with a typical ependymal epithelium (Fig. 3b). An increase of oligodendroglial cells could also observed in some areas, as well as blood vessels forming convolutions similar to an angioma.

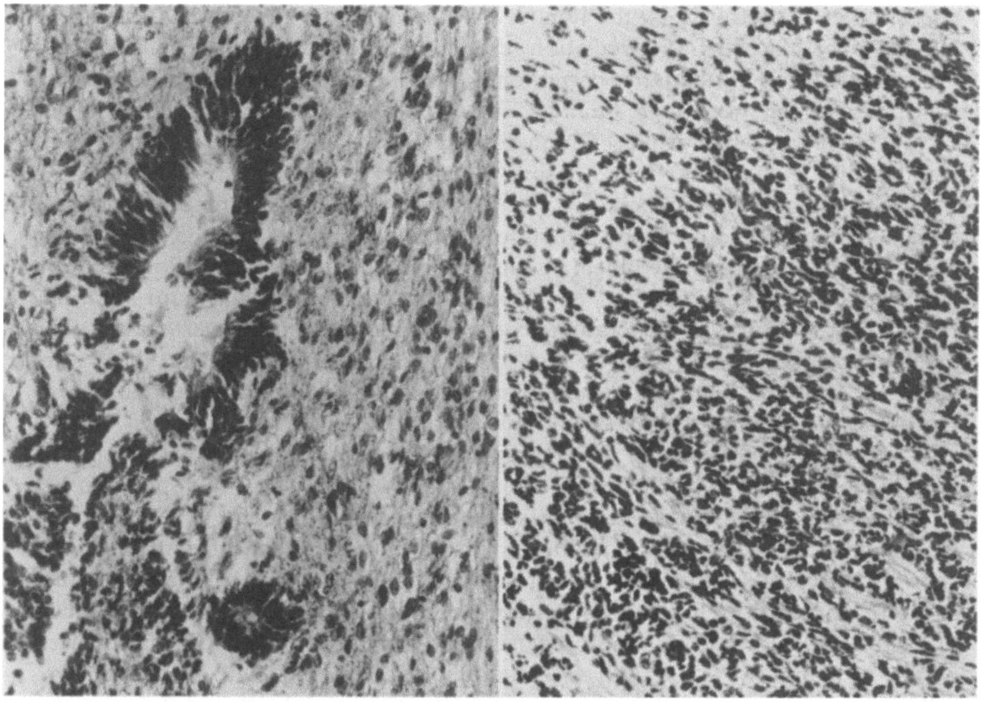

a b

Fig. 3. a A highly cellular tumour of small cells. The nuclei are sometimes carrot-shaped, forming distinctive pseudorosettes. HE, × 120. **b** Elongated space the wall of which is covered with a typical ependymal epithelium. HE, × 250

Within the cortex the migration of the nerve cells had not yet terminated. In the cerebellum the outer germ layer was still preserved. Apart from these signs of immaturity no further indications of malformation could be recognised.

Discussion

Teratomas do not have a uniform picture in the CT-scan. Often parts with negative density predominate. The different types of tissues present within a teratoma such as cartilage and bone tissue, already cause high density values in the plain scan. For this reason measurements in different parts of the tumour show a wide range of densities [7]. After injection of contrast medium an evident increase of density within the malformation tumour often occurs especially if there is a malignant degeneration.

In our case the CT-scan showed some special features which complicated the diagnosis and which could only be clarified by necropsy.

The teratoma consisted of several nodules. The tumour had grown from the midline into both hemispheres. The diencephalon and the midbrain were infiltrated and completely destroyed by the tumour and therefore they were not visible in the CT-scan. The blocked CSF circulation resulted in an extreme hydrocephalus, both internal and external; the latter corresponds with the frontal and occipital fluid-filled cavities which were seen in the CT-scan. The accumulation of fluid in the subarachnoid space had displaced both hemispheres aside, so that it appeared like a malformation of the brain in the CT-scan.

The origin of the teratoma could not be clarified. The sella turcica was not suspicious. The pineal could not be identified, so it could not be decided whether the tumour had started from the pineal and had grown from the diencephalon into both hemispheres, or whether it had developed from the floor of the third ventricle. Histological structures of the teratoma corresponded with all three germ layers. The major part of the tumour showed higher somatical differentiation, but there were abundant masses of neuroectodermal tissue within the tumour and exceptionally in the infiltrated diencephalon. Landrieu et al. [8] give a description of cytoarchitectonic features within the tumour similar to those of the normal developing neocortex. They did not believe – as Vraa-Jensen [13] did – that this specimen belonged to the residual central nervous system structures, which had undergone a developmental arrest in maturation. In our case the development of immature stem cells into a neuroblastoma-like tumour or a medulloblastoma is of interest because of the rapid growth of the tumour and its malignancy. A differentiation of the embryonal neuroepithelial tissue into ependymomatous structures had been reported by several authors [4, 9, 11]. The combination of a germinoma with the typical two-cell pattern and a teratoma is very frequent [10], but we did not find it in our material. The mixed histological pattern of the tumour demonstrates the multipotentiality of the stem cells [2, 6].

Summary

In a premature male infant a massive midline intracranial teratoma was observed with infiltration in both hemispheres. In the CT-scan the cranial cavity was filled by several nodules with hypodense and hyperdense areas. Liquid filled cavities were visible frontally and occipitally. No brain structures could be identified. By light microscopy the tumour contained tissues of all three germ layers. In the infiltrated and destroyed diencephalon the tumour corresponded with a neuroblastoma or a medulloblastoma. Some parts were differentiated into an ependymoma. The mixed histological pattern of the teratoma demonstrates the multipotentiality of the stem cells.

References

1. Arita, N., Ushio, Y., Abekura, M., Koshino, K., Hayakawa, T.: Embryonal carcinoma with teratomatous elements in the region of the pineal gland. Surg. Neurol. *9*, 198–202 (1978)
2. Borit, A.: Embryonal carcinoma of the pineal region. J. Path. (Edinb.) *97*, 165–168 (1969)

3. Camins, M. B., Takeuchi, J.: Normotopic plus heterotopic atypical teratomas. Child's Brain *4,* 151–160 (1978)
4. Finck, F. M., Antin, R.: Intracranial teratoma of the newborn. Amer. J. Dis. Child *109,* 439–442 (1965)
5. Herrschaft, H.: Die Teratome des Zentralnervensystems. Dtsch. Z. Nervenheilk. *194,* 344–365 (1968)
6. Jellinger, K., Minauf, M., Kraus, H., Sunder-Plassmann, M.: Embryonales Carcinom der Epiphysenregion. Acta neuropath. (Berl.) *15,* 176–182 (1970)
7. Kazner, E., Wunsch, S., Grumme, T., Lanksch, W., Stochdorph, O.: Computertomographie intrakranieller Tumoren aus klinischer Sicht. Berlin, Heidelberg, New York: Springer Verlag 1981
8. Landrieu, P., Goffinet, A., Caviness, V., Lyon, G.: Formation of "Neo-cortex" in a congenital human teratoma. Acta Neuropathol. (Berl.) *55,* 35–38 (1981)
9. Rubinstein, L. J.: Tumours of the central nervous system. Armed Forces Institute of Pathology, Washington DC 1972
10. Tekeuchi, J., Mori, K., Moritake, K., Tani, F., Waga, S., Handa, H.: Teratomas in the suprasellar region: Report of five cases. Surg. Neurol. *3,* 247–254 (1975)
11. Tamura, H., Kury, G., Suzuki, K.: Intracranial teratomas in fetal life and infancy. Obstet. Gynec. *27,* 134–141 (1966)
12. Tobo, M., Sumiyoshi, A., Yamakawa, Y.: Sellar teratoma with melanotic progonoma. A case report. Acta Neuropathol. (Berl.) *55,* 71–73 (1981)
13. Vraa-Jensen, J.: Massive congenital intracranial teratoma. Acta. neuropath. *30,* 271–276 (1974)

The Isolated Fourth Ventricle: Review of Current Concepts and Report on Three Cases in Children

E. Mahlmann, D. Voth, and M. Schwarz

The phenomenon of a congenital cystic dilatation of the fourth ventricle, recognised at the end of the 19th century, is a well-defined morphological and clinical entity known as the Dandy-Walker syndrome. The progress of neuroradiological diagnosis and neurosurgical treatment of hydrocephalus and tumours of the posterior fossa led to the recognition of a secondary, non-congenital dilatation of the fourth ventricle as a specific clinical syndrome, frequently associated with signs of a posterior fossa mass. This was first called the 'Post-operative Dandy-Walker syndrome' [13, 19], 'double compartment hydrocephalus' [3], 'cystic transformation of the fourth ventricle' or 'trapped fourth ventricle' [26]. The term 'isolated fourth ventricle', introduced by Hawkins [8] allows a precise definition, as it is used by Scotti et al. [20].

The term 'isolated fourth ventricle' implies a morphological or functional stenosis of the aqueduct of Sylvius and the foramina of Luschka and Magendie which separates the fourth ventricle from the supratentorial compartment and the subarachnoid space. The lack of resorption of the CSF continually produced by the chorioid plexus leads to an accumulation of intraventricular fluid. The ventricle expands with pressure on the surrounding structures, namely the cerebellum, brainstem and tentorium and this may result in clinical signs of a posterior fossa mass.

There are different aetiological causes for this syndrome. Some aspects of pathogenesis can be based on experimental and clinical findings on secondary stenosis or obstruction of the aqueduct and the outlets of the fourth ventricle.

The length of a normal aqueduct is 11–20 mm, and the cross section varies between 0.2 and 1.8 mm^2 [4, 17]. In no case is the post mortem appearance representative for intravital stenosis, which depends on actual pressure relationships.

Besides congenital (hereditary?) stenosis, forking or membranous occlusion of the aqueduct, direct compression and local inflammatory reactions can lead to a secondary stenosis of the aqueduct [21]. Compression can be caused by mid-line tumours (pinealoma, corpus callosum lipoma and brain stem tumours) or downward herniation of the temporal lobe by a supratentorial mass or a hydrocephalic lateral ventricle. Malabsorption of CSF in the cisterna ambiens can lead to additional external pressure. Raised CSF pressure proximal and distal to a stenosis may result in a membranous septum [25] of the aqueduct. An expanding mass in the posterior fossa (e.g. tumour, or arachnoid or Dandy-Walker cyst) can induce an aqueduct stenosis by upward herniation of the upper cerebellar vermis. The reversibility of such a mechanism has been described by Raimondi in 1969 [15] and was called 'dynamic block' by Jacubowski [9].

Besides a direct mechanical obstruction of the aqueduct by clotted blood or other material like cholesterin crystals originating from a craniopharyngioma, an inflammation of the ependymal layer can lead to a stenosis [10, 16, 22]. Other causes are mumps and other viruses, bacterial infection (e.g. following shunt therapy or ventricular taps), or noninfective lesions of ependyma by intraventricular blood and distension of ependymal cells by CSF under raised pressure [15]. The corresponding histological findings are subependymal gliosis and 'aqueductuli' which are separated by gliosis [22].

The second condition for isolation of the fourth ventricle is a functional insufficiency of the foramina of Luschka and Magendie. It is not a morphological proven obstruction, but rather an imbalance between intraventricular CSF production and ventricular outflow via the basal cisterns which is decisive. (There are proven cases of Dandy-Walker syndrome, where the outlets of the fourth ventricle have been found definitely open [7, 2].) The reduced CSF resorption is caused mainly by arachnoiditis, induced by different pathogenetic factors: purulent meningitis, spontaneous and traumatic subarachnoid haemorrhage [11, 19]. Both are possible complications of posterior fossa operations, ventricular taps and shunt-therapy with multiple revisions. The importance of these factors was first described by Scatliff [19] who established the term 'post-operative Dandy-Walker syndrome' [13, 18, 19]. Once an imbalance between CSF production and outflow from the fourth ventricle has occurred, a progressive dilatation of the fourth ventricle can perpetuate itself by compression of basal cisterns and stenosis of the aqueduct by transtentorial herniation of the upper cerebellar vermis.

This development can be of importance in two different groups of patients:

- a lateral ventricle shunt is performed for a communicating hydrocephalus (or a Dandy-Walker syndrome or in a case of posterior fossa tumour), the CSF pressure in the supratentorial compartment is reduced and the still elevated pressure in the fourth ventricle can lead to a secondary aqueduct stenosis.
- repeated revisions of shunt therapy in a hydrocephalus with primary aqueduct stenosis can be complicated by meningitis or minor subarachnoid haemorrhage, causing impairment of outflow of CSF from the fourth ventricle.

The isolation of the fourth ventricle is a consequence of both these pathological conditions.

Clinical signs are mainly those of a posterior fossa mass: cerebellar ataxia, impaired coordination, nystagmus and disturbance of ocular movement. The patient's complaints are often diffuse headache, vertigo and recurrent vomiting. Pre-existing neurologic deficits can deteriorate, but even asymptomatic progress has been reported [20]. Signs of increased intracranial pressure are usually absent. In cases of shunt therapy the shunt proves to be intact. The literature contains altogether about 30 cases, mainly children [5, 8, 12, 13, 15, 20]. We want to contribute three cases as examples of a different origin of an isolated fourth ventricle:

- a child with a cerebellar midline tumour (ependymoma)
- a child with internal hydrocephalus after meningitis
- a child with occipital meningocele and cystic transformation of a congenital wide fourth ventricle.

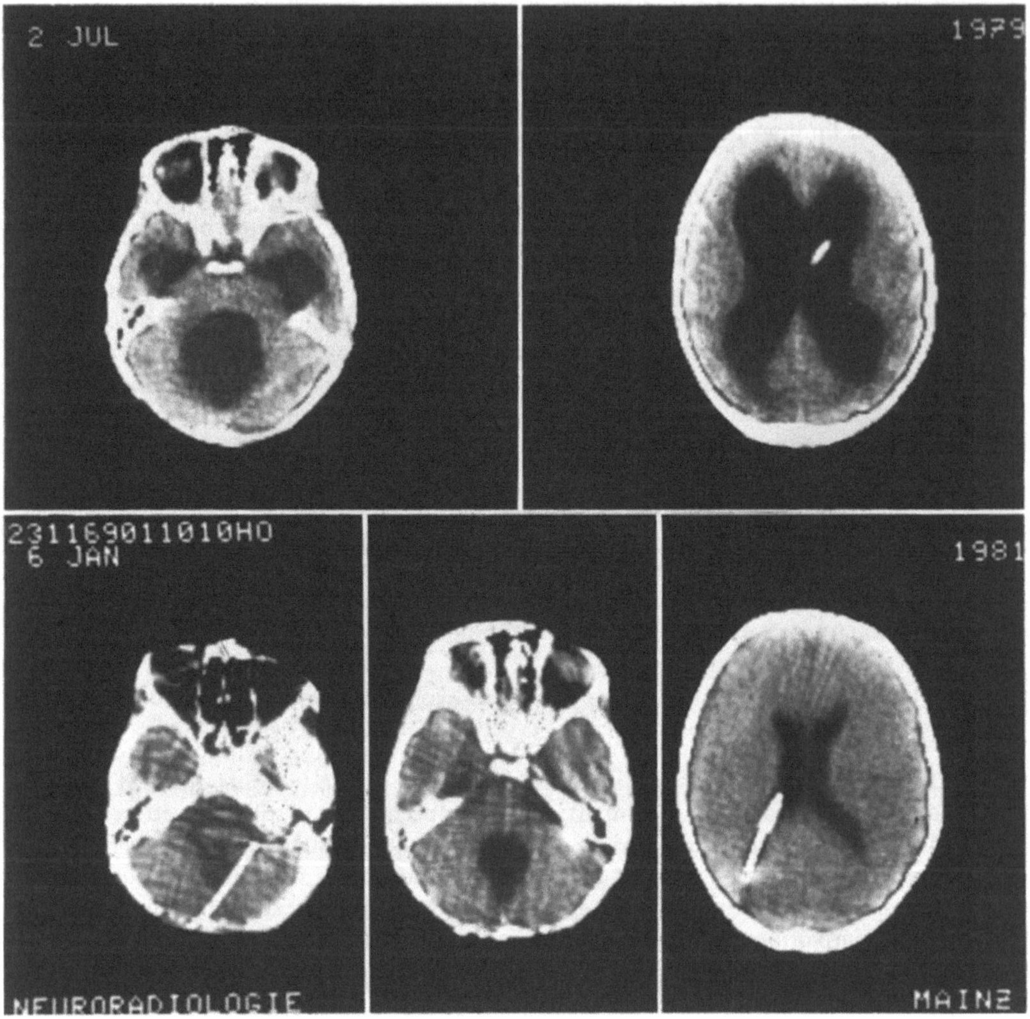

Fig. 1. *Above:* Postoperative cystic dilatation of the fourth ventricle (Ependymoma). *Below:* Decrease of dilatation after shunting of the fourth ventricle

Case 1. A nine-year-old boy complained about diffuse headache and showed progressive ataxia of gait and recurrent vomiting. On admission he had papilloedema. CT and ventriculography were performed and showed a midline cerebellar tumour with obstructive hydrocephalus. The tumour was removed and proved to be an ependymoma. A ventriculo-peritoneal shunt was performed. The post-operative course was satisfactory and the ataxia receded. After an interval of six months, there was again deterioration with nystagmus and cerebellar ataxia but no headache. CT controls showed a progressive dilatation of the cystic fourth ventricle. After a separate atrial shunting the ataxia receded again leaving only slight residual symptoms. CT showed a significantly smaller fourth ventricle (Fig. 1).

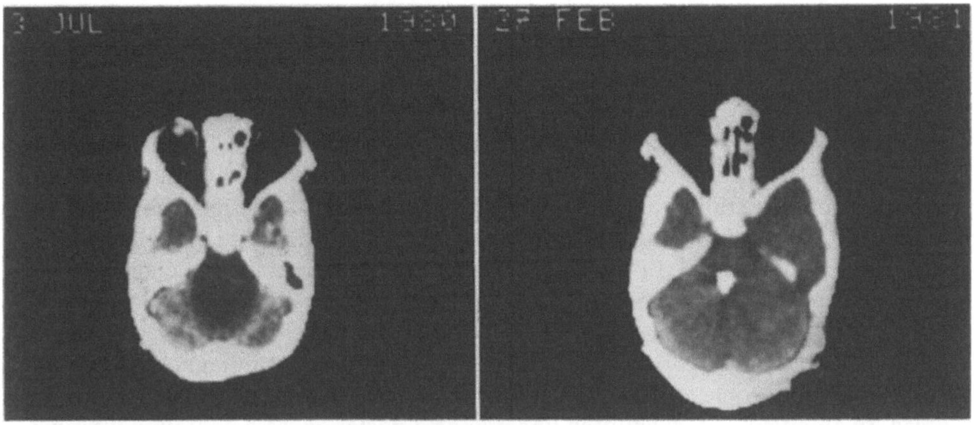

Fig. 2. *Left:* Lateral shunting of hydrocephalus internus following meningitis. Dilatation of the fourth ventricle is persistent. *Right:* The fourth ventricle becomes smaller after selective shunting. Revision of lateral ventricle shunt

Case 2. A premature female of the 24th week showed various postnatal complications: postpartum asphyxia, a hyaline membrane syndrome, cardiac arrest, enterococci sepsis and meningitis, intracerebral haemorrhage and convulsions.

An internal hydrocephalus developed and was treated with a ventriculo-atrial shunt that had to be revised once. At the age of two the girl had mental retardation, a spastic syndrome involving all four limbs; she could sit erect but could not walk. At this time, headache and vomiting began and she assumed an opisthotonic posture. CT demonstrated a dilatation of the fourth ventricle and a normal sized supratentorial compartment. Metrizamide given intrathecally did not pass from the basal cisterns into the fourth ventricle. A selective peritoneal shunting of the fourth ventricle was performed. At operation extensive arachnoidal adhesions were found in the basal cisterns and further downwards. Post-operative CT demonstrated a return to normal of the fourth ventricle. There was no further history of vomiting or opisthotonic episodes [2] (Fig. 2).

Case 3. A male newborn had an occipital meningocele about 4 cm in diameter at a basal fissure of the occipital squama. CT demonstrated the hypodense meningocele and a rather wide fourth ventricle. After resection of the sac, an incipient internal hydrocephalus necessitated a lateral ventriculo-atrial shunt that was later converted to a peritoneal shunt. Subsequent CT-controls showed a progressive cystic dilatation of the fourth ventricle in association with a clinical deterioration and the development of a spastic syndrome. Metrizamide given intrathecally stayed outside the fourth ventricle. After an anastomosis between the fourth and right lateral ventricle with a ventricle catheter and low pressure valve was performed, the spasticity receded and the fourth ventricle became smaller again.

Discussion

Symptoms and signs in the cases reported were impressive but not specific: ataxia, nystagmus, spasticity and headache and recurrent vomiting can be interpreted as consequences of a posterior fossa lesion in general. As a specific cause we can assume that post-operative and post-meningitic arachnoid adhesions impaired the outflow of CSF from the fourth ventricle in cases 1 and 2 and that an aqueduct stenosis developed in case 3. In all cases, CT was decisive in making the diagnosis. We have tried to prove separation of the fourth ventricle by intraventricular and intrathecal injection of metrizamide, which did not enter the enlarged fourth ventricle. Following Scotti et al. [20], contrast studies are not essential for diagnosis, when the dilated fourth ventricle is clearly visible and the supratentorial ventricles are not enlarged. In about 20% of all children undergoing a posterior fossa operation we saw a transient dilatation of the fourth or all ventricles, so that close observation of clinical progress and a CT is necessary (H. Stein, [23]). Differential diagnosis from porencephalic, extra-axial cysts, post-operative defects or cystic astrocytomas usually requires no other method than CT [1, 6, 20, 24, 26].

The treatment of a hydrocephalic and isolated fourth ventricle that is causing symptoms has to be operative. A direct reopening of the fourth ventricle into the basal cisterns requires a rather extensive exposure and is in danger of causing a postoperative arachnoiditis. Shunt systems can be fitted as a separate peritoneal (or atrial) CSF shunt from the fourth ventricle, in connection with a pre-existing lateral ventricle shunt or as a valve-less connection (interventriculostomy) between the fourth and a lateral ventricle. These techniques are afflicted with the known complications of shunt systems. Another possible way to re-establish CSF flow might be by placing a catheter leading from the fourth ventricle into the cervical CSF space, but there are no personal or published experiences yet available.

Summary

The isolated fourth ventricle is a cystic dilatation of the fourth ventricle caused by a functional occlusion of the aqueduct of Sylvius and the foramina of Luschka and Magendie, secondary to a hydrocephalus treated by shunting of the lateral ventricles or operative exploration of the posterior fossa. Current concepts of pathogenesis are reviewed and reports of three patients are given. The predominant signs of the posterior fossa are nonspecific. Computed tomography is essential for diagnosis and leads to differentiation from other space-occupying lesions of the posterior fossa. Treatment consists in the shunting of the fourth ventricle and different techniques are discussed.

References

1. Archer, C. R., Darwish, H., Smith, K.: Enlarged cisterna magna and posterior fossa cysts simulating Dandy-Walker-Syndrome on computed tomography. Radiology *127,* 681–686 (1978)
2. Brown Joe R.: The Dandy-Walker Syndrome. In: Vinken, P. J. and Bruyn, G. (eds.), Handbook of clinical Neurology, Vol. 30, p. 623–646 Amsterdam 1977
3. DeFeo, D., Foltz, El.: Double compartment hydrocephalus in a patient with cysticercosis meningitis. Surg. Neurol. *4,* 247–251 (1975)
4. Emery, J. L., Staschak, M.: The size and form of the cerebral aqueduct in children. Brain *95,* 591–598 (1972)
5. Foltz, El., Shurtleff, D. B.: Conversion of communicating hydrocephalus to stenosis or occlusion of the aqueduct during ventricular shunt. J. Neurosurg. *24,* 520–529 (1966)
6. Haller, J. S., Wolpert, S. M.: Cystic lesions of the posterior fossa in infants. Neurology *21,* 494–506 (1971)
7. Hart, M. N., Malamud, N., Ellis, W. G.: The Dandy-Walker Syndrome. Neurology *22,* 771–780 (1972)
8. Hawkins, J. C., Hoffmann, H. J.: Isolated fourth ventricle as a complication of ventricular shunting. J. Neurosurg. *49,* 910–913 (1978)
9. Jakubowski, J., Jefferson, A.: Axial enlargment of the third ventricle and displacement of the brain stem in benign aqueduct stenosis. J. Neurol. Neurosurg. Psychiatr. *35,* 114–123 (1972)
10. Johnson, R. T.: Hydrocephalus and viral infections. Develop. Med. Child Neurol. *17,* 807–816 (1975)
11. Juhl, J. H., Wesenberg, R.: Radiological findings in congenital and acquired occlusions of the foramina of Magendie and Luschka. Radiology *86,* 801–813 (1966)
12. Kaufman, B., Weiss, M. H.: Effects of prolonged cerebrospinal fluid shunting on the skull and brain. J. Neurosurg. *38,* 288–297 (1973)
13. Mclauri, N. R., Ford, L. E.: Obstruction following posterior fossa surgery: the post-operative Dandy-Walker Syndrome. Johns Hopkins Med. J. *122,* 309–318 (1968)
14. Paraicz, E.: Membranverschluß des Aquaeductus Sylvii. Zentralblatt für Neurochirurgie *31,* 235–245 (1970)
15. Raimondi, A., Samuelson, G., Yarzagaray, L., Norton, Th.: Atresia of the foramina of Luschka and Magendie. J. Neurosurg. *31,* 202–216 (1969)
16. Raimondi, A., Clark, S. J., Mclone, D. G.: Pathogenesis of aqueductal occlusion in congenital murine hydrocephalus. J. Neurosurg. *45,* 66–77 (1976)
17. Salam, M.: Stenosis of the aqueduct of Sylvius. In: Vinken, P. J., Bruyn, G. (eds.), Handbook of clinical neurology, Vol. 30, Amsterdam 1977, 609–622
18. Sanchis, J., Bordes, M.: Distension of the operative site after posterior fossa surgery. Acta neurochirurg *40,* 243–251 (1978)
19. Scattliff, J. H., Kummer, A. J.: Cystic enlargment and obstruction of the fourth ventricle following posterior fossa surgery: the post operative Dandy-Walker Syndrome. Am. J. Roentgen. *88,* 536–542 (1962)
20. Scotti, G., Musgrave, M., Fitz, Ch., Harwood-Nash, D.: The isolated fourth ventricle in children: CT and clinical review of 16 cases. Am. J. Roentgen. *135,* 1233–1238 (1980)
21. Shellshear, I., Emery, J. L.: The tectum and the aqueduct of Sylvius in hydrocephalus unassociated with myelomeningocele. Develop. Med. Child Neurol. 17 supp. *35,* 26–34 (1975)
22. Shellshear, I., Emery, J. L.: Gliosis and aqueductule formation in the aqueduct of Sylvius. Develop. Med. Child Neurol. 18 supp. *37,* 22–28 (1976)
23. Stein, B. M., Tenner, S. M., Fraser, R.: Hydrocephalus following removal of cerebellar astrocytomas in children. J. Neurosurg. *36,* 763–768 (1972)
24. Tal, Y., Freigang, B., Dunn, H. G., Durity, F. A., Moyes Moyes, P. D.: Dandy-Walker Syndrome: Analysis of 21 cases. Develop. Med. Child Neurol. *22,* 189–201 (1980)
25. Williams, B.: Is aqueduct stenosis a result of hydrocephalus? Brain *96,* 399–412 (1973)
26. Zimmerman, R. A., Bilaniuk, L. T., Gallo, E.: Computed tomography of the trapped fourth ventricle. Am. J. Roentgen. *130,* 503–506 (1978)

Follow-Up Findings with CT Scan and Ventriculography After Radiotherapy of Inoperable Midline Tumours in Childhood

H.-J. König and H. Altenburg

The diagnosis and operative treatment of midline tumours of the brain may be a difficult problem for the neuroradiologist and the neurosurgeon.

To answer the question, if operation is possible or if radiotherapy or chemotherapy is required, different diagnostic procedures have to be performed. In particular CT scans, but also angiography, and in certain cases positive ventriculography have to be done [1, 5].

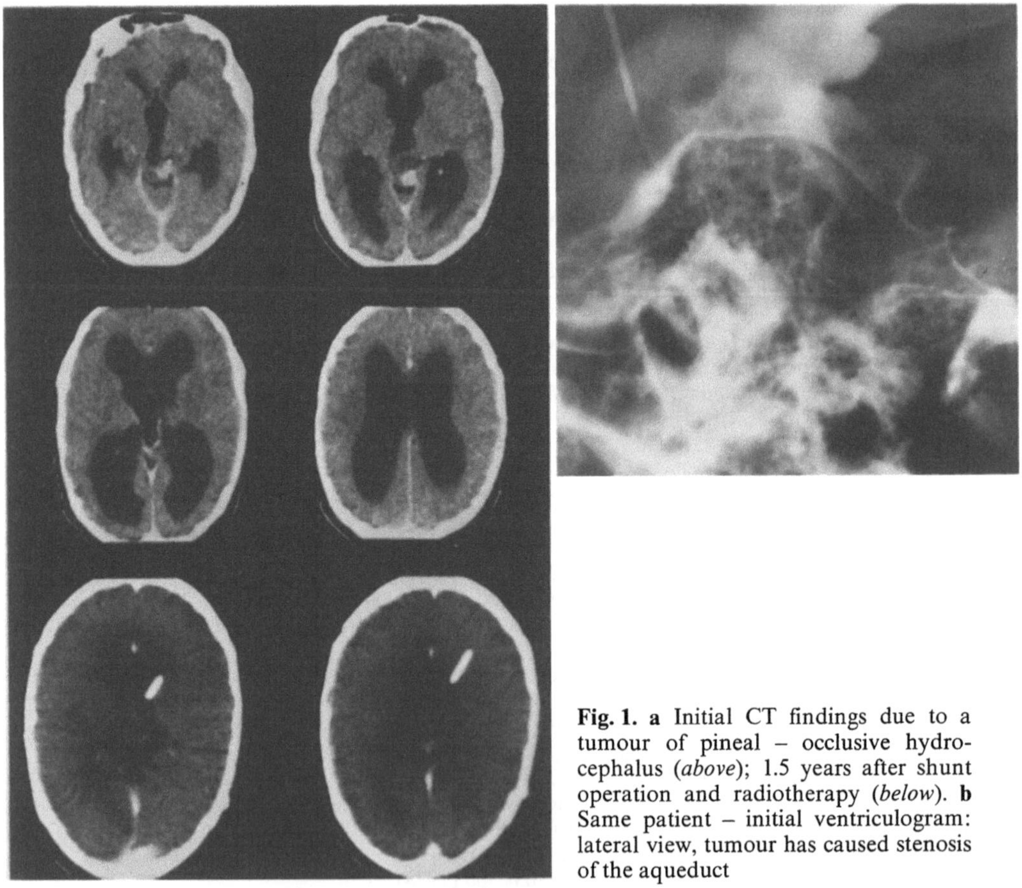

a b

Fig. 1. a Initial CT findings due to a tumour of pineal – occlusive hydrocephalus (*above*); 1.5 years after shunt operation and radiotherapy (*below*). **b** Same patient – initial ventriculogram: lateral view, tumour has caused stenosis of the aqueduct

According to the site of the tumour, the indications for operation may be difficult to estimate. Infiltrating tumours are excluded as far as possible from operative treatment, by most neurosurgical departments.

Any operation in the midline of the brain carries with it a high risk for the life of the patient or of postoperative neurological deficit.

Operation is indicated in benign tumours growing within the ventricles or in those showing cystic components or showing no effects from radiotherapy. If there is no indication for operation, radiotherapy combined with polychemotherapy is usually done [6]. Raised CSF pressure is controlled by a shunting operation or drainage in order to avoid obstructive hydrocephalus. Dexamethasone is given for a long time (Fig. 1).

The success of treatment can be shown by ventriculography [7]. There is no longer any obstruction of the cerebrospinal fluid pathways and the outline of solid tumour is no longer present in the aqueduct and ventricles [1, 5].

Nowadays CT scan is of great importance in the diagnosis and follow-up of midline tumours [2]. In some cases the CT findings are complemented by ventriculography, especially if the indications for operation must be reconsidered after radiotherapy has not produced any effect [1, 6, 7].

Conclusion

A decision about the operative treatment of midline tumours can only be taken after complete diagnostic procedures. During and after treatment its success is controlled by CT scan. In some cases ventriculography has to be added in order to answer specific questions. Regrowth of tumours can be detected early by this means.

References

1. Altenburg, H., Walter, W.: Value of central ventriculography with Dimer-X in the differentiation between cerebellar tumours and caudal brain stem tumours before and after radiation therapy of so-called inoperable midline tumours. Adv. in Neurosurg. *5,* 155–158 (1978)
2. Gardeut, D., Nachanakian, A., Millard, J. C., De Gennes, J. L., Turpin, G.: The value of computerized tomography in the exploration and surveillance of diencephalic tumours. Nouv. Presse Med. *7,* 2231–2233 (1978)
3. Hara, M., Takenchi, K.: A temporal study of survival of patients with pontine gliomas. J. Neurology *216,* 189–196 (1977)
4. Kretzschmar, K., Aulich, A., Schindler, E., Lange, S., Grumme, T., Meese, W.: The diagnostic value of CT for radiotherapy of cerebral tumours. Neuroradiology *14,* 245–250 (1978)
5. Kunze, St., Schiefer, W.: Ventrikulographie mit positiven Kontrastmitteln bei raumfordernden Prozessen der Mittellinie und im Bereich der hinteren Schädelgrube. Radiologie *9,* 495–499 (1969)
6. Pertuiset, B., Visot, A., Metzger, J.: Diagnosis of pinealoblastomas by positive response to Cobalt-therapy. Acta Neurochir. *34,* 151–152 (1976)
7. Suzuki, J., Hori, S.: Evaluation of radiotherapy of tumours in the pineal region by ventriculographic studies with iodized oil. J. Neurosurg. *30,* 595–603 (1969)

Discussion

P. Gutjahr (Mainz) referring to the paper by *K. Kretzschmar (Mainz)* stated that there was an apparent discrepancy between the results he had described and those mentioned on the same and the following day, from the neurosurgical clinic and the children's clinic, because Kretzschmar's investigations only include those patients who had CT examinations pre-operatively and postoperatively in the Neuroradiology department. These, however, are only a part of the total patient material.

K. J. Zülch (Cologne) referred to a patient of *Kretzschmar (Mainz)* in whom a glioblastoma multiforme developed after radiation of a craniopharyngioma which had been subtotally removed. He asked what evidence was available which could possibly support the genesis of this glioblastoma as a second tumour induced by the radiotherapy. In his reply Kretzschmar stated that the possible connection had to be discussed, but however there was no definite proof.

P. Gutjahr (Mainz) reported two further observations from his clinical material in whom likewise, gliomas developed after radiation to the head. One case had a glioblastoma multiforme and the other an astrocytoma. Here, the striking concidence needs to be stressed, without there being any definite evidence about the connection.

Bohl (Mainz), Kretzschmar (Mainz) and *K. J. Zülch (Cologne)* all touched on the problem of giving radiation without any histological findings. *J. M. Schröder (Aachen)* also pointed out, that from the neuropathological point of view it could not be regarded as sensible to give radiation without a definite diagnosis of tumour with histological reports. He referred to a meeting in which were reported lesions which had been erroneously interpreted as tumours and then radiated.

D. Voth (Mainz) referring to the papers by *S. Wende* et al. and by *Altenburg* et al. stated his view about the neurosurgical aspects of ventriculography with positive contrast medium, in supratentorial lesions, namely that it did not provide any additional information over and above the CT findings. This held good even for extracerebellar lesions in the posterior fossa, for instance lesions in the cerebello-pontine angle. The indications for performing ventriculography have become so drastically reduced by the CT scan, that only occasionally are there special questions which need to be answered by this investigation. Even in these few cases, CT after the intrathecal injection of contrast medium is just as valuable and is attended by less risk. At the present time, in his view as a neurosurgeon, there remains a definite indication for performing ventriculography in one case only. This is in cerebellar midline tumours, where the relationship to the floor of the fourth ventricle is not clear. Here the ventriculogram can occasionally allow one to express a clear opinion as to whether the tumour is infiltrating the floor of the fourth ventricle or if it is merely lying on the floor. This question is not important as far as the size of the tumour and its precise diagnosis are concerned, but may be so for the actual operative procedure. The answer to this question is, in his opinion, the only remaining indication for ventriculography with positive contrast medium. In any case the latest generation of CT apparatus, with or without the addition of intrathecal contrast medium, will probably answer this question as well.

E. Kazner (Berlin) said that in his opinion ventriculography is superfluous. It should be during the operation, when enucleating the tumour in the fourth ventricle, that one determines whether or not the hind brain is infiltrated.

K. Schürmann (Mainz) considered that the neurosurgeon needs more information than the doctor who is purely concerned with diagnosis in a detached way, more precisely the neuroradiologist. The desire for more information is the reason why the neurosurgeon makes every effort to utilize as wide a range as possible of available diagnostic procedures.

S. Wende (Mainz) indicated that in his opinion ventriculography had no advantage as regards locating a tumour in the supratentorial or infratentorial cavity or even regarding the type diagnosis, which improves on the information supplied by the CT scan. On the other hand the desire of the neurosurgeon for maximal information is understandable, so that occasionally the use of this investigation may be approved of.

Evolutional, Developmental, and Clinical Aspects of Brain Stem Organisation

P. GLEES

The human brain stem (rhombencephalon and mesencephalon) shows the basic features of vertebrate brain organisation and the developmental phases in ontogeny repeat largely the evolutionary stages of vertebrates. In the following the rhombencephalon, the hindbrain vesicle, will be considered. This hindbrain vesicle, the cranial extension of the neural tube and frontal to the spinal cord contains like the spinal cord nerve cell columns of motor and sensory properties. These neurons are topographically however in a different position from their spinal counterparts. This shift in position is due to the opening of the spinal cord into the IV. ventricle and

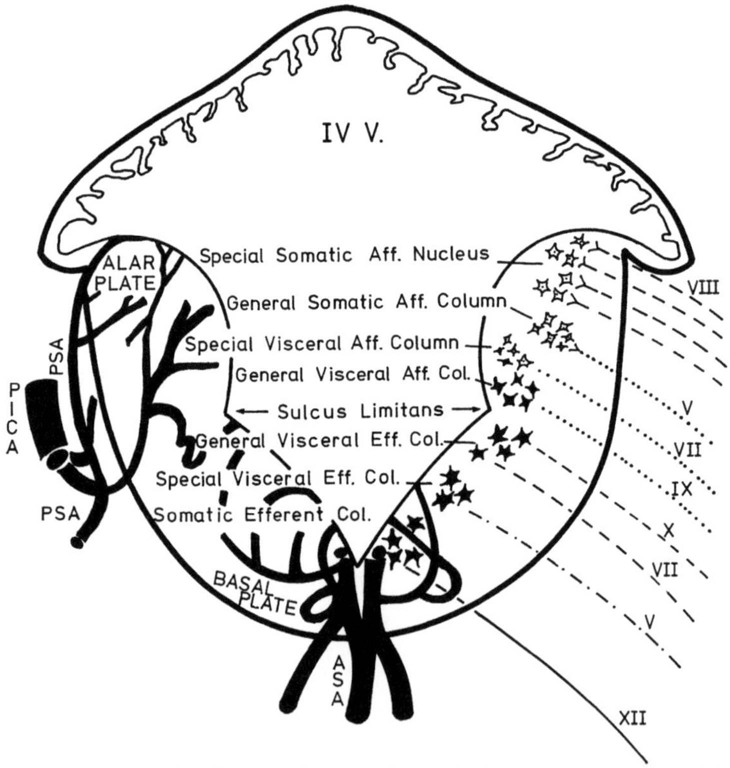

Fig. 1. A composite diagram showing the evolutionary organisation of the rhombencephalon. On the right side, the distribution of cranial nerve nuclei, on the left the vascular supply. *ASA* Vertebral arteries and medial branches from spinal arteries; *PSA* posterior spinal artery; *PICA* posterior inferior cerebellar artery supplying lateral and dorso-lateral areas

the addition of special afferent and efferent neurons (Fig. 1). This arrangement can be found in all vertebrates but obviously with some variation due to the changed mode of life during the evolutionary process.

Thus if we compare a sagittal section through the head of an early human embryo with an elasmobranch embryo we see clearly the basic vertebrate pattern in both (Fig. 2a, b). Even with the radical change in peripheral supply regions – e.g. the change from external gill breathing to internal lung oxygenation, the vagal nerve nuclear position in the medulla remains.

As the brain stem is clearly recognizable early on in fetal life and bases on firm evolutionary principles it houses the important cranial nerves and centres for respiration, heartbeat and digestion functions of the foregut derivatives (Fig. 3). Due to these functions the brain stem becomes a regulative centre for important vital maintenance of body functions. Even with subsequent cortical development impressive both in size and importance, loss of brain stem function means loss of life, not only the loss of certain cranial nerve supply regions. The reason is the irreparable neuronal loss of the reticular system, with its far reaching ascending and descending connections dispersed in the nerve fibre matrix of the brain stem. This system was first recognized and investigated closely by Magoun and his school (c.f. Glees 1957, 1961). Magoun not only clarified the importance of the reticular neurons for muscle tone but stressed also the importance for the maintenance of the state of conscious awareness and attention. Due to this new concept the cerebral cortex has been put into a role of a filing cabinet or reference library depending for its proper function on the brain stem.

The nuclei of the brain stem stretch from the lowest level of the brain stem where the hypoglossal nucleus lies at the commencement of the IV. ventricle and as far cranial as the oculomotor nuclei in the midbrain. Only brain sections in a longitudinal or sagittal plane demonstrate sufficiently the considerable longitudinal extension of cranial nerve nuclei in contrast to the convential transverse plane. The topography of the nuclei is based on a modified developmental arrangement of the embryonic spinal cord divided in a dorsal sensory and a ventral motor lamina centered around the spinal canal. This canal opens at medullary level shifting the nuclei of the sensor or alar lamina laterally (see Fig. 1) including the special nerve nuclei for the special senses excluding of course optic and olfactory channels which are not true cranial nerves but brain tracts coming from forward positions of embryonic brain vesicles.

The cranial nerves are most useful clinically for assessing brain stem functions, not only for initiating and testing reflex action of a particular cranial nerve but allowing indirectly a proof of the presence of sufficient blood supply for total brain stem function needed particularly for the maintenance of consciousness. The irreversible loss of brain stem function or brain stem death is clinically identical with brain death even if the EEG might initially show some residual activity. The present view taken by British neurologists is illustrated in Fig. 4 and Tables 1 and 2, kindly given to me by Dr. C. Pallis.

The role of the cerebral cortex for the organisation of the brain stem: This aspect can be studied in early fetal stages of brain development, when in the third and fourth month the cerebral hemispheres expand first posteriorly and then swing forward temporally. The telencephalic vesicles fuse essentially medially

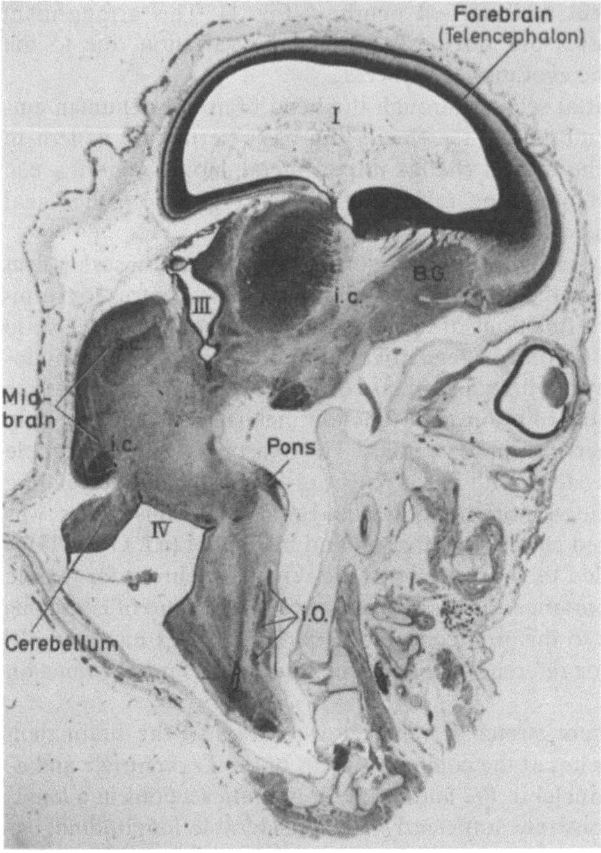

a

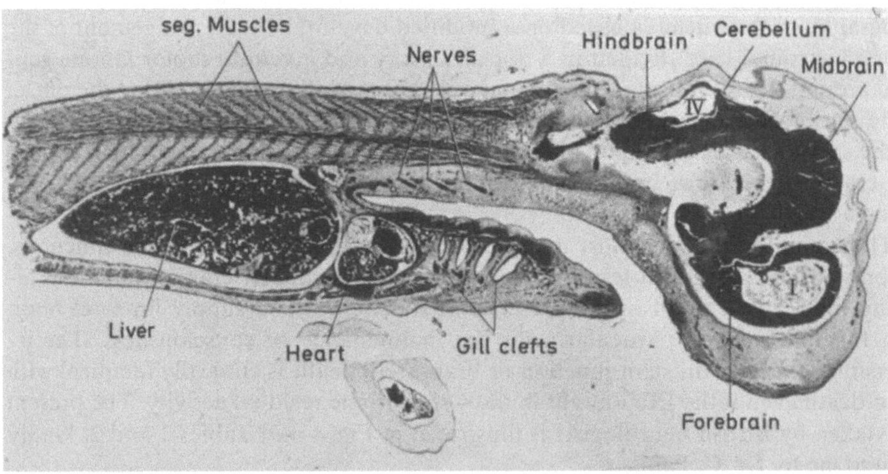

b

Fig. 2. a Sagittal section through the head of a human embryo (about 12 weeks) illustrating the marked advance of the brain stem development in contrast to the late development of the telencephalon. **b** This sagittal section through an elasmobranch (cartilagenous fish) illustrates a comparative stage in evolutional terms in a species where the midbrain will keep entirely its dominant role in contrast to man

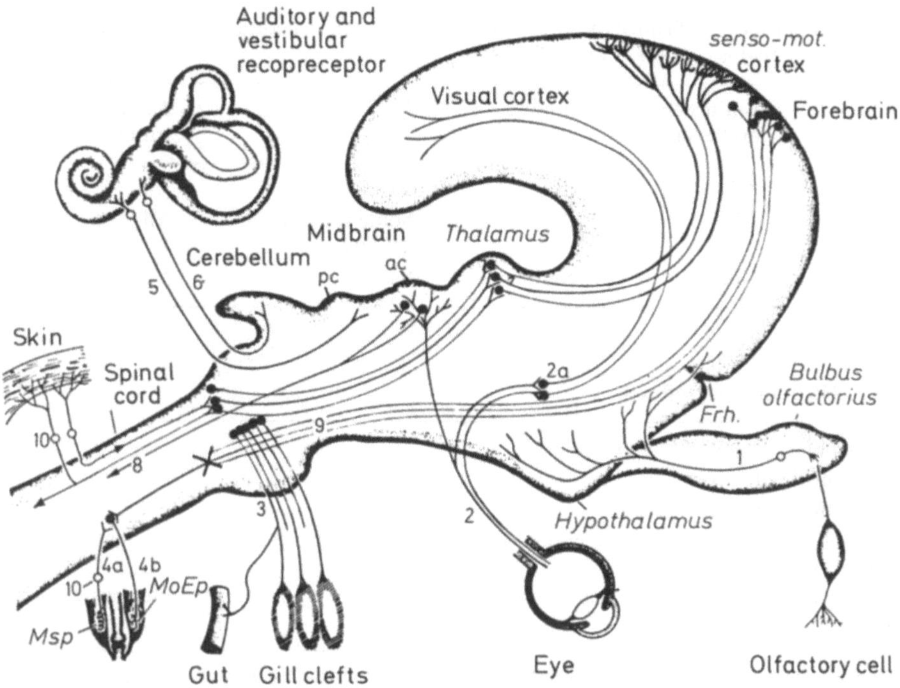

Fig. 3. Composite diagram illustrating the evolutionary history of vertebrates culminating in the dominating development of the cerebral cortex in mammals. A step initiated by the arrival of proprioceptive and exteroceptive impulses at cortical level, followed by visual input and the descend of a motor cortical control system. *1* Olfactory tract, *2* optic tract, *2a* visual pathway relay, *3* gill nerves and nerve to foregut (vagus), *4a* somato-sensory nerve, *4b* somato-motor nerve, *5* cochlear division, *6* vestibular division, *7* posterior column relay, *8* tecto-spinal tract, *9* pyramidal tract, *10* spinal ganglion, *Frh* Fissura rhinalis, *Msp* muscle spindle, *MoEp* motor endplate. (Modified from Glees [8])

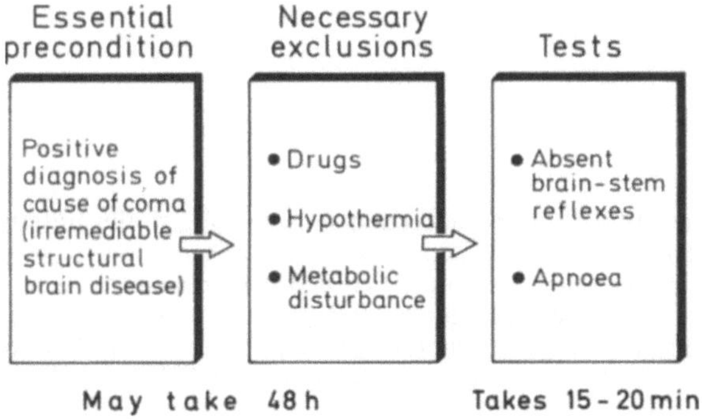

Fig. 4. The road to brain stem death

Table 1. Prognostic significance of brain stem death (known, structural brain disease, no drug-induced cases). [Pallis C (1981) Lancet I: 379]

Number of cases	Brain stem areflexia	Apnoea	EEG	Asystole within days
> 1000	All	All	'Isoelectric'	All
147	All	All	Some residual activity	All
16	None	None	'Isoelectric'	None

Table 2. No brain stem reflexes

1. No pupillary response to light
2. No corneal reflex
3. No vestibulo-ocular reflexes
4. No motor responses within the cranial nerve distribution in response to adequate stimulation of any somatic area
5. No gag reflex or reflex response to bronchial stimulation by suction catheter passed down trachea

- All brain stem reflexes must be absent, before brain stem death can be diagnosed
- No oculo-cephalic reflexes. Testing not specifically required in U. K. Code. Much time saved if tested first. If present: patient clearly not brain stem death

Fig. 6. Transverse section, diagrammatically, of the brain section shown in Fig. 5, illustration of the area of fusion between telencephalon and diencephalon. *1 a, b* cerebral hemisphere, *2* corpus callosum, *3* choroid plexus entrance, *4* nucleus caudatus, *5* cortico-thalamic and thalamo-cortical fibres, *6, 7, 11* lentiform nucleus, *8* nucleus amygdalae, *9* thalamus, *10* hypothalamus, *12* stria medullaris, *13* stria terminalis, *14* fornix, *15* choroid plexus, *16* vessels of choroid plexus (III., V.), *17* cortico-fugal fibres, *18 (X)* line of fusion between telencephalon and diencephalon ►

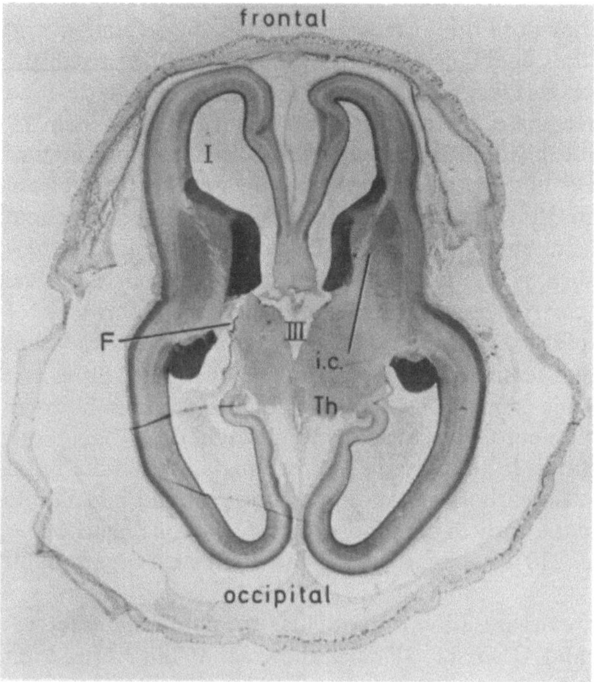

Fig. 5. Horizontal section through the foetal brain showing on the left side the area of fusion (*F*) between telencephalon and diencephalon (*Th*). *I* Lateral ventricle, *III* third ventricle, *i.c.* internal capsule

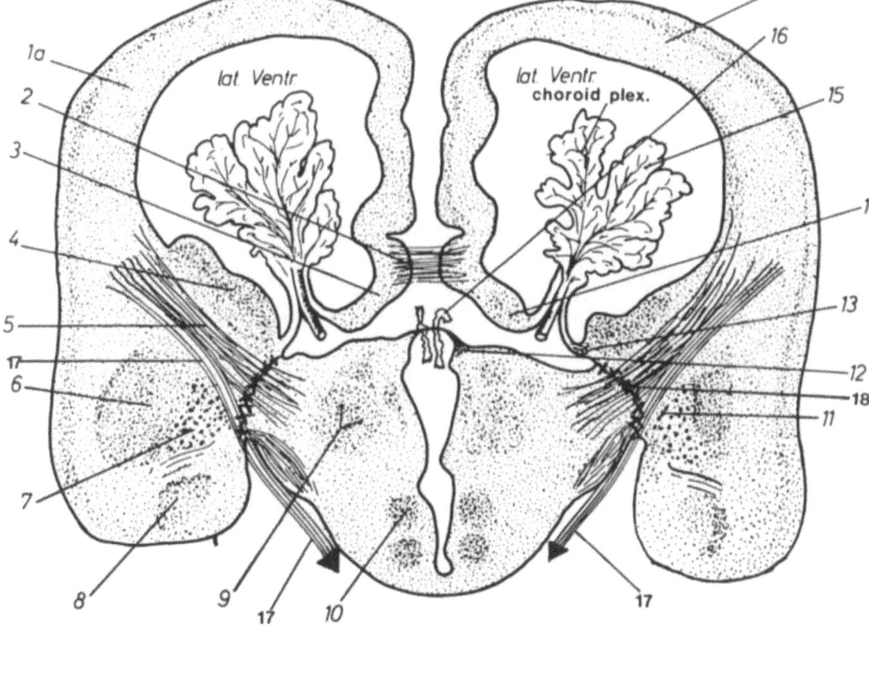

Fig. 6

with the thalamus in an anterior-posterior direction bringing diencephalon and telencephalon in close contact thus enabling fibres from the thalamus to reach the cortex and vice versa. Only when this fusion is achieved cortical fibres can descend to lower levels (Figs. 5, 6). When these descending fibres reach the brain stem by keeping a ventral course without invading the already fully organised and mature midbrain and medulla. The nuclei of the brain stem receive their cortical input from fibres ascending from the ventrally situated cortico-mesencephalic, pontine and pyramidal tract fibres. This means the cortico-subcortical fibres establishing new synapses with relevant nuclei, such as the pontine nuclei, do not alter anymore the basic architecture. This can be clearly shown in a case of a hydrocephalus which I was able to study, where the rapidly expanding hemispheres prevented their fusion with the diencephalon and thus the ventral downgrowth of the cortico-fugal fibres and the ingrowth of the cortico-thalamic connections. Sections of the brain stem however reveal a fully developed fibre and neuronal pattern of organisation (Fig. 7). Not only the absence of cortico-fugal fibres in this case of hydrocephalus shows the brain stem organisation to be intact, also early degeneration of one pyramid in infantile hemiplegia, long standing traumatic cortical damage, or removal of one hemisphere with a long survival period (Glees 1979) appear leaving the brain stem organisation unaltered (Fig. 8).

Concerning cortico-fugal fibre organisation in particular the pyramidal tract, recent experiments by Dawnay and Glees [1–3] have shown that the fibres from physiological subdivisions of the motor cortex in the monkey when reaching the brain stem are not segregated in distinct bundles related to these subdivisions. This

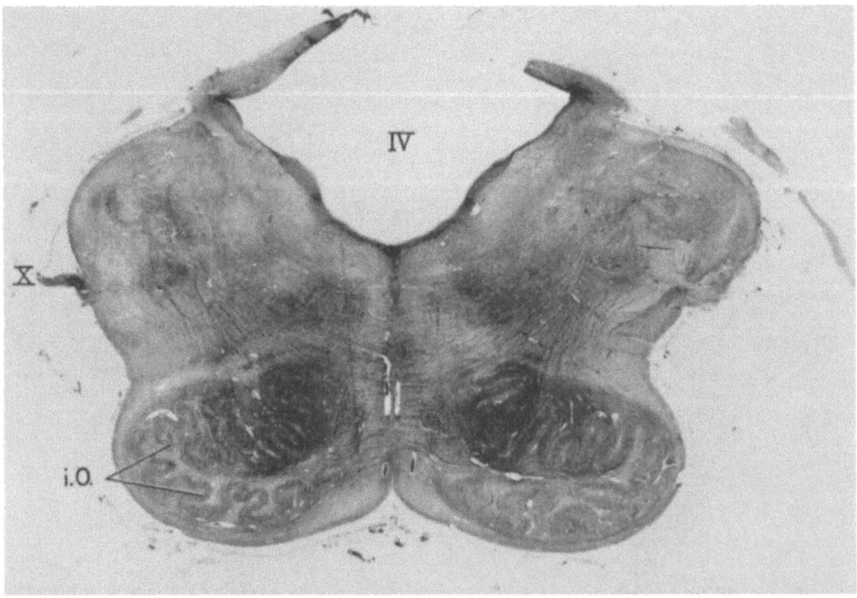

Fig. 7. Medulla of a hydrocephalic brain, in which the fusion between telencephalon and diencephalon did not take place (see text). The structure of the rhombencephalon is normal, apart from the missing pyramids. *i.O.* Inferior olive, *X* vagus, *IV* IVth ventricle (Glees method)

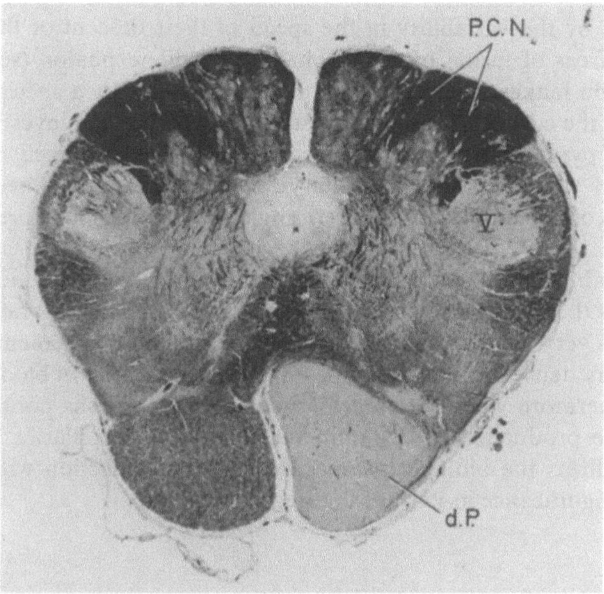

Fig. 8. Transverse section through the lower medulla at the level of Goll and Burdach (posterior column nuclei). The degeneration of one pyramid (*d.P.*) for one year has not altered the basic structure of the medulla, e.g. compare the size of the trigeminal nucleus (*V*) on both sides, or the posterior column nuclei (*P.C.N.*)

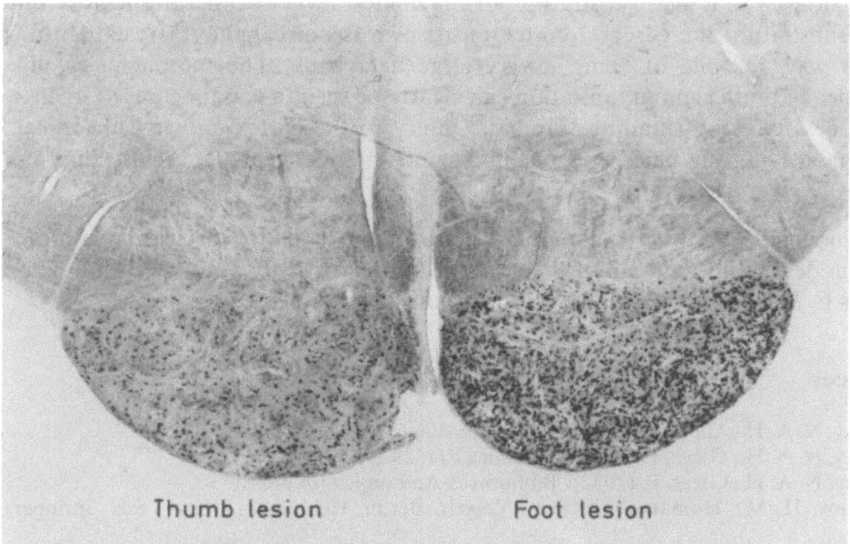

Fig. 9. A cross-section of a monkey's medulla (MCLCG 1). Both pyramids show fibre degeneration, caused by a lesion in the left thumb area of the motor cortex affecting the left pyramid. A lesion in the right foot area of the motor cortex resulting in fibre degeneration in the right pyramid. Note that neither lesion caused circumscribed bundled fibre degeneration, in fact thumb and foot fibres intermingle in their descending course

behaviour can be explained by the variability in the speed of their descent or the hazards in penetrating the areas of fusion of telencephalon and diencephalon (see Figs. 1, 5, 6). This observation makes any suggestion of fibre guidance by a special set of "knowing fibres" from the cortex invalid. At this stage of experimental investigations we believe that the pyramidal tract fibres become progressively mixed in their descending course and when reaching medullary levels degenerating fibres from the thumb subdivision of the motor cortex intermingle freely with foot fibres (Fig. 9).

While the location of brain stem nuclei was already been well described in admirable detail by Jacobson [9], recent highly successful vascular injections of brain stem by Duvernoy [4] give a very clear topography of their neuronal arrangements as these are supplied by a very dense capillary bed in contrast to the paucity of blood supply of fibre tracts. Furthermore when viewing the nucleus pigmentosus pontis coerulei, concerned with the production of dopamin the richness of capillaries is especially startling and confirms the biological importance of its connection with the caudate nucleus and its significance in Parkinson disease.

Summary

For evolutionary, ontogenetic and physiological reasons brain stem organisation is well established before the cerebral cortex matures and reaches a certain dominance. One must assume that the integrating and regulating power of the brain stem produces a corresponding level of awareness and integrated activity which feeds the cerebral cortex with a vital substratum for the highest level of consciousness. Without this substratum the cerebral cortex on its own is not capable of reacting in a conscious way, in spite of being a very large data bank. The morphological independence of brain stem organisation can clearly be seen in certain cases of hydrocephalus or after long-standing traumatic injury to the cortex and its subcortical connexions leaving the basic mesencephalic and rhombencephalic architecture intact.

Acknowledgment. I wish to thank Dr. Christopher Pallis for discussing with me brain stem death and the loan of the relevant tables. Mr. J. F. Crane for photography, Miss E. Rohde and Mrs. F. Glees for technical assistance.

References

1. Dawnay, N. A. H., Glees, P.: J. Anat. *133,* 124–126 (1981 a)
2. Dawnay, N. A. H., Glees, P.: Acta Anatomica *111,* 29–30 (1981 b)
3. Dawnay, N. A. H., Glees, P. (1982): Bibliotheca Anatomica (in press)
4. Duvernoy, H. M.: Human Brain Stem Vessels, Berlin, Heidelberg, New York: Springer 1978
5. Glees, P.: Morphologie und Physiologie des Nervensystems. Stuttgart: Thieme 1952
6. Glees, P.: Experimental Neurology. Oxford: Clarendon Press 1962
7. Glees, P.: In: Histopathological technic and practical histochemistry. p. 617. Ed. R. D. Lillie 1965
8. Glees, P.: Gehirnpraktikum. Stuttgart, New York: G. Fischer 1976
9. Jacobsohn, L.: Über die Kerne des menschl. Hirnstammes. Akad. der Wissenschaften, Berlin 1909

Standard Techniques and Microsurgical Procedures in the Removal of Supratentorial and Infratentorial Tumours

D. Voth

Godlee and Bennett appear to have been the first surgeons who marked the beginning of glioma surgery by the removal of a glioma from a young man in the year 1884. Then a few years later other surgeons such as Horsley and McEwen in Great Britain, Krause and von Bergmann in Germany and Keen in the USA ventured to perform such procedures which, with the absence at that time of any ancillary diagnostic measures, represented no small risk. Between 1900 and 1913 Cushing had operated on 194 tumours: he developed a number of the familiar techniques that are still used even today, and also introduced the endothermy in 1926 [2a, 2b].

Parallel with this there was the striking development of diagnostic procedures, which extend from the use of ventriculography and encephalography by Dandy (1918), angiography by Moniz (1928), through electroencephalography by Berger (1930) up to the methods of measuring cerebral blood flow, isotope procedures, echoencephalography and finally what is indeed the most important discovery of recent decades, computer assisted tomography (CT).

Standard Techniques for the Removal of Supratentorial and Infratentorial Tumours

Supratentorial tumours are exposed by means of an osteoplastic craniotomy, whose size can be adapted to the particular lesion. After opening the dura, the cerebral cortex is inspected and assessed by palpation. With malignant gliomas arterialisation of the venous blood may be observed, oligodendrogliomas can produce changes in the cortex which give an appearance of pseudogyri, while cysts in a tumour betray themselves by palpation, and also by bulging under the cortex, which may alter its outline.

After marking out the line of resection with the endothermy and, at the same time dealing with the pial vessels, the strip retractors are introduced into the depths, the tumour freed on all sides and removed (Fig. 1). All visible vessels are dealt with by electrocoagulation. The line of demarcation from the healthy, normal tissue can usually be seen, but can also be checked by palpation, although this is not always very obvious. Often, if a glioma is confined to a single lobe it is possible to remove it completely by a routine lobectomy, up to the healthy tissue. However, one has to be careful to preserve important parts of the brain such as Broca's or Wernicke's area (Figs. 2, 3).

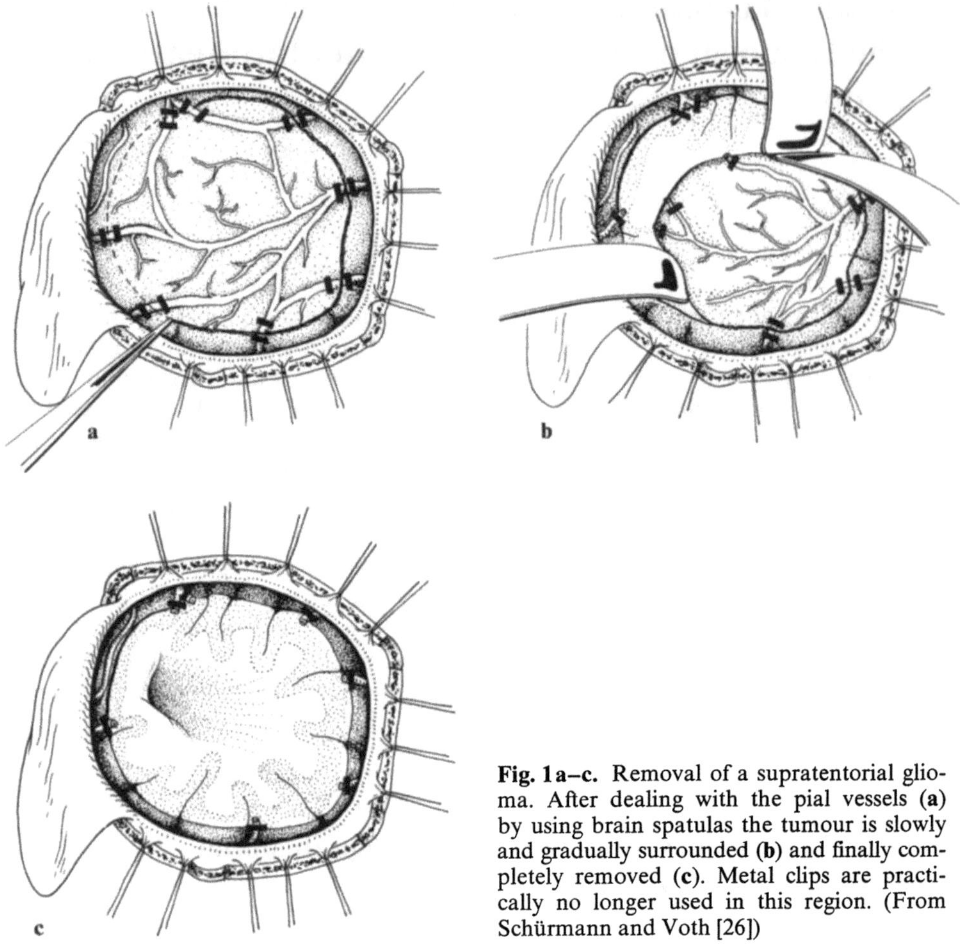

Fig. 1a–c. Removal of a supratentorial glioma. After dealing with the pial vessels (**a**) by using brain spatulas the tumour is slowly and gradually surrounded (**b**) and finally completely removed (**c**). Metal clips are practically no longer used in this region. (From Schürmann and Voth [26])

Infratentorial tumours are generally exposed by a craniectomy of the posterior fossa. In children it is better to make the midline incision S-shaped, in contrast to the incisions usually used in adults. After exposure of the operation field one can obtain a general view of the site and extent of the lesion. By entering the posterior end of the fourth ventricle its cavity can be inspected. Any deformity of the structures in its floor, and particularly a displacement of the midline sulcus, suggests the presence of a deep-seated tumour. Tumours confined to one hemisphere can usually be enucleated after dealing with the pial vessels in the same way that one deals with gliomas in the cerebral hemisphere. It is possible to resect the caudal and central portion of the cerebellum without serious sequelae, as ataxia follows principally after removal of the rostral part of hemisphere. A complete resection of the lower and medial portion of the hemisphere usually means the removal of tissue near the vermis or the cerebellar peduncles. The extent of any particular resection is naturally planned according to the size of the lesion. Tumours within the fourth ventricle are

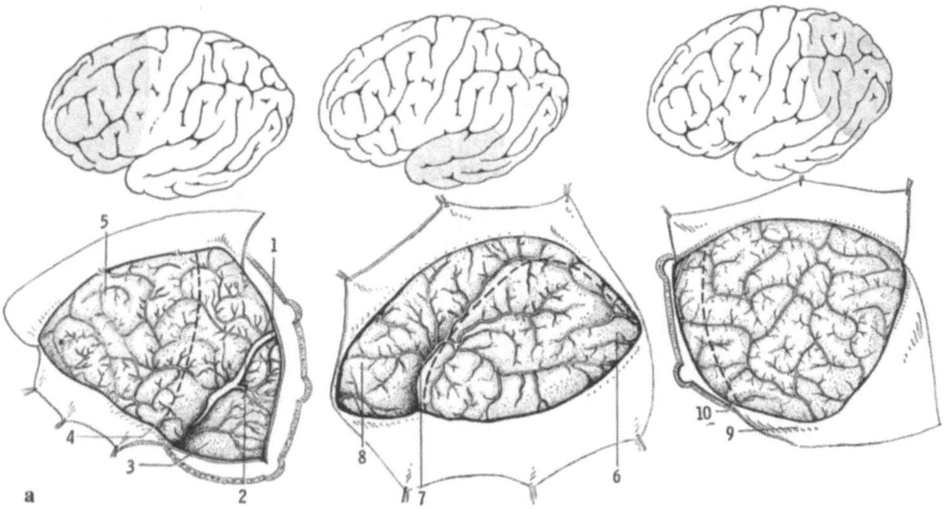

a

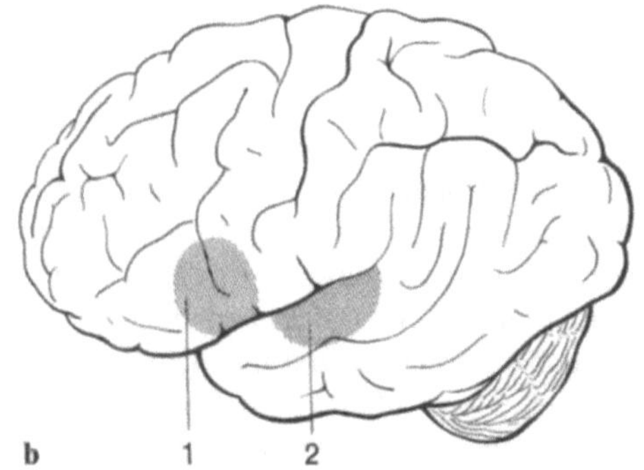

b

Fig. 2. **a** Lines for resection of a lobe. The part which is to be resected is shown stippled. The particular operation site corresponds to the sketch but for the operator it is, of course, turned around through 180 degrees. *1* Sylvian fissure, *2* Sylvian vein, *3* left temporal lobe, *4* line of incision, *5* left frontal lobe, *6* temporal lobe, *7* sylvian fissure, *8* frontal lobe, *9* dura mater, *10,* line of resection. **b** The *hatched area* must be preserved in the dominant hemisphere because this involves Broca's (*1*) and Wernicke's area (*2*). (From Schürmann and Voth [26])

exposed by splitting the vermis and are then removed. If a cystic tumour is found, room can be created by tapping the cyst. With all tumours which are confined to the cerebellar hemispheres an attempt should be made to remove them completely. If the tumour extends into the floor of the fourth ventricle or into the midbrain, it is only possible to perform a subtotal removal, the extent of which must be judged on the result of a rapid histological report [27]. With a medulloblastoma it is unreasonable to press on and perform as complete a resection as possible.

Great care must be exercised when using the endothermy near the floor of the fourth ventricle, as the heat may produce localised damage to vital structures; this applies equally to any mechanical handling with retractors or forceps.

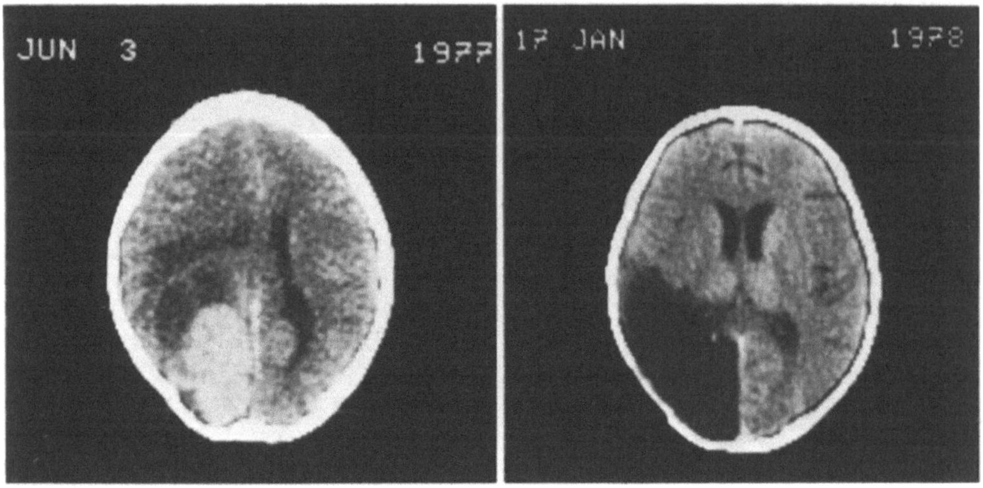

Fig. 3. Appearance shown in the CT after an extensive occipital lobe resection for an ependymoma. The child has been free of recurrence for four years

After the initial exposure of the cerebellum we proceed to inspect its surface. A hemisphere lesion may already be suspected, especially if cysts are present. Herniation of one or both tonsils, with localised circulatory disturbances provide valuable evidence of raised intracranial pressure. If no hemisphere lesion can be seen, the tonsils protected by cotton wool patties should be retracted, first of all by two dissectors and then by two spatulas and the posterior end of the fourth ventricle inspected (Fig. 8). In this way intraventricular tumours are unlikely to be overlooked. Particular attention should be paid to the contours of the floor of the fourth ventricle, as deformities of the otherwise symmetrical structures can easily be recognised. A further hint may be a displacement from the midline of the median sulcus. If the search for the tumour is still unsuccessful the vermis should be split. This allows one to inspect the upper end of the fourth ventricle as far as the aqueduct. If there is a midline lesion the tumour can as a rule be recognised as one looks into the fourth ventricle after retracting the tonsils.

If there is actual involvement of the vermis, one goes in as far as possible on each side of the portion infiltrated with tumour, otherwise the vermis is split in the midline (Fig. 4). The tumour is then revealed. If it proves to be firmly attached to the floor of the fourth ventricle total removal is impossible. However, in every case subtotal removal is recommended. If it can be mobilised, it is carefully separated from the floor of the fourth ventricle with cotton wool and then followed to its point of attachment. Vessels entering the tumour from its immediate neighbourhood are dealt with by using the endothermy. Particular attention should be paid to the choroidal arteries which are often involved in the blood supply of such lesions. If the tumour is firm enough it can be held with tissue forceps. If its point of origin is in the region of the peduncle or the floor of the ventricle a total removal is impossible and should definitely not be attempted. Many soft and necrotic tumours usually

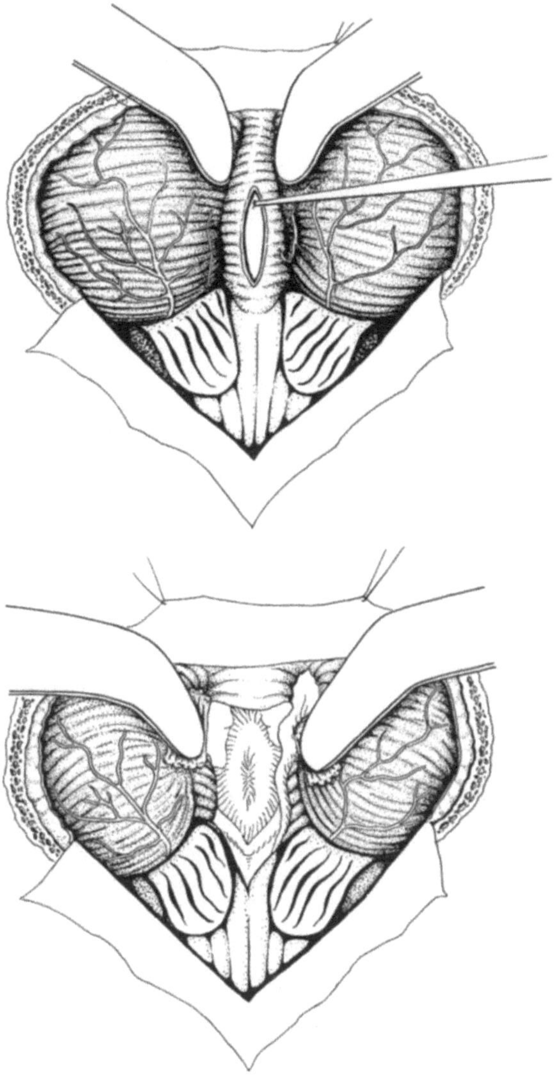

Fig. 4. Splitting of the vermis to expose the fourth ventricle. (From Schürmann and Voth [26])

medulloblastomas and glioblastomas can occasionally be removed by using the sucker. Their complete removal is, without exception, impossible. The nature of the tumour should be determined during the operation by a rapid section or smear. After removal of the tumour, great care and patience must be exercised in securing haemostasis as even slight postoperative bleeding can have disastrous results in this region. With a lesion in the hemispheres the pial vessels are first coagulated, as in the cerebral hemispheres, after which the larger vessels can be dealt with. The tumour can then be carefully removed with the narrow brain spatulas right up to the healthy tissue.

Historical Retrospect on the Development of Microneurosurgery

While the use of the operating microscope in ear nose and throat surgery and ophthalmology by Holmgren [10] as well as Nylen (1921/22) had already been anticipated by the use of magnification, using magnifying spectacles [25, 33], its use in the field of neurosurgery took an astonishingly long time. In 1923 Holmgren had already substituted a binocular microscope for the monocular instrument of his predecessors. Hinselmann [9] introduced microscopic colposcopy in the field of gynaecology. In the field of ophthalmology we must mention the important work of Perrit [20], Barraquer [2] and de Voe [28] as representative figures from a much larger group.

After the pioneer work of House [11] in the treatment of acoustic neurinomas, several neurosurgeons eventually grasped the possibilities of magnification and coaxial illumination [12, 15, 23, 24]. Parallel with this went the development of special microinstruments [12, 32] as well as the use of bipolar coagulation [16, 5]. Quite quickly the microscope was adopted in the surgery of peripheral and cranial nerves and vascular surgery. It was also used in all transventricular, trans-sphenoidal, transmastoid and translabyrinthine procedures, that is to say in all operations with a narrow and deeply situated field.

Finally it became an almost indispensible appliance in nearly all difficult procedures, especially in operations in the posterior fossa, midline lesions such as craniopharyngiomas, pituitary tumours, pinealomas and in aneurysm surgery. It also proved advantageous in operations on the spinal cord and even in simpler procedures such as herniated intervertebral discs.

The advantage of the microscope rests in providing an optimal magnification, excellent illumination and a stereoscopic view. It also enables one to document the operative findings with the 35 mm camera, or the film camera, as well as by video recorder. Finally we may complete the picture here by mentioning the use of the laser in association with the microscope.

The importance of microsurgery for our speciality is so great that each year we are able to run a most successful week's course for thirty participants with lectures and practical work on animals.

Delays in the Development of the Microscope and of the Appropriate Instrumentarium

While the use of the monocular and binocular microscope took place relatively early the principle of coaxial illumination proved to be a very significant advance. The particular field of vision in the microscope was intensively and optimally illuminated and the lighting follows all movements of the microscope.

Microscopes from several manufacturers have been used in the field of neurosurgery. Apart from the apparatus made by Zeiss, which was already developed in 1952 and has since then been continuously improved, other models made by other firms have appeared in the meantime. Each particular microscope has its own particular advantages. The models vary from those on a moveable stand to those mounted in the ceiling. Finally there are compact units manufactured, consisting of an operation stool/chair with numerous control facilities and incorporating its own microscope. Its various functions can be controlled by hand, by foot switch or by a mouth control.

Parallel to this technical perfection has gone the development of the special microsurgical instruments, so that now these are being supplied by numerous firms, in good quality and very practical forms. Details are only of interest to the surgeon. The use of bipolar coagulation and the laser has already been mentioned.

Microneurosurgery in Supratentorial Tumours

The principle domain of microneurosurgery in supratentorial tumours is undoubtedly in dealing with the midline lesions such as craniopharyngioma, pinealoma and chordoma, all of which are extracerebral lesions. On the other hand, in the removal of intraventricular tumours (Fig. 5) the microsurgical approach has proved to be extremely sensible and useful. The approach takes place by a transventricular exposure of the tumour, made in such a way that the incision is not in an eloquent area of the cortex. Figure 6 shows the CT appearance before and after the resection of an intraventricular astroblastoma. It is also important that we are able to intervene in the region of the rostral basal ganglia, so that these structures no longer constitute an absolute limit. With more than a few of these tumours, such as *as-*

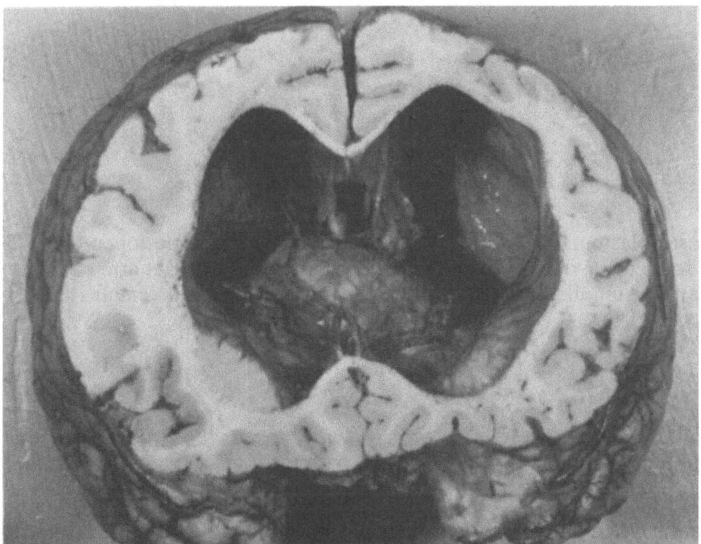

Fig. 5. Post-mortem specimen of an intraventricular tumour, which had produced an obstructive internal hydrocephalus, by blocking the foramina of Monro

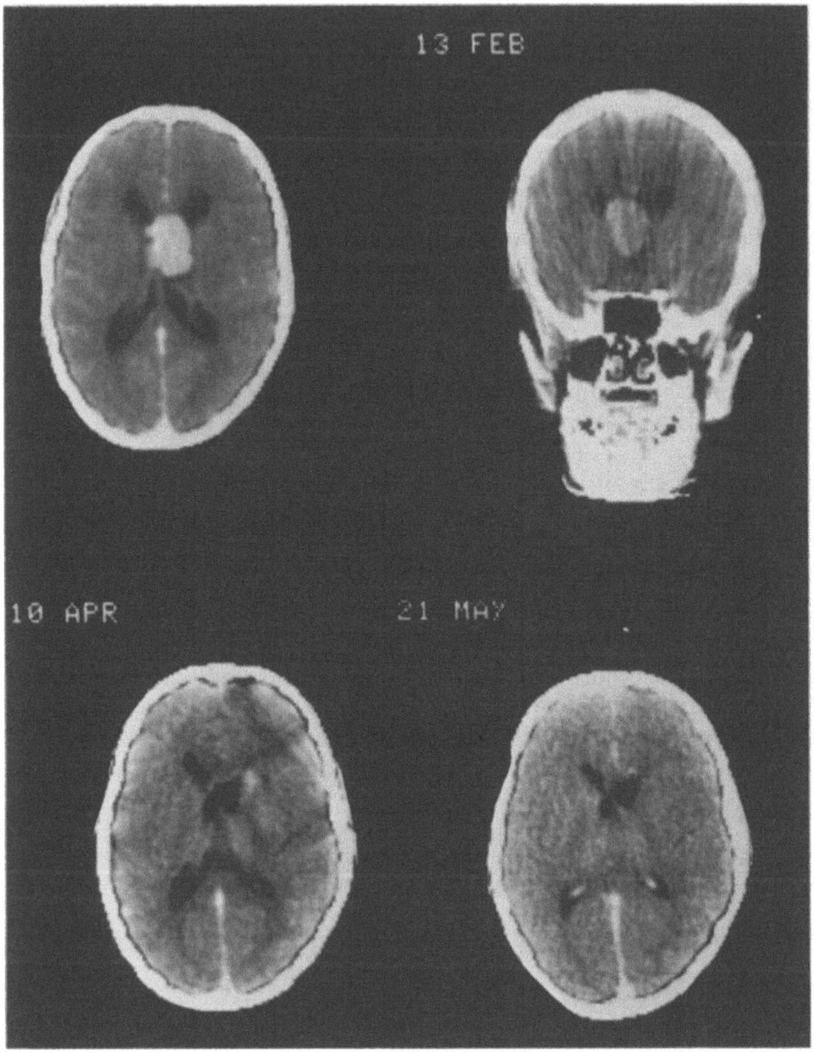

Fig. 6. Intraventricular astroblastoma (III) in a 14-year-old girl. The first postoperative CT (10th April) still showed some reactive changes in the region of the right frontal horn, but these had completely disappeared a month later (21st May). Meanwhile the child remains free of recurrence after two years

troblastoma, giant cell astrocytoma and *pilocytic (piloid) astrocytoma* complete extirpation is possible. Even *ependymomas* can quite often be resected by a transventricular or a combined approach. As the classical but nevertheless rare lesion with an intraventricular location the choroid plexus papilloma should also be mentioned, as its extirpation likewise proved to be very satisfactory. Finally, this is of value also for space-occupying lesions which are only partially intraventricular, as for instance the case shown in Fig. 7 with a pilocytic astrocytoma.

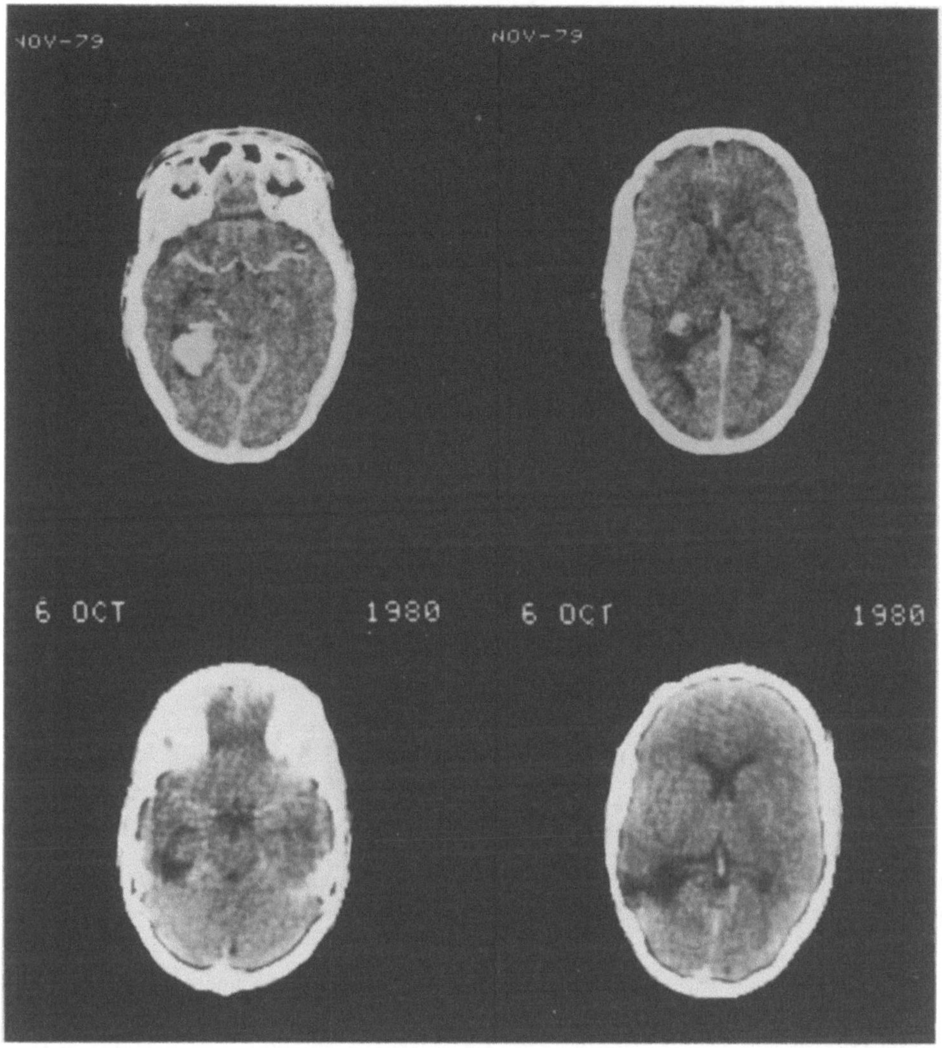

Fig. 7. Pilocytic astrocytoma (I) of the left trigone region in a girl, now 17 years old; pre-operative (November, 1979), and almost one year after the operation (6. 10. 80). The child has had no neurological abnormality

The Value of Microneurosurgery in Infratentorial Lesions

Posterior fossa operations are pre-eminently the province for microsurgical procedure. Here it proved to be of such general value that we carry out all interventions with the microscope. The patients are in a sitting position, but to avoid possible air embolus they are often placed in a position markedly on their side. It is essential to

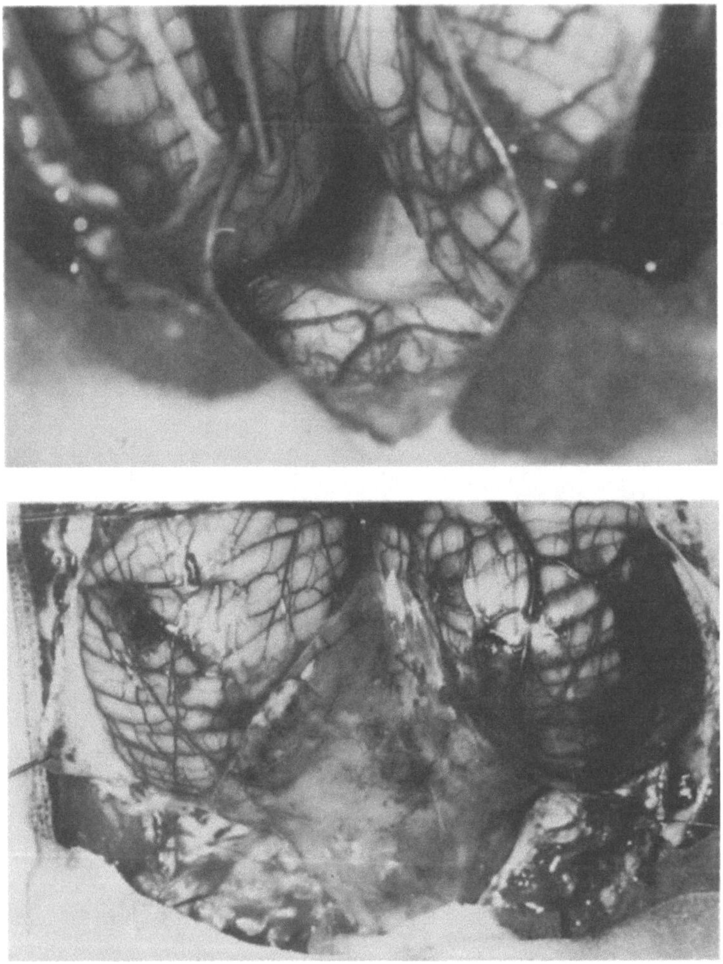

a

b

Fig. 8. a Widely open entrance to the fourth ventricle in a case of arachnoid cyst. Here, access to the rhomboid fossa should present no problems. **b** Medulloblastoma bursting out from the fourth ventricle between the cerebellar tonsils in a six-year-old boy. Here, the usual access to the rhomboid fossa is obstructed by tumour. It is safer not to try and make a way through the tumour tissue but after splitting the vermis to expose its upper part from above and to remove it from above downwards. In this way it is easier to avoid any damage to the hindbrain

use a monitor which operates on the Doppler principle as an indicator of air embolism. The youngest child we have operated on in this position was three months old.

Histologically we find that unfortunately the *medulloblastoma* is the most frequent tumour, followed by *pilocytic astrocytoma* and *ependymoma.*

We make the exposure either with a midline or an S-shaped incision; this allows an adequate exposure even with very large tumours. When the dura has been opened we place the microscope in position, so that with patients in the sitting position the line of vision is horizontal. Purely hemisphere tumours, as for instance the pilocytic astrocytomas can often be seen and removed without exposure of the fourth ventricle. Medulloblastomas and ependymomas which almost always show a close relationship to the fourth ventricle, are first of all approached between the cerebellar tonsils and the rhomboid fossa is displayed from below upwards. If it appears that the tumour has not infiltrated the floor of the ventricle but is only pressing on it, small strips of cotton wool can be gently introduced between the tumour and the rhombencephalon, after which the vermis can be split until the lesion becomes visible. Its definitive removal is then possible and should pose no problems (Fig. 8a, b). Resection can be undertaken without hesitation in the cerebellar hemispheres, nevertheless we try to spare the rostral quadrants if at all possible on account of the disturbances of equilibrium which are otherwise likely to occur.

If the tumour is infiltrating the cerebellar peduncle it can, even in these cases be removed below the level of the rhomboid fossa, at least this holds true for the middle cerebellar peduncle. In general, however, the resection should end at the level of the floor of the rhomboid fossa. Generally in operations on the cerebellar hemispheres it holds good that even more extensive resections can be functionally compensated for after some time.

If the tumour is infiltrating the rhombencephalon first of all the maxim holds good that the level of the floor of the fourth ventricle marks the limits of resection in the direction of the rhombencephalon (Fig. 9). Although we may overstep these limits in suitable cases under the microscope, we must certainly reckon on cranial nerve deficits. On account of the position of the nuclei here we may damage, above all, the abducens, and less commonly the hypoglossal, (trigonum hypoglossi). The facial nerve can be damaged in the region of the facial eminence, where the fibres are close under the surface. With the microscope it is no problem to identify the various structures such as the calamus scriptorius, obex, the area postrema, the ala cinerea, the striae medullares and the colliculus facialis, but it may be that the contours of the rhomboid fossa are markedly changed because of the tumour tissue. Although the CT scan certainly has priority in diagnosis, it seems to us in these cases that ventriculography with positive contrast medium can give information from time to time, which is not entirely without value for the surgeon (1, 13, 29).

If the tumour is already infiltrating the hindbrain opposite the tonsils (Figs. 8b, 9) it is not reasonable to approach it from below. In these cases the ventriculogram gives us the information as to whether we have to deal with obstructed, dilated fluid pathways, possibly the rostral end of the fourth ventricle. If this is the case, the surgeon can expose the tumour without any trouble by splitting the vermis and deal with it from above downwards (Fig. 9). With the present-day improvements in CT scanning the indications nowadays for a ventriculography with positive contrast medium are drastically falling off and in the future it may well be dispensed with altogether.

It is essential to take notice of the blood supply [3, 17] when operating in the posterior fossa. Although an injury of the anterior inferior cerebellar artery (AICA) was previously more to be feared in a cerebello-pontine angle tumour than with a hemisphere lesion, at least lesions of the more important vessels are possible by carelessness. For instance one should look out for the posterior part of the posterior inferior cerebellar artery (PICA) lateral to the caudal portion of the rhomboid fossa. In medulloblastomas and plexus papillomas also, the cerebello-pontine angle can

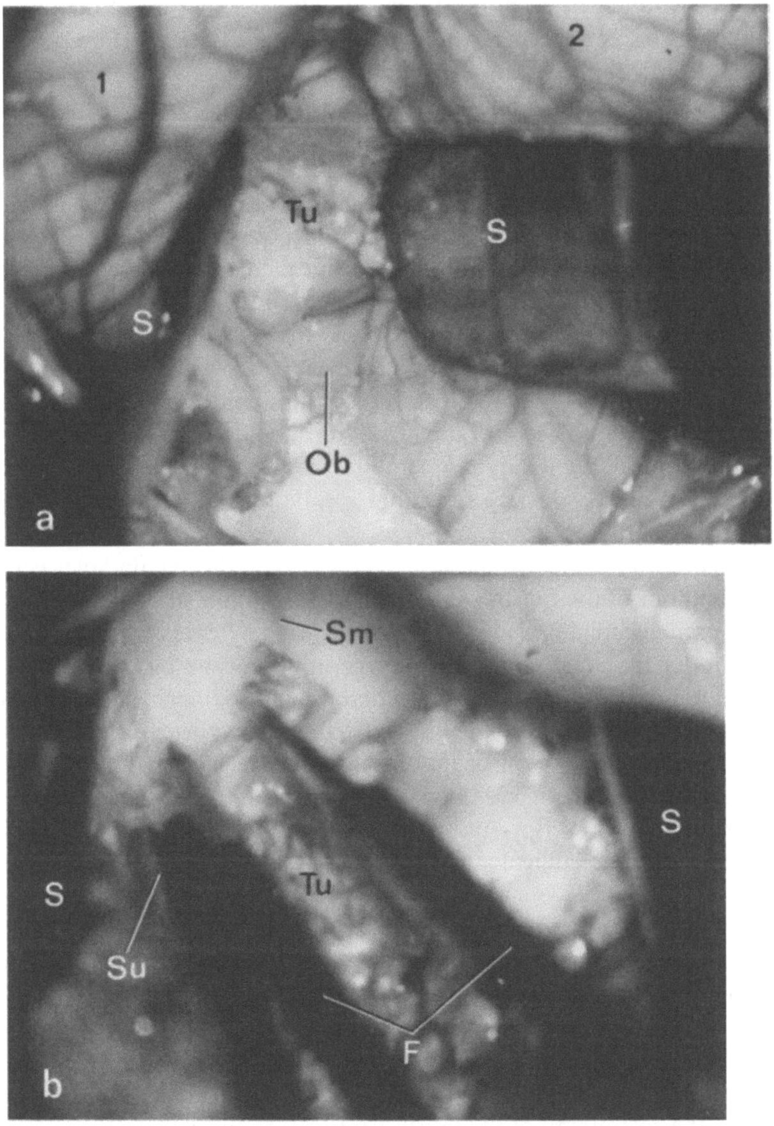

Fig. 9a, b. Tumour infiltration of the hindbrain by a medulloblastoma (four-year-old boy). After splitting the vermis the rostral part of the tumour was mobilised to expose the floor of the fourth ventricle. Portion of an operation film. **a** After partial division of the vermis and retraction of both cerebellar hemispheres (*1, 2*) with two brain spatulas (*S*) the tumour (*Tu*) becomes visible. The posterior portion of the fourth ventricle with the obex (*Ob*) is still not infiltrated by tumour. **b** At a later stage of the operation the blocked rostral portion of the ventricle is exposed; the median sulcus (*Sm*) is visible in the centre. Between the two spatulas (*S*) the tumour (*Tu*) is exposed and then with bipolar coagulation (*F* forceps) and by using the irrigating sucker (*Su*) it is carefully separated from above downwards off the floor of the fourth ventricle

sometimes be involved, if the tumour makes its way to the outside through the lateral recess; here most meticulous care must be taken of the AICA with its various, and functionally very important branches.

Results and Discussion

Among the *tumours of the brain stem* especially the medulla and the pons, there are a few that are definitely primarily inoperable, for instance the gliomas diffusely involving the hindbrain. In appropriate cases a tumour which is projecting into the rhomboid fossa, can be partially removed so that firstly the patency of the CSF pathways can be ensured and secondly it is possible to make an exact histological classification of the tumour. Also, in these cases the insertion of a Leksell drain is indicated.

However, a proportion of these tumours is operable, as they appear to be relatively sharply demarcated from the normal tissue and can be microsurgically removed without too severe sequels for the patient. In these cases, particularly the benign gliomas, an attempt at a total removal should be made. These tumours often reveal themselves in the ventriculogram by the irregular nodular contours in the floor of the fourth ventricle.

Apart from those tumours which are diffusely growing in the hindbrain and are not removable, an operative exposure should be undertaken in all cases. Even if total removal or a significant reduction in the size of the tumour is not possible, the information about the actual nature of the tumour is of great importance in planning the subsequent treatment. In addition, an assessment of the prognosis is easier under such conditions, a point of view which gains importance in relation to the family background of the little patient.

In all these operations the main advantage of the microsurgical technique is the good identification of normal and pathological structures, and the possibility of identifying and sparing even the finest vessels and nerves. We are in a position to carry out a more complete, more precise and gentle removal of the tumour [14, 21, 22, 32].

If a complete resection under the microscope is not successful, because the lesion is infiltrating the hindbrain too extensively, it is still worth while to remove the maximum amount possible. Particularly with medulloblastomas, and to a lesser extent with ependymomas, combined radiotherapy and chemotherapy after a partial operative removal, still show quite impressive temporary or even lasting results [4, 6, 7, 8, 21].

The Leksell drain which we put in when the indications are appropriate has already proved valuable as a relatively safe procedure. By using the microscope it is possible to introduce the catheter under direct vision and without risk into the aqueduct and push it onwards into the anterior horn (see p. 216, 283). If one considers the development of operative mortality, for instance in posterior fossa tumours, defined as the death rate up to six weeks postoperatively, it will be noticed straight away that the mortality in the 1960's was alarmingly high. Its drop in the last few years to values between 0 and 5% can certainly be attributed to a number of factors, among which certainly microsurgical techniques occupy no small part. Besides the more gentle operation technique there is also a modification of the procedure in the sense of a maximal resection, if a total removal is not possible, which is certainly of great importance.

It should be emphasised that even in the future, and despite any technical progress the particular brain structures will still represent an absolute limit for any operative procedures. It remains to be seen whether any refinements of technique and new procedures will open up fresh possibilities. Still, the very marked and gratifying drop in the operative mortality has shown that undoubted progress can be made.

Summary

Although the extracerebral midline lesions (pinealomas, craniopharyngiomas, pituitary adenomas) can be regarded as the main domain of microneurosurgery, this technique is also capable of offering great advantages in intraventricular and paraventricular tumours. To a still greater extent this holds good for posterior fossa tumours (medulloblastoma, ependymoma, pilocytic astrocytoma, plexus papilloma, epidermoids, etc). It is here that the use of the operating microscope and a suitable technique has led to a drastic fall in the operative mortality.

References

1. Agnoli, A., Eggert, H. R., Zierski, J., Seeger, W., Kirchoff, D.: Diagnostische Möglichkeiten der positiven Ventrikulographie. Acta Neurochir. *31,* 227–243 (1975)
2. Barraquer, J. I.: The microscope in ocular surgery. Amer. J. Ophthal. *42,* 6–11 (1956)
2a. Cushing, H.: Macewen memorial lecture on the meningiomas arising from the olfactory groove and their removal by the aid of electro surgery. Lancet *1,* 1329–1339 (1927)
2b. Cushing, H.: Electrosurgery as an aid to the removal of intracranial tumours. With a preliminary note on a new surgical current generator (by W. T. Bovie) Surg. Gynac. & Obst. *47,* 751–784 (1928)
3. Gerald, B., Wolpert, S. M., Haimovici, H.: Angiographic anatomy of the anterior inferior cerebellar artery. Am. J. Roentgenol. *118,* 617–621 (1973)
4. Gold, J. A., Smith jr., K. R.: Childhood brain tumours: A 15-year survey of treatment in a University Pediatric Hospital. South. Med. J. *68,* 1337–1344 (1975)
5. Greenwood, J. jr.: Two point coagulation. A new principle and instrumentation for applying coagulation current in neurosurgery. Am. J. Surg. *50,* 267–271 (1940)
6. Gutjahr, P., Voth, D.: Erfolgreiche Medulloblastom-Therapie – und danach? Adv. Neurosurg. *5,* 257–258 (1978)
7. Gutjahr, P., Voth, D.: Treatment and prognosis of childhood brain tumours: experience with 140 cases. Verhdlg. Dtsch. Krebsges. *2,* 434–435 (1979)
8. Gutjahr, P., Voth, D., Neidhardt, M.: Ergebnisse der kombinierten Behandlung (Operation, Radio- und Chemotherapie) bei 132 Kindern mit primären ZNS-Tumoren. Therapiewoche *28,* 4346–4352 (1978)
9. Hinselmann (1925) zitiert nach Grünberger, V. und Ulm R.: Diagnostische Methoden in der Geburtshilfe und Gynäkologie. Georg Thieme Verlag, Stuttgart 1968

10. Holmgren, G.: Some experiences in surgery of otosclerosis. Acta oto-laryng. (Stockh.) *5*, 460–466 (1923)
11. House, W. F.: Surgical exposure of the internal auditory canal and its contents through the middle cranial fossa. Laryngoscope *71*, 1363–1385 (1961)
12. Jacobsen, J. H., Suarez, E. L.: Microsurgery in anastomosis of small vessels. Surg. Forum *11*, 243–245 (1960)
13. Kazner, E., Aulich, W., Grumme, T.: Results of computed axial tomography with infratentorial tumours. In: Cranial computerized Tomography (Ed. Lanksch-Kazner). Berlin-Heidelberg-New York: Springer-Verlag 1976
14. Koos, W. Th., Böck, F. W., Spetzler, R. F.: Clinical microneurosurgery. Stuttgart: Georg Thieme Verlag 1976
15. Kurze, T., Boyle jr., J. B.: Extradural intracranial (middle fossa) approach to the internal auditory canal. J. Neurosurg. *19*, 1033–1037 (1962)
16. Malis, L. I.: Bipolar coagulation in microsurgery. In: Microvascular Surgery, Ed. by R. M. P. Donaghy und M. G. Yasargil, pp. 126–130 Stuttgart: Georg Thieme Verlag 1967
17. Naidich, T. P., Kricheff, I. I., George, A. E., Lin, J. P.: The anterior inferior cerebellar artery in mass lesions. Preliminary findings with emphasis on the lateral projection. Radiology *119*, 375–383 (1976)
18. Nylen, C. D.: The microscope in aural surgery, its first use and later development. Acta otolaryng. (Stockh.) Suppl. *116*, 226–240 (1954)
19. Olivecrona, H.: The surgical treatment of intracranial tumours. In: Olivecrona/Tönnis "Handbuch der Neurochirurgie" Vol. IV, pp. 1–301, Berlin-Heidelberg-New York: Springer Verlag 1967
20. Perritt, R. A.: Recent advantages in corneal surgery. Amer. Acad. ophthal. oto-laryng. Course Nr. 288 (1950)
21. Pia, H. W.: Komplikationen infratentorieller Eingriffe im Kindesalter. Z. Kinderchir. *12*, 181–186 (1973)
22. Rand, R. W.: Microneurosurgery. 2nd. ed. Saint Louis: C. V. Mosby Company 1978
23. Rand, R. W., Kurze, T.: Microneurosurgical resection of acoustic tumours by a transmeatal posterior fossa approach. Bull. Los Angeles Neurol. Soc. *30*, 17–20 (1965)
24. Rand, R. W., Jannetta, P. J.: Microneurosurgery for aneurysms of the vertebral basilar enterial system. J. Neurosurg. *27*, 330–335 (1967)
25. Bohr, M. von, Stock, W.: Über eine achromatische Brillenlupe schwacher Vergrößerung. Klin. Mbl. Augenheilk. *51*, 206–213 (1913)
26. Schürmann, K., Voth, D.: Neurochirurgie. In: Baumgartl, Kremer, Schreiber (Ed.) „Spezielle Chirurgie für die Praxis", Vol. I/2, p 831–1019, Stuttgart: Georg Thieme Verlag 1975
27. Seeger, W.: Microsurgery of the brain. Wien-New York: Springer Verlag 1980
28. Voe, A. G. de: Microsurgery. Highlights Ophthal. *7*, 212–219 (1964)
29. Voth, D., Hey, O., Nakayama, N., Emmrich, P.: Die kontinuierliche Registrierung des intrakraniellen Druckes im Rahmen der pädiatrischen Intensivmedizin. In: P. Emmrich (Ed.): „Pädiatrische Intensivmedizin", Bd. *3*, S. 104–109. Stuttgart: Georg Thieme Verlag 1977
30. Voth, D., Schwarz, M., Hüwel, N., Mahlmann, E.: Shunt therapy in medulloblastoma? Acta Neurochir. *56*, 278–279 (1981)
31. Voth, D., Schwarz, M.: New Light on the technique and indication for ventriculo-cisternal drainage according to Leksell (Interventriculostomy). Neurosurg. Rev. *4*, 179–184 (1981)
32. Yasargil, M. G.: Microsurgery applied to neurosurgery. Georg Thieme Verlag, Stuttgart und Academic Press, New York-London (1969)
33. Zehender, W. von: Beschreibung der binocularen Cornea-Lupe. Klin. Mbl. Augenheilk. *25*, 496–507 (1887)

Additional Operative Procedures (Shunt Systems, Leksell and Torkildsen Drainage)

M. Schwarz and D. Voth

Introduction

Nowadays in children the diagnosis of brain tumour is usually made by computer tomography. The site of the tumour, i.e. its immediate relationship to the adjacent structures, decides its primary operability, subtotal resection or necessary palliative operation such as, a shunt operation. Not infrequently the clinical symptoms are predominantly the result of interference with the CSF pathways.

According to the severity of the obstructive internal hydrocephalus and the clinical findings a relieving operation is necessary. The simplest procedure which can be carried out on severely affected patients, even under local anaesthesia, is the insertion of an *external ventricular drain* attached to a system controlled by a valve. At the same time continuous ventricular pressure measurements can be made.

Ventriculo-Atrial and Ventriculo-Peritoneal Shunts

As with childhood hydrocephalus not caused by tumour the well known shunt procedures are the method of choice. Early papers [1, 2] report on a striking drop in the mortality, as a result of primary shunting in obstructive hydrocephalus caused by space-occupying lesions in the posterior fossa.

Both procedures, the ventriculo-atrial and the ventriculo-peritoneal shunt are quite familiar as regards their technical details.

In many neurosurgical clinics both shunt procedures are preferred to open ventricular drainage. If a suitable valve is used after putting in a primary shunt, the intracranial pressure will return to normal. A further advantage will be seen that after primary shunt implantation the patient can be mobilised postoperatively and intensive physiotherapy and rehabilitation can be given.

Temporary postoperative pressure crises, which can often develop between the second and fourth postoperative days after a successful tumour operation, are avoided by a functioning shunt system [6]. The number of local postoperative complications, such as CSF fistula is reduced. If, after the histological findings it is considered necessary to give radiotherapy the oedema induced by this can lead once more to disturbances of the CSF circulation through obstruction of the aqueduct.

In considering the acceptability and complications of shunt systems it appears to us that the indications for primary shunt operations are doubtful. According to investigations by Fuchs [3] a shunt operation is necessary in only 70% of patients after removal of a tumour, Schafer and Lapras [13] after probing the aqueduct and fixing a catheter going down as far as the cisterna magna have only implanted a shunt system in three of fifty tumour patients. In our clinic in recent years out of fifty-four patients with tumours of the posterior fossa eight patients were treated with a shunt on account of persisting internal hydrocephalus.

Apart from this it is well known that aqueduct stenosis can be produced by a shunt system and hence shunt dependency induced; further neurosurgical complications are decompression effusions and subdural haematoma.

Shunt Complications

The study initiated by Wüllenweber in 1976 in which nine German clinics collaborated, collected 1612 patients, who had been treated with ventriculo-atrial or ventriculo-peritoneal shunt, irrespective of their basic disease. Altogether 24% of these patients treated by an atrial shunt and 31% treated by a peritoneal shunt had to be revised. The principle reasons for the revision of the peritoneal shunt were local infection, deconnection, peritoneal adhesions and malabsorption of the fluid. In seems important in this respect to point out that in patients who were primarily treated with an atrial shunt, shunt insufficiency developed in 48% in the first year and in 20% in the second year; with the peritoneal shunt these results were 60% in the first and 12% in the second year [10, 14].

With large tumours in the upper part of the vermis or tumours which have grown into the tentorial hiatus and displaced the midbrain an upward tentorial pressure cone can result from a sudden decompression of an obstructive hydrocephalus with a shunt. Midbrain compression syndromes are also very prominent.

Lesions of the quadrigeminal plate show themselves essentially by disturbances of ocular co-ordination, vertical upward ocular spasms and later paresis of vertical gaze. Further increases of tone develop in the lower extremities with positive pyramidal signs, later extensor spasms of the lower limbs and flexor postures in upper limbs, going on later to disturbances of consciousness and finally coma.

Up to now we have been able to observe one case of commencing upward herniation. A further problem with shunts is the possibility of metastases from a medulloblastoma, which has been described not only with atrial but also with peritoneal drainage. Altogether since 1973 more than sixty cases have been reported [8].

Ventriculocisternal Drainage (Torkildsen)

A further shunting procedure is ventriculocisternostomy introduced by Torkildsen in 1939 [15]. The indication for this is inoperable tumours of the brain stem, the pineal region, tumours of the basal ganglia and thalamus and tumours of the third ventricle with obstruction of the foramina of Monro. This procedure is significantly more time-consuming and the complication rate is correspondingly higher [1]. In a survey by Grote [4] which comprises altogether 239 cases, there were 12.6% intracranial haemorrhages occurring during the operation and 43.6% postoperative complications. Prominent are local infections in 3.7%, CSF fistulas in 8.1% and meningitis in 10%. Shunt insufficiency was reported in 5.5%.

In our clinic between 1975 and 1981 we performed the Torkildsen procedure twenty-one times as a palliative operation. In one case revision was needed on account of a CSF fistula. In another patient with a basal ganglia and thalamic tumour the control CT scan showed a persistent internal hydrocephalus and furthermore the optic fundi showed papilloedema, so a ventriculo-peritoneal drain was inserted in addition. We have not encountered any severe problems with wound healing which have necessitated revision or removal of the drainage. For slow growing tumours which are producing an obstructive hydrocephalus, as compared with the other shunt procedures, ventriculocisternostomy is a significantly safer method and guarantees the patient a long survival, as late complications and insufficiency are rare.

Interventriculostomy (Leksell)

The modified interventriculostomy of Leksell has only recently been described. Up to now in our clinic we have put in twenty-five Leksell drains without complications. In considering the malignant tumours of the posterior fossa this type of internal drainage seems to us to be the most favourable [11, 16, 17]. In four cases we have observed fleeting internuclear ocular palsies, although it is not clear that these have been caused by the insertion of the drain or by the original operative manipulations. From time to time there is difficulty in advancing the catheter into the anterior horn of the lateral ventricle, so that in three cases the tip of the catheter remained in the third ventricle (see p. 283).

Recommendations for Shunt Treatment and Summary

In posterior fossa tumours first of all primary decompression and continuous pressure measurement is carried out through a right frontal burr-hole. After three to four days treatment with high doses of Dexamethazone, total removal or a maximal resection of the tumour is carried out. Particularly, however, in medulloblastomas or other malignant tumours with a considerable likelihood of recurrence, a Leksell drain is put in at the time of operation. The ventricular drain remains in for a maximum of up to the fourth postoperative day, according to the clinical state of the child and pattern of the intracranial pressure tracings. Should the first postoperative CT control show that the hydrocephalus is static or even progressing then a shunt operation is absolutely necessary.

References

1. Abraham, J., Chandy, J.: Ventriculo-atrial shunt in the management of posterior fossa tumours. J. Neurosurg. *20,* 252–253 (1963).
2. Elkins, C. W., Fonseca, J. E.: Ventriculovenous anastomosis in obstructive and acquired communicating hydrocephalus. J. Neurosurg. *18,* 139 (1961).
3. Fuchs, E. C.: Quantitative CSF drainage in cases of posterior fossa tumors. Advanc. Neurosurg. *5,* 211–215 (1978).
4. Grote, E., Zierski, J., Klinger, M., Grohmann, G., Markakis, E.: Complications following ventriculocisternal shunt. Advanc. Neurosurg. *6,* 10–16 (1978).
5. Hekmatpanah, J., Mullan, S.: Ventriculocaval shunt in management of posterior fossa tumours. J. Neurosurg. *26,* 609–613 (1967).
6. Hemmer, R., Haensel-Friedrich, G., Friedrich, H.: The value of pre-operative shunt in posterior fossa tumours. Mod. Probl. Paediat. Vol. *18,* 48–50 (1977).
7. Hemmer, R., Mohadger, M., Schiefer, K.: Untersuchungen zur cerebralen Dysregulation bei Tumoren der hinteren Schädelgrube mit Hydrocephalus occlusus. Neurochirurgia *17,* 96–106 (1974).
8. Hoffmann, H. J., Hendrick, E. B., Humphrey, R. P.: Metastasis via ventriculoperitoneal shunt in patient with medulloblastoma. J. Neurosurg. *44,* 562–566 (1976).
9. Jane, J. A., Kaufmann, B., Nulsen, F.: The role of angiography and ventriculovenous shunting in the treatment of posterior fossa tumours. Acta. neurochirurg. *28,* 13–28 (1975).
10. Leem, W., Miltz, H.: Complications following ventriculoatrial shunts in hydrocephalus. Advanc. Neurosurg. *6,* 1–5 (1978).
11. Leksell, L.: A surgical procedure for atresia of the aqueduct of Sylvius. Acta. Psychiatr. (Kobenh.) *24,* 559–568 (1949).
12. Richard, K. E.: Long-term measuring of ventricular CSF pressure with tumours of the posterior fossa. Advanc. Neurosurg. *5,* 179–183 (1978).
13. Schafer, M., Lapras, C., Ruf, H.: Catheterization of the aqueduct in certain lesion of the posterior fossa. Advanc. Neurosurg. *5,* 216–219 (1978).
14. Strahl, E. W., Liesegang, J., Roosen, K.: Complications following ventriculoperitoneal shunts. Advanc. Neurosurg. *6,* 6–9 (1978).
15. Torkildsen, A.: A new palliative procedure in cases of inoperable occlusion of the Sylvian ductus. Acta. Chir. Scand. *82,* 177–185 (1939).
16. Voth, D., Schwarz, M.: New light on the technique and indication for ventriculocisternal drainage according to Leksell (interventriculostomy). Neurosurg. Rev. *4,* 179–184 (1981).
17. Voth, D., Schwarz, M., Hüwel, N., Mahlmann, E.: Shunt therapy in medulloblastoma? Adv. Neurosurg. *10,* (1982).

The Significance of Continuous Recording of Intracranial Pressure in Children with Brain Tumours

M. Brock and H.-J. Schmitz

The intracranial space is filled to capacity with fluids – blood and cerebrospinal fluid (CSF) – and brain parenchyma, all of which are nearly incompressible. Only reciprocal changes in the volume of these constituents are possible without alteration of the total volume. This concept, known as the Monro-Kellie doctrine, dates back to 1824. Such reciprocal changes are the basis for a compensatory mechanism which finds its expression in the intracranial pressure/volume relationship. Increased intracranial pressure results when an addition to the intracranial volume by increase of one constituent exceeds the compensatory capacity provided by displacement of one or both of the others. This may lead to a reduction in cerebral perfusion pressure below the autoregulatory level and, eventually, to cerebral vasomotor paralysis [1] accompanied by brain ischaemia and cerebral oedema [11].

To detect and treat these changes in due time, continuous recording of cerebral metabolic parameters (blood flow, blood volume, oxygen and glucose consumption) would be the method of choice. Monitoring of these figures, however, is technically difficult and time-consuming. On the other hand, observation of clinical signs alone is misleading, and their severity does not correlate with the extent of the rise in ICP.

However, as continuous recording of ICP is nowadays technically easy and reliable, it has become a routine procedure. Although invasive, its risks are amply outweighed by its value for the patient. In general, and also for paediatric purposes, two methods are used for continuous recording of ICP. Increasing experience has led to the development of specific indications for each of these methods.

Recording of cerebrospinal fluid pressure (CSFP) by means of a ventricular catheter was described by Lundberg [13] and Janny [10]. This method also permits pressure-controlled CSF drainage, and is indicated in the presence of hydrocephalus whether it is obstructive, congenital or due, for instance, to obstruction of the CSF pathways by a posterior fossa tumour. It is also the method of choice when drainage of bloody CSF is indicated. A specially developed catheter provided with a 3-way tap permits simultaneous recording of ICP (Statham PD 23) and CSF drainage. For drainage, we are presently using a disposable system (Manufacturer: Cordis, Eckrath). As this system still presents some practical drawbacks, a new one is being developed at present.

The rate of drainage is regulated according to the individual needs as proposed by Pampus in 1953 and 1961 [15, 16]. In cases of obstructive hydrocephalus, ICP is gradually reduced to physiological values by progressively lowering the drainage level before operation, in order to avoid abrupt "decompression".

In the presence of pathological pressure waves or wide variations in CSFP, drainage also contributes to stabilization of pressure [4] and probably improves cerebral blood flow (CBF). Furthermore, the decrease in the amplitude of CSF pulsations during open drainage (Fig. 1) indicates a favourable influence on the pressure/volume relationship.

In the immediate postoperative phase, pressure recording proceeds for 24–48 hours *without* CSF-drainage in order to control the efficacy of the operation. If indicated CSF drainage may be started again, otherwise, the ventricular catheter is simply withdrawn.

A drawback of CSFP recording and drainage is infection. In our experience [17] meningitis occurs in 2% while a raised CSF cell-count is detectable in about one third of the patients.

Recording of *epidural pressure* is indicated whenever any increase in ICP is not due to hydrocephalus, when the ventricles are not enlarged and no CSF drainage is envisaged. The epidural technique is the method of choice in cases of craniocerebral trauma. Various procedures have been suggested [3, 5, 6, 7, 20, 21]. Particularly for children, however, the screw-type transducers have proved inadequate. Coplanarity is difficult to achieve with such screw-transducers (thin skull, open fontanelles, etc.) as pointed out by several authors [14, 18, 19].

The fibre-optic system (Manufacturer: Ladd Co.) described by Levin in 1977 [12] and the Gaeltec ICT/b pressure transducer (Manufacturer: Gaeltec LTD., Dunvegan, Isle of Skye, Scotland) (Fig. 2) are the most suitable for the recording of epidural pressure in children. The advantage of both systems is that the pressure transducer is introduced into the epidural space, thus eliminating the problem of fixation to the child's skull. We prefer the Gaeltec ICT/b transducer. It is sterilized in ethylene oxide for 14 days or in formalin gas for 24 hours. The pressure sensor is

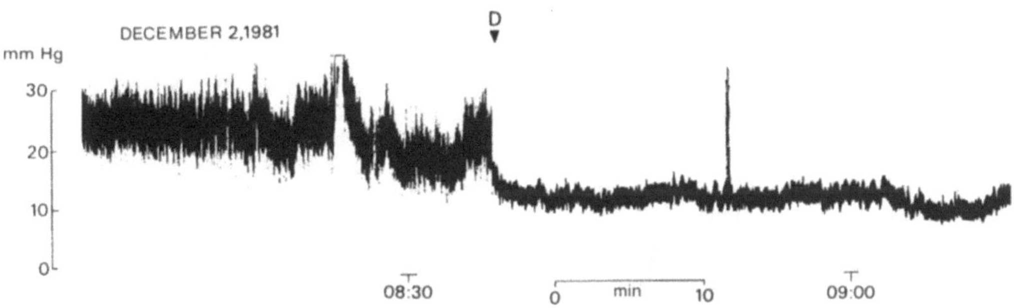

Fig. 1. Reduction of intracranial pressure and CSF pulse amplitude by open ventricular drainage

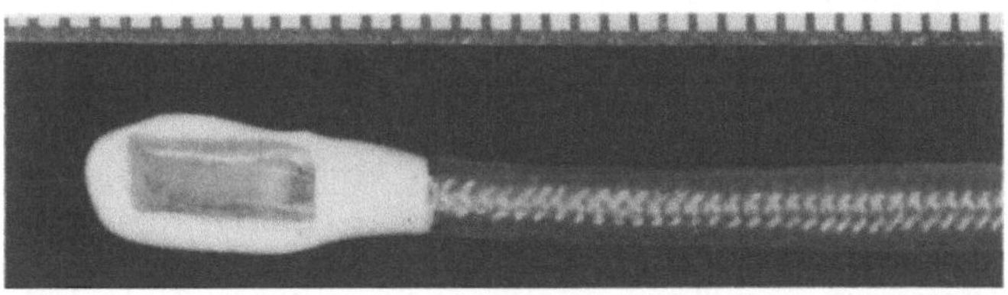

Fig. 2. Pressure transducer Gaeltec ICT/b from below (pressure-sensitive membrane in contact with the dura). Scale in millimeters

implanted in the operating theatre through a 12 mm burr-hole, usually in the right frontal region. The dura is freed from the calvarium for 2–3 cm with the dissector. The bony edges of the burr-hole are smoothed with a rongeur in order to prevent damage to the sensor at the time of its withdrawal. The pressure transducer is gently introduced between dura and calvarium, with the pressure sensing diaphragm facing the dura. The wound is closed and the cable of the transducer fixed to the skin by one suture. In vivo zeroline calibration is possible and is performed at least once a day. At the end of the recording period, the transducer can be easily removed like a drain, by gentle traction. The ICT/b transducer can be reused after cleansing, checking the tightness of the system, re-zeroing and re-calibration. In paediatric neurosurgery, and in the absence of hydrocephalus, epidural measurement is mainly indicated in cases of cranial trauma. Routine epidural pressure recording before elective surgery is rare in children, unless the operation has to be postponed despite increased ICP. Under such circumstances epidural recording serves to monitor the conservative management of the raised ICP.

On the other hand, in the postoperative phase, epidural pressure monitoring is used more frequently [2].

Lumbar CSFP measurement [9] and drainage has not been used in our series. This method is contraindicated in the presence of expanding intracranial lesions and hinders mobilization and management of the children.

References

1. Alexander, S. G., Lassen, N. A.: Cerebral circulatory response to acute brain disease. Anaesthesiology *32,* 60–67 (1970).
2. Beks, J. W. F., Journee, H. L., Albarda, S., Flanderijn, H.: The significance of ICP-monitoring in the post-operative period. In: Intracranial Pressure III, Beks, J. W. F., Bosch, D. A., Brock, M. (eds.), pp. 251–254. Berlin, Heidelberg, New York: Springer 1976.
3. Beks, J. W. F., Albarda, S., Gieles, A. C. M., Kuypers, M. H., Flanderijn, H.: Extradural transducer for monitoring intracranial pressure. Acta Neurochirurgica *38,* 245–250 (1977).
4. Brock, M., Wigand, H., Zillig, C., Zywietz, C., Mock, P., Dietz, H.: The effect of dexamethasone on intracranial pressure in patients with supratentorial tumors. In: Pappius, H. M., Feindel, W. (eds.): Dynamics of Brain Edema, pp. 330–336. Berlin, Heidelberg, New York: Springer 1976.
5. Brock, M., Diefenthäler, K.: A modified equipment for the continuous telemetric monitoring of epidural pressure. In: Brock, M., Dietz, H. (eds.) pp. 21–26. Berlin, Heidelberg, New York: Springer 1972.
6. Dorsch, N. W. C., Symon, L.: A practical technique for monitoring extradural pressure. J. Neurosurg. *42,* 249–257 (1975).
7. Gobiet, W., Bock, W. J., Liesegang, J. et al.: Longtime monitoring of epidural pressure in man. In: Intracranial Pressure: Experimental and clinical aspects. Brock, M., Dietz, H. (eds.) pp. 14–17. Berlin, Heidelberg, New York: Springer 1972.
8. Gobiet, W., Bock, W. J., Liesegang, J., Grote, W.: Experience with an intracranial pressure transducer readjustable in vivo – technical note – J. Neurosurg. *39,* 272–276 (1974).
9. Hartmann, A.: Continuous monitoring of CSF pressure in acute subarachnoid hemorrhage. In: Intracranial Pressure IV, Shulman, K., Marmarou, A., Miller, J. D., Becker, D. P., Hochwald, G. M., Brock, M. (eds.) pp. 220–228. Berlin, Heidelberg, New York: Springer 1980.
10. Janny, P.: La pression intracranienne chez l'homme. Méthode d'enregistrement – étude de ses variations et de ses rapports avec les signes cliniques et ophthalmologiques. Thèse de Paris (1950).

11. Klatzo, I., Wiesniewski, H., Steinwall, D.: Dynamics of cold injury edema. Brain Edema, Ed. I, Klatzo, J., Seidelberger, F. (eds.). New York: Springer 1967.
12. Levin, A. B.: The use of a fibre-optic intracranial pressure monitor in clinical practice. Neurosurg. *1,* 266–271 (1977).
13. Lundberg, N.: Continuous recording and control of ventricular fluid pressure in neurosurgical practice. Acta psychiat. neurol. scand. *36,* (Suppl. 149): 1–193 (1960).
14. Majors, R., Schettini, A., Mahig, J., Nevis, A. H.: Intracranial pressures measured with the coplanar pressure transducer. Med. & Biol. Eng. *10,* 724–733 (1972).
15. Pampus, F.: Zur Technik der Ventrikeldrainage. Zbl. Neurochir. *13,* 219–223 (1953).
16. Pampus, F.: Die Indikationen zur Anwendung der Ventrikeldrainage. Zbl. Neurochir. *21,* 216–221 (1961).
17. Pöll, W., v. Waldthausen, W., Brock, M.: Infection rate of continuous monitoring of ventricular fluid pressure with and without open cerebrospinal fluid drainage. In: Advances in Neurosurgery 9. Schiefer, W., Klinger, M., Brock, M. (eds.) pp. 363–366. Berlin, Heidelberg, New York: Springer 1981.
18. Schettini, A., Walsh, E.: Simultaneous pressure-depth measurement of the intracranial system epidurally. In: Intracranial Pressure II, Lundberg, N., Ponten, U., Brock, M. (eds.) pp. 397–402. Berlin, Heidelberg, New York: Springer 1975.
19. Schmitz, H.-J.: Critical evaluation of ICP-measurement using transducers which are screwed into the cranial bone. In: Advances in Neurosurgery 9. Schiefer, W., Klinger, M., Brock, M. (eds.) pp. 367–373. Berlin, Heidelberg, New York: Springer 1981.
20. Vries, J. K., Becker, D. P., Young, H. F.: A subarachnoid screw for monitoring intracranial pressure – technical note – J. Neurosurg. *39,* 416–419 (1973).
21. Yoneda, S., Matsuda, M., Shimizu, Y., Handa, J., Handa, H., Oda, F., Matsuo, K., Taguchi, N.: SFT – a new device for continuous measurement of intracranial pressure. Surg. Neurol. *1,* 13–15 (1973).

Preoperative and Postoperative Intensive Care and Oedema Therapy

J. Otte, P. Emmrich, and G. Meinig

Introduction

78% of our child patients with brain tumours showed signs of raised intracerebral pressure on first admission to the department. They were thus endangered patients who require subtle diagnosis. We should like to describe our therapeutic procedure in the preoperative and postoperative phase and to report on typical problems and complications.

We have therefore evaluated in terms of various criteria the progress of all 113 children who were operated on for a brain tumour during the last eight years.

Patient Material, Plan of Treatment

The tumours of the CNS observed are broken down in Table 1 according to their diagnosis. A classification in terms of topographical criteria has been chosen. Preoperative diagnostics clarifies the tumour localization and establishes the indication for surgery and its strategy. If symptoms of raised ICP are shown preoperatively, first of all continuous intraventricular pressure measurement (IVP) is carried out besides the obligatory dexamethasone therapy in the dosage 16–25 mg/m² body

Table 1. Tumours of CNS (1973 – 1981) $n = 113$

A. *Infratentorial*	*n*	B. *Supratentorial*	*n*
1. Cerebellar, IV. ventricle		1. Chiasma-sella region	
Medulloblastoma	23	Craniopharyngioma	17
Astrocytoma	19	Opticus glioma	6
Ependymoma	2	2. Cerebrum, midbrain	
Haemangioblastoma	2	Astrocytoma	15
Oligodendroglioma	1	Glioblastoma multiforme	3
Plexus papilloma	2	Ependymoma	2
2. Pons-, brain stem tumours	12	Teratoid	1
		Undifferentiated	2
C. *Tumours of spinal cord*	4	Arachnoidal sarcoma	1
		Pinealoma	1

surface area in four single doses in an existing disorders of CSF circulation. The measurement was carried out via a frontal borehole [13]. Therapeutic relief of CSF pressure in pressure peaks is possible with an additional system [19]. Ventriculography can also be carried out for diagnostic purposes via the indwelling catheter. After normalization of the intraventricular pressure, which is achieved after about two to three days by repeated withdrawals of CSF and by the dexamethasone therapy which has been started, extirpation of the tumour is then aimed for. Postoperatively, the children are ventilated for 12 to 48 hours with a volume-controlled respirator; hyperventilation is attained. The dexamethasone therapy is continued postoperatively. The intraventricular pressure measurement is registered postoperatively when it had been commenced preoperatively or on occurrence of an additional problem. The patients are sedated with barbiturates and lytic mixture. The patient can be moved to a general ward when the vital functions are stable and the intraventricular pressure has normalized.

Results

The tumour was totally or partially resected in 105 of the 113 children. A Torkildsen drainage was applied in eight children because of an inoperable brain stem tumour.

Preoperative Symptoms of Intracranial Pressure Increase

At the time of inpatient admission, 78% of the children showed symptoms of raised brain pressure (Table 2). Above all the children with tumours of the posterior cranial fossa and the brain stem showed signs of raised intracranial pressure.

Table 2. Tumours of CNS (1973 – 1981) $n = 113$

		Signs of initially elevated brain pressure	IVP measurement	
			preop.	postop.
A. *Infratentorial*				
Medulloblastoma	(n=23)	23	21	13
Astrocytoma	(n=19)	18	14	14
Pons-, brain stem	(n=12)	10	2	–
Other	(n= 7)	6	4	4
B. *Supratentorial*				
Craniopharyngioma	(n=17)	12	2	–
Opticus glioma	(n= 6)	–	–	–
Midbrain-, cerebrum	(n=25)	20	6	3

Preoperative Measurement of Intraventricular Pressure

Continuous measurement of intraventricular pressure was indicated when the children showed symptoms of a raised intracranial pressure and when disturbances of CSF circulation were present in addition. Preoperative pressure measurement was performed in a total of 44% of the children (Table 2). Most measurements were performed in tumours of the posterior fossa. Tumours in this location very frequently bring about a compression of the aqueduct with consequent hydrocephalus occlusus due to their growth. The duration of the preoperative pressure measurement was roughly equally long in all children. It averaged 69 hours. The preoperative normalization of the pressure curve indicated the correct time for tumour extirpation.

Postoperative Intraventricular Pressure Measurement

Postoperative pressure measurement was performed in 30% of the children. The pressure was measured an average of 62 hours after operation in the children with medulloblastomas. In the children with cerebellar astrocytomas, it was measured an average of 56 hours after operation. The postoperative pressure normalization constitutes the indication for discontinuation of pressure measurement.

Postoperative Controlled Hyperventilation

An average respirator treatment of 24 hours was carried out in 18 of the 23 children with medulloblastoma and in 20 of the remaining 26 children with tumours of the posterior cranial fossa. The period of mechanical ventilation in the children with brain stem tumours and supratentorial tumours greatly differed depending on their individual situation.

Problems and Complications (Table 3)

Of the 90 children with tumours of the CNS, two children died during the observation period (Table 3). A three-year-old child with a very large glioblastoma multi-

Table 3. Tumours of CNS (1973 – 1981), $n = 113$. Postoperative complications

	n
1. Exitus letalis	2
2. Infections – meningitis	4
sepsis	1
3. CSF fistulae	4
4. Epidural haematoma	1
5. Secondary aqueduct stenosis	3

forme in the region of the basal ganglia was already comatose on admission and died from the direct consequences of infiltrative tumour growth 22 days after inpatient admission after a partial tumour resection had been performed for palliative and diagnostic reasons. An 11-year old boy died of the consequences of meningitis and crisis rises in brain pressure a few days after removal of a medulloblastoma. Four further children contracted meningitis postoperatively. It is worth mentioning that continuous measurement of intraventricular pressure had been performed in only one of these children. In two children with postoperative meningitis, the occurrence of CSF fistulae had to be regarded as the cause of this infection. CSF fistulae were observed in two further children. One child contracted staphylococcal sepsis postoperatively; the child had a central venous catheter.

A recraniotomy because of an epidural haematoma in the area of the surgery had to be performed in one child. In three children with malignant cerebellar tumours, crisis rises in brain pressure occurred in the postoperative phase in consequence of secondary aqueduct stenosis. In these children, shunt systems were applied for relief of pressure. A diabetes insipidus was observed in all children with craniopharyngiomas.

Discussion

Our experience in the treatment of children with brain tumours shows that a focal point of therapy must be consistent treatment of an increased intracranial pressure. If possible, an anti-oedema therapy should be commenced first of all before tumour extirpation in the presence of brain pressure symptoms. The wellknown therapeutic principles for treatment of raised brain pressure [1, 5, 6, 8, 9] require control based on objective monitoring data. Continuous measurement of intraventricular pressure proves to be an excellent technique [18, 19] which should be applied if possible in every case of disturbed CSF circulation. The possibility of therapeutic and diagnostic CSF sampling renders this technique superior to other methods, e.g. epidural pressure measurement [7, 9], at least in tumour patients [19]. This can be illustrated with an example: a seven-year-old girl was admitted with signs of raised brain pressure. Ophthalmologically, congestion papillae of four diopters were shown on both sides, the child showed ataxia and tendency to fall to the left. In the computer tomogram of the skull, a large cerebellar tumour with occlusion hydrocephalus was detected. The pressure relief performed immediately via a frontal borehole led to rapid improvement of the clinical picture. A continuous measurement of intraventricular pressure followed. First of all, the curve course showed a distinctly pathological basic pressure of over 30 mmHg (see Fig. 1 a). Demonstration of plateau waves was to be evaluated as typical sign of the pathological intracranial pressure elevation. By repeated therapeutic CSF sampling via an additional system, dangerous pressure peaks were prevented. By the simultaneously commenced dexamethasone therapy, an additional lowering of pressure was attained. After about three days, the brain pressure was markedly lower (see Fig. 1 b), and pathological values were only shown briefly. At this time, the tumour extirpation could be per-

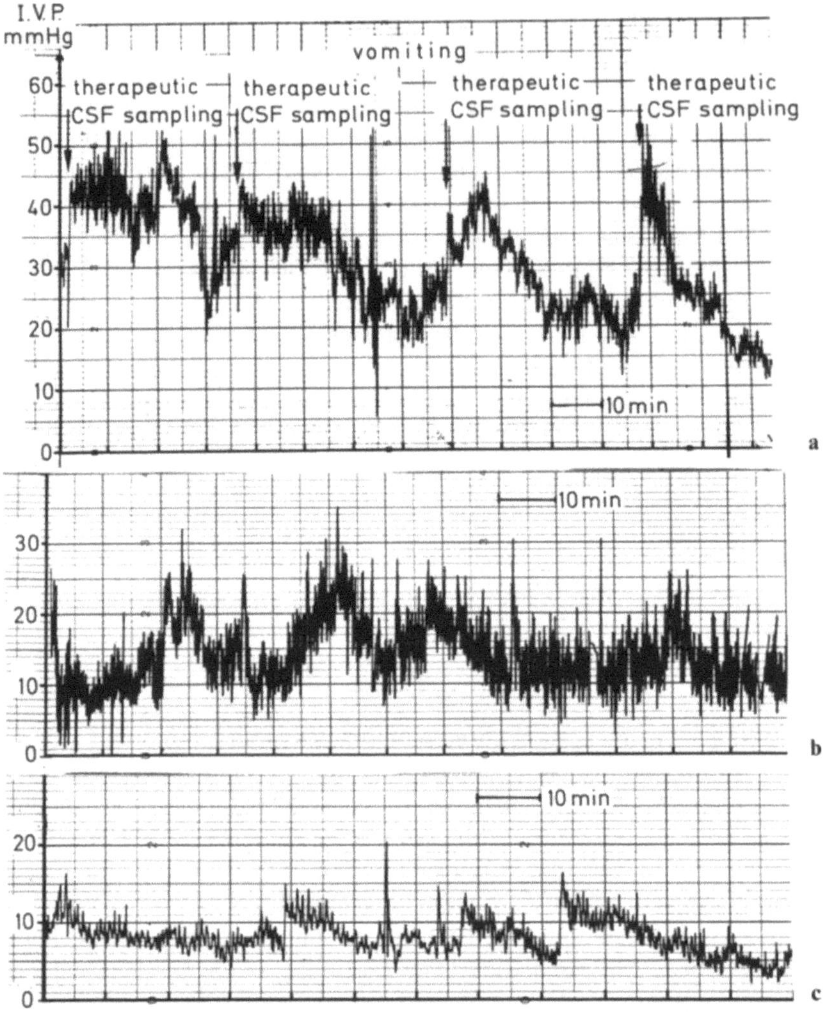

Fig. 1a, b. Preoperative brain pressure measurement. **a** The curve course showed a distinctly pathological basic pressure of over 30 mmHg. Demonstration of plateau waves was to be evaluated as typical sign of the pathological intracranial pressure elevation. By repeated therapeutic CSF sampling dangerous pressure peaks were prevented. **b** After about three days, the brain pressure was markedly lower by the dexamethasone therapy and by repeated therapeutic CSF sampling. **c** Postoperative brain pressure measurement. Three days postoperatively the pressure curve showed a normal course. The basic pressure was markedly under 15 mmHg

formed without danger. Three days postoperatively, a proper CSF circulation was demonstrated (see Fig. 1c), the pressure curve showed a normal course, and the basic pressure was markedly under 15 mmHg.

A raised risk of infection is not to be expected in the pressure measurement when strict hygienic guidelines are observed. We observed a meningitis in one child after extirpation of medulloblastoma and continuous intraventricular pressure measurement over several days. In the remaining four children with postoperative meningitis, no pressure measurements were performed. The practice of some centers, who first of all apply a shunt system for relief of pressure in children with tumours of the posterior cranial fossa and disturbed CSF circulation before tumour extirpation [2] is avoided if possible at our hospital. There is danger of metastasis and generalization of medulloblastomas via such shunt systems [3, 4, 11, 12, 17]. We observed a pulmonary metastasis of a medulloblastoma even in a 12-year-old boy. The child had been given a ventriculoatrial drainage because of a disturbed CSF circulation. On the other hand, there is always a potential danger of insufficiency in shunt systems which necessitates a fresh operation. An additional problem results from the subsequent therapy in malignant tumours. The question is still unclarified as to whether a raised rate of complications in the patients with a shunt system is present or is to be expected during radiotherapy with 50–60 Gy. We observed during radiotherapy and cytostatic therapy serious infectious complications which required removal of this reservoir in two children in whom Ommaya reservoirs had been implanted. Our therapeutic procedure in children with tumours of the posterior cranial fossa and simultaneous disturbed CSF circulation appears to us to be the better form of treatment. The principle of open CSF drainage in combination with continuous intraventricular pressure measurement permits control of the brain oedema therapy on the basis of objective data. During the tumour operation, it is of course very important to create a free CSF circulation if application of a shunt system is to be avoided. In some cases, it has proved effective to apply a lamellar catheter through the aqueduct. A free CSF circulation is ensured by this measure. A secondary aqueduct stenosis, which can occur in radiotherapy by postoperative swelling or in consequence of an oedema, is thereby effectively prevented. We have not yet observed complications due to this drainage system.

References

1. Batzdorf, U.: The management of cerebral edema in pediatric practice. Pediatrics *58,* 78–87 (1976).
2. Bongartz, E. B., Nau, H. E., Bamberg, M., Bayindir, C., Grote, W.: Concerning the question of total tumour removal in medulloblastoma in view of new postoperative techniques in radiotherapy. In: Advances in Neurosurgery 7, hrsg. von Marguth, F., Brock, M., Kazner, E., Klinger, M., Schmiedek, P., p. 108, Berlin, Heidelberg, New York: Springer 1978.
3. Brutschin, P., Cülver, G. J.: Extracranial metastases from medulloblastomas. Radiology *107,* 359–362 (1973).
4. Chu, J. Y.: Metastatic medulloblastoma simulating acute leukemia. J. Pediat. *94,* 921–923 (1979).
5. Faupel, G., Reulen, H. J., Müller, D., Schürmann, K.: Dexamethason bei schweren Schädel-Hirn-Traumen. Akt. traumatol. *8,* 265–281 (1978).
6. Fuhrmeister, U., Berndt, S. F.: Pathophysiologie, Klinik und Therapie des Hirnödems. Dtsch. Ärztebl. *73,* 1601–1607 (1976).
7. Gaab, M. R., Sörensen, N.: Extradurale Langzeit-Messung des intrakraniellen Druckes in der Pädiatrie. Kinderarzt *11,* 11–20 (1980).
8. Girke, W., Lieske, V.: Pathophysiologie und Therapie des Hirnödems. Med. Klin. *69,* 1–11 (1974).
9. Gobiet, W.: Intensivtherapie nach Schädel-Hirn-Trauma 2. Auflage, Berlin Heidelberg, New York: Springer 1979.

10. Hirsch, J. F., Renier, D., Czernichow, P., Benveniste, L., Pierre-Kahn, A.: Medulloblastoma in Childhood. Survival and functional results. Acta Neurochirurgica *48*, 1–15 (1979).
11. Hoffmann, H. J., Hendrick, E. B., Humphreys, R. P.: Metastases via ventriculo-peritoneal shunt in patients with medulloblastoma. J. Neurosurg. *44*, 562–566 (1976).
12. Kessler, L. A., Dugan, P., Concannon, J. P.: Systemic metastases of medulloblastoma promoted by shunting. Sur. Neurol. *3*, 147–152 (1975).
13. Lundberg, N.: Continous recording and control of ventricular fluid pressure in neurosurgical practice. Acta psychiat. scand. (Suppl. 149) *36*, 1–193 (1960).
14. Lundberg, N., Troupp, H., Lorin, H.: Continous recording of the ventricular fluid pressure in patients with severe acute traumatic brain injury. J. Neurosurg. *22*, 581–590 (1965).
15. Mealy, J., Hall, P. V.: Medulloblastoma in children. Survival and treatment. J. Neurosurg. *46*, 56–64 (1977).
16. Neidhardt, M. et al.: Therapiestudie Medulloblastom 1980 der Gesellschaft für Pädiatrische Onkologie e. V. (see p. 349–353).
17. Thomas, P. R. M., Duffner, P. K., Cohen, M. E., Sinks, L. F., Cameron, T., Freeman, A. I.: Multimodality therapy for medulloblastoma. Cancer *45*, 666–669 (1980).
18. Troupp, H., Vapalathi, M.: Ventricular fluid pressure in children with severe brain injuries. In: Schürmann, K., Brock, M., Reulen, H. J., Voth, D. (Eds.): Advances in Neurosurgery *1*, p. 62–67. Berlin, Heidelberg, New York: Springer 1973.
19. Voth, D., Hey, O., Nakayama, N., Emmrich, P.: Die kontinuierliche Registrierung des intrakraniellen Druckes (intraventrikuläre Druckmessung) im Rahmen der pädiatrischen Intensivmedizin. In: Pädiatrische Intensivmedizin: Symposion Mainz 1975, p. 104–109. P. Emmrich (Ed.) Stuttgart: Thieme 1977.

Therapy of Peritumoural Brain Oedema

G. MEINIG

In more extensive earlier publications [1, 2, 3], we have attempted to quantify the effect of anti-oedema therapy in adult brain tumour patients. We should like to summarize some clinical aspects and consequences for oedema therapy.

There are various areas of anti-oedema therapy in brain tumour patients:

1) Preoperative treatment and preparation
2) Postoperative and also intraoperative therapy (see J. Otte et al., pp. 222–228)
3) Long-term therapy in inoperable patients.

The dosage and duration of therapy vary very substantially in view of the different objectives. The individual situation also always requires individual therapy.

A central concern is always the restoration of a disturbed brain function. The consciousness situation can already be appreciably improved within hours under dexamethasone, whereas other symptoms (e.g. hemiparesis symptoms) frequently regress very much more slowly and also incompletely.

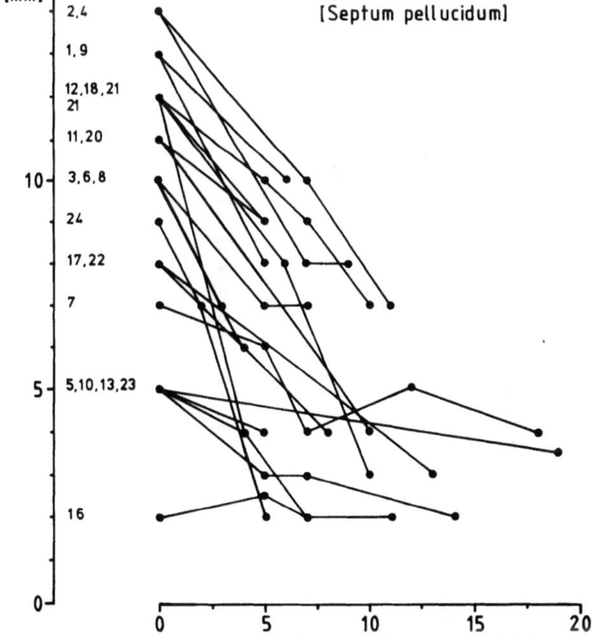

Fig. 1. Reduction of midline shift during combination therapy with dexamethasone and furosemide

It is no less important to reduce the increasing volume due to brain oedema, to reduce the size of the oedema area and thus to diminish the midline displacement, Reopening of the ventricular system and the cisternae must be made possible, the intracranial pressure must be lowered and finally (as a consequence) the cerebral blood flow must be improved.

The reduction of oedema is especially important for preoperative preparation. However, in contrast to the frequently very rapid regression of the neurological symptoms, reduction of peritumoural oedema always takes place only with a very substantial delay and is practically always incomplete. The oedema area, which we have measured planimetrically, often only regresses within weeks despite combination therapy with furosemide. Accordingly, the midline displacement also shows a delayed reduction (Fig. 1).

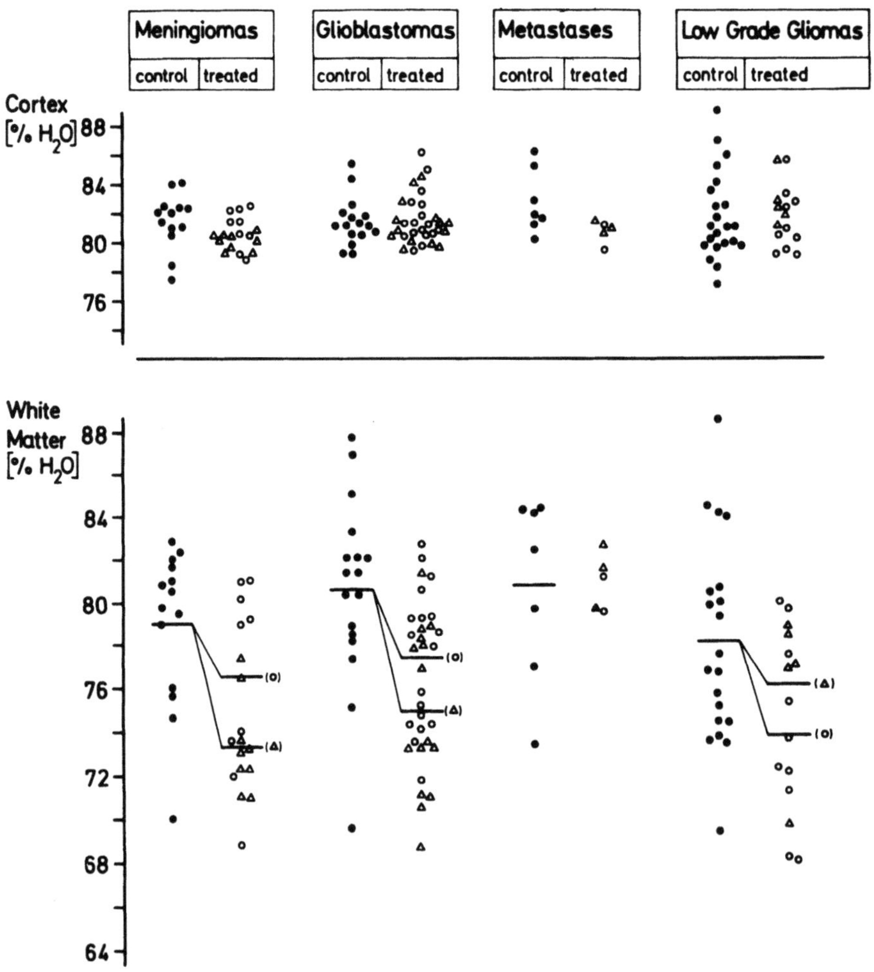

Fig. 2. Correlation of the result of anti-oedema therapy with the nature of respective brain tumours. • Untreated, ○ pretreated with dexamethasone, △ pretreated with dexamethasone and furosemide

Table 1. Water and electrolyte content in peritumoural cerebral cortex and white matter in groups I to V

Measurement[a]	I	II	III	IV	V
Cerebral cortex					
H_2O	81.83 ± 0.30 (61)	81.31 ± 0.34 (29)	81.57 ± 0.47 (12)	81.98 ± 0.72 (11)	81.11 ± 0.26 (34)
Na	348 ± 12.60 (50)	334.90 ± 20.30 (27)	369.70 ± 38.60 (11)	357.20 ± 32.40 (11)	304.80 ± 13.70 (33)
Cl	301.10 ± 18.80 (13)	299.00 ± 27.20 (25)	345.80 ± 37.90 (11)	369.60 ± 34.60 (11)	324.00 ± 23.10 (33)
K	440.60 ± 13.70 (49)	457 ± 18.10 (27)	477.90 ± 30.80 (11)	496.80 ± 15.50 (11)	484.90 ± 8.40 (33)
White matter					
H_2O	79.61 ± 0.54 (61)	76.43 ± 0.80 (29)	75.95 ± 0.89 (12)	75.02 ± 1.46 (11)	75.24 ± 0.64 (34)
Na	389.33 ± 18.80 (47)	343.41 ± 23.37 (28)	350.12 ± 26.61 (12)	232.61 ± 36.46 (10)	306.92 ± 18.91 (33)
Cl	359.44 ± 27.32 (12)	304.85 ± 16.66 (26)	345.44 ± 37.08 (12)	335.65 ± 39.28 (10)	364.29 ± 26.55 (33)
K	272.32 ± 9.01 (48)	259.31 ± 13.97 (28)	260.68 ± 17.01 (12)	224.77 ± 9.50 (10)	212.47 ± 6.11 (33)

Note: Means ± SEM; number of patients in parentheses.

[a] H_2O results in milligrams per cent, and electrolytes in milliequivalents per kilogram dry weight.

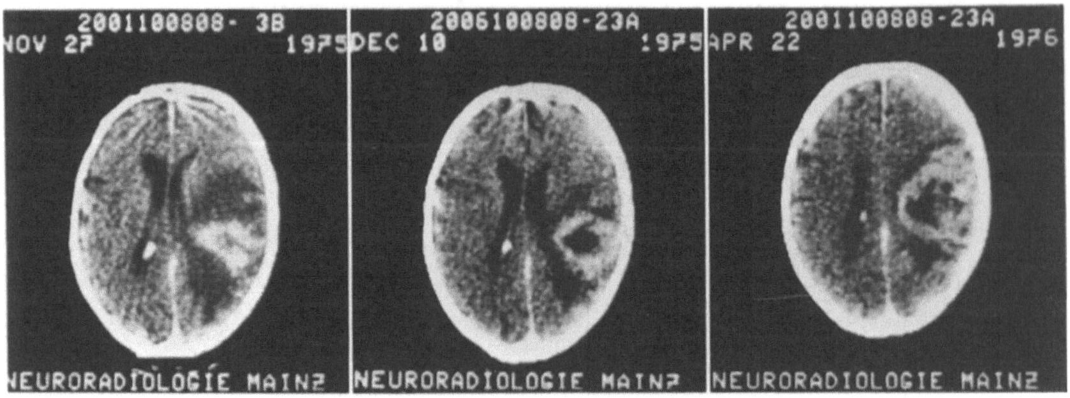

Fig. 3. Long-term CT study. Initially the patient received the combination therapy over a period of 2 weeks, and later he received 9 mg dexamethasone over a period of several months

Whereas the water content of the peritumoural brain cortex alters only slightly under the anti-oedema therapy, the white matter (Table 1) shows a reduction of the water content by about 2.5% after 4 to 6 days of dexamethasone treatment. On average, the water content was raised peritumourally by about 10% in nontreated patients. After dexamethasone treatment of 3×8 mg i.m., a reduction by just under 3% can be attained. After combination therapy with dexamethasone and furosemide, the water content is reduced by 4.5%. The same effect as that of the 4–6 day treatment with combination therapy can be attained within about 3 to 4 weeks by a long-term therapy with dexamethasone 4×4 mg per day on its own. This means that under these conditions we can reduce the water content by at most roughly half.

In consequence of our CT and tissue investigations, we have no misgivings about carrying out a preoperative treatment over 1 to 2 weeks when there is a large space occupation due to the oedema. We are keen on using the combination with furosemide, possibly only temporarily.

Figure 2 shows that the result of therapy varies depending on the kind of tumour. In the glioblastomas, we have attained a reduction of the water content by 6%.

Whereas the main objective of preoperative preparation is the reduction of the space occupation due to the oedema, in long-term treatment of brain tumour patients which cannot be operated on, highest priority is given to eliminating the neurological symptoms as far as possible, i.e. in order to render the patient subjectively healthy. The commencement of therapy may be identical with preoperative therapy. After regression of the clinical symptoms, especially when an impending incarceration is eliminated, the dosage can frequently be drastically reduced. The furosemide should be reduced as rapidly as possible (e.g. to 2×4 mg dexamethasone p.o.).

The patient (Fig. 3) received the combination therapy for barely two weeks and later received 9 mg dexamethasone p.o. In the initial phase, the patient was unconscious and had a severe left hemiparesis. After a few hours, the patient was completely awake and the hemiparesis disappeared within three days. In the ambulant checkups carried out at long intervals, he did not show any neurological deficits over about 9 months, although the tumour size had considerably increased.

It may be noted that we have tried out the 4 mg Decadron or 4 mg Fortecortin tablet without disadvantages and with good efficacy in many hundreds of patients in the meantime. We routinely administered 20 mg p.o.

References

1. Meinig, G., Aulich, A., Wende, S., Reulen, H. J.: Resolution of peritumoral brain edema following combination therapy with dexamethasone and furosemide. Adv. Neurosurg. *4*, 207–211 (1976)
2. Meinig, G., Aulich, A., Wende, S., Reulen, H. J.: The effect of dexamethasone and diuretics on peritumoral brain edema: Comparative study of tissue water content and CT. In: Dynamics of Brain Edema. Pappius, H. M., Feindel, W. (eds.), pp. 301–305. New York: Springer 1976
3. Meinig, G., Reulen, H. J., Simon, R. S., Schürmann, K.: Clinical, Chemical and CT Evaluation of Short-Term and Long-Term Antiedema Therapy with Dexamethasone and Diuretics. Adv. Neurology, Vol. 28: Brain Edema. J. Cervós-Navarro, Ferszt, R. (eds.), pp. 471–488, New York: Raven Press 1980

CT-Sterotactic Biopsy of Brain Tumours

F. MUNDINGER

In every case of an unverified, progressive intracranial lesion its nature should be histologically confirmed whether it is a neoplasm or otherwise. This applies whatever its location, and whether there are solitary or multiple lesions. This is essential before the planning of any conservative or radiation treatment. The exception to this is when an open exploratory operation is primarily indicated, during the performance of which adequate biopsy material can be obtained for conventional histological examination. This holds true even today, when modern computer tomographic devices guarantee improved differential diagnosis. Experience with CT has proved, after the initial phase of the first few years, that as a result of misinterpretation of the CT scan diagnostic errors can occur and, as a result of this the selection of the wrong treatment or even the failure to achieve a cure.

The clinician cannot but be dismayed when, for example, he sends a patient for percutaneous radiation with the diagnosis of "ring" glioblastoma, on the basis of a solitary deep-seated round focus with a ring structure, and later on the autopsy shows an abscess which could have been drained and rinsed out by stereotactic puncture, and treated successfully with antibiotics. On the other hand, in cases of lesions in the brain stem, pons, the basal ganglia or the cerebral white matter close to the midline, there is a considerable risk of causing severe functional deficits, when obtaining biopsy material by means of an open operation, the so-called exploratory craniotomy.

Nowadays stereotactic biopsy should be the method of choice as it avoids the above-mentioned risks, and rules out the danger of uncertainty, as for example, mistaking small foci. Furthermore it eliminates the possibility of error inherent in freehand puncture. With this method tissue can be obtained with 1 mm precision from foci larger than 7 mm in diameter and can be histologically compared with the surrounding tissue. Treatment can be decided upon immediately, even if the intra-operative examination of a smear preparation has still to be completed (together with Metzel [12]. I introduced this method into our stereotactic technique, in the early 1960's.)

This means for example, that in cases of inflammatory, necrotic foci or systemic diseases conservative treatment can be started. In one case of cerebellar necrosis, a young girl was spared an exploration of the posterior fossa and a partial cerebellar resection. In other cases, as soon as the localized pilocytic astrocytoma of the brain stem, pons or the basal ganglia is confirmed, interstitial radiotherapy can be performed immediately by permanently implanting a radionuclide (such as iridium-192 or iodine-125) [8, 11, 12] or, in cases where there is a cyst, a catheter for drainage can be implanted [8] (Fig. 1a).

In the case of a more malignant glioma, it can be established intraoperatively whether the combination of brachy-radiotherapy with percutaneous irradiation is indicated or the latter alone (cf. p. 247). For a deep-seated intraventricular, dysontogenetic tumour, an ependymoma, or a meningioma, microsurgical total resection can subsequently be aimed for. In such cases percutaneous irradiation, which affects the tumour itself far less than the rest of the brain, is not indicated. Particularly in cases of deep-seated, non-resectable tumours, the evaluation of the cases treated solely with conventional irradiation suffers from the lack of histological confirmation, so that benign cysts, haematomas, low-grade gliomas, dermoids, teratomas, etc., cannot be recognized among expanding and displacing lesions which are radiated as tumours. Naturally they show good long term results, although they could have and should have been treated by operation or local radiotherapy with good palliative or curative results.

The stereotactic biopsy of intracranial lesions has proved to be a successful method of examination [4, 8, 10, 12, 14, 15, 18, 19]. One of the advantages of this method is that the focus to be punctured can be reached exactly, to the nearest millimetre with a thin needle or a biopsy probe. Any previously selected point or focus, whether intracranial, intracerebral, or intracerebellar, can be stereotactically punctured from any point on the surface of the skull. Careful selection of the angle of puncture and its adjustment to the location of the focus to be punctured ensures the protection of functionally important areas and larger vessels. The risk of functional damage is thus reduced to a minimum.

The biopsy material is usually taken along the puncture tract. Specimens are taken continuously, beginning in the healthy tissue, through the pathological tissue to the other side, into reactively changed or healthy tissue. A morphological picture can thus be provided at the same time. This procedure has a further advantage in that it takes in the infiltration zone of tumours, which escapes every other diagnostic method.

Stereotactic biopsy, particularly of multiple foci, was first made more simple and more reliable by computerstereotaxy, as we developed it together with Birg [9, 3] from 1970 on, using a modification of the stereotactic device of Riechert and Mundinger [16] (Fig. 1 b). Computer stereotaxy has furthermore broadened the range of indications in functional stereotactic neurosurgery. Multiple biopsy specimens can be obtained through a small burr-hole (6 mm diameter) with various approach angles, all of which is calculated beforehand by computer. For lesions in both hemispheres, a bilateral burr-hole is necessary.

Target points for stereotactic biopsy used to be localized by using invasive neuroradiological techniques such as pneumo-encephalography, ventriculography, arteriography (because of calcification in the plain x-ray), or scintigraphy. Radionuclide-scintigraphy, in particular, made it possible to locate to the nearest millimetre nuclidestoring foci and determine their size, as our numerous biopsy controls carried out at that time confirm.

Computed tomography (CT), without a doubt, further improved the stereotactic technique of biopsy, even when the first generation devices were still being used. With the aid of a graphic or mathematical procedure, the CT-focus is transferred from the axial CT-layers on sagittal and coronal planes onto the plain x-ray scans, in which the target point and optimum angle of access are determined. We worked

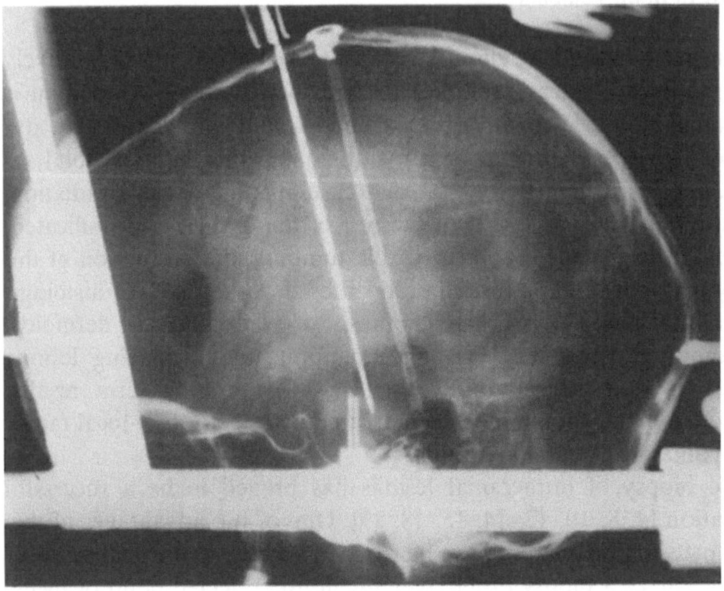

a

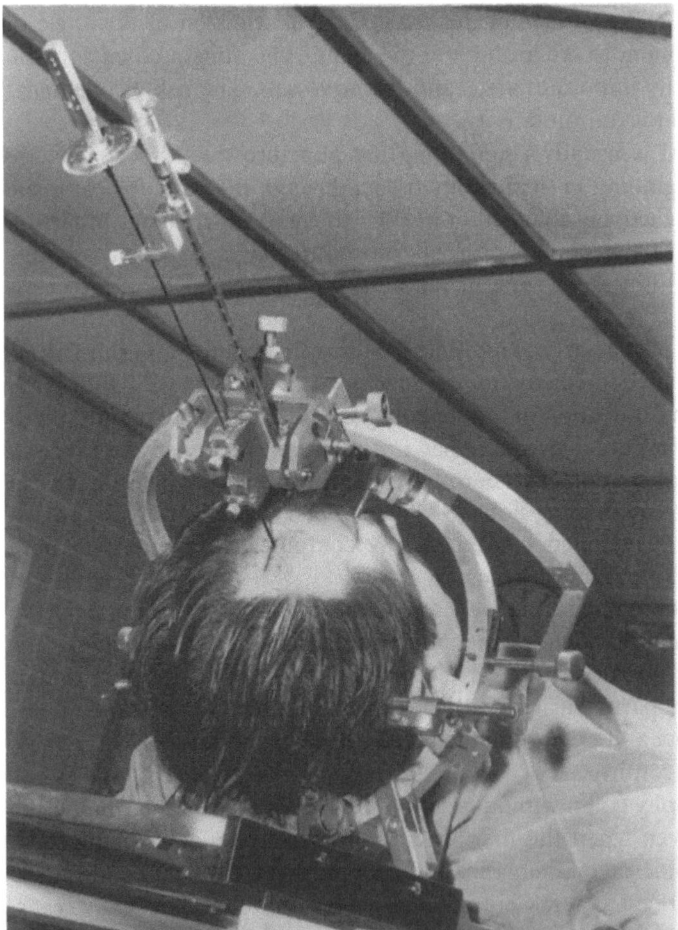

b

out this transferral method together with Birg and Krebber [2]. Another method was followed in which x-ray nuclide plates having x-ray contrast markings are set on the target device frames for CT, whereby the focus is indirectly established on the sagittal and coronal planes. These methods also made it possible – if in a roundabout way – to locate the foci.

The decisive breakthrough was the recent direct integration of computed tomography into the computer-stereotaxy-method. This achieved an extraordinary simplification of the method together with a target precision of 1 mm. This technique, which I also developed together with Birg [3, 10] and which has been named computed tomography-stereotaxy (CT-stereotaxy), will be briefly described below.

CT-Localization Technique

Our method is based on the fact that with modern CT-scanners it is possible to take directly from the CT scans the coordinate information necessary for the stereotactic operation. Furthermore, the target points can easily be determined with our stereotactic device, for it is one of the very few on the market today that works on the polar coordinate principle. The device can be adapted with no difficulty to any CT device that has a large opening (gantry = > 40 cm). The target point is given in cartesian spatial coordinates. The O-point of the coordinate system represents the centre of the base ring, which is secured on the head. It is only necessary to make the centre of the base ring coincide with the O-point of the coordinate system of the commercial tomograph gantry opening and to establish the x-axis position. No change had to be made to our stereotactic device.

Procedure

The patient's head, on which the stereotactic base ring has been secured, is scanned in the CT gantry. For this purpose, we have constructed a holder which makes it possible to achieve an exact relation between the coordinates represented on the scanner and the zero-point of the stereotactic base ring, or to convert the CT coordinates into the base ring coordinates. This is carried out using a frontal and sagittal scout view CT scan. With a gantry angle of 0° and a distance between layers of 1.5–10 mm, CT scans are taken parallel to the stereotactic base ring. The lowermost CT section is thereby situated on the zero plane of the stereotactic ring. Thin sections of 0.5–5 mm are taken in the area of the relevant structures (tumour, etc.) in

Fig. 1. a S.B., 11 years. Cystic pilocytic astrocytoma in the region of brain stem and pons. The stereotactically implanted catheter for repuncture is situated in the cystic portion (filled with air); the biopsy probe is in the solid tumour (in front of the cystic part). Twenty-one injections of interferon were administered locally in two series, through this cannula. **b** K.A. Stereotactic device (Riechert and Mundinger, computer modification by Mundinger and Birg). The target arch is secured on the base ring. The probe lies in the target point

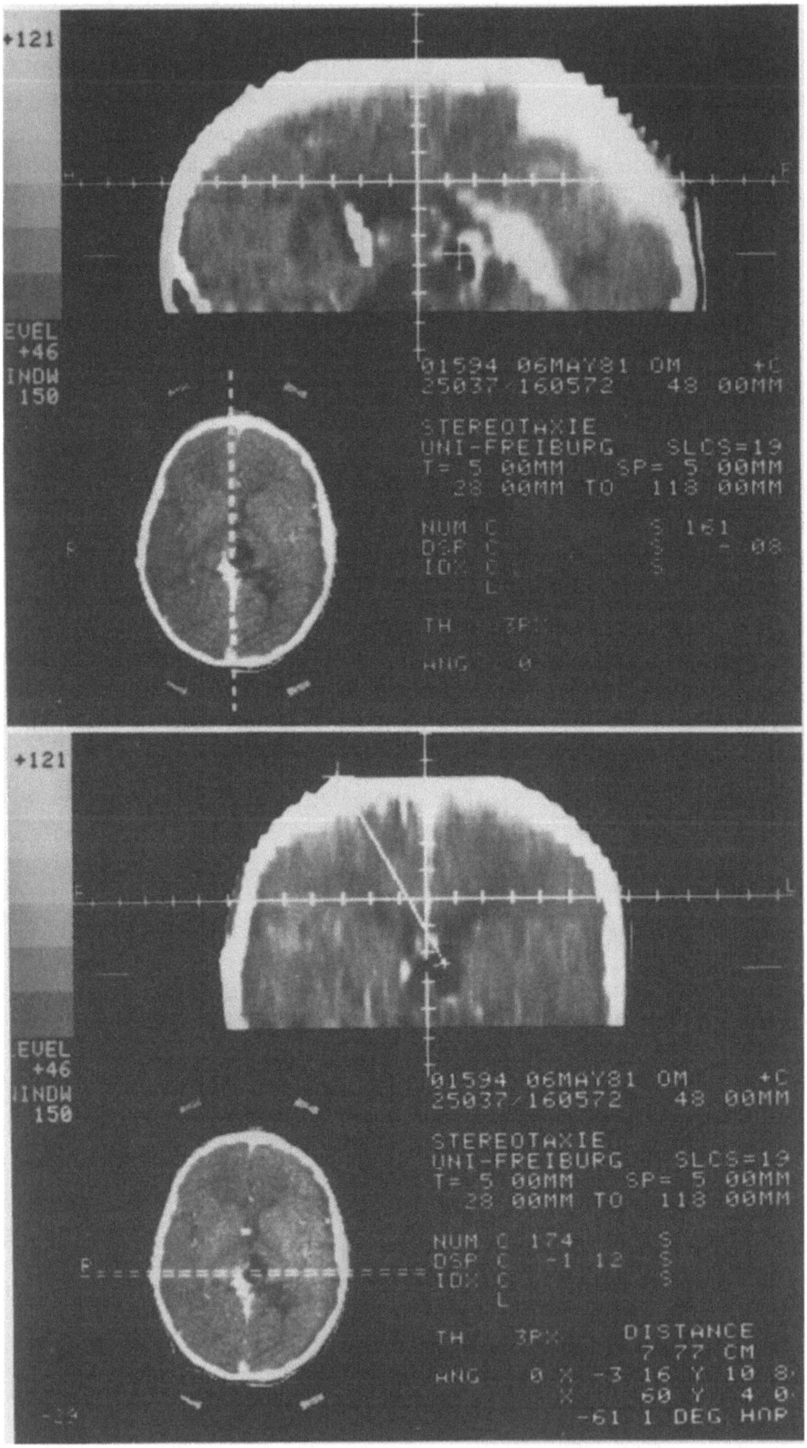
+121
EVEL
+46
INDW
150
01594 06MAY81 OM +C
25037/160572 48 00MM
STEREOTAXIE
UNI-FREIBURG SLCS=19
T= 5 00MM SP= 5 00MM
28 00MM TO 118 00MM
NUM C S 161
DSP C S - 08
IDX C S
L
TH 3PX
ANG 0
+121
EVEL
+46
INDW
150
01594 06MAY81 OM +C
25037/160572 48 00MM
STEREOTAXIE
UNI-FREIBURG SLCS=19
T= 5 00MM SP= 5 00MM
28 00MM TO 118 00MM
NUM C 174 S
DSP C -1 12 S
IDX C S
L
TH 3PX DISTANCE
7 77 CM
ANG 0 X -3 16 Y 10 8
X 60 Y 4 0
-61 1 DEG HOR

a

b

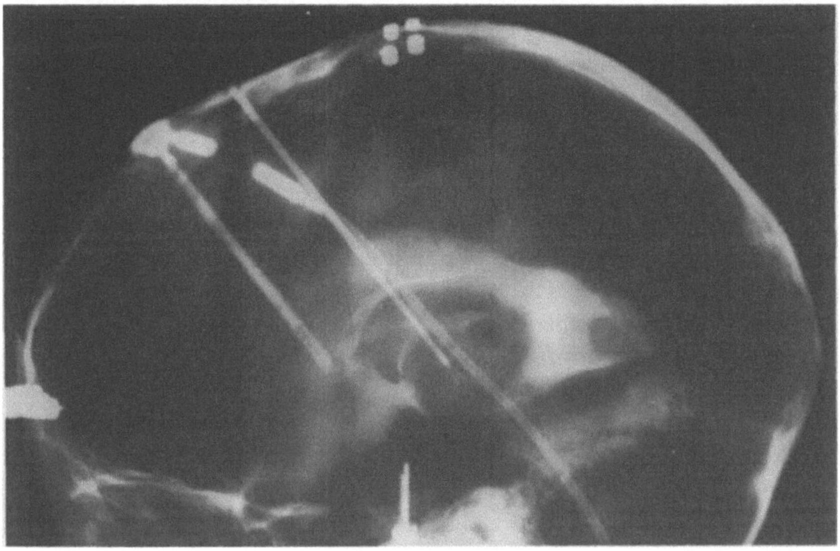
c

Fig. 2a–c. R.W., 9 years. Dermoid. **a** CT-stereotaxy: the coronal reconstruction shows in the area of the posterior third ventricle, a focus having sharp margins and surrounded by calcification in the dorsal portion. For the stereotactic CT biopsy, the centre of the focus is determined as the target point. With the CT computer, the coordinate axes x, y and z of the target point are calculated after the access angle to the target point and to the site of the burr-hole has been established. **b** Coronal reconstruction. Hypodense focus taken again as target point. The burr-hole site and electrode approach are determined with the CT-computer. **c** Lateral x-ray. Intraventricular dermoid: with the CT stereotactic method, a Rickham catheter with reservoir was first inserted in the anterior horn of the lateral ventricle and ventriculography was then performed. The intraventricular tumour contour is clearly demonstrated. The target point of the biopsy was the centre of the tumour. The biopsy probe lies exactly at the previously calculated point in the centre. Since the smear preparation showed the growth to be a microsurgically resectable intraventricular dermoid, only a ventriculo-atrial shunt was completed during the operation. The dermoid was later completely resected by microsurgery

order to facilitate reconstruction in the coronal and sagittal plane. The sagittal and coronal reconstructions are calculated using pixel sizes of approximately 1–3 = 1.1–3.3. For purposes of time and protection from radiation, these reconstructions are confined to the target area.

Evaluation

The one or more target points for biopsy (and also for the draining of cysts and for the implantation of catheters and radioactive isotopes for radiotherapy) are measured using the CT computer or an external computer. The x and y coordinates are each taken from the respective axial CT scans. The z coordinate is given by the position of the section relative to the middle of the base ring (= 0). If the software for reconstruction is available, the target point of the sagittal and coronal (vertical) reconstructions is taken from the thin section scan.

The coordinates of the point for making the burr-hole are measured either in the scout view scan (y and z coordinates in the sagittal, x coordinate in the coronal scan) or by extrapolation to the skull using a second target point taken from the sagittal and coronal reconstruction. The selection of probe access can also be integrated here in terms of its angle to the target point (Fig. 2a, b).

All the coordinate information for the stereotactic puncture with the aid of CT is thus at hand. The settings for the computer-stereotaxy device are calculated using the coordinate information. The stereotactic computer programme can be integrated into the CT computer software. For aseptic reasons, the operation take place in the operating theatre and the CT is therefore available for other patients.

Our CT stereotactic biopsies performed to date (643 cases up to Feb. 28, 1981) show that the target points determined by CT stereotaxy can in fact be morphologically reached with a probe exactness of less than 1 mm. This precision is increased, first of all, by the fact that the anatomical and pathological structures are directly measured and, secondly, that the coordinates of the target point are determined directly with the CT computer. Any further transferal procedure, such as ventriculography or angiography, or a special frame construction to mark the CT section is not necessary.

Materials and Method

For biopsy we use a set of cannulas, each of which consists of two cannulas with one having a smaller diameter so that it can be slid inside the other. For example, the cannula used for the brain midline area has a diameter of only 1.2 mm. The biopsy forceps, which is 0.8 mm in diameter, is introduced through the inside cannula (Fig. 2c). Two claw-like jaws of the forceps take hold of the tissue and snip it off. The amount of tissue is 1–3 mm^3. These forceps jaws have a head piece with millimetre intervals (up to 30 mm) without having to follow it with the outer cannula, which is secured in the guide rail of the stereotactic device. Thus in areas with a concentration of neuronal structures or in central areas such as the diencephalon, mesencephalon, and brain stem, the biopsy can be performed safely and with little risk of tissue damage.

In the sagittal and coronal reconstruction (thin sections) the angle of puncture is selected in such a way that, in cases of spherical lesions, the biopsy forceps can be

Fig. 3a, b. A.Z., 13 years. **a** CT with enhancement: pilocytic astrocytoma (optic nerve glioma) with considerable suprasellar extension and progressive development. The parents would not consent to an open operation. Stereotactic biopsy to confirm the diagnosis and for interstitial radiotherapy. The extension of the markedly hyperdense tumour is shown in the sagittal reconstruction. The clinoid process on the left is partially destroyed. The glioma shows suprasellar extension, has compressed the third ventricle, and completely fills the basal cisterns. It has enclosed the carotid siphon and extends as far as the sphenoid sinus. **b** Widening of the sella and the sella opening. The biopsy probe (0.8 mm in diameter) with opened jaws is in the anterior part of the tumour (= later anterior implantation point for iodine-125 permanent implantation (see text, p. 247)

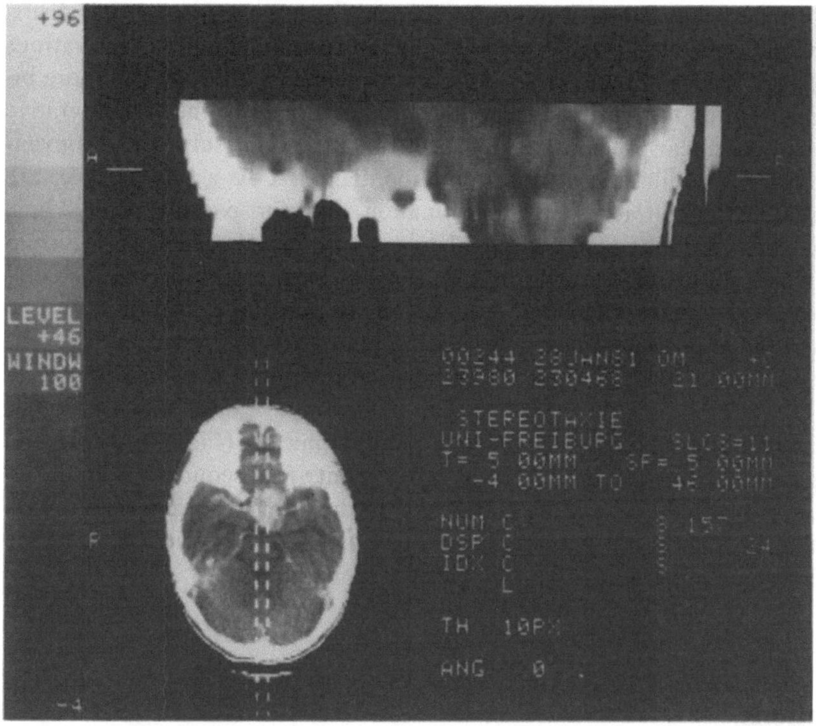
+96
LEVEL
+46
WINDW
100
STEREOTAXIE
UNI-FREIBURG
NUM
DSP
IDX
TH 10PX
ANG 0

a

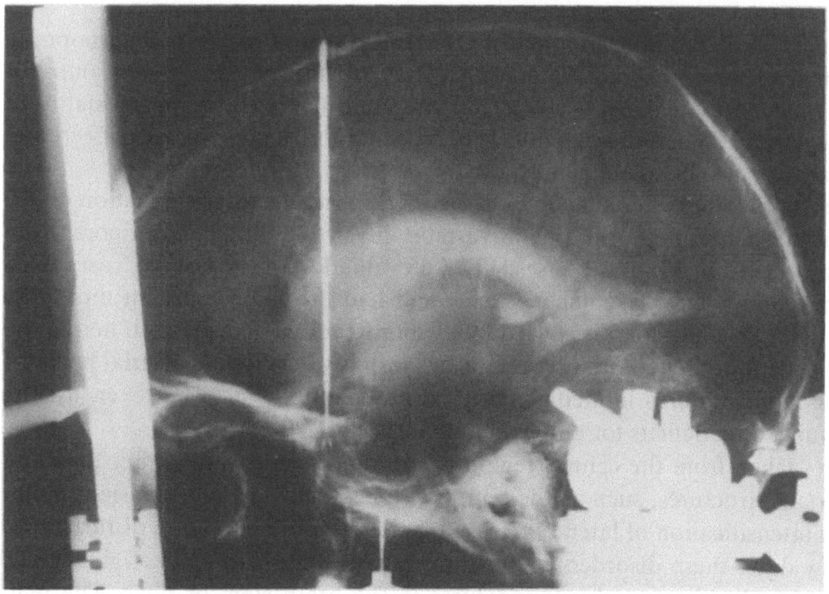

b

introduced into the centre, in cylindrical lesions along the axis of the cylinder, and in cases of geometrically more complicated lesions – also in terms of a later distribution of the radionuclide for radiotherapy – the forceps can be put into the various areas at different angles of puncture. If we obtain an average of 6–10 and more biopsy specimens from the various areas it facilitates not only the intraoperative examination of the smear preparation [1, 5, 6, 7, 17] but also the subsequent conventional histological examination in confirming the diagnosis. As a rule, samples are taken alternately for intraoperative examination and for paraffin embedding. Stereotactic biopsy is done in the peripheral areas of the focus in cases of a recurrent tumour or where progressive growth of the focus has been established in the computer tomogram (e.g., after interstitial radiotherapy or percutaneous irradiation), to examine the residue of tumours left after operation or parts of a recurrent tumour, and for the purpose of making a distinction between tumours and radiation necrosis.

The recording of the biopsy track is done radiographically (Figs. 2c, 3a, b) and by inserting a small silver clip or wire at the target point, if subsequently no radioactive seeds are implanted to mark the biopsy site. In the latter case, however, the diameter of the clip should not be more than a few tenths of a millimetre, since the metal artefact would otherwise affect the interpretation of the CT.

Complications

Using modern localization techniques of CT stereotaxy and regularly incorporating cerebral angiography to avoid puncturing vessels (of the sylvian vessel group, for example) or deep cranial nerves, etc., has dramatically reduced the mortality of stereotactic biopsy. When the patient's general condition is poor, atlases of cerebral angiography can also be of help and spare the patient the angiography.

The mortality of our stereotactic biopsies is 1.3%. In an earlier evaluation of 302 patients in my department, the operative mortality was still 2.3%. Temporary deterioration occured in 3% of the cases [13]. An evaluation of the last 582 cases (Oct. 81) that had undergone stereotactic biopsy and had the same transient morbidity was only 1.4%. This mortality is caused by the nontreatable oedema with herniation of the brain stem in the tentorial fissure or by a rapidly developing arterial haemorrhage. The latter requires immediate surgical evacuation, which, however, usually results in functional deficits for any patient that survives.

Biopsies taken from the central region or from motor tracts and other functionally important structures, such as the temporal lobes, can lead to a transient motor or sensory intensification of latent pareses, to aphasia or organic brain disturbances. After a few days, these disorders either disappear or return to their original state. The same complications apply to punctures in the brain stem or pons. The temporary functional deficits are caused by an intensification of perifocal oedema and microhaemorrhages, as our CT controls show. In my opinion, the small number of transient functional deficits and the low mortality rate present no contraindication, if one considers the diagnostic and therapeutic advantages.

Number of Patients and Results

Table 1 gives the number of stereotactic biopsies that were carried out. Some of them were followed immediately by interstitial, intracavitary radiotherapy, catheter implantation for drainage, cyst or abscess puncture, or – as in one case – by the direct instillation of interferon into a fibrillary pilocytic brain stem astrocytoma (see Fig. 1 a).

Table 2 shows the histological diagnoses obtained from the intracranial tumours. Biopsies were also taken for functional operations, e.g., to examine the striate catecholamine metabolism.

From Table 3 it can be seen that the number of operations performed each year increased considerably after the introduction of computed tomography and in particular, of CT-stereotaxy. (The evaluations were carried out together with K. Wei-

Table 1. Non-functional indications for stereotactic neurosurgery (1952 – 1981)

	No. of cases
Diagnostic biopsy	1665
Interstitial radiotherapy of inoperable tumours	813
Interstitial local radiotherapy	270
Intracavitary radiotherapy	20
Drainage procedures (arachnoid cysts, abscess)	61
Local application of Interferon	1
Ventriculocisternostomy	13
Combined open-stereotactic procedures (in AV-malformations, pituitary adenomas, cerebral haematomas, foreign bodies)	122
Total	2965

Table 2. Stereotactic biopsy, followed by interstitial radiotherapy procedures (1952 – 1981)

Glioblastoma	177
Astrocytoma	408
Oligodendroglioma	94
Ependymoma	29
Pinealoma	17
Meningioma	16
Metastases	20
Sarcoma	11
Pituitary adenoma	246
Craniopharyngioma	22
Other lesions	41
Hypophysectomy	56
Pallidotomy	21
Total	1158

Table 3. CT-controlled stereotactic brain biopsy

	No. of cases
1977 (Sept. – Dec.)	23
1978	125
1979	111
1980	147
1981	191
Total	597

gel). The results of our cases, along with a comparison of the intraoperative diagnosis in a smear preparation (paraffin embedding) with conventional histological examination, are compiled in an article in this book by P. Kleihues (p. 247). We would like to take this opportunity to thank Dr. Kleihues and his colleagues for their outstanding collaboration. The neuropathologist must be present at the intraoperative examination and has a decisive say in the therapeutic decision: for example, in the case of a tumour, depending on its nature, whether a long or short course of radiotherapy is to be started immediately, or, in the case of a resectable tumour (ventricular tumour, for instance), if the stereotactic operation should end with the biopsy and later an open surgical intervention be performed. In the case of a non-tumourous lesion, such as a necrotic or inflammatory focus, the operation is likewise terminated and the appropriate conservative therapy started.

Summary and Indication

The modern technique of stereotactic biopsy and the results and indications based on 1665 cases are presented. By incorporating computed tomography into the computer stereotactic procedure (CT-stereotaxy), the site of the biopsy and its coordinates can, for the first time, be determined directly and anatomically. The target precision is better than 1 mm and there are fewer complications associated with the operation (transient morbidity 3%, mortality 1.1%). Solitary and multiple foci and those lying in both hemispheres are biopsied with a biopsy forceps (0.8 mm in diameter) through a small burr-hole (7 mm in diameter). The approach is adapted to the shape of the focus.

Since the classification and the nature of the lesion is usually established intraoperatively by the smear preparation, it can be decided right away whether, for example, radiotherapy should be started immediately during the same operation or whether the lesion should be resected by open operation. A stereotactic biopsy has no effect on the subsequent microsurgical resection of benign tumours (e.g., intraventricular tumours, ependymomas). The histologically confirmed indication is an advantage for the surgical procedure. The percutaneous irradiation therapy of malignant tumours is also carried out after the indication has been histologically confirmed, whereby benign cysts, necroses, low-grade gliomas, or inflammatory foci, etc., can be excluded. Abscesses and cysts are punctured immediately following the biopsy and, if necessary, drained with stereotactically implanted catheters. Inflammatory degenerative diseases are differentially diagnosed and are given conservative therapy. Aneurysms and vascular deformities are a contra-indication – another reason why angiography, apart from its role in reducing the risk of puncture, is absolutely indispensable before stereotactic biopsy is performed.

Our experiences have shown that stereotactic biopsy is a method that offers significant diagnostic and therapeutic advantages and, at the same time, relatively little risk.

References

1. Badt, B.: Mikroskopische Schnelldiagnose bei hirnchirurgischen Eingriffen. Zentralbl. Neurochir. *2,* 123 (1937).
2. Birg, W., Krebber, L., Mundinger, F.: Ein einfaches Verfahren für die Übertragung von Tomographie-Scan-Schichten auf das Röntgenbild, insbesondere für die funktionelle Neurochirurgie. Fortschr. Neurol. Psychiat. *47,* 637–640 (1979).
3. Birg, W., Mundinger, F.: Direct target point determination for stereotactic brain operations from CT-data and the calculation of setting parameters for polar-coordinate stereotactic devices. Proc. 8th Meeting World Soc. Stereotactic and Functional Neurosurgery, Part III, Zürich 1981, Appl. Neurophysiol. *45,* 387–395 (1982).
4. Heath, R. G., John, S., Foss, O.: Stereotaxic biopsy: A method for the study of discrete brain regions of animals and man. Arch. Neurol. *4,* 291 (1961).
5. Kautzky, R.: Die Schnelldiagnose intracranieller Erkrankungen mit Hilfe des supravital gefärbten Quetschpräparats. Virchows Arch. Path. Anat. 320–495 (1951).
6. MacMenemey, W. H.: An appraisal of smear-diagnosis in neurosurgery. Am. J. Clin. Pathol. *33,* 471 (1960).
7. Morris, A. A.: The use of the smear technique in the rapid histological diagnosis of tumours of the central nervous system: Description of a new staining method. J. Neurosurg. *4,* 497–504 (1947).
8. Mundinger, F.: Die stereotaktische interstitielle Therapie nicht resezierbarer intracranieller Tumoren mit Ir-192 und Jod-125. In: Kombinierte chirurgische und radiologische Behandlung maligner Tumoren. Wannemacher, M., Schreiber, H. W., Gauwerky, F., pp. 90–112, München: Urban & Schwarzenberg 1981.
9. Mundinger, F.: Implantation of Radioisotopes (Curietherapie) In: Textbook of Stereotaxy of the Human Brain. Ed.: Schaltenbrand/Walker, pp. 410–445, Stuttgart: Thieme 1982.
10. Mundinger, F., Birg, W.: CT-Aided Stereotaxy for Functional Neurosurgery and Deep Brain Implants. Advances in Neurosurgery *10,* Berlin, Heidelberg, New York: Springer 1981.
11. Mundinger, F., Hoefer, T.: Protracted long-term irradiation of inoperable midbrain tumours by stereotactic Curietherapy using Iridium-192. Acta Neurochirurg. Suppl. *21,* 93–100 (1974).
12. Mundinger, F., Metzel, E.: Interstitial radioisotope therapy of intractable diencephalic tumors by the stereotaxic permanent implantation of iridium-192. Including Bioptic Control. Conf. neurol. *32,* 195–202 (1970).
13. Ostertag, Chr. B., Mennel, H. D., Kiessling, M.: Stereotactic biopsy of brain tumors. Surg. Neurol. *14,* 275–283 (1980).
14. Pecker, J., Scarabin, J.-M., Vallee, B., Bruchner, J.-M.: Treatment in tumours of the pineal region: Value of stereotaxic biopsy. Surg. Neurol. *12,* 341 (1979).
15. Riechert, T., Giesinger, M. A., Mölbert, E.: Biopsien während stereotaktischer Operationen beim Parkinsonsyndrom. Neurochirurgia *10,* 106–118 (1967).

16. Riechert, T., Mundinger F.: Beschreibung und Anwendung eines Zielgerätes für stereotaktische Hirnoperationen (II. Modell). Acta Neurochir. *33*, 308 (1955).
17. Shetter, A. G., Bertuccini, T. V., Pittman, H. W.: Closed needle biopsy in the diagnosis of intracranial mass lesions. Surg. Neurol. *8*, 341 (1977).
18. Sugita, K., Mutsuga, N., Takaoka, Y., Hirota, T., Shibuya, M., Doi, T.: Stereotaxic exploration of para-third ventricle tumours. In Proceedings of the 6th Symposium of the International Society of Research in Stereoencephalotomy, part II. Tokyo (1973) Convin. Neurol. *37*, 156 (1975).
19. Waltregny, A.: Apport des méthodes steréotaxiques dans le diagnostic et le traitement des tumeurs cérébrales. Ann. Radiol. *19*, 241 (1976).

Diagnostic Potential of Stereotactic Biopsy of Brain Tumours. A Report of 400 Cases

M. KIESSLING, J. ANAGNOSTOPOULOS, G. LOMBECK, and P. KLEIHUES

Introduction

Biopsies taken by stereotactic techniques require diagnostic decisions based on the microscopic examination of minute tissue samples. To avoid a two-stage stereotactic operation, rapid diagnosis is essential for making decisions about treatment in the case of brain tumours suitable for consecutive interstitial radiotherapy [3, 4, 10, 11]. The problem for the pathologist is mostly one of receiving multiple minute fragments from different parts of the lesion, with the demand for instant diagnosis. The small amount of tissue is an essential limitation for the use of frozen sections.

Stereotactic biopsy samples are, however, suitable for the preparation of smears stained with methylene-blue, a method which has been repeatedly proposed for rapid diagnosis or as a screening test during neurosurgical operations [2, 5, 7–9, 11]. The present report deals with the validity of morphological diagnosis on stereotactic brain tumour biopsies and the correlation of diagnoses obtained from smear preparations and paraffin-embedded sections.

Materials and Methods

The present series of 400 patients is restricted to cases in which a stereotactic biopsy was performed to confirm or rule out a clinically suspected intracranial neoplastic lesion. Depending on the size of the lesion, two to ten biopsies were taken stepwise at distances of 5 to 10 mm with a stereotactic biopsy forceps (manufactured by F. L. Fischer, Co., Freiburg, F.R.G.). The resulting amount of biopsy material was approximately 1 mm^3 per biopsy site.

In all cases the final neuropathological diagnosis was the result of two different diagnostic procedures: – rapid diagnosis by cytological analysis of smear preparations during the operation, was followed by histological examination of serial paraffin sections obtained from additional stereotactic specimens.

For cytological analysis, biopsy material was placed on glass slides, gently spread out with needles, stained with methylene-blue and slightly pressed with a coverslip. After microscopic examination smear preparations were photographed for the records. Additional stereotactic samples were processed for the preparation of conventional paraffin-embedded sections.

Results and Discussion

Data on the age distribution of patients undergoing stereotactic operation and a comparison with biopsies taken by open operation, are summarized in Fig. 1. Comparative evaluation of 400 (stereotactic operation) and 3565 (open surgery) cases revealed a generally earlier occurence of stereotactic biopsies with a peak incidence in the first and second decade. The percentage of patients under 20 years was more than twice as high in the stereotactic group as in the craniotomy group. Within the third and fourth decades the relative number of patients was similar in both groups. At a higher age, the frequency of open operation cases largely outnumbered that of stereotactic biopsies.

The prevalence of stereotactic biopsies in the lower age groups is mainly due to the high incidence of deep-seated low grade astrocytomas in children and younger individuals [13]. Since these tumours are often located close to midline structures and are considered inoperable [12], stereotactic biopsy is indicated in order to achieve classification and grading of the lesion before appropriate radiotherapeutic measures are taken.

The majority of biopsied lesions were located supratentorially (Table 1). The cerebral hemispheres were the site most frequently involved (44%) with a marked predilection for functionally important hemispheric regions such as the central region and the speech area. Second in frequency were locations close to midline structures such as the basal ganglia and the hypothalamus (23% and 10% respectively) followed by the midbrain-pineal region (9.5%). Cerebellum and brain stem were rarely encountered sites, as were intraventricular tumours and extracerebral lesions at the base of the skull.

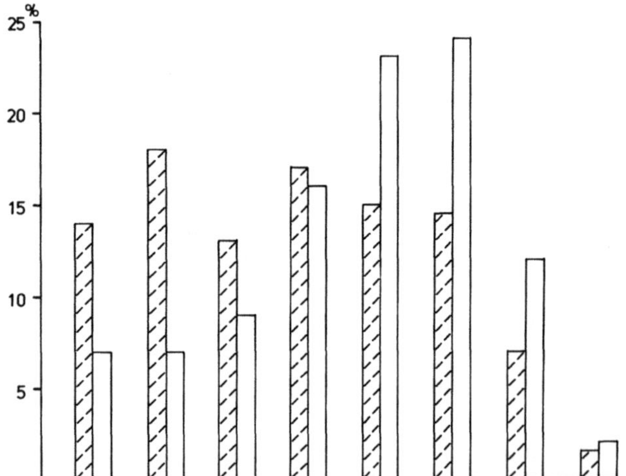

Fig. 1. Comparative age distribution of patients undergoing stereotactic brain tumour biopsy (400 cases, *hatched columns*) and of patients with biopsies taken by open surgical intervention (3565 cases, *open columns*)

Marked differences between stereotactic biopsies and biopsy material obtained from open surgical intervention were also observed when the type and incidence of the lesions were evaluated (Table 2). The incidence of astroglial tumours was much higher in the stereotactic group than in exploratory and therapeutic craniotomies (47% and 14% respectively). This was particularly true for pilocytic astrocytomas,

Table 1. Site of biopsied lesions

Supratentorial	85%
– Hemispheres	44%
– Basal ganglia	23%
– Diencephalon	10%
– Ventricles	4%
– Base of skull	4%
Infratentorial	15%
– Midbrain-pineal region	9.5%
– Pons-medulla	4.5%
– Cerebellum	0.75%
– Ventricle	0.25%

Table 2. Frequency distribution of tumour types

	Stereotactic biopsy (400 cases)	Open operation (3565 cases)
Astrocytic tumours	189 (47%)	506 (14%)
– Pilocytic astrocytoma	70 (17.5%)	219 (6%)
– Astrocytoma	68 (17%)	219 (6%)
– Anaplastic astrocytoma	31 (8%)	63 (2%)
Oligodendroglial tumours	21 (5%)	255 (7%)
– Oligodendroglioma	18 (4.5%)	147 (4%)
– Anaplastic oligodendroglioma	2 (0.5%)	87 (2%)
– Mixed oligo-astrocytoma	1 (<1%)	21 (1%)
Ependymoma	9 (2%)	96 (3%)
Plexus papilloma	4 (1%)	11 (1%)
Glioblastoma	64 (16%)	490 (15%)
Medulloblastoma	1 (<1%)	113 (3%)
Neurinoma	–	317 (9%)
Meningioma	5 (1%)	755 (21%)
Lymphoma	2 (0.5%)	57 (2%)
Germinoma	11 (3%)	17 (1%)
Teratoma	3 (1%)	
Craniopharyngioma	12 (3%)	71 (2%)
Pituitary adenoma	2 (0.5%)	376 (11%)
Chordoma	1 (<1%)	35 (1%)
Metastatic tumours	10 (2.5%)	243 (7%)
Unclassified tumours	11 (3%)	68 (2%)

which accounted for 17.5% of all biopsied lesions and thus represent the most frequent tumour type in our series. Grade II astrocytomas and anaplastic astrocytomas were also more frequent in stereotactic biopsies when compared to open surgery (17% against 6% and 8% against 2% respectively), whereas the incidence of neuroepithelial tumours other than astrocytomas was similar in both groups. Stereotactic biopsy material showed a low incidence of neurinomas and meningiomas (1%) due to their extracerebral, easily accessible location. This is similarly true for pituitary adenomas (0.5% in stereotactic biopsies against 11% in open operations). In contrast, germ cell tumours – due to their predilection for the midbrain-pineal region – were four times more frequent in the stereotactic group.

After combined cytological and histological examination, in 320 (80%) out of 400 stereotactic biopsies a definite tumour diagnosis including tumour type and ap-

Table 3. Diagnostic potential of stereotactic brain tumour biopsies (smear preparations + paraffin-embedded sections)

Tumour + tumour type + approximate grading	80%
Tumour clinically suspected, but not confirmed	11%
Glioma without grading	6%
Tumour (unclassified)	3%

Table 4. Accuracy of stereotactic diagnosis

Clinical follow-up	Confirmation	Radiation necrosis (no tumour)	Diagnostic errors
– Subsequent open operation	10	1	3
– Recurrence (additional stereotactic biopsy)	20	5	3
– Recurrence	3	–	–
Autopsy	8	2	1

Table 5. Correlation of diagnoses obtained from smear preparations and paraffin sections

Smear diagnosis confirmed		77%
Lack of correlation		8%
– Difference in tumour type	3.5%	
– Difference in grading	3.5%	
– Presence of tumour	1%	
No discrepancy, no confirmation (sampling error, border zone, necrosis)		15%
– Diagnosis from smear preparation only	14%	
– Diagnosis from paraffin section only	1%	

proximate grading was made (Table 3). In an additional 44 cases (11%) a clinically suspected neoplastic lesion was definitely ruled out by the combination of both procedures. In 24 cases (6%) a glioma was diagnosed but precise grading was not possible. In the remaining 12 cases (3%) the presence of a tumour was confirmed, but tissue samples available were insufficient for histopathological classification.

Data on the accuracy and reliability of stereotactic diagnoses as verified by clinical follow-up or autopsy (56 cases) are summarized in Table 4. Combined stereotactic diagnoses were confirmed by subsequent therapeutic craniotomy, additional biopsies of recurrent tumours or autopsy in 41 cases. In eight cases radiation necrosis and absence of a tumour was demonstrated after interstitial radiotherapy of previously diagnosed neoplastic lesions. Diagnostic errors were encountered in seven cases. However, in four of these, the apparent discrepancy was probably related to progressive increase in malignancy during the time interval between the two biopsies.

Stereotactic biopsy was followed by interstitial radiotherapy in 240 cases (60%). In 236 cases (59%) interstitial implantation of isotopes was performed in a one-stage operation, i.e. a positive diagnosis was established exclusively by cytological examination during the operation. In only four cases (1%) additional histological evaluation was considered necessary before any treatment.

To estimate the diagnostic relevance of smear preparations the correlation of diagnoses obtained from smear preparations and paraffin-embedded sections was evaluated (Table 5). Results showed a confirmation of the cytological diagnosis by subsequent histological examination of additional samples in 308 cases (77%). The cytological diagnosis had to be substantially changed in 32 cases (8%). A discrepancy related to tumour type or grading was present in 28 cases (3.8% each). A diagnostic error in smear preparations concerning the presence of tumour tissue occurred in four cases (1%). In 60 cases (15%) the verification of one part of the diagnosis was not possible. This was predominantly due to sampling errors. In these cases the biopsy material of one of the two methods employed contained a border zone of the lesion or consisted only of necrotic or haemorrhagic areas.

Because of their uniform architecture, well-differentiated gliomas are easily recognizable in smear preparations. Even minute tissue samples are usually representative of the entire neoplasm. The fibre network is clearly visible in smear preparations and is a useful feature in the diagnosis of pilocytic and fibrillary astrocytomas (Fig. 2a). In constrast, tissue architecture is much less preserved in smears of anaplastic gliomas. They are predominantly composed of individual polygonal cells and thus may be confused with malignant epithelial neoplasms (Fig. 2b). Because of the heterogeneous structure of malignant neuroepithelial tumours with extensive central necrosis and only a small rim of solid neoplastic tissue, sampling errors are more frequent but can partly be avoided by close cooperation between the neuropathologist and the neurosurgeon (Fig. 3).

The vast majority of non-glial tumours was also found to exhibit typical cytological features in smear preparations from stereotactic biopsies and allowed a specific diagnosis with sufficient reliability. In particular, lesions such as craniopharyngiomas in otherwise inaccessible sites, are easily recognized in smears if bands or clusters of large regular epithelial cells with well-defined plasma membranes and small eccentric nuclei are present. Smear preparations of germinomas which most

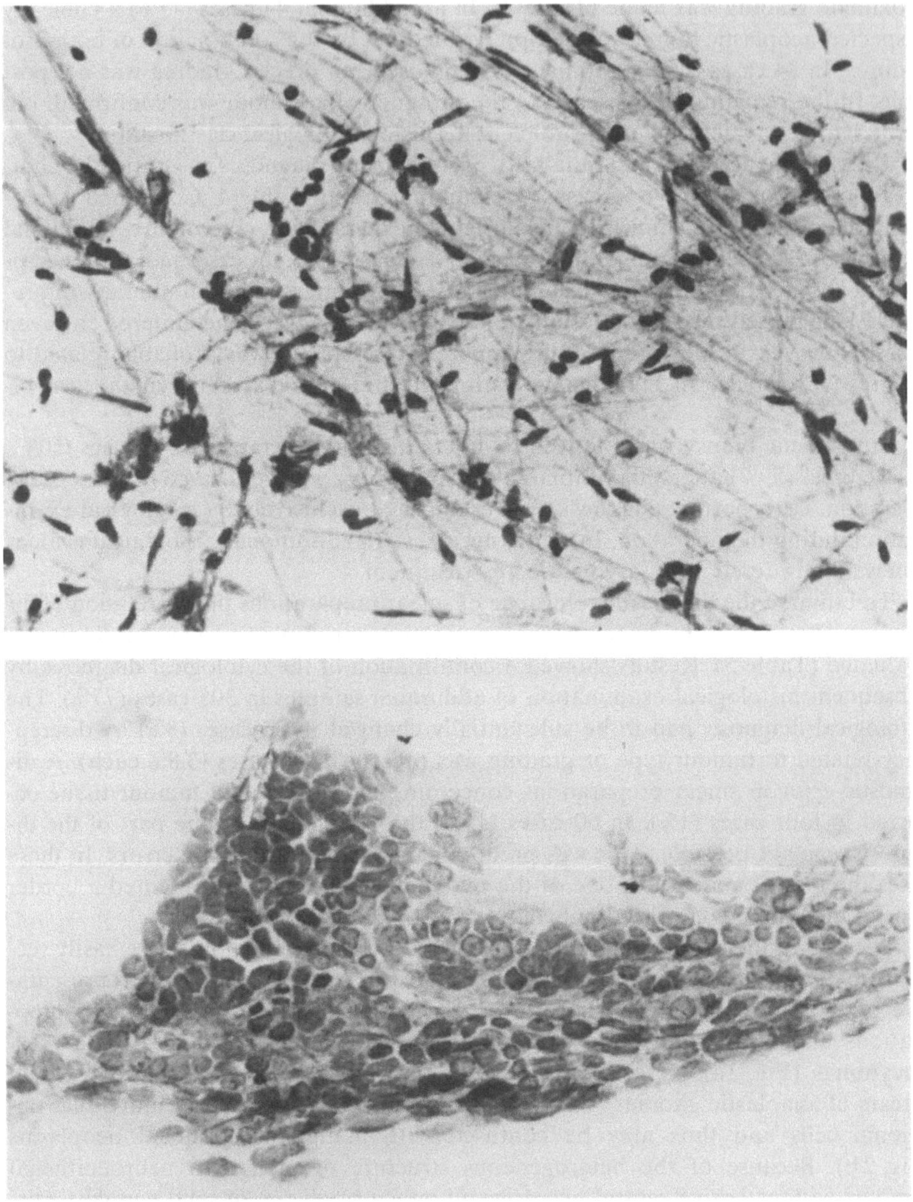

a

b

Fig. 2. **a** Smear preparation of a pilocytic astrocytoma with typical bipolar cell shape, regular elongated nuclei and tapering processes forming a prominent network of densely packed fibres, ×250. **b** In contrast, smears of anaplastic astrocytomas are often composed of cells with pseudoepithelial morphological features, ×250

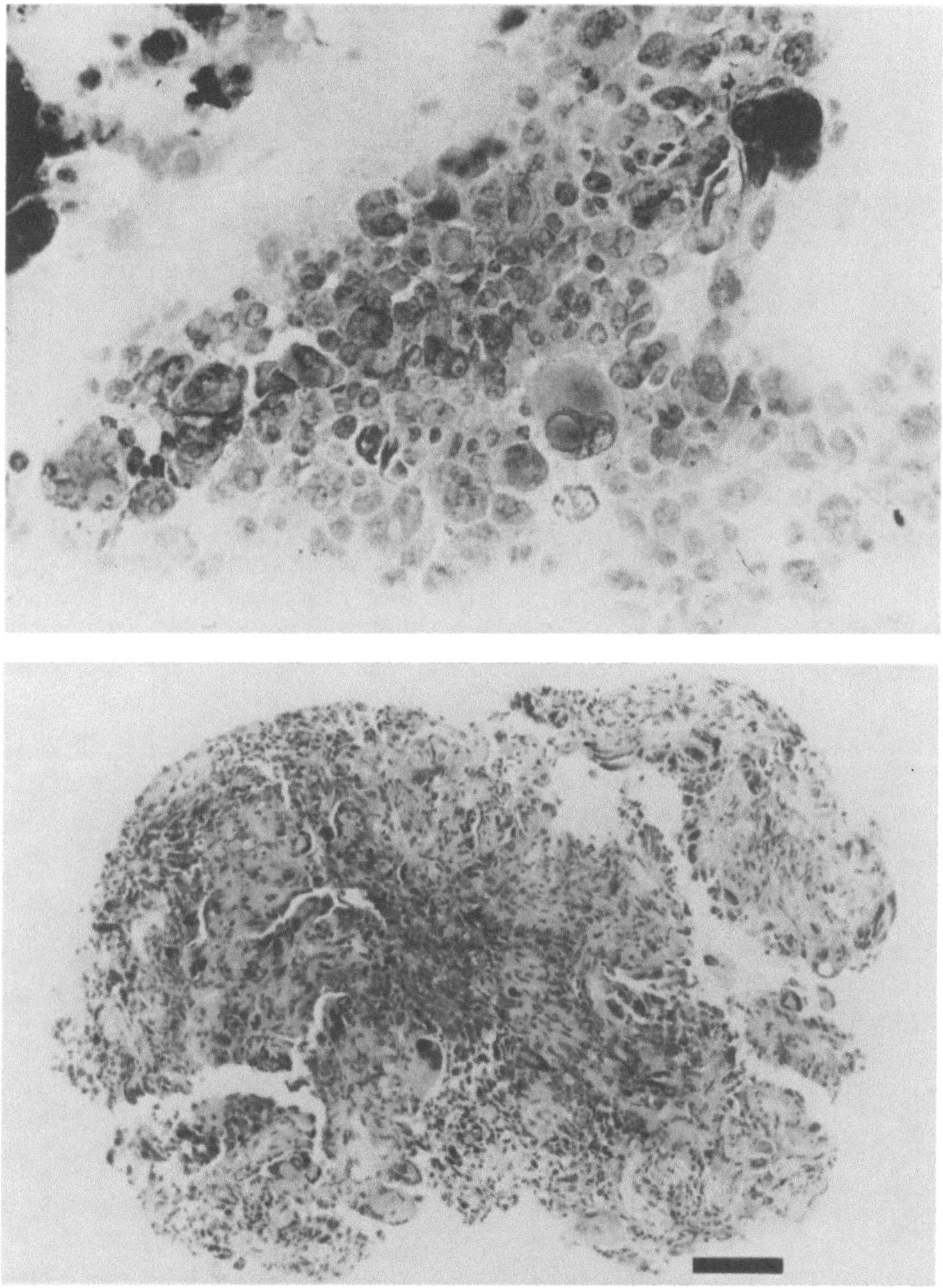

a

b

Fig. 3. a Smear preparation of a giant cell glioblastoma exhibiting marked cellular pleomorphism, ×250. **b** Photomicrograph of the corresponding paraffin-embedded tissue section illustrating the size of a stereotactically removed tissue sample. The horizontal bar corresponds to 0.1 mm (H & E)

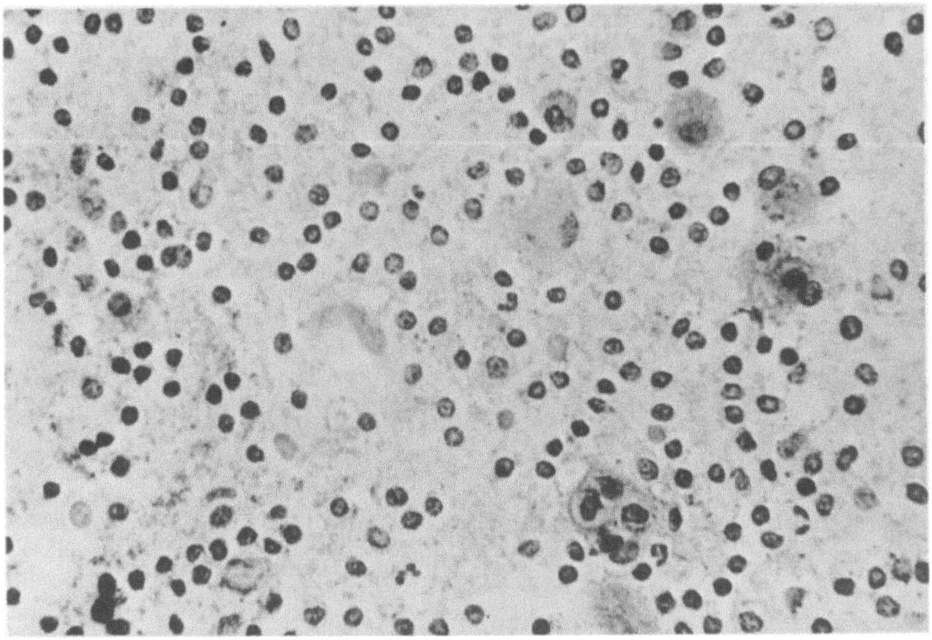

a

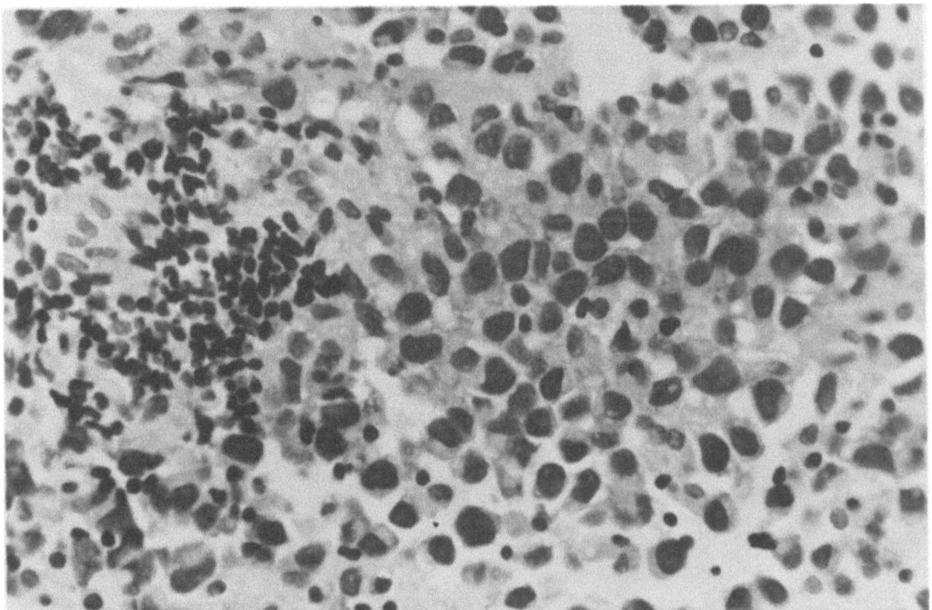

b

Fig. 4. a Smear preparation of a germinoma demonstrating the characteristic cytological features with two distinct cell types and lack of any transitional cellular elements, ×250. **b** Detail of the corresponding histopathologic picture of an additional paraffin-embedded tissue specimen obtained by stereotactic operation, ×250

commonly occur in the pineal region often allow an instant diagnosis based on the characteristic "two-cell-type" of these neoplasms (Fig. 4). Large spheroidal cells with central nuclei and clear-cut cell membranes are intermingled with numerous small lymphoid elements. No transitional forms are seen between these two cell types. Smears of epidermoids display typical crystalloid plates of cholesterin, which are no longer visible after the chemical procedures of paraffin embedding.

A more extensive description of the cytology of tumours affecting the central nervous system has recently been given elsewhere [1, 6, 11].

Conclusions and Summary

The validity of morphological diagnosis on stereotactic brain tumour biopsies was investigated by a retrospective evaluation of 400 cases. Combined cytological (smear preparations) and histological examination of stereotactic biopsy samples revealed the nature of the lesion in 366 cases (91%). In the remaining 34 cases (9%), the presence of a tumour was confirmed but the available tissue samples were not sufficient for an unequivocal classification of the neoplasm. To estimate the diagnostic relevance of smear preparations for rapid diagnosis during stereotactic operations, the correlation of findings obtained from smears and paraffin-embedded sections was reviewed. A confirmation of the cytological diagnosis was found in 308 cases (77%). Lack of correlation was present in 32 cases (8%). In the remaining 60 cases the verification of one of the two methods employed did not yield conclusive results probably due to sampling errors.

The small amount of tissue in individual samples obtained by stereotactic biopsy is an essential limitation for the pathological diagnosis. In the large majority of our cases, however, stereotactic biopsy provided sufficient information for a differentiated typing of brain tumours after combined cytological and histological examination. In most cases which called for an instant diagnosis, smear preparations were found to yield correct classification of the biopsied lesions with sufficient reliability to allow for decisions regarding treatment.

The present results support the stereotactic approach for brain biopsies if open surgical intervention involves a considerable risk for the patient. It is the method of choice for obtaining histological evidence of lesions in otherwise inaccessible or functionally inoperable sites and in cases of multiple small intracerebral neoplasms of unknown aetiology.

References

1. Adams H., Graham D. I., Doyle D.: Brain Biopsy. The smear technique for neurosurgical biopsies. London: Chapman and Hall 1981
2. Badt B.: Mikroskopische Schnelldiagnose bei hirnchirurgischen Eingriffen. Zentralbl. Neurochir. *2*, 123–139 (1937)
3. Conway L. W., O'Foghludha F. T., Collins, S. F.: Stereotactic treatment of acromegaly. J. Neurol. Neurosurg. Psychiat. *32*, 48–59 (1969)

4. Conway, L. W.: Stereotaxic diagnosis and treatment of intracranial tumours including an initial experience with cryosurgery for pinealomas. J. Neurosurg. *38,* 453–460 (1973)
5. Eisenhardt, L., Cushing, H.: Diagnosis of intracranial tumours by supravital technique. Am. J. Pathol. *6,* 541–552 (1930)
6. Jane, J. A., Yshon, D.: Cytology of tumours affecting the nervous tissue. Springfield (Ill.): Charles C. Thomas 1969
7. Kautzky, R.: Die Schnelldiagnose intracranialer Erkrankungen mit Hilfe des supravital gefärbten Quetschpräparates. Virchows Archiv Path. Anat. *320,* 495–500 (1951)
8. Marshall, L. F., Adams, H., Doyle, D., Graham, D. I.: The histological accuracy of the smear technique for neurosurgical biopsies. J. Neurosurg. *39,* 82–88 (1973)
9. McMenemey, W. H.: An appraisal of smear-diagnosis in neurosurgery. Am. J. Clin. Pathol. *33,* 471–479 (1960)
10. Mundinger, F., Ostertag, Ch. B., Birg, W., Weigel, K.: Stereotactic treatment of brain lesions. Biopsy, interstitial radiotherapy (Iridium-192 and Jodine-125) and drainage procedures. Appl. Neurophysiol. *43,* 198–204 (1980)
11. Ostertag, Ch. B., Mennel, H. D., Kiessling, M.: Stereotactic biopsy of brain tumours. Surg. Neurol. *14,* 275–283 (1980)
12. Roberson, C., Till, K.: Hypothalamic gliomas in children. J. Neurol. Neurosurg. Psychiat. *37,* 1047–1052 (1974)
13. Russell, D. S., Rubinstein, L. J.: Pathology of tumours of the nervous system, pp. 150–152, London: Edward Arnold 1977

Internal Shunt or Perioperative Pressure-Controlled Ventricular Fluid Drainage (C-VFD) in Children and Juveniles with Infratentorial Tumours

K. E. RICHARD, R. HELLER, and R. A. FROWEIN

In the last two decades opinions have differed concerning the technique of prophylaxis of postoperative CSF circulation disturbances in patients with infratentorial tumours. The advocates of temporary perioperative external ventricular fluid drainage (C-VFD) [1, 8, 9, 11–13, 15, 17] are opposed to those authors who demand preoperative implantation of an internal shunt system [1–3, 5, 6, 10]. Recently Albright [2] pointed out that as yet there have been no investigations as to whether C-VFD or internal shunt is the better method of treatment.

Material

From 1973–1980 we treated 85 children and juveniles with an infratentorial space-occupying lesion. There were 21 patients with medullublastoma, 19 patients with astrocytoma, 5 patients with cystic lesions, 4 patients with neurinomas and 14 patients with brain stem tumours of unknown histological diagnosis. 19 patients remained without C-VFD or internal shunt. 33 patients received C-VFD, either pre-, post-, or perioperatively. In the latter cases the ventricular fluid pressure (VFP) was monitored simultaneously. In 33 patients an internal shunt was inserted either pre- or postoperatively.

Results

In the 3 treatment groups – i.e. patients with neither drainage nor shunt, patients with C-VFD and patients with internal shunt – rates of mortality, survival and frequency of complications were compared (Table 1).

In the first group of patients without drainage or shunt, the postoperative or intraoperative *mortality rate* was strikingly high: 58%. By contrast, mortality in patients with a C-VFD was 6%, in patients with an internal shunt 36%. The relatively high mortality rate of the 3rd group is due to the high proportion of inoperable brain stem lesions with a postoperative mortality rate of 57% (Mortality = fatal outcome during inpatient treatment).

Table 1. Posterior fossa tumours (children and juveniles)

Mode of treatment	No.	†	Intra-op. Early p. op. death	↑	Free of compl.	Complications: CSF fistula	CSF-infection/ sepsis	Post-op. intracran. hypoten.	Tumour haemorrh.	Subdural hygroma (Haema-toma)	Collapse of ventricles	Miscell. complic.
No drainage/ no shunt	19	11 (58%)	10 (53%)	8 (42%)	7 (88%)	1 (12%)	–	–	–	–	–	–
External drainage												
pre-op.	5	–	–	5	2	–	–	–	–	–	–	–
post-op.	9	–	–	9	8	–	–	–	–	–	–	–
peri-op.	19	2	1	17	14	2 (SH)	2	–	–	–	–	2
S	33	2 (6%)	1 (3%)	31 (94%)	24 (77%)	2 (6%)	2 (6%)	–	–	–	–	2 (7%)
Internal shunt [V-A/V-P]												
pre-op.	8	1	–	7	3	–	1	4	–	2+(1)	–	1
post-op.	11	3	–	8	3	1	3	2	–	2+(1)	3	1
Brain stem tumours	14	8	6	6	–	–	1	2	2	–	–	2
S	33	12 (36%)	6 (19%)	21 (64%)	6 (29%)	1 (5%)	5 (24%)	8 (38%)	2 (10%)	6 (29%)	3 (14%)	4 (19%)
Total	85	25 (29%)	17 (20%)	60 (71%)	37 (62%)	4 (7%)	7 (12%)	8 (13%)	2 (3%)	6 (10%)	3 (5%)	5 (8%)

Table 2. Prognosis of infratentorial tumours in children and juveniles without external drainage or without internal shunt system (group 1): Survivors; deaths "Sudden death" = term used by H. Cushing (1930/31). It means acute deterioration with fatal outcome in the early postoperative period

Site of tumour	Σ	↑	†	"Sudden death"
Hemisphere	6	5	1	(1)
(cyst. tu.)	(4)	(4)		
Vermis	7	2	5	(4)
4th Ventricle	3	1	2	(2)
Cereb.-pont. angle	1	–	1	(1)
Brain stem	2	–	2	(2)
Σ	19	8	11	(10)

10 out of 11 patients of the first group died in the early postoperative period of the first week, frequently after an acute respiratory paralysis, or even intraoperatively (4 patients) (Table 2).

In the first group 5 out of 6 patients with cystic brain tumours survived without complications, but only 2 of 7 patients with solid tumours of the vermis and only 1 of 3 patients with tumours in the fourth ventricle (Table 2). The few children with tumours in the cerebellopontine angle and in the brain stem who received no drainage all died postoperatively (Table 2).

Table 3. CSF-infection/sepsis

	No.	Infection (no. of pats.)	Pleocytosis (no. of pats.)	Duration of drainage (days)	
				$\bar{x}$	mx
External drainage					
pre-op.	5	–	2	2.8	4
post-op.	9	–	4	4.8	8
peri-op.	17	2	5	8.4	25
Total	31	2 (6%)	11 (35%)	6.7	25
Internal shunt				Manifestation (day post-op.)	
pre-op.	7	1	–	21	
post-op.	8	3	–	10, 13, 300	
brain stem	6	1	4	1	
Total	21	5 (24%)	4 (19%)		

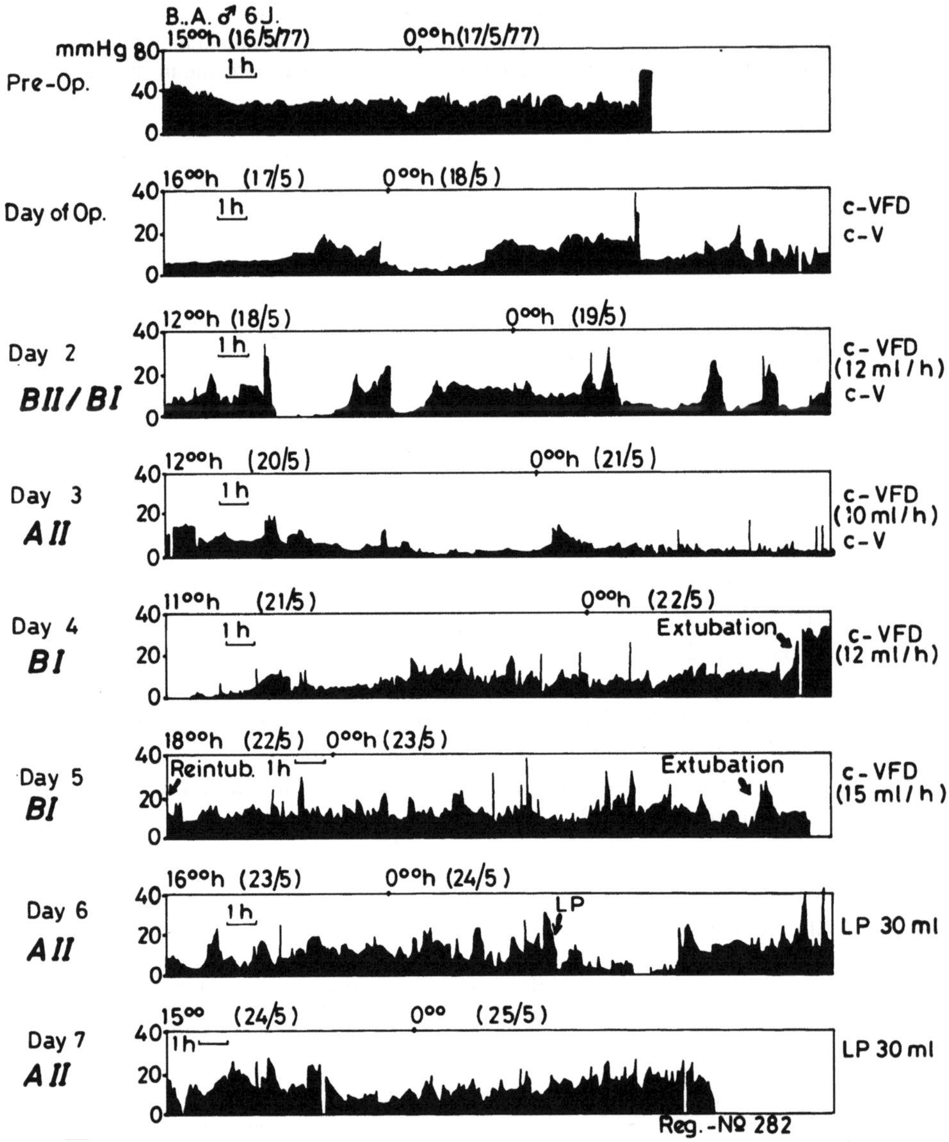

Fig. 1. Typical pre- and postoperative behaviour of ventricular fluid pressure (VFP) in a 6-year-old boy with an astrocytoma of the cerebellar hemisphere. Under continuous pressure-controlled ventricular fluid drainage (C-VFD) and continuous ventilation (C-V) fluctuating values of VFP in the normal range. Immediately after extubation steep pressure increase to pathological level (day 4). On day 6 stopping of C-VFD. After lumbar puncture VFP drops to low values for 3 to 4 hours

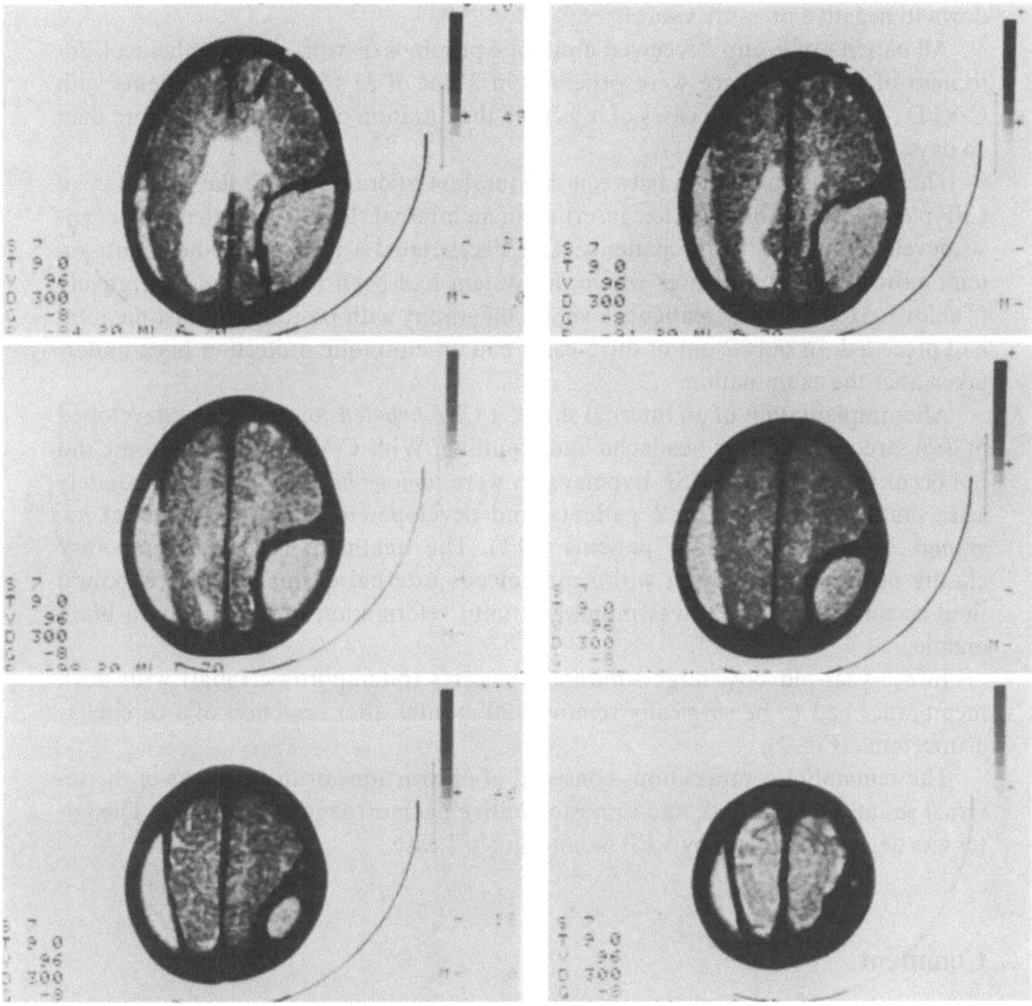

Fig. 2. Computer tomogram of the skull in a 3-year-old boy with bilateral supratentorial empyemas in the subdural space. Diagnosis 20 months after resection of a cerebellar astrocytoma

Continuous VFP monitoring showed acute pressure *increases* both preoperatively, during induction of anaesthesia, and in the early postoperative period of the first week, if C-VFD was interrupted, especially in cases with difficulties in respiration (Fig. 1).

In one patient, there were also long periods of B-waves after implantation of a ventriculo-atrial shunt system, which pointed to a malfunction of the system.

With C-VFD the postoperative course was more frequently free of *complications* than in patients with an internal shunt (Table 1). Two of the externally drained patients developed a *CSF-fistula* in the area of operation; therefore the insertion of an internal shunt was necessary. A fistula which continued in spite of the internal shunt only closed after lumbar drainage for several days with drastic lowering of VFP down to negative pressure values.

All patients of group 2 received antibiotic prophylaxis with chloramphenicol. *Infections* of the CSF space were observed in 2 out of 31 (6%) of the patients with C-VFD (Table 3). In both cases of infection, the duration of drainage was more than 14 days.

There was also a relation between the duration of drainage and the frequency of CSF pleocytosis (Table 3). After insertion of an internal shunt, CSF infection or sepsis developed in 24% of the patients. This necessitated a removal of the shunt system, most frequently in cases where the system had been inserted postoperatively (Tables 1, 3). In all these patients a ventriculography with positive contrast medium had preceded. In only 2 out of the 5 cases had an antibiotic protection been undertaken after the examination.

After implantation of an internal shunt, a *CSF hypotension* syndrome developed in 38%, accompanied by headache and vomiting. With C-VFD, this syndrome did not occur. The effects of CSF hypotension were *tumour haemorrhages* immediately after shunt implantation in 2 patients, and development of uni- or bilateral *hygromas* or *haematomas* in 6 patients (29%). The treatment used was temporary closure of the internal shunt with simultaneous external drainage of the subdural fluid accumulations. VFP was monitored until reformation of the collapsed brain mantle.

In a 3-year-old boy, large subdural abscesses (bitemporo-occipital) with thick membranes had to be surgically removed 20 months after resection of a cerebellar astrocytoma (Fig. 2).

The remaining complications consisted of obstructions or dislocations of the internal shunts in 4 patients, and in postoperative haemorrhage in 2 patients. The latter was detected early on by VFP monitoring in 1 case.

Comment

There is basic agreement in the modern literature that an infratentorial space-occupying lesion should not be operated on without preliminary reduction of an elevated VFP and that postoperative VFP-increases as a result of CSF absorption disturbances have to be prevented. For this purpose selected methods of a temporary C-VFD or internal shunts each have their specific advantages, and also their risks which should not be overlooked.

The *temporary C-VFD* offers the possibility of continuous perioperative VFP monitoring [11–13]. An obstruction of the drainage system can be detected early on by the increase in intracranial pressure. After normalization of the CSF circulation the C-VFD could generally be removed between the 3rd and the 7th postoperative day [12, 13].

This method bears a risk of infection between 2 and 10% [8, 9, 11, 12, 15, 16, 18]. Complications such as 'upward herniation' [6, 10] or tumour bleedings [17] as a result of an abrupt lowering of the VFP are probably avoidable by C-VFP. This occurred in 2 patients after insertion of an internal shunt.

The *internal shunt* has the advantage of a quick mobilization of the patient. Specific dangers include the CSF hypotension syndrome [4, 10] with collapse of ventricles and development of subdural hygromas or subdural haematomas [10], which have to be operated on. None of the systems used nowadays affords sufficient protection against this complication [4], which amounts to 8% in Raimondi's large material [10]. As a cause of the high infection rate in our patients with internal shunts for all of these the preceding ventriculography with positive contrast medium without sufficient antibiotic protection has to be discussed. The percentages given by other authors range from 2 to 11 % [1, 13], and are therefore no lower than in patients with C-VFD.

With such a low incidence of complications and with the possibility of simultaneous regulation of pressure, a C-VFD is therefore seen to be preferable. In the choice of the various drainage methods, the type and the position of the space-occupying lesion can be decisive. C-VFD is suitable for solid, removable lesions of the cerebellum and the vermis, requiring a period of drainage of no more than seven days. With cystic lesions, no postoperative drainage is generally required.

The indication for the implantation of an internal shunt system is given in the following cases: inoperable tumours of the brain stem with hydrocephalus; only partially removable tumours of the 4th ventricle and cerebello-pontine angle; rare cases of continued disturbance of CSF circulation after operations on tumours of the cerebellum or brain stem.

References

1. Abraham, J., Chandy, J.: Ventriculo-atrial shunt in the management of posterior fossa tumours. J. Neurosurg. *20,* 252–253 (1963)
2. Albright, L., Reigel, D. H.: Management of hydrocephalus secondary to posterior fossa tumours. J. Neurosurg. *46,* 52–55 (1977)
3. Böhm, B., Mohadjer, M., Hemmer, R.: Preoperative continous measurements of ventricular pressure in hydrocephalus occlusus with tumors of the posterior fossa: the value of ventricular-auricular shunt. Adv. Neurosurg. *5,* 194–198 (1978)
4. Gruss, P., Gaab, M., Knoblich, O. E.: Disorders of CSF-circulation after interventions in the area of the posterior cranial fossa with prior shunt operation. Advances in Neurosurg. *5,* 199–202 (1978)
5. Hekamatpanah, J., Mullan, S.: Ventricular caval shunt in the management of posterior fossa tumors. J. Neurosurg. *26,* 609–613 (1967)
6. Hoffman, H. J., Hendrick, E. B., Humphreys, R. P.: Metastasis via ventriculoperitoneal shunt in patients with medulloblastoma. J. Neurosurg. *44,* 562–566 (1976)
7. Kessler, L. A., Dugan, P., Concannon, J. P.: Systemic metastases of medulloblastoma promoted by shunting. Surg. Neurol. *3,* 147–152 (1975)
8. Lundberg, N., Kjällquist, A., Kullberg, G., Pontén, U., Sundbärg, G.: Non-operative management of intracranial hypertension. In: Advances and Technical Standards in Neurosurgery. Eds. H. Krayenbühl et al. (pp. 1–60) Wien, New York: Springer 1974
9. Pertuiset, B., Van Effenterre, R., Horn, Y.: Temporary external valve drainage in hydrocephalus with increased ventricular fluid pressure. Acta Neurochir. *33,* 173–181 (1976)
10. Raimondi, A. J., Tadaneri, T.: Hydrocephalus and infratentorial tumours. Incidence, clinical picture, and treatment. J. Neurosurg. *55,* 174–182 (1981)
11. Richard, K. E.: Liquorventrikeldruckmessung mit Mikrokatheter und druckkontrollierte externe Liquordrainage. Acta Neurochir. *38,* 73–87 (1977)
12. Richard, K. E.: Long-term measuring of ventricular fluid pressure with tumours of the posterior fossa. Adv. Neurosurg. *5,* 179–185 (1978)

13. Richard, K. E., Frowein, R. A., Vanner, G. K.: Ventricular fluid pressure in posterior fossa tumours of childhood. Mod. Probl. Paediat. *18*, 35–39 (1977)
14. Sayers, M. P.: Shunt complications. Clin. Neurosurg. *28*, 393–400 (1976)
15. Shalit, M. N., Ari, Y. B., Eynan, N.: The management of obstructive hydrocephalus by the use of external continuous ventricular drainage. Acta Neurochir. *47*, 161–172 (1979)
16. Smith, R. W., Alksne, J. F.: Infections complicating the use of external ventriculostomy. J. Neurosurg. *44*, 567–570 (1976)
17. Vaquero, J., Cabezudo, J. M., De Sola, R. G., Nombela, L.: Intratumoral hemorrhage in posterior fossa tumours after ventricular drainage. Report of two cases. J. Neurosurg. *55*, 390–396 (1981)
18. Wyler, A. R., Kelly, W. A.: Use of antibiotics with external ventriculostomies. J. Neurosurg. *37*, 185–187 (1972)

Indications and Experiences with the Ommaya-Reservoir for Treatment of CNS Neoplasms in Childhood

K. Roosen, W. Havers, and J. Schaaf

The following case history demonstrates in an exemplary manner the advantages and disadvantages of the CSF-reservoir system published by Ommaya in 1963 [8]:

In 1974, an 11-year-old girl, suffering from acute lymphatic leukaemia (ALL), developed a symptomatic, non-resorptive, communicating hydrocephalus. A ventriculo-atrial CSF-drainage-system (PHD) had to be inserted. During the following 36 months 13 recurrences of the leukaemic meningiosis were treated with Methotrexate and Cytosinarabinoside, administered intrathecally. The cytostatic drugs were injected into the frontal subcutaneous pump-device of the PHD.

After 86 punctures an infection with Staphylococcus epidermidis occurred. After treatment of the bacterial meningitis implantation of a contralateral Ommaya-System (O.S.). Because of left-sided focal Jacksonian epilepsy the position of the Ommaya device was corrected. Until the child's death 11 months later intrathecal cytostatic therapy with a total of 59 punctures was well tolerated without any complications.

By now 11 children aged from 2 to 11 years, have been treated in a similar way for different diseases of the CNS (Table 1):

Table 1. Diseases (n = 11)

Meningiosis	
Acute lymphatic leukaemia (ALL)	4
Non-Hodgkin's lymphoma (NHL)	3
Acute myeloid leukaemia (AML)	1
CNS tumours	
Craniopharyngioma	1
Cystic spongioblastoma	1
Reticular sarcoma	1

Eight patients were suffering from a leukaemic meningiosis. On three occasions an Ommaya-device was implanted for drainage of recurring, expanding tumour-cysts after previous operations on intracranial tumours.

Following Bleyer et al. [2], Galicich and Guido [5], Goedhart [6] und Spiers [13] the right frontal position of the reservoir is preferred. As shown in Fig. 1 a semicircular incision with its base facing medially is used; by interruption of afferent sensory fibres nearly painless punctures in the partly or completely analgesic skin flap become possible. The burr-hole is situated in the typical parasagittal, precoronal site. The correct intraventricular position of the cannula tip is always checked intraoperatively by fluoroscopy after injection of contrast medium into the reservoir.

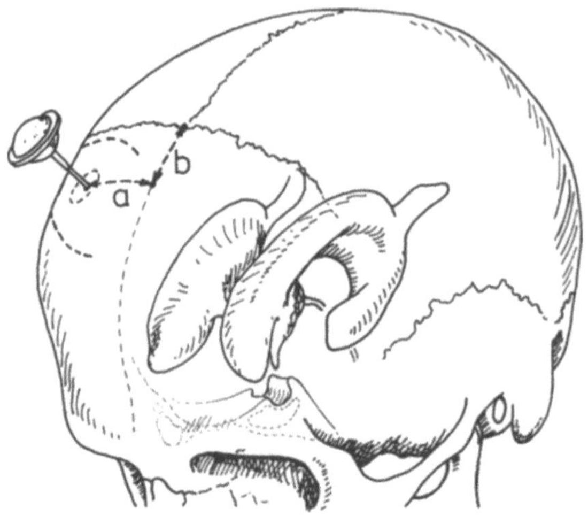

Fig. 1. AP-view of Ommaya reservoir system to be implanted

The time of insertion varied: in the case of four children it was done after the first manifestation of the meningiosis but with the other children after the second or third recurrence. In the three cases of CNS neoplasms the recurred tumours with expanding cysts were regarded as inoperable; the time interval between the first surgical intervention and the recurrence varied between 5 months and 2½ years.

Figs. 2a and b demonstrate the frequency of reservoir punctures per patient; in Fig. 2a in relation to the primary disease. In cases of leukaemia (ALL + AML = acute lymphatic and acute myeloid leukaemia; NHL = Non-Hodgkin-Lymphoma) diagnostic and therapeutic CSF punctures were distinguished. In the latter case, ventricular CSF was always taken out of the reservoir before giving the cytostatic drug, in order to control the therapeutic effect. The number of punctures ranged from 2 to 86 per subcutaneous silastic reservoir.

The number of CSF punctures after insertion of the O.S. until the end of life is shown in Fig. 2b. The low frequency of two and five punctures in the cases of leukaemic meningiosis is to be accounted for the complications of a haemorrhage and a bacterial sepsis, that will be explained later. In another case, in which the O.S. was used only seven times, the parents asked that any therapy should be stopped because of the fatal prognosis of the disease. Reservoirs with drainage function were

Table 2. Complications (4 patients)

Insertion	
Focal fits	1
Intracerebral haemorrhage	1
CSF fistula	1
Misplacement of catheter	1
Use	
Infections (Staph. epid. and aureus)	2

evacuated only in accordance with clinical symptoms of raised intracranial pressure and enlargement of tumour cysts, demonstrated in the CT-scan.

Besides the two complications mentioned above – Jacksonian focal seizures (because of incorrect operative technique) and inoculation of Staphylococcus epidermidis after three years treatment in our first patient – a seven-year-old boy, suffering from AML with a manifest meningiosis, developed a clinically silent haemorrhage in the right frontal lobe. At the time of surgical intervention plasmatic and

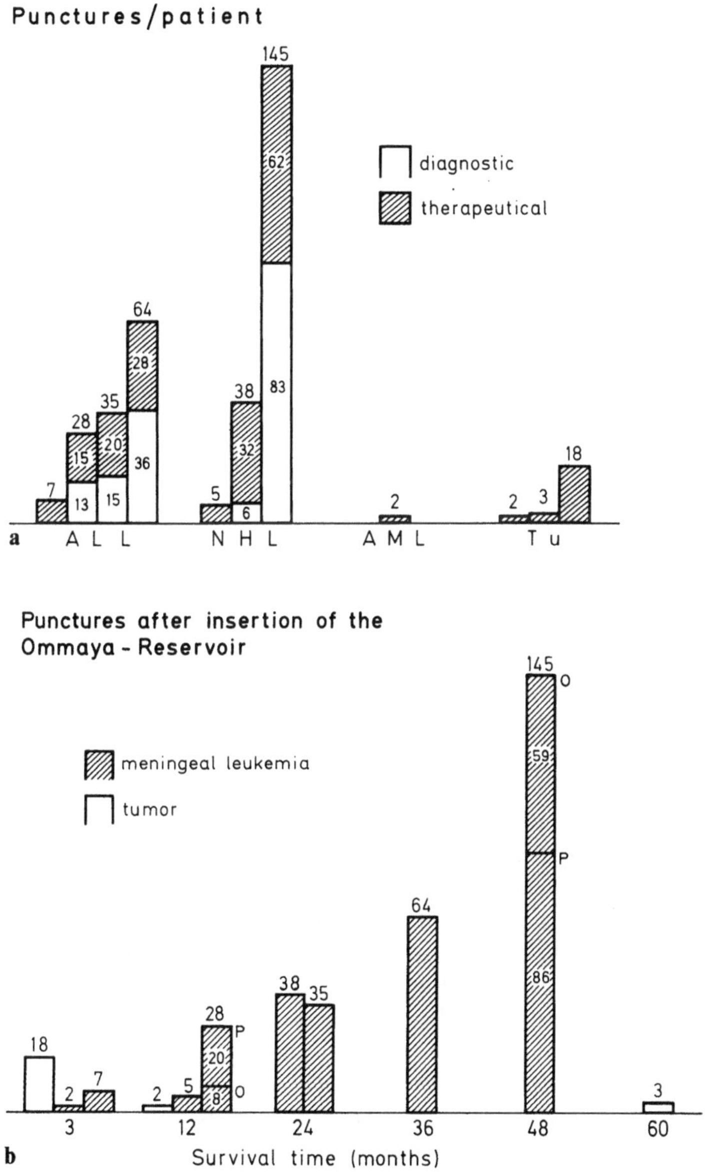

Fig. 2. a Use of the Ommaya system in treatment of leukaemic and tumours CNS diseases. **b** Number of punctures and survival-time after insertion of the O.S. *O* Ommaya system; *P* pump of PHD

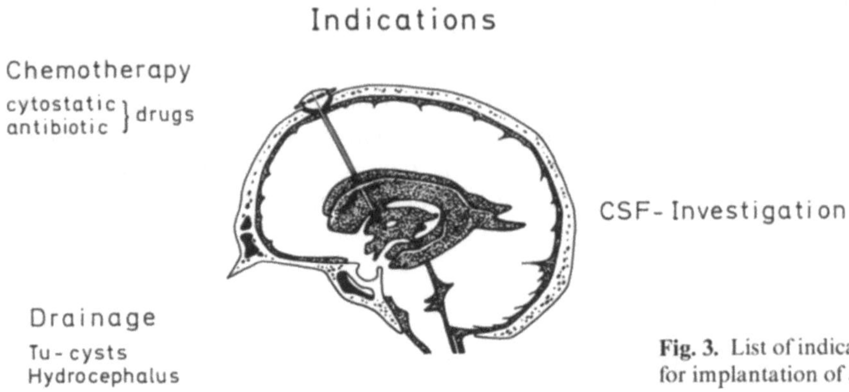

Fig. 3. List of indications for implantation of an O. S.

corpuscular coagulation were intact. The CT-scan was initiated three days after insertion of the O. S., because blood-clots were recovered when trying to obtain ventricular CSF through the reservoir. Ten days later the patient died with the symptoms of an acute recurrent haemorrhage; the AML had proved to be resistant to systemic therapy. Whether the bleeding was caused by leukaemic meningiosis or by the surgical procedure is not clear.

The CSF fistula developed 20 days after implantation. An attempt to close the fistula and the wound failed. In consequence of the massive CSF-production a ventricular-atrial-anastomosis was inserted three weeks later, which made it possible to continue intraventricular cytostatic treatment without any complications for another year. The cause of this avoidable complication was too large a dural and arachnoidal incision; furthermore the skin-flap was too small and produced too much tension on the edges of the wound.

After two intraventricular doses of methotrexate the expected recovery of the NHL-meningiosis in a ten-year-old girl failed to appear. An X-ray two months later showed the tip of the cannula to be misplaced in the midline fissure. After changing the O. S. and correcting the position of the drain and after three cytostatic injections, a Staphylococcus aureus infection developed 16 days later with clinical signs of meningitis. The Ommaya-device was removed and the infection was cleared up. We try to avoid such incidents by means of intraoperative fluoroscopy and particular attention to sterile conditions during the use of the device.

The necrotizing methotrexate-leucencephalopathy, mentioned in the literature [2, 9, 11, 13] was not seen by us, although all children after skull radiation with 1800 to 2500 rad were treated with MTX for the following nine months to three years.

Summarizing the information from the Anglo-American literature and our own experiences based on the 11 patients described above, one child with ventriculitis, and in 12 adults with haematological diseases and CNS neoplasms – the following possible indications for the use of an O. S. can be listed (Fig. 3).

The O. S. permits an easy, nearly painless and safe repeated withdrawal of CSF and administration of chemotherapeutic drugs [1, 2, 3, 5, 9, 10–13]. Water-soluble contrast media or isotopes can be injected if necessary for diagnostic reasons [2, 6, 7, 9]. Relief of expanding cysts [4, 6, 7, 8, 9] and local treatment of bacterial and fungal ventricular infections are possible [3]. The complication rates described vary between 10 and 50 per cent. With attention to the technical problems and under strict indications it can be brought down to 10 per cent [2, 7, 12].

The majority of the O.S. inserted by us, were implanted at a time when leukaemic meningiosis was noticed more often and could only be efficiently influenced by intraventricular administration of cytostatic drugs [1, 10–13]. Because of the more aggressive character of today's systemic chemotherapy it is seen less frequently. If a recurrent meningiosis develops in spite of or during systemic therapy, the advantages of the O.S. should be considered in the programme of treatment, especially in childhood, since in accordance with our experiences, the childrens' quality of life can be considerably improved by avoiding repeated painful lumbar or cisternal punctures.

References

1. Blasberg, R. G., Patlak, C. S., Shapiro, W. R.: Distribution of methotrexate in the cerebrospinal fluid and brain after intraventricular administration. Cancer Treat. Rep. *61,* 633–641 (1977)
2. Bleyer, W. A., Pizzo, Ph. A., Spence, A. M., Platt, W. D., Benjamin, D. R., Kolins, J., Poplack, D. G.: The Ommaya-Reservoir. Newly recognized complications and recommendations for insertion and use. Cancer *41,* 2431–2437 (1978)
3. Diamond, R. D., Bennett, J. E.: A Subcutaneous reservoir for intrathecal therapy of fungal meningitis. New Engl. J. Med. *288,* 186–188 (1973)
4. Fox, J. L.: Intermittent drainage of intracranial cyst via the subcutaneous Ommaya reservoir. J. Neurosurg. *27,* 272–273 (1967)
5. Galicich, J. H., Guido, L. J.: Ommaya device in carcinomatous and leukemic meningitis. Surg. Clin. North Am. *54,* 915–922 (1974)
6. Goedhart, Z. D.: Het Ommaya system. Ph. D. Thesis. Leiden (1978)
7. Goedhart, Z. D., Hekster, R. E. M., Matricali, B.: Neurosurgical and neurological applications of the Ommaya reservoir system. Adv. Neurosurg. *6,* 45–47 (1978)
8. Ommaya, A. K.: Subcutaneous reservoir and pump for sterile access to ventricular cerebrospinal fluid. Lancet *2,* 983–984 (1963)
9. Ratcheson, R. A., Ommaya, A. K.: Experience with the subcutaneous CSF reservoir. New Engl. J. Med. *279,* 1025–1031 (1968)
10. Shapiro. W. R., Young, D. F., Mehta, B. M.: Methotrexate: Distribution in cerebrospinal fluid after intravenous, ventricular and lumbar injections. N. Engl. J. Med. *293,* 161–166 (1975)
11. Shapiro, W. R., Posner, J. B., Ushio, Y., Chernik, N. L., Young, D. F.: Treatment of meningeal neoplasms. Cancer Treatm. Rep. *61,* 733–743 (1977)
12. Spiers, A. S. D., Firth, J. L.: Treating the nervous system in acute leukaemia. Lancet *1,* 433 (1972)
13. Spiers, A. S. D.: Chemotherapy of acute leukaemia. Clin. Haematology *2,* 127–164 (1972)

Indications for the Trans-Sphenoidal Approach to Craniopharyngioma Operations in Youth and Childhood

E. HALVES and N. SÖRENSEN

Despite the significant progress which has been made in the field of radiological diagnosis, of improvement in operating technique, and, in the treatment with hormone substitution of children suffering from craniopharyngioma, even very experienced neurosurgeons have failed, so far, to reduce the rate of recurrence to below 25%, although the attempt was made to remove the tumour entirely [8, 9, 10, 11, 14, 15]. As tumours usually develop in a widespread way in the extrasellar area, the classical subfrontal approach has been modified in diverse ways [14, 15, 19]. This approach has been developed in order to ensure that the entire tumour can be removed from the surrounding neurovascular structures.

Despite the above-mentioned measures, because of the anatomical structures of the base of the skull and the basal sectors of the brain blind spots remain, which make a direct view impossible. The same applies to the floor and walls of a grossly enlarged sella which has been found to be present in a relatively large number of the cases examined [15]. The trans-sphenoidal approach offers potentially the most effective conditions for ensuring that the entire mass of craniopharyngioma tissue is removed from this area.

As we achieved good results with this approach when dealing with pituitary adenomas of the same size, using the endoscopic operation technique [2], we started operating in craniopharyngiomas in this way in February 1977 [3, 4]. Since then we have operated on seven children and a youth suffering from craniopharyngioma, by the transnasal approach.

We operated on our first patient in a two-stage operation (primarily transnasal). We left, though, at this point some tumour tissue in the frontal sinus cavernosus angle, which we would now in the light of our further experience, try to remove. Thanks to a second operation 2½ years later and postoperative irradiation, there has not been a clinical or a radiological relapse, up to the present date (a further two years).

The solid portion of another patient's tumour caused the sella to widen slightly and later a large supra-sellar cyst formed. This cyst continued to refill over a period of a few months, despite three subfrontal operations. Not until craniopharyngioma tissue, surrounded by bone, had been removed from the floor of the sella and from the sphenoid sinus by a transnasal operation, did the patient remain free of symptoms (period of observation 4½ years).

The attempt to arrest the course of the illness by extirpation of the solid basal part of the tumour in another child, a girl had proved to be in vain previously. She had already undergone, four years earlier, two subfrontal operations on a large cystic craniopharyngioma. In the space of two years another two large cysts had formed.

We also intended operating by the two-stage primary transnasal approach on a tumour, whose solid intrasphenoidal part was clearly larger. As unexpectedly the cyst, which reached far into the supra-sellar area, came easily away, it was entirely removed with the help of an endoscope. A subfrontal extirpation would possibly have avoided the eye muscle impairment, which is still apparent as a fusion weakness today, 2½ years later.

In the case of the transnasal operations on three further patients with intrasellar-intrasphenoidal tumour growth no problems arose (periods of observation: 1, 3, and 4 years, respectively).

Only one of these seven patients with intrasphenoidal tumour has not had to undergo hormonal replacement treatment. In none of these patients is the vision severely limited; they have developed well, psychologically and intellectually.

We took mainly the computerized tomography and the lateral X-ray as the basis for our decision, as to which approach to choose. Craniopharyngiomas with little or no intrasellar component, are operated on primarily by the subfrontal approach. When a greater enlargement of the sella is diagnosed and a complete removal of the tumour is uncertain or impossible, the next step taken is the transnasal exploration. Purely intrasellar-intrasphenoidal tumours and others with a large proportion within these structures are operated exclusively or primarily transnasally.

When primarily subfrontal operated craniopharyngiomas recur the basal part of the tumour can easily be reached; however, only exceptionally can a radical operation be accomplished transnasally.

Undoubtedly the operation-microscope and endoscope offers the best possible and safest means of identifying and extirpating craniopharyngioma tissue.

It is obvious that the contents of a widened sella cannot be seen with the help of a microscope by the subfrontal approach because of the anatomical structure of the base of the skull. This was the reason why we chose the transnasal approach for this stage. It also offered a safe exposure of the medial walls of the cavernous sinus, of the floor of the sella and of the bony structures of the sphenoid. It also enables a better separation of the portions of the pituitary gland still remaining, and of its stalk from the tumour, or – if all goes well – its preservation [15].

Contrary to a pituitary adenoma with suprasellar or retrosellar extension, tissue cannot be extirpated transnasally from these areas without greater risk in the case of a craniopharyngioma. As the subfrontal approach does not offer an unlimited vision there is either the possibility of operating without visual control or through the corpus callosum or the 3rd ventricle.

When a transnasal operation takes place, one should ensure a generous removal of the bone within the sphenoid basally and laterally. In doing so one can ensure that the tumour can be safely removed, from the bony structures and also from the walls of the cavernous sinus with the aid of the microscope (and perhaps with an endoscope). However, if it is firmly adherent, to the carotid artery, extirpation is impossible; but tissue, which has infiltrated the cavernous sinus, can be reached from the subfrontal approach. When dissecting the upper layers of the tumour one should note carefully whether the diaphragma sellae is perforated. If the tumour has extended beyond this, the attempt to pull it downwards endangers the surrounding neuro-vascular structures. Parts of the tumour, which are encapsulated and have

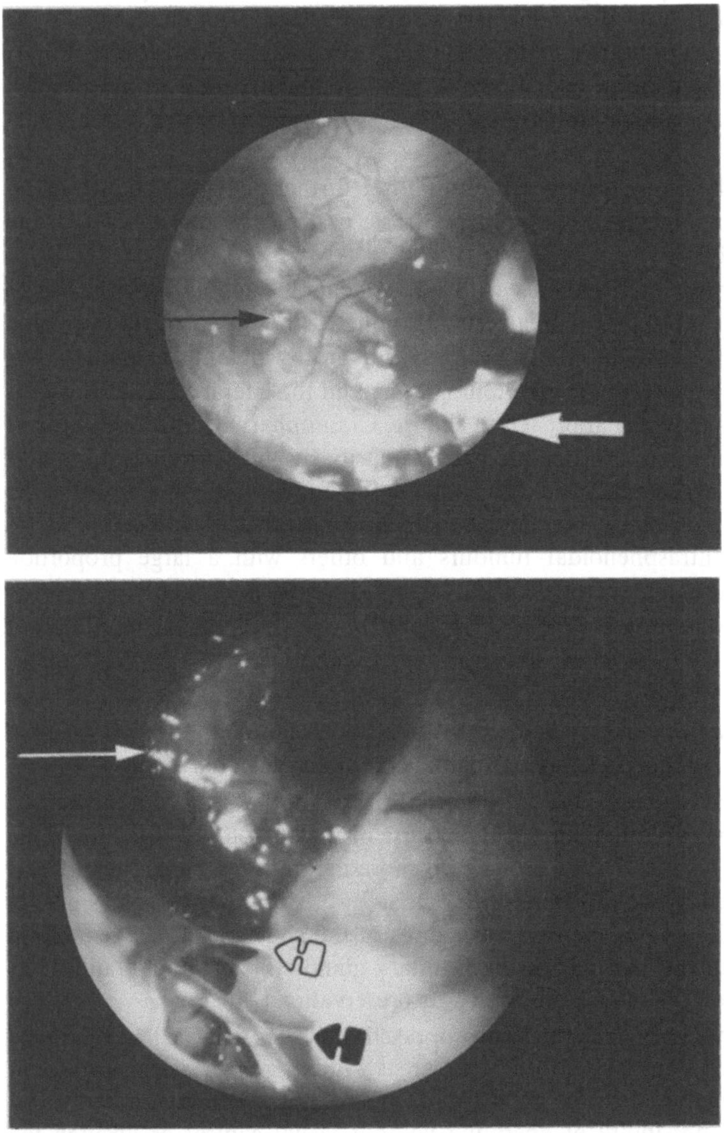

a

b

Fig. 1. Endoscopic photographs of the inner (**a**) and outer (**b**) layer of a cystic craniopharyngioma. Calcified tumour tissue (→), vascular (⏩) and fibrous (⇨) neurovascular adhesions with the tumour

scarcely spread beyond the sella, or of a thinwalled cyst, can – if necessary – be dissected and removed extracapsularly with the endoscope.

The opening of the arachnoid should be accepted as a calculated risk, as this step increases the degree of safety of extirpation; to close it is relatively simple.

The same applies to a tumour which has grown into the pituitary stalk or which originated there, where a subarachnoidal separation must take place.

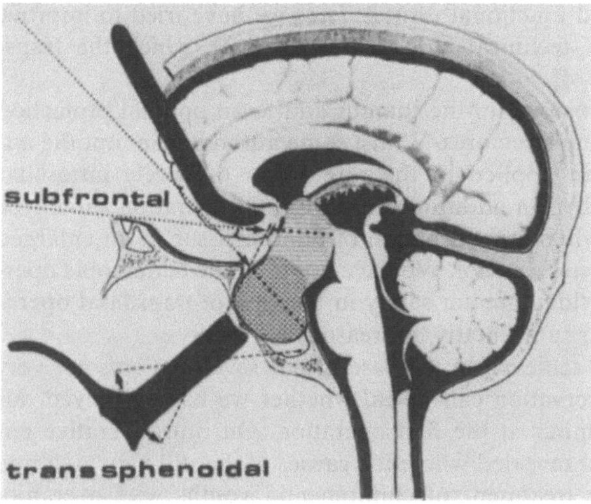

Fig. 2. Blind spots within the enlarged sella and in the suprasellar and retrosellar region (....) with the subfrontal approach. The trans-sphenoidal approach allows a wide look into the tumour (- - →) but excision should not exceed the dotted area without extratumoural visual control

Discussion

In numerous postoperative check-ups of children, who had undergone a craniopharyngioma operation, the attempt has repeatedly been made to reach a consensus, as to how this group of patients should be treated [1, 7, 9, 10, 14, 15, 16, 19]. Due to the special situation of the development in childhood and the possible rapid growth of these tumours in childhood and early youth [13, 16] it is of particular significance to develop appropriate treatment; this, however, involves many problems. The principal methods of treatment vary between a conservative partial removal [11] followed by postoperative radiotherapy [13] – and the general attempt to achieve a radical tumour removal [9, 10, 14, 17].

However, an examination of the cases treated reveals that the best results making use of modern diagnosis, operation techniques and pharmacological treatment [9, 10, 16] in the treatment of children and youth can be achieved in the long run, if every attempt has been made to remove the tumour totally at the time of the first operation. It is impossible even for highly experienced neurosurgeons to be certain during the operation that the attempt to remove the tumour totally has been successful [1, 12].

It is equally uncertain which cell structures of the tumour may cause a recurrence of growth [12, 14, 16]. Perhaps in the future computerized tomographical examinations of the growth of a tumour will be able to answer some of these questions. Experience has taught us that almost exclusively the first operation offers us the optimal chance to remove a craniopharyngioma totally [9, 10, 12, 14, 16, 19], and in so doing to achieve good functional results. Thus we have tried to improve this method by the use of all technical aids at our disposal, which the transsphenoidal approach offers [2, 3, 4].

This applies to the radical removal of the tumour and to an optimal protection of the function of the surrounding structures. Whilst some authors point out the advantage of this approach, when applied to the rarer form of purely intrasellar growth [5, 6, 7, 15], we think that, in addition the subfrontal operation should be followed by a transnasal one, when an extirpation of tumour tissue in an enlarged sella cannot take place under visual control. We have not used the endoscopic operative technique, which has provided greater safety in the case of transnasal operations, when exposing the tumour subfrontally, for reasons of sterility.

Even if the results we have achieved in the case of our seven patients are very favourable, only long term observation can reveal whether we have achieved our aim of removing the entire tumour at the first operation. Our intraoperative endoscopic check-ups have at least revealed where the causes of the still very high rate of recurrence in the operative treatment of children and youths with a craniopharyngioma could possibly lie.

References

1. Bartlett, J. R.: Craniopharyngiomas – a summary of 85 cases. J. Neurol. Neurosurg. Psychiat. *34,* 37–41 (1971)
2. Bushe, K.-A., Halves, E.: Modifizierte Technik bei transnasaler Operation der Hypophysengeschwülste. Acta Neurochir. (Wien) *41,* 163–175 (1978)
3. Halves, E., Bushe, K.-A.: Transsphenoidal operation on craniopharyngiomas with extrasellar extensions. Acta Neurochir. Suppl. *28/2,* 362 (1979)
4. Halves, E.: Die ergänzende transsphenoidale Operation bei Kraniopharyngiomen im Kindes- und Jugendalter. Neurochirurgia *23,* 71–79 (1980)
5. Hamberger, C. A., Hammer, G., Norlen, G., Sjögren, B.: Surgical treatment of craniopharyngioma. Acta oto-laryng. *52,* 285–292 (1960)
6. Hamer, J.: Removal of craniopharyngioma by subnasal-transsphenoidal operation. Neuropädiatrie *9,* 312–319 (1978)
7. Hardy, J., Vezina, J. L.: Transsphenoidal neurosurgery of intracranial neoplasma. Adv. Neurol. *15,* 261–273 (1976)
8. Hoff, J. T., Patterson jr. R. H.: Craniopharyngiomas in children and adults. J. Neurosurg. *36,* 299–302 (1972)
9. Hoffman, H. J., Hendrick, E. B., Humphreys, R. P., Buncie, J. R., Armstrong, D. L., Jenkin, R. D. T.: Management of craniopharyngioma in children. J. Neurosurg. *47,* 218–227 (1977)
10. Humphreys, R. P., Hoffman, H. J., Hendrick, E. B.: A long-term postoperative follow-up in craniopharyngioma. Child's Brain *5,* 530–539 (1979)
11. Kahn, E. A., Gosch, H. H., Seeger, J. F., Hicks, S. P.: Forty-five years experience with the craniopharyngiomas. Surg. Neurol. *1,* 5–12 (1973)
12. Katz, E. L.: Late results of radical excision of craniopharyngiomas in children. J. Neurosurg. *42,* 86–90 (1975)
13. Kramer, S.: Craniopharyngioma. The best treatment is conservative surgery and postoperative radiation therapy. In: Morley, Current controversies in neurosurgery: pp 336–343. Philadelphia: Saunders 1976
14. Matson, D. D., Crigler, J. F.: Management of craniopharyngioma in childhood. J. Neurosurg. *30,* 377–390 (1969)

15. Rougerie, J.: What can be expected from the surgical treatment of craniopharyngiomas in children. Child's Brain *5,* 433–449 (1979)
16. Shapiro, K., Till, K., Grant, D. N.: Craniopharyngiomas in childhood. J. Neurosurg. *50,* 617–623 (1979)
17. Shillito, J.: The treatment of craniopharyngiomas of childhood. In: Morley, Current controversies in neurosurgery. pp 332–335. Philadelphia: Saunders 1976
18. Svien, H. J.: Surgical experiences with craniopharyngiomas. J. Neurosurg. *23,* 148–155 (1965)
19. Sweet, W. H.: Radical surgical treatment of craniopharyngioma. Clin. Neurosurg. *23,* 52–79 (1976)

Which Considerations Determine the Choice Between the Subfrontal and Trans-Sphenoidal Approach to Tumours of the Sellar Region in Youth and Childhood?

W. ISCHEBECK, S. MÜLLER, and W. BRAUN

As tumours of the sellar region in infancy and youth we find mainly craniopharyngiomas, gliomas of the optic nerve and pituitary adenomas. Although computerized tomography (CT), more refined endocrinological laboratory studies and advanced microsurgical technique have already accomplished a lot, there are still many unsolved problems.

The hypothalamic crisis during or after an operation and the problem of incomplete removal i.e. recurrence of these tumours are the reasons that Olivecrona [4] found in his cases and in 1967 he still had a mortality of over 70%.

In connection with our subject we want to emphasize that there must be more tumours of the sellar region in youth than we can estimate on the basis of the small number of children we operate on. If we find those tumours during the early twenties often a normal development of puberty has not taken place in those patients. Therefore we want to put great emphasis on the possibility that in cases where normal puberty development has not occurred, this may well be caused by a tumour of the sellar region.

There are mainly three ways of operating on those tumours:

1) the subfrontal approach,
2) the trans-sphenoidal approach,
3) a combination of both.

We need not point out that nowadays CT gives us the best possibility of diagnosing sellar tumours from the topographical point of view. If the tumour growth is largely parasellar and/or retrosellar we should choose the subfrontal route. With this type of approach we can see the optic nerves with the frontal part of the chiasm and the carotid arteries. A lesion of the frontal lobe and the olfactory nerves can mostly not be avoided. Most dangerous is the fact that we cannot see the border between tumour and the hypothalamic region which can cause great danger. The slightest irritation of the hypothalamus can be irreparable. The conflict between total removal of a tumour and these problems very often cannot be solved.

The indication for using the transnasal-trans-sphenoidal route in our opinion is the growth of tumour in the sella itself and in the suprasellar region. The angle by which we approach the sella is of great importance. We thus have the chance to extirpate under direct vision the tumour itself and even calcified structures which are in intimate relation with the hypothalamus. We therefore think that the transethmoidal approach has no advantage.

As an example we wish to mention the case of a young woman in her early twenties who had had amenorrhoea from her thirteenth year onwards. We found a craniopharyngioma with a calcified capsule which could be removed during the operation using the trans-sphenoidal route. The CT showed no recurrence after two years and a diabetes insipidus stopped after a few months.

Even with children we prefer the incision right through the nose instead of the sublabial incision. Then we follow the transseptal-trans-sphenoidal approach. The nose is so extensible that the view is wide enough through the speculum. The supporting structures of the nose have to be kept intact because the growth of the nose should not be disturbed. Postoperatively the children feel better because the lips are not swollen and there is no sublabial wound.

Very often an urgent indication for the operation on these tumours is advanced visual disturbance. Again and again the patients are coming late because they tolerate them so long.

It is nearly always possible to free the optic nerves from pressure with the aid of this operation. If we do not succeed, contrary to our expectation with the total removal of the tumour using the trans-sphenoidal approach, we have the great advantage that a newly developing cyst can be punctured under X-ray control, because the route to the sella has already been opened up.

As an example: we operated on an eight-year-old boy with a cystic craniopharyngioma with very severe visual disturbances. After the trans-sphenoidal operation the vision and the visual fields became normal in a short time. The CT-control showed a normal situation. Seven months later he was again admitted with visual disturbances. We punctured the newly developed cyst with good result. Later we were able to perform the subfrontal operation with less danger because the hypothalamus was not under pressure.

The trans-sphenoidal approach gives us the possibility of complete removal of tumour of the sellar region. Naturally recurrence cannot always be avoided, but the same is true for the subfrontal approach. If there is no chance from the beginning to remove the tumour completely through the trans-sphenoidal route we perform the subfrontal operation. If possible we do not want to submit patients especially children to a second operation.

Although there is the danger of rhinorrhoea and inflammation, we think that the transnasal-trans-sphenoidal approach can be a great advantage in the surgical treatment of sellar tumours. We see no indication for performing the two approaches in one operation at the same time.

References

1. Ganzer, U., Ischebeck, W.: Der transseptale-transsphenoidale Zugang bei der Hypophysektomie – eine gemeinsame Aufgabe des Otologen und Neurochirurgen. Laryng. Rhinol. *58*, 795–800 (1979)
2. Guiot, G.: Considerations on the surgical treatment of pituitary adenomas. In: Treatment of pituitary adenomas (Fahlbusch, R., Werder, K. v., eds.) p. 202–218 . Stuttgart: G. Thieme 1878
3. Landolt, A. M., Strebel, P.: Technique of transsphenoidal operation for pituitary adenomas. In: Advances and Technical Standards in Neurosurgery Vol. *7*, 119–177 (Krayenbühl, H., ed.). Wien, New York: Springer 1980
4. Olivecrona, H.: The surgical treatment of intracranial tumours. In: Handbuch der Neurochirurgie Vol. IV/4, p. 277–301. Berlin, Göttingen, Heidelberg: Springer 1967

The Influence of Different Antihypertensive Drugs on Intracranial Pressure

J. HIDDING, C. PUCHSTEIN, and H. VAN AKEN

Introduction

The methods for inducing a systemic reduction of blood pressure, of establishing a bloodless surgical field, and optimal conditions for neurosurgery were described as early as 1917 by H. W. Cushing [4]. New techniques permitted one to reduce significantly the duration of the procedure, the operative blood loss, and the resulting morbidity and mortality rates.

Blood pressure may be reduced by chemical agents with either direct or indirect influence on the vascular wall. In neurosurgery special care is necessary to avoid pressure peaks in patients with space-occupying intracranial lesions, and during the surgical approach to intracranial aneurysms. Disturbances of the autoregulation of cerebral blood supply are apt to impair severely both normal and damaged cerebral tissue [8, 10]. Under elevated arterial pressure, failure of the blood-brain barrier may result in focal loss of plasma from the vessels with subsequent cerebral oedema [15, 17]. It appears worth while to correlate the sequelae of systemic pressure reduction with regard to possible alterations of intracranial pressure. In our study, intracranial pressure changes were recorded under antihypertensive medication with Hydralazine and Labetalol, respectively.

Materials and Methods

Animals: 2 groups of 6 mongrel dogs, body weight 27–33 kg
Premedication: Thalamonal 0.15 ml/kg b.w.
Initial sedation: Piritramide 1 mg/kg, Pancuronium bromide 0.1 mg/kg b.w.
Maintenance of narcosis: Piritramide 0.5 mg/kg, Pancuronium bromide 0.06 mg/kg b.w.

Ventilation by tracheal intubation with 30% O_2, 70% nitrous oxide. Hyperventilation by constant pCO_2 of 28–30 mm Hg. Blood pressure was measured within the femoral artery, intracranial pressure was measured through a burrhole and catheter introduced into the lateral ventricle. Cardiac output was measured by thermodilution with a SWAN-Ganz catheter.
Administration of tested drugs: Hydralazine 0.5 mg/kg i.v. Labetalol bolus of 100 mg, subsequent infusions to a maximum of 600 mg.

Results

Sedation was stabilized for 30 minutes before the intravenous administration of Hydralazine (0.5 mg/kg). Heart rate (HF), blood pressure (BP), cardiac output (CO) and intracranial pressure (ICP) were continuously monitored. The maximum alterations of these four values are shown on Table 1. We noted a slight increase of heart rate and cardiac output, while blood pressure values decreased by approximately 15%. There is a remarkable rise of intracranial pressure after Hydralazine, which attains its maximum 10 minutes after the injection.

Labetalol was administered to the second group of dogs in a bolus of 100 mg per animal. Fig. 1 shows that the immediate result is a reduction of blood pressure by 15%. A reduction of mean pressure values by 30% was recorded after 300–400 mg Labetalol, but higher doses were ineffective in producing stronger reductions. Intra-

Table 1. Effect of Hydralazine on haemodynamics and on intracranial pressure (ICP) in dogs. (no=6, $\bar{M} \pm S_D$)

HF	77 ± 9	86 ± 8	$p<0.002$
BP	133 ±26 syst.	115 ±19	$p<0.01$
	74 ±11 diast.	65 ± 8	$p<0.01$
CO	5.9 ± 0.6 l/min	7.2 ± 0.6	$p<0.001$
ICP	11,67± 1.21 mm Hg	23.67± 1.21	$p<0.001$

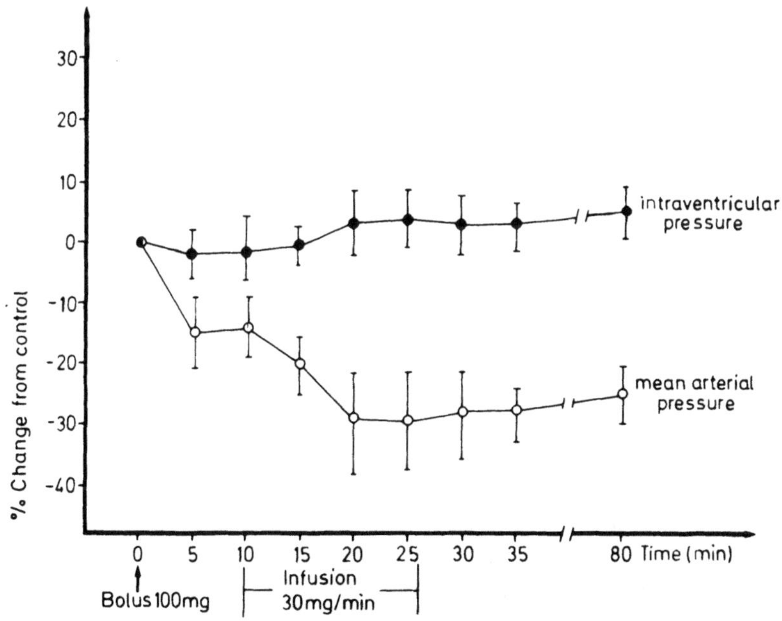

Fig. 1. Effect of Labetalol on intracranial pressure and on mean arterial pressure. Labetalol was given as bolus of 100 mg, then as infusion of 30 mg per minute to a total of 600 mg. (Values are mean v., ±SEM, n=6)

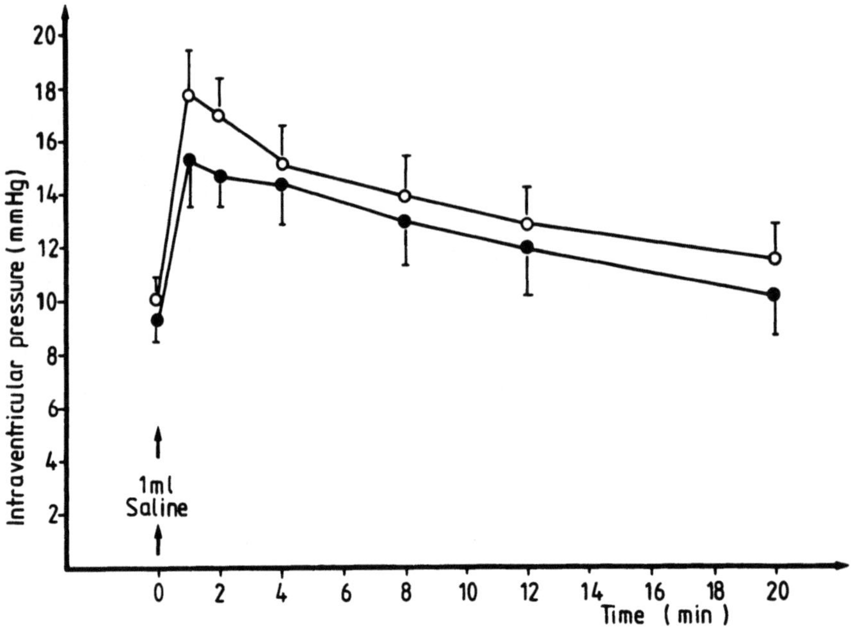

Fig. 2. Effect of Labetalol on intracranial compliance in anaesthesized dogs. Ventricular pressure response before and after Labetalol infusion. (Values are mean v., ±SEM, n=6)

cranial pressure remained largely constant throughout the entire period of observation.

Figure 2 shows a comparison of intracranial compliance, tested by injecting 1 ml saline into the ventricle. The ventricular pressure response showed no significant change before and after Labetalol.

Discussion

The controlled balance of vascular hypotension and cranial pressure is an important neurosurgical problem. Johnson [9] had been the first to introduce sodium nitroprusside as an antihypertensive drug in 1929. Moraca et al. [12] reported in 1962 about successfully controlled hypotension in neurosurgical operations. The immediate relaxation of the vascular musculature is liable to induce not only peripheral reduction of pressure, but also an increase in cerebral blood volume, rising intracranial pressure, and a deterioration of intracranial compliance [3, 18]. During the postoperative period uncontrolled hypotension was recorded as a rebound effect [2, 26].

Hydralazine was shown in our study to increase intracranial pressure severely during its antihypertensive action. This effect involves a considerable risk in the surgical approach to space-occupying intracranial lesions, i.e. it is apt to produce a deterioration in the pre-operative status of the patient. In a recent publication [5]

Hydralazine had been recommended for preventing hypertension during intubation. Referring to the results of other authors [11] and of our own study, the use of Dihydralazine is certainly contraindicated in neurosurgical patients with space-occupying intracranial lesions, or in the surgical treatment of intracranial aneurysms prior to opening the dura mater.

Labetalol, a combined alpha- and beta-blocker, is now available for rapid reduction of blood pressure by decreasing the peripheral vascular resistance (alpha blocking) and simultaneous prevention of reflex tachycardia (beta blocking) [1, 7, 14, 19]. It was introduced into clinical practice for the intraoperative control of hypertensive crises during the surgical approach to intracranial aneurysms [11].

Labetalol is in fact an anti-hypertensive drug capable of maintaining constant intracranial pressure under reduction of blood pressure by up to 30%. Intracranial compliance was equally unaffected by the influence of Labetalol. The drug was, however, ineffective in reducing blood pressure by more than 30%.

In the surgical management of patients with increased intracranial pressure the use of an antihypertensive drug without effect on intracranial pressure – such as Labetalol – is obviously recommended, especially prior to the surgical access to the dura mater. As soon as the dura is opened, controlled hypotension can be achieved by more potent anti-hypertensive drugs such as NNP, NTG or Hydralazine.

References

1. Brittain, R. T., Levy, G. P.: A review of the animal pharmacology of Labetalol, a combined alpha- and beta-adreno-receptor-blocking drug. Br. J. Clin. Pharmacol. *3,* 681–694 (1976)
2. Cottrell, J. E., Illner, P., Kittay, M. J., et al.: Rebound hypertension after sodium nitroprusside-induced hypotension. Clin. Pharmacol. Ther. (in press)
3. Cottrell, J. E., Patel, K., Ransohoff, I. R. et al.: Intracranial pressure changes induced by sodium-nitroprusside in patients with intracranial mass lesion. J. Neurosurg. *48,* 329–331 (1978)
4. Cushing, W. W.: Tumours of the nervus acusticus and the syndrome of the cerebello-pontine angle. Philadelphia: W. B. Sauders 1917
5. Davies, M. J., Cronin, K. D., Cowie, R. W.: The prevention of hypertension at intubation. Anesthesia *36,* 147–152 (1981)
6. Gupta, B., Cottrell, J. E., Rappaport, H. et al.: Nitroglycerine raises intracranial pressure. J. Neurosurg. (submitted)
7. Hansson, L., Hänel, B.: Labetalol, a new alpha- and beta-adrenoreceptor-blocking agent in hypertension. Br. J. Clin. Pharmacol. *3,* 763–764 (1976)
8. Huse, K.: Die kontrollierte Hypotension mit Nitroprussid-Natrium in der Neuroanaesthesie. Anaesth. Wieder-Belebung H. 107. Berlin, Heidelberg, New York: Springer 1977
9. Johnson, C. C.: The action and toxicity of sodium nitroprusside. Arch. intern. Pharmacodyn. *35,* 480 (1929)
10. Langfitt, T. W., Weinstein, J. D., Kassel, N. F.: Cerebral vasomotoric paralysis produced by intracranial hypertension. Neurology *15,* 761–765 (1965)
11. Lüben, V., Rieder, W., Zierski, G., Hempelmann, G.: Hämodynamische Untersuchung von Labetalol zur intraoperativen Therapie hypertoner Krisen in der Chirurgie zerebraler Aneurysman. Anaesth. Intensivther. Notfallmed. *16,* 184–187 (1981)
12. Moraca, P. P., Bitte, E. M., Hale, D. E., Wasmuth, C. E., Pontasse, E. F.: Clinical evaluation of sodium nitroprusside as a hypotensive agent. Anesthesiology *23,* 193 (1962)
13. Nickerson, M., Ruedy, J.: Antihypertension agents and the drug therapy of hypertension. In: Goodman, L. and Gilman: The Pharmacological Basis of Therapeutics, 5th Edition

14. Richards, D. A.: Pharmacological effects of Labetalol in man. Br. J. Clin. Pharmacol. *3*, 721–724 (1976)
15. Skinhoj, E., Strandgaard, S.: Pathogenesis of hypertensive encephalopathy. Lancet 1973/I, 461–463
16. Spring, A., Spring, G., Kirchner, E.: Postoperative Blutdruckreaktionen nach neurochirurgischen Operationen nach Hypotension. Anaesth. Intensivther. Notfallmed. *15*, 1–6 (1980)
17. Strandgaard, S., McKenzie, E. T., Sengupta, D.: Upper limit of autoregulation of cerebral blood flow in the baboon. Circ. Res. *34*, 435–440 (1974)
18. Turner, J. M., Powell, D., Gibson, R. M.: Intracranial pressure changes in neurosurgical patients during hypotension induced with sodium nitroprusside or trimetaphan. Br. J. Anaesth. *49*, 419–426 (1977)
19. Williams, L. D., Murphy, M. J., Parsons, V.: Labetalol in severe and resistant hypertension. Br. J. Clin. Pharmacol. *8*, 143–147 (1979)

Ventriculocisternostomy by the Method of Leksell – Indications, Technique, and Results

D. VOTH, K. SCHÜRMANN, and M. SCHWARZ

Introduction

Obstructive hydrocephalus is a frequent accompaniment of space-occupying lesions in the posterior fossa [6, 7, 8, 18]. The best treatment consists of relieving the acute pressure symptoms before the tumour operation, by means of a preliminary ventricular drainage, or by the insertion of a ventriculo-peritoneal or ventriculo-atrial shunt system. After the removal of the tumour the problem of interference with the fluid pathways can again develop, on account of a recurrence of the tumour or secondary aqueduct stenosis. In such cases a further operation is often necessary. Because of this we have adopted a drainage procedure which remains free of complications and spares the child any further operations, because in general it remains trouble-free. In addition it does not involve the risk of a dissemination of tumour cells through the blood stream or intraperitoneally, by means of the shunt. These requirements are met by using Leksell's technique of ventriculo-cisternostomy [1, 2, 14, 15, 17, 26].

Material and Methods

The use of the Leksell drainage requires opening of the posterior fossa, splitting of the vermis and a direct exposure of the posterior end of the aqueduct. In the cases described here this was almost always preceded by the complete extirpation or a maximal resection of the existing infratentorial tumour. The only exceptions were those cases with cysts or a membranous occlusion of the aqueduct. As a modification of the original technique we use the Portnoy flanged catheter [19]. This is passed through the aqueduct under direct vision using the microscope and its flanged portion is then placed in the anterior horn of the ventricle. No difficulties have been experienced in this atraumatic introduction of the catheter under direct vision. The distal end of the catheter is then inserted into the cervical subarachnoid space at the level of the second cervical vertebra. With this technique it is unnecessary to fix it in any way and we have not found that it has slipped in any case. In all cases the insertion of the catheter follows the extirpation of the tumour.

We have now used this modification of the Leksell drainage in twenty-five patients. Our material is made up as follows: Thirteen patients with medulloblastoma (nine boys, four girls), five with piloid astrocytoma (three boys, two girls), four with ependymoma (two boys, two girls) and also three patients with other conditions, including a mesencephalic cyst, an arachnoid cyst in the fourth ventricle and a membranous obstruction of the aqueduct.

At present the longest period of follow-up is almost six years. It has not been necessary to carry out any sort of revision in any patient.

Results

The use of this form of drainage does not present any significant difficulties, with a direct demonstration of the often dilated aqueduct under the microscope. The cath-

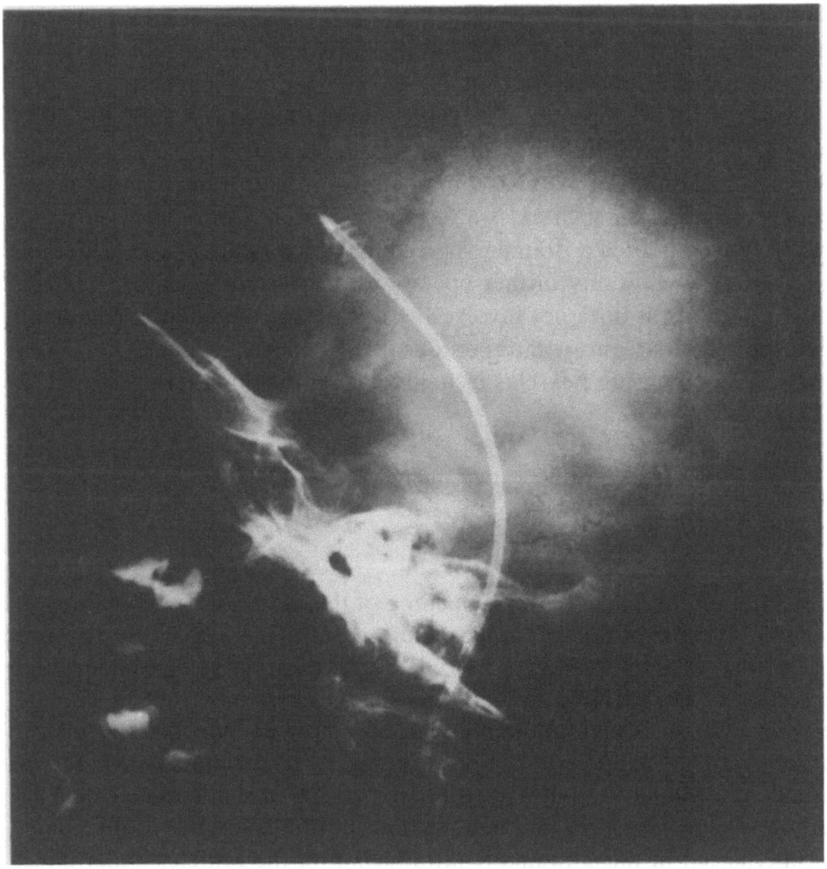

Fig. 1. The lateral radiograph shows the position of the drain and its course from the anterior horn of the ventricle to the cervical subarachnoid space

Fig. 2. Leksell-drainage in a four-year-old boy with a medulloblastoma, shown before the operation, and also the appearance at follow-up, six months after the operation. The CT scans show the course of the catheter above and below the tentorium. In the later CT controls the size of the ventricles has returned almost to normal, and this is associated, so far, with very satisfactory clinical progress

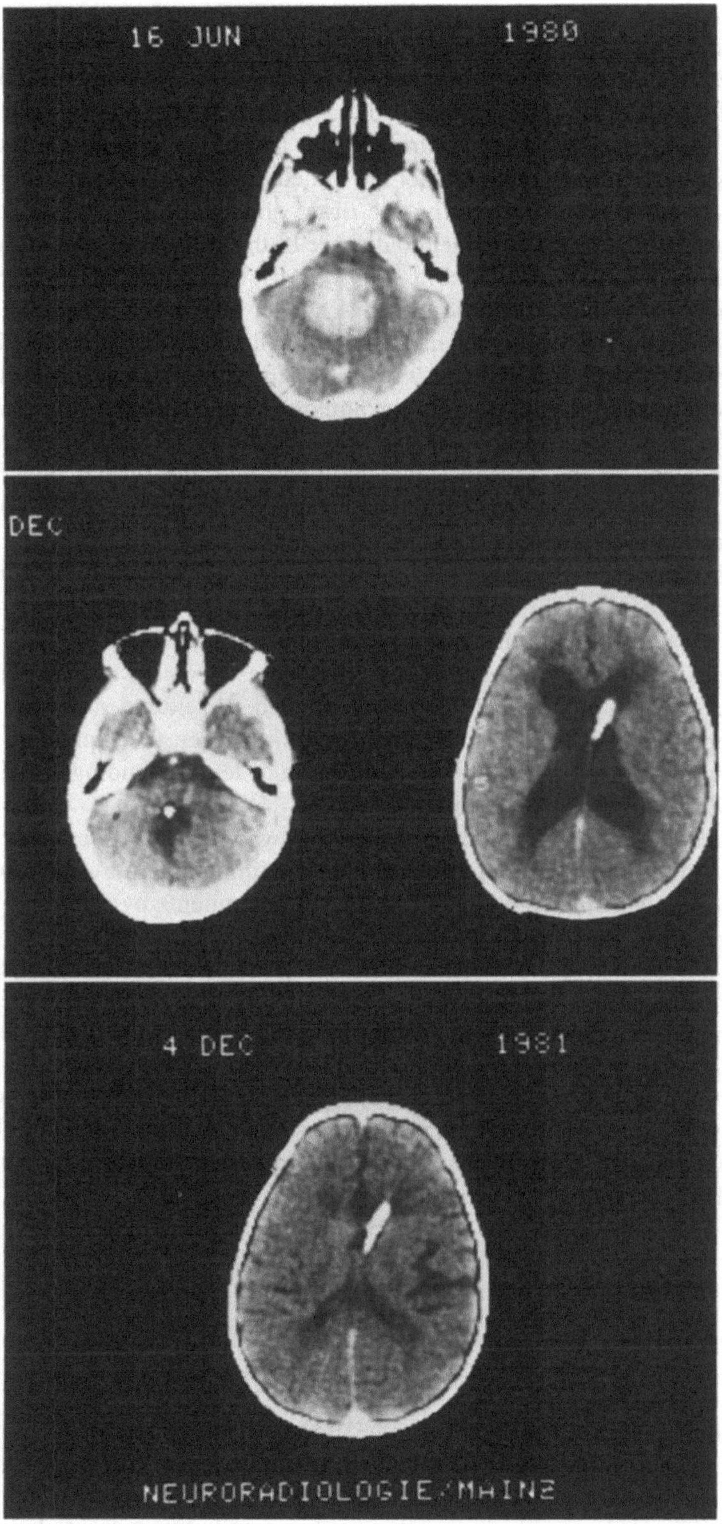
16 JUN
1980
DEC
4 DEC
1981
NEURORADIOLOGIE/MAINZ

eter, without any stylet, must be carefully introduced with a forceps, until a resistance is felt. If the catheter is introduced for about 4–6 cm from the posterior end of the aqueduct it is fairly certain that it will have reached the anterior horn of one of the lateral ventricles. An X-ray control (Fig. 1) proved unnecessary at the time, as an increased resistance, with kinking of the catheter and formation of a loop, became immediately apparent. After cutting the distal end of the catheter to the correct length it was placed in the subarachnoid space of the cervical region, at the level of the second or third cervical vertebra (Fig. 1). Any fixation of the catheter is quite unnecessary, as the flanged portion of the catheter which has been advanced into the anterior horn of the ventricle ensures that it will not be displaced. We have seen the catheter displaced distally in only two cases, in both of which it had proved impossible to advance the catheter into the anterior horn of the ventricle. However, it was seen in the CT control that the umbrella-like flanges of the catheter were held at the upper end of the aqueduct and this prevented any further downward displacement. In spite of the fact that the catheter was not in the desired position the drainage continued to function and remained trouble-free.

We have not seen any *acute side-effects* which could definitely be attributed to the drainage. In all, four children presented temporary disturbances of co-ordination, associated with impairment of eye movements and double vision. These lasted for a maximum of five days and were regarded as *mesencephalic disturbances.* In all these cases the tumour which had been removed also extended upwards as far as the mid-brain, so that these disturbances could have been the expression of the lesion produced by the tumour and also of the brain oedema extending into this region. They were all completely reversible.

The *reliability of the functioning* of the drain was excellent. We have not seen a single case of failure. This applies not only to the immediate post-operative period, in which *continuous intraventricular pressure* measurements by Lundberg's method [16, 24] gave precise data about the pressure relationships, but also to the entire period of observation up to a maximum of six years, which is well documented by computer-tomography and its evidence regarding the size of the ventricles (Fig. 2). If there should be a recurrence of the tumour in the region of the fourth ventricle the tube continues to function quite unimpaired, even though the catheter has been partially surrounded by tumour. The survival time of our patients was influenced in different ways by the type of tumour, as for instance in the group of medulloblastomas with recurrences. In spite of this, none of these patients again developed an obstructive hydrocephalus.

Discussion

Among additional measures which can be used in the treatment of space-occupying lesions in the posterior fossa in children, the treatment of obstructive hydrocephalus must be regarded as one of the most important. The ventriculo-atrial and ventriculo-peritoneal shunts which are often used as a palliative measure before the actual removal of the tumour, seem to us to be ineffective and dangerous, as on the one hand they involve the danger of a generalized dissemination of the tumour ([12] and one personal observation), and on the other hand they are very susceptible to disturbances of various kinds [4, 5, 9, 10, 11, 13, 20, 21, 22, 25]. Because of this a *preliminary external ventricular drainage* is definitely more effective (and desirable) before the operation [23, 24].

Postoperatively a shift of the aqueduct can develop as a result of brain oedema, or also from a reactive gliosis. In addition, secondary atresias of the aqueduct are a well-recognized sequel to a supratentorial shunt ([3], see pp. 180–185). Finally, a recurrence can lead to the development of a hydrocephalus, once again. The Leksell-drainage allows us to avert this additional strain on the patient [27].

The indications for the use of a Leksell-drainage are as follows:

1) An infratentorial tumour extending to the lower end of the aqueduct, which leads one to expect that postoperatively there will be stenosis or displacement of the aqueduct, as a result of oedema or gliosis.

2) If there seems to be the danger of a recurrence of the tumour, either because of a sub-total removal or, even when there has been a complete extirpation, but the lesion is highly malignant.

3) As dissemination of the tumour through the shunt system has been described in the case of medulloblastoma, and we have ourselves had experience of such a case, we consider that such types of shunt are contraindicated and we much prefer the Leksell type of drainage.

4) The usual shunt systems require revision in a high proportion of cases, whereas the Leksell-drainage is very reliable and is comparable with the Torkildsen procedure.

5) A ventriculo-atrial or ventriculo-peritoneal shunt placed supratentorially can lead to a secondary atresia of the aqueduct and also, in rare cases, to the syndrome of an "isolated fourth ventricle" (see pp. 180–185). This complication can be prevented by the ventriculo-cisternostomy of Leksell.

References

1. Dandy, W. E.: The diagnosis and treatment of hydrocephalus resulting from strictures of the aqueduct of Sylvius. Surg. Gyn. Obstet. *31*, 701–704 (1969)
2. Elvidge, A. R.: Treatment of obstructive lesions of the aqueduct of Sylvius by interventriculostomy. J. Neurosurg. *24*, 11–23 (1966)
3. Foltz, E. L., Shurtleff, D. B.: Conversion of communicating hydrocephalus to stenosis or occlusion of the aqueduct during ventricular shunt. J. Neurosurg. *24*, 520–529 (1966)
4. Forrest, D. M., Cooper, D. G. W.: Complications of a ventriculo-atrial shunt: A review of 455 cases. J. Neurosurg. *29*, 506–512 (1968)
5. Gardner, P., Schoenbaum, S. D., Shillito, J.: Infections of cerebrospinal fluid shunts: epidemiology, clinical manifestations, and therapy. J. Infect. Dis. *131*, 543–552 (1975)
6. Gutjahr, P., Voth, D., Neidhardt, M.: Ergebnisse der kombinierten Behandlung (Operation, Radio- and Chemotherapie) bei 132 Kindern mit primären ZNS-Tumoren. Therapiewoche *28*, 4346–4352 (1978)
7. Gutjahr, P., Voth, D.: Erfolgreiche Medulloblastomtherapie – und danach? Adv. Neurosurg. *5*, 257–258 (1978)
8. Gutjahr, P., Voth, D.: Treatment and prognosis of childhood brain tumors: Experience with 140 cases. Verhdlg. Dtsch. Krebsges. *2*, 434–435 (1979)

9. Hakim, S., de la Roche, F. D., Burton, J. D.: A critical analysis of valve shunts used in the treatment of hydrocephalus. Dev. Med. Child Neurol. *15,* 230–255 (1973)
10. Hemmer, R.: Complications of atrial-ventricular shunts and their prevention. Kinderchirurgie *5,* 10–24 (1967)
11. Ignelzi, R. J., Kirsch, W. M.: Follow-up analysis of ventriculo-peritoneal and ventriculo-atrial shunts for hydrocephalus. J. Neurosurg. *42,* 679–682 (1975)
12. Kessler, L. A., Dugan, P., Concannon, J. P.: Systemic metastases of medulloblastoma promoted by shunting. Surg. Neurol. *3,* 147–152 (1975)
13. Leem, W., Miltz, H.: Complications following ventriculo-atrial shunts in hydrocephalus. Adv. Neurosurg. *6,* 1–5 (1978)
14. Lapras, C., Poirier, N., Deruty, R., Bret, P., Joyeux, O.: Le cathétérisme de l'aqueduct de Sylvius. Neuro-Chir. *21,* 101–109 (1975)
15. Leksell, L.: A surgical procedure for atresia of the aqueduct of Sylvius. Acta Psychiatr. (Københ.) *24,* 559–568 (1949)
16. Lundberg, N.: Continuous recording and control of ventricular fluid pressure in neurosurgical practice. Acta psychiat. Scand. (Suppl. 149) *36,* 1–193 (1960)
17. Norlen, G.: Contribution to the surgical treatment of inoperable tumors, causing obstruction of the Sylvian aqueduct, Acta psychiatr. (Københ.) *24,* 629–637 (1949)
18. Otte, J., Emmrich, P., Schwarz, M., Voth, D., Gutjahr, P.: Zur postoperativen Behandlung von Kindern mit Tumoren des ZNS. In "Pädiatrische Intensivmedizin" *8,* Georg Thieme Verlag, Stuttgart (1982), (in press)
19. Portnoy, H. D.: New ventricular catheter for hydrocephalic shunts. J. Neurosurg. *34,* 702–703 (1971)
20. Steinbock, P., Thomson, G. B.: Complications of ventriculo-vascular shunts: Computer analysis of etiological factors. Surg. Neurol. *5,* 31–35 (1976)
21. Strahl, E. W., Liesegang, J., Roosen, K.: Complications following ventriculo-peritoneal shunts. Adv. Neurosurg. *8,* 6–9 (1978)
22. Voth, D.: Nuklearmedizinische Funktionsprüfung ventrikulo-atrialer und ventrikulo-peritonealer Anastomosen. Klinische Wertung. Pädiatr. Nuklearmed. *1,* 40–45 (1979)
23. Voth, D., Nakayama, N.: Ein neues ventilgesteuertes System für die präliminare Ventrikeldrainage (Technische Beschreibung und klinische Erfahrungen). Neurochirurgia *19,* 196–201 (1976)
24. Voth, D., Hey, O., Nakayama, N., Emmrich, P.: Die kontinuierliche Registrierung des intrakraniellen Druckes (Intraventrikuläre Messung) im Rahmen der pädiatrischen Intensivmedizin. Pädiatr. Intensivmed. (Ed.: P. Emmrich), Georg Thieme Verlag, Stuttgart, 104–109 (1977)
25. Voth, D.: Über die körperliche Belastbarkeit von Kindern mit einem Shuntsystem zur Behandlung des Hydrocephalus internus. Sozialpädiatrie *4,* 315–320 (1982)
26. Voth, D., Schwarz, M.: New light on the technique and indication for ventriculo-cisternal drainage according to Leksell (Interventriculostomy). Neurosurg. Rev. (1981)
27. Voth, D., Schwarz, M., Hüwel, N., Mahlmann, E.: Shunt therapy in medulloblastoma? Acta Neurochir. *56,* 278–279 (1981)

Discussion

K. Schürmann (Mainz) referring to the paper by *P. Glees (Cambridge)* stated that the angioarchitecture of the brain stem displayed the nuclei and tracts very well.

P. Glees (Cambridge) agreed with the observation, remarking that the angioarchitecture in a certain sense reflected the cytoarchitecture of the particular area of the brain. Referring to the question from *K. Schürmann (Mainz)* about the development of such fibre systems, such as the spino-thalamic tract *Glees* pointed out that one had assumed that for instance in the regeneration of the optic nerve in amphibians, which led to very well ordered connections between the retina and the midbrain, there are certain "Lock"-mechanisms which attract the sprouting fibres. After this the idea developed that just a few fibres acted *quasi* as pathfinders and gave signals to the neighbouring fibres, in order that they would develop further in a certain direction. This idea no longer seems to be correct. In the investigations on regeneration of the optic nerve one sees much more that the optic nerve occupies the entire terminal territory in a diffuse manner and that all the fibres which do not belong to a particular connecting point just disappear. To what extent these concepts play any part, for elaborately constructed systems such as in mammals, is not known for certain.

Bohl (Mainz) mentioned the vascular injections which had been shown and asked to what extent during development the vascularisation could be influenced or controlled. As an example he mentioned a vascular adaptation in congenital heart defects.

Glees (Cambridge) was not able to make any specific comment on this and referred to the vascular studies of Duvernoy (1970).

D. Voth (Mainz) asked if with large craniopharyngiomas a large bifrontal craniotomy was preferred similar to that recommended by Raimondi, or else a bilateral craniectomy. *Koos (Vienna)* replied that in certain cases he preferred to trephine bilaterally. He thought that the extensive exposure associated with bilateral bone flaps was too much of a strain in young children.

K. Schürmann (Mainz) in expanding on the remarks of *Koos* pointed out that modifications of the incision and the exposure should be adapted to each individual case. It was possible in relatively large lesions, by suitably adapting the incisions to facilitate the operation to a considerable degree, and also reduce the risk for the patients.

A question from the "floor" asked if it were not sensible to process the biopsy material not only in paraffin, but to fix some of it in glutaraldehyde and make semi-thin sections. *P. Kleihues (Freiburg)* replied that in certain cases, besides formalin fixed material embedded in paraffin he fixed some in glutaraldehyde for the purpose of semi-thin sections, as well as for electronmicroscopy. Nevertheless he emphasized that in the majority of cases no additional information worth mentioning could have been achieved by this. In most cases the effort was not worth while.

D. Müller (Hamburg) emphasized that use of the rapid smear technique is a great advantage in intra-operative diagnosis. These preparations are suitable for rapid guidance, nevertheless in addition routine sections are necessary for the final classification of a tumour.

P, Kleihues (Freiburg) confessed that originally he had been very sceptical about the technique of rapid smear preparations. He confessed that quite quickly it leads to results which depend on the extent of the experience of the investigator. A disadvantage however, is that no special stains are possible.

G. Argyropoulos (Graz) commented on the importance of the laser, which in combination with microsurgery, greatly facilitated the removal of intramedullary tumours or those infiltrating the rhombencephalon.

K. Schürmann (Mainz) commented that the blind puncture of tumours had often been unsatisfactory, not only as regards obtaining positive specimens, but also as regards the interpretation of the microscopic findings.

With regard to that *P. Kleihues (Freiburg)* said that they worked in close cooperation with the neurosurgeons, so that usually the majority of biopsy specimens were examined immediately in the form of smear preparations. In this way one could carry out during the operation an immediate evaluation of the stereotactic or radiological localisation of the tumour. This procedure certainly takes a lot of time, but in Kleihues' opinion it represents a really decisive improvement in diagnosis.

Koos (Vienna) speaking as a neurosurgeon and *Ebhardt (Cologne)* as a neuropathologist were in agreement on this subject.

Habermalz (Berlin) asked to what extent basal ganglia tumours were resectable. *Voth (Mainz)* and *Koos (Vienna)* as neurosurgeons replied to the effect that in a proportion of tumours, for instance in the hind brain or else in the thalamus, total removal was possible with the aid of the microscope. They pointed out certain neuroradiological criteria which would help to distinguish between those gliomas of the brain stem and other gliomas which could be partly or completely extirpated.

E. Halves and *W. Ischebeck* replied to a question from *D. Voth (Mainz)* stating that they had a lower age limit for the trans-sphenoidal approach in children, if using the speculum bilaterally meant destruction or coagulation of the turbinates. The youngest child in the material of Halves was an eight-year-old youngster, in whom this approach had presented no problems.

W. Ischebeck (Wuppertal) further pointed out that the freeing of the capsule of a craniopharyngioma or a large pituitary by a high pressure lumbar injection, is a relatively good possibility. Naturally there is not the same safety with this technique as with mobilization of the capsule under direct vision. However, definite dangers do undoubtedly exist, particularly with craniopharyngiomas, which are closely attached to their surroundings and in which by these procedures haemorrhages may be caused.

Both speakers gave their opinion on a question from *Argyropoulos (Graz)* regarding to what extent complications develop in the nasal mucous membrane, from using this approach. It was stated that complications such as ozoena were extremely rare. Ischebeck, in his material, had not seen a case of ozoena and merely two cases of atrophic rhinitis. Halves mentioned a single case of ozoena among 150 patients, and this developed in an old woman who already showed extensive destruction of the nasal skeleton.

The Radiosensitivity of the Infant Brain

W. Hinkelbein and M. Wannenmacher

With the fractionated radiotherapy usually given today we know the threshold of tolerance of various human organs and tissues against megavoltage photons, and in relation to the varying biological efficacy of other types of rays given, although restrictions have to be made here. Figure 1 shows this, in reference to Rubin and Casarett [34]. The brain is missing from this schedule, as unfortunately it has not so far been possible to fix an equivalent tolerance dose for it.

Since the first descriptions in the thirties of delayed radionecrosis of the brain we know that the human brain is not at all the radioresistant organ it had been considered to be until then. Apart from these late necrotic changes we know today about other cerebral radioreactions which occur earlier. The clinical picture of radiation-induced cerebral lesions ranges from an asymptomatic state through reversible dysfunctions up to very rare deleterious syndromes with a fatal outcome.

The acute radioreaction of the human brain occurs during irradiation with high single doses, and is manifested by sudden severe headache, lethargy, vomiting and

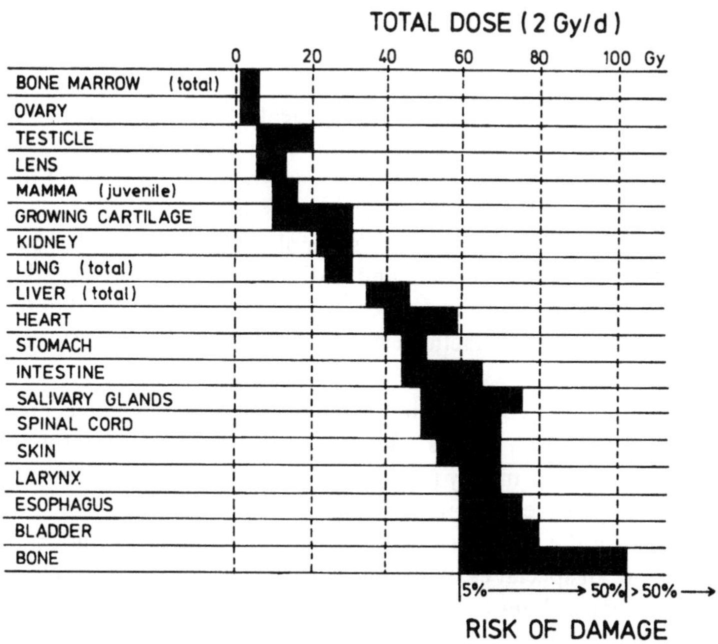

Fib. 1. Tolerance doses of human organs and tissues on fractionated megavoltage x-ray therapy. After Rubin and Casarett [34]

possibly with papilloedema, and with bulging of the fontanelle. It depends on an increase of intracranial pressure, and is often characterized as "radiation oedema". This definition is an unfortunate choice because most possibly it is a combined effect with a perifocal oedema of the tumour or a postoperative wet brain plus radiation effect. In experiments on animals, no cerebral oedema can be caused purely by cerebral irradiation with a solitary dose up to 20 Gy. By low initial dose irradiation, the increase of pressure may usually be avoided, if need be, it can be treated quickly with corticosteroids. The early changes seem to be marked anatomo-pathologically by capillary lesions and perivascular inflammation, and are thus connected with disorders of the blood-brain barrier [37]. The descriptions of the macro-pathological as well as of the histo-pathological x-ray changes are obtained from animal experiments, and can only be transferred to human conditions to a limited extent. Firstly they are often based on experiments with essentially higher irradiation doses than those normally used in radiotherapy; secondly, most of the studies were carried out without fractionation or, at best, with very few fractions. It is not sufficiently known how far the radiosensitivity of those animal brains examined is similar to human conditions. Adequate knowledge of the pathological anatomy of radiation effects on the human brain only exists for delayed radiation necrosis and for the infantile subacute necrotising leukoencephalopathy.

The radiogenic CNS changes which become manifest after the end of radiotherapy are classified into so-called "early-" and "late"-delayed reactions. The early subacute reactions cause symptoms some weeks to months after the end of treatment. We must also mention here the, certainly very rare, clinical picture described by Rider in 1963 [33], with nausea, vomiting, cerebellar ataxia, dysarthria and dysphagia, horizontal nystagmus, and a positive Romberg sign. Normally, these symptoms recede within 2–3 months. Similar observations have been reported by Hoffman [17]. These changes are interpreted as a consequence of demyelination. Usually, the symptoms disappeared completely, and the patients seem to remain without subsequent pathological findings. Isolated cases of death have been reported [23]. In these cases, disseminated foci of demyelination with central necrosis and petechial haemorrhages were found. Additional single cases with obscure cerebral haemorrhages, and syndromes similar to late radionecrosis have been seen. The clinical picture described as post-irradiation- or as somnolence syndrome also belongs to the so-called "early"-delayed reactions, and is discussed later. As far as the latency period is concerned, the subacute leukoencepalopathy should be added here. The symptoms of the "early"-delayed reactions can sometimes be favourably influenced by corticosteroids [42].

The true late radiation-induced complication of the brain ("late"-delayed reaction) is the late radionecrosis which occurs after an interval of many months to years. The symptoms are irreversible, mostly progressive, and most often indicate an intracranial mass. Often the outcome is fatal, especially if the delayed necrosis, because of its symptoms and with the tentative diagnosis of recurrence of a tumour, is treated by further irradiation. In special cases superficial areas of necrosis can be removed by excision [53]. As regards long-term survivors, late cerebral radionecrosis is a very rare complication. By far, the majority of the cases described occurred after an extremely high dose, and date back to an era where the quality, technique and planning of irradiation did not allow one to give the dose homogeneities and isodose distributions needed. Numerous detailed descriptions have been given of the patho-morphology of the cerebral radionecrosis, e.g. by Zülch [53]. Characteristically the white matter is predominantly affected. It has been demonstrated in animal experiments that there are also clear morphological changes during the latent interval [24]. Today the discussion of the pathogenetic mechanism of late radionecrosis is still a subject of controversy. Certainly the vascular changes play an important part, similar to other late radiation effects. These changes become more and more significant, especially with the growing latency period. Many examiners maintained that there was a definite vascular cause as shown by degenerative and proliferative changes in the vascular wall [16]. Contrary to that, a direct effect on the

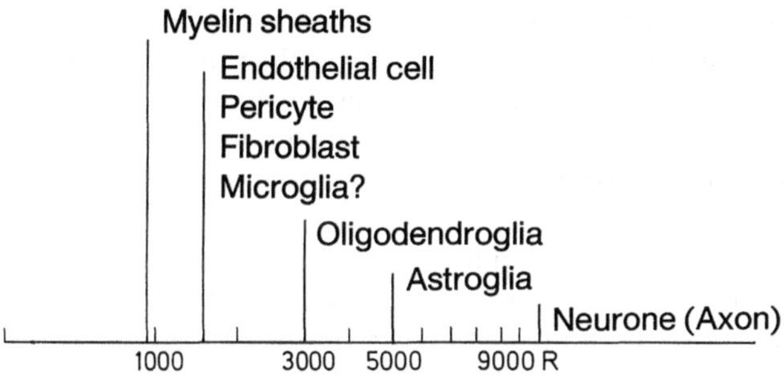

Fig. 2. Radiosensitivity of different components of brain tissues related to conventional single-dose irradiation (primary, rapidly developing severe lesions). After Schmitt [38]

glial cells has been noted [52]. Today we consider that both primary lesions play a part in the development of the attack caused by radiation [38]. In addition, other pathogenetic principles have been, and are still being discussed, such as an oedematous necrosis, a secondary antigen-antibody reaction like an autoaggressive mechanism after myelolysis [53], or a viral cause [6] in the sense of viral activation or modification or even of a "viral genesis" induced by radiation, and a primary myelin sheath lesion [38]. Figure 2 shows the different radiosensitivity of the various components of the CNS, as described by Schmitt [38].

As the latest possible radiation effect on the brain, with a latent interval of ten or more years, the question of radiation-induced malignant tumours has to be discussed. Sarcomas of the menginges after irradiation of the brain [20], and sarcomatous parts after irradiation of pituitary tumours [45] have seldom been mentioned; nevertheless, pituitary adenomas occasionally seem to form sarcomatous parts without irradiation [45].

Even now, the question of a varying radiosensitivity of different areas of the brain cannot be answered finally. Possibly there is a greater sensitivity of the brain stem, and of other midline structures [18]. In any case, midline lesions seem to develop symptoms more often and more seriously, and they seem to have a more unfavourable prognosis. Considering the radiosensitivity of the brain, we must also take into consideration that many of the cases studied have been treated with chemotherapy which might possibly have a toxic effect on the CNS itself, or intensify the radiotoxicity [4]. In general, the interactions between chemotherapy and radiotherapy are still not sufficiently clarified. Other factors which may perhaps lower the cerebral tolerance are existing meningitis and other CNS infections, a manifest diabetes mellitus, possibly a hypercorticism (Cushing's syndrome), or a long-standing arterial hypertension [12], as well as a cerebral oedema [4]. Late necrosis, being favourably influenced by a wet brain, might be prevented in these cases by administration of steroids during the treatment. As to irradiation techniques, the size of the irradiated cerebral volume is of great importance [2], the diseases in question normally require an exposure of the whole brain, at least a great deal of the tumour dose, so that in practice the relation to the field size is not of great significance. It is different when choosing the kind of radiation. So far, our report only applies to photons and high-energy electrons. Still there are only few observations regarding the use of rays with higher LET. Concerning their use on the brain, the therapeutic range of fast neutrons seems to be lower than that of photons. This means that compared with photons, although neutrons have a better effect on brain tumours, they cause unacceptable damages in the surrounding brain tissues [5]. Other heavy particles also seem to have the potential for producing severe damage.

Efforts to find the tolerance dose of the human brain from particulars in the literature about radionecrosis had been made earlier; however, they did not manage to get halfway to the exact doses, as nothing was known about biologically equivalent effective doses with varied fractionation. Several attempts were made to apply the so-called NSD-conception of Ellis [11] to the brain. The conditions at the skin, however, upon which the NSD-formula is based, cannot easily be transmitted to other tissues. In 1975, Wara et al. [48] found other exponents for the lung, and they found out that their formula was more precise for the spinal cord than the Ellis formula. The studies of van der Kogel [21] and White [50] also led to a correction of the exponents for the spinal cord. These results have been transferred to the brain by Sheline [42], emphasizing the great significance of fractionation, as compared to the total duration of treatment. Trott [46], also arrived at a good description of the clinical data with these exponents, and concluded that in the treatment of glioblastomas the healing and damaging rate were equal and that in irradiation of glioblastomas the dose is inadequate. Hornsey [19] found a higher exponent for fractionation in rat brains, too. Evaluating 29 patients with cerebral necrosis or lesions of the optic nerve, who had been treated with fractionated megavoltage photons or electrons, Pezner and Archambeau [30] found a formula of quite similar exponents. It allows one to estimate the risk of radionecrosis in fractionated cerebral irradiation (Fig. 3). However, it seems to be too early to give an exact tolerance dose in the sense of Fig. 1. Certainly the brain tolerates doses equal to those given to the skin, if there is a sufficiently high fractionation. Thus late necrosis with fractionated megavoltage irradiation and total doses of 60 Gy are extremely rare today. Even after total irradiation of the brain with local saturation up to 80 Gy, Salazar [36] did not find any cerebral necrosis in the normal brain tissue but often in the area of the tumour combined with a recurrence.

These results, of course, cannot lightly be transferred to the infantile brain. The process of maturation of the human brain with increase of the glial and vascular system, and with completion of the myelinisation extends to about the fifth year of age when the myelinisation is being completed, but the greatest amount occurs up to the

Biol. equivalent-doses for the brain		
Ellis [11]	TD = NSD (ret)	$\times N^{0.24} \times T^{0.11}$
Sheline [42]	TD = neuret	$\times N^{0.44} \times T^{0.06}$
Pezner [30]	TD = btu	$\times N^{0.45} \times T^{0.03}$
Hornsey et al. [19]	TD = "NSD"	$\times N^{0.38} \times T^{0.02}$

Fig. 3. The Ellis formula [11] (*N*ominal *S*tandard *D*ose) compared to the equivalent doses of the brain. Sheline's [42] "neuret" formula is based on the radiosensitivity of the spinal cord, Pezner's [30] brain tolerance unit (*btu*) on late human radionecrosis of the brain and Hornsey's modified "NSD" formula [19] from experimental work in rats. *N* Number of fractions, *T* total treatment time, *TD* total dose

end of the second year of age [3]. Although the recuperative capacity of the glial and vascular system is presumably higher than that of adults, and although there are better possibilities for functional compensation, we may not ignore any longer that the still developing infantile brain is more sensitive to irradiation than the adult [3, 25].

As mentioned in the beginning, apart from the previously described radiation effects, we can observe in children the somnolence syndrome, and the subacute disseminated necrotising leukencephalopathy. The somnolence syndrome which is often characterized as post-irradiation syndrome, was first described by Druckmann in 1929 [8]. The latency period is four to nine weeks after the end of radiotherapy of the cranium [13], and is characterized by sudden symptoms of lethargy or somnolence, sickness with vomiting and eventually diarrhoea and irritability. After a period from four [7] to about 38 days [13], the symptoms recede spontaneously. Neurological focal symptoms are regularly lacking [13]. Changes in the EEG can be usually found, mostly as slight generalized changes, followed by paroxysmal dysrhythmia and general changes of a medium degree. They are supposed to be reversible, although they do not disappear simultaneously with the clinical improvement [13]. Wehinger [49] even reported about the retroregression of pathological changes in the EEG with children with acute lymphoblastic leukaemia after having been treated with radiotherapy to the CNS. Authors report very differently, but it is generally noticed that it seems to arise more often in children with ALL who have undergone a "prophylactic" irradiation of the CNS than it arises after irradiation of a tumour, although the doses normally are lower. The statements regarding the prophylaxis of meningeosis range between 0% [49] to 79% [13], yet the majority lie between 21 and 66% [7, 28].

No relationship with the intrathecal administration of methotrexate can be stated [13]; the incidence is higher as the fractionation of irradiation is lower [28]. The greater frequency in the low dosed prophylaxis of meningiosis must be interpreted as referring to a sensitisation by preceding poly-chemotherapy. The dependence of cerebral dysfunctions arising later, on somnolence syndromes which had been presumed by Ch'ien et al. [7], must be verified. A temporary disorder of myelin synthesis is thought to be the cause [13].

A much more substantial and serious disease with an often fatal outcome is the subacute disseminated necrotising leukoencephalopathy. Up to now, it has been interpreted exclusively in connection with the "prophylactic" CNS-irradiation of the ALL and malignant lymphomas, and after intraventricular infusion of methotrexate with tumours of the posterior cranial fossa [41]. These changes are definitely connected with the administration of methotrexate, which also involves children with ALL and malignant lymphomas. Price and Jamieson [32] found them in 5.6% of the children who had had high intravenous doses of methotrexate after CNS-irradiation, in which presumably the blood-brain barrier had been altered [27]. Nevertheless, this had been seen likewise in the course of the CNS-prophylaxis [35], indeed, such changes have been reported just after administration of methotrexate only, without irradiation [26]. With necrotising leukoencephalopathy, the radiotherapy produces at most a favourable effect, and any dependance on radiation dose and fractionation has not been noticed.

Changes in the sense of mineralising microangiopathy and dystrophic calcifications must possibly be seen in close connection with leukoencephalopathy and the administration of methotrexate [42]. They were also detected by computed tomography in children with ALL [29], mostly without symptoms. In addition we can see ventricular and sulcal dilatations in the CT-scan as well as widenings of the interhemispheric cleft and of the subarachnoid spaces similar to a cerebral atrophy [29]. Changes in the CT-scan can very often be observed, nevertheless, studies with an adequate number of patients and initial CT-scans are still lacking. Such changes are particularly said to be observed after radiotherapy only [51].

Changes of the cerebrospinal fluid such as a pleocytosis and and increase of protein [47] have been described repeatedly in CNS-prophylaxis, but these might be due to intrathecal cytostatic administration [15]. Raised basic myelin has also been detected in the spinal fluid of patients with leukoencephalopathy [14]. EEG-changes after irradiation are much rarer than morphological changes in the late phase, especially if we disregard the preventive CNS-therapy.

In recent years, many authors pointed to radiogenic, hypothalamic or pituitary dysfunction, first of all to those of the STH-secretion [40], often not influencing the growth of the children. Such disturbances have been reported very rarely in adults. They were observed only after administration of higher doses during the irradiation of cerebral tumours, and do not usually appear after preventive CNS-therapy [39].

The question of late neuropsychological changes in children after cerebral irradiation is much more difficult. They are quite often observed with long-term surviving children after radiotherapy of cerebral tumours, whereas the combined effect of tumourous damage, operative trauma and radiation effect must be assumed and, in addition to that, cytostatic chemotherapy must be considered as an additional cause. Spunberg et al. [44] controlled 14 surviving children with cerebral tumours who had been irradiated during the especially vulnerable stage, that is before the end of the second year of age; eight of them had no abnormal neurological findings, 12 had a Karnofski index of 70 or better, six were without findings in the psychological examination, two showed only a slight retardation, and 11 were educable.

Other authors, too, reported similar favourable analyses, referring to the bad prognosis of the basic disease [1, 3]. There were also sporadic reports about possible psychological alterations with children after "prophylactic" cerebral irradiation [47]. On the other hand, Soni [43] did not corroborate this, in retrospective and prospective studies. In follow-up examinations of children with ALL, Eiser [10] found retardation in those patients who were under five years of age at the time of irradiation. These delays are said to be more frequent if the cerebral irradiation follows shortly after the poly-chemotherapy (within two months of the diagnosis), than if the interval is longer (at least six months after diagnosis) [9]. A possible effect of chemotherapy must not be ignored. As to children with developmental disturbances and psychological defects, we must always consider a direct psychic alteration, caused by the therapeutic manipulations themselves [31]. An eventual alopecia and the reaction of the environment upon the sick child must also be considered. An increase of late necrosis in children with the usual fractionated megavoltage therapy given today, has not been published.

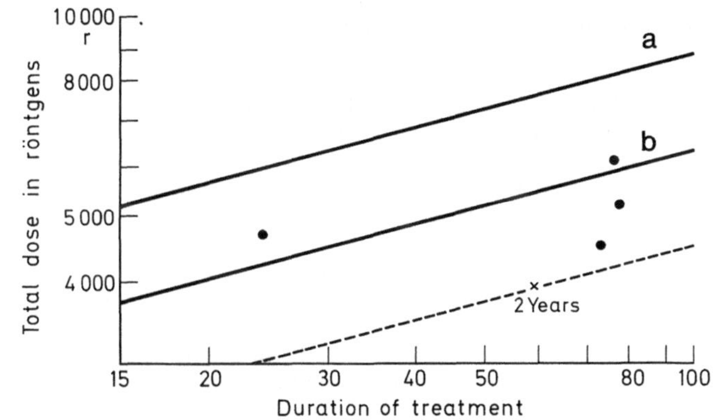

Fig. 4. Strandquist's dose-time diagram. Above line a, the risk of cerebral radionecrosis is high, below line b, no radionecrosis was seen in adults. The four points indicated long-term surviving children without necrosis lesions, concluding that line b is also good for children. The dotted line is the lowest dose level of a radionecrosis, seen in a child aged 2 (Lindgren [25])

There are not sufficient facts available to evaluate the biologically equivalent doses for the infantile brain, that is up to the age of five, but especially up to two years of age. Strandquist's curve, mentioned by Lindgren in 1974 [25] – Fig. 4 – may give certain evidence for finding out the tolerance dose, although considerable radio-biological reservations are to be made. Following curve b, it suggests that no late necrosis is to be expected in children although of course this does not apply to children under two years of age.

Summarizing we can say that, as regards children older than five years, the radiotolerance of the brain corresponds to that seen in adults. In trying to avoid late radiogenic effects, and without being able to exclude those with absolute certainty, today's usual fractionated dosage schedules proved to be good in the treatment of infantile cerebral tumours with about 50% of the adult dose for children under three years of age, and about 75% of it for children under five. If we treat with a combination of radio- and chemotherapy, or if very high doses are required, the number of fractions has to be increased in the first place. Concerning children with ALL, the prognosis has improved so considerably since the combined CNS-prophylaxis was introduced that, with regard to the increasing number of surviving children, we must think of a reduction in treatment to avoid possible late damage [22]. Before however we risk having a possibly larger number of recurrences by reducing the radiation dose, the increase in the number of fractions is more important. Yet we must be careful of irradiation given with more than one fraction per day [42], as at present, its effects cannot be estimated. In addition the question of an eventual reduction of the methotrexate dose should be considered.

References

1. Abramson, N., Raben, M., Cavanaugh, P. J.: Brain tumours in children – Analysis of 136 cases. Radiology *112,* 669–672 (1974)
2. Berg, N. O., Lindgren, M.: Relation between fieldsize and tolerance of rabbit's brain to roentgen irradiation (200 KV) via a slit-shaped field. Acta Radiol. (N.S.) *1,* 147–168 (1963)
3. Bloom, H. J. G., Wallace, E. N. K., Henk, J. M.: The treatment and prognosis of medulloblastoma in children. Am. J. Roentgenol. *105,* 43–62 (1969)
4. Burger, P. C., Mahaley, M. S. Jr., Dudka, L., Vogel, F. S.: The morphologic effects of radiation adminstered therapeutically for intracranial gliomas. Cancer *44,* 1256–1272 (1979)
5. Catterall, M., Bloom, H. J. G., Ash, D. V., Walsh, L., Richardson, A., Uttley, D., Gowing, N. F. C., Lewis, P., Chaucer, B.: Fast neutrons compared with megavoltage x-rays in the treatment of patients with supratentorial glioblastoma: a controlled pilot study. Int. J. Radiat. Oncol. Biol. Phys. *6,* 261–266 (1980)
6. Caveness, W. F., Kemper, Th. L., Vernon, K. L.: Is an infections agent involved in the delayed effects of CNS irradiation? VIII. INt. Congr. of Neuropathology, 1.–7. Sept., Budapest (Abstracts pp 49–51) Vol. 1, pp 83–95, 1975. Amsterdam: Elsevier 1974
7. Ch'ien, L. T., Aur, R. J. A., Stagner, S., Cavallo, K., Wood, A., Goff, J., Pitner, S., Hustu, H. O., Seifert, M. J., Simone, J. V.: Long-term neurological implications of somnolence syndrome in children with acute lymphocytic leukemia. Ann. Neurol. *8,* 273–277 (1980)
8. Druckmann, A.: Schlafsucht als Folge der Röntgenbestrahlung. Beitrag zur Strahlenempfindlichkeit des Gehirns. Strahlenther. *33,* 382–384 (1929)
9. Eiser, Ch.: Intellectual abilities among survivors of childhood leukemia as a function of CNS irradiation. Arch. Dis. Child. *53,* 391–395 (1978)
10. Eiser, Ch., Lansdown, R.: Retrospective study of intellectual development in children, treated for acute lymphoblastic leukemia. Arch. Dis. Child. *52,* 525–529 (1977)
11. Ellis, F.: Dose, time and fractionation: a clinical hypothesis. Clin. Radiol. *20,* 1–7 (1969)
12. Franke, H. D.: Die Strahlenempfindlichkeit des Nervensystems. In: Braun, H., Heuck, F., Ladner, H.-A., Messerschmidt, O., Musshoff, K., Streffer, Ch.: Strahlenempfindlichkeit von Organen und Organsystemen der Säugetiere und des Menschen. Strahlenschutz in Forschung und Praxis, Bd. XIII, p. 173. Stuttgart: G. Thieme 1973
13. Freeman, J. E., Johnston, P. G. B., Voke, J. M.: Somnolence after prophylactic cranial irradiation in children with acute lymphoblastic leukemia. Br. Med. J. *4,* 523–525 (1973)
14. Gangji, D., Reaman, G. H., Cohon, S. R., Bleyer, W. A., Ladisch, S., Poplack, D. G.: Elevated basic myelin protein in the cerebrospinal fluid of acute lymphoblastic leukemia patients with leukoencephalopathy. Proc. Amer. Assoc. Cancer Res. a. Amer. Soc. Clin. Oncol. *20,* 353–355 (1979)
15. Haghbin, M., Tan, C. T. C., Clarkson, B. D., Mike, V., Burchenal, J. H., Murphy, M. L.: Treatment of acute lymphoblastic leukemia in children with prophylactic intrathecal methotrexate and intensive systemic chemotherapy. Cancer Res. *35,* 807–811 (1975)
16. Haymaker, W.: Delayed radionecrosis of the brain in monkeys. J. Neuropath. exp. Neurol. *27,* 118–131 (1968)
17. Hoffman, W. F., Levin, V. A., Wilson, C. B.: Evaluation of malignant glioma patients during the postirradiation period. J. Neurosurg. *50,* 624–628 (1979)
18. Holdorff, B.: Radiation damages to the brain. In: Vincken, P. J., Bruyn, G. W. (eds.): Handbook of clinical neurology, vol. 23. Amsterdam: North-Holland Publ. Co., 1975
19. Hornsey, S., Morris, C. C., Myers, R.: The relationship between fractionation and total dose for x-ray induced brain damage. Int. J. Radiat. Oncol. Biol. Phys. *7,* 393–396 (1981)

20. Hustu, H. O., Aur- R. J. A., Verzosa, M. S., Simone, J. V., Pinkel, D.: Prevention of central nervous system leukemia by irradiation. Cancer *32,* 585–597 (1973)
21. Kogel, van der A. J.: Late effects of radiation on the spinal cord. Publication of The Radiobiological Institute TNO Rijswijk, The Netherlands, 1979, pp. 118–121
22. Lampert, F.: Kombinationschemotherapie und Hirnschädelbestrahlung bei 530 Kindern mit lymphoblastischer Leukämie. Dtsch. Med. Wschr. *25,* 308–312 (1977)
23. Lampert, P. W., Davis, R. L.: Delayed effects of radiation on the human central nervous system. "Early" and "late" delayed reactions. Neurology *14,* 912–917 (1964)
24. Lierse, W., Franke, H.: Ultrastrukturelle Veränderungen am Gehirn des Meerschweinchens und der Ratte während der Latenzzeit der Strahlenreaktion. Fortschr. Röntgenstr. *112,* 151–160 (1970)
25. Lindgren, M.: Strahlentherapie der Tumoren im Kindesalter. Strahlenther. *147,* 109–116 (1974)
26. Liu, H. M., Maurer, H. S., Vongsrivut, S., Conway, J. J.: Methotrexate encephalopathy: A neuropathologic study. Human Pathol. *9,* 635–648 (1978)
27. Meadows, A. T., Evans, A. E.: Effects of chemotherapy on the central nervous system, a study of parenteral methotrexate in long-term survivors of leukemia and lymphoma in childhood. Cancer *73,* 1079–1086 (1975)
28. Parker, D., Malpas, J. S., Sandland, R., Sheaff, P. C., Freeman, J. E., Paxton, A.: Outlook following "somnolence syndrome" after prophylactic cranial irradiation. Br. Med. J. *4,* 554–559 (1978)
29. Peylan-Ramu, N., Poplack, D. G., Pizzo, P. A., Adornato, B. T., Di Chiro, G.: Abnormal CT-scans of the brain in asymptomatic children with acute lymphocytic leukemia after prophylactic treatment of the central nervous system with radiation and intrathecal chemotherapy. N. Engl. J. Med. *298,* 815–818 (1978)
30. Pezner, R. D., Archambeau, J. O.: Brain tolerance unit: a method to estimate risk of radiation brain injury for various dose schedules. Int. J. Radiat. Oncol. Biol. Phys. *7,* 397–402 (1981)
31. Poehler, A., Riedesser, P., Jobke, A., Wannenmacher, M.: Psychische Aspekte der Strahlenbehandlung von Kindern und Jugendlichen. Klin. Pädiat. *193,* 184–188 (1981)
32. Price, R. A., Jamieson, P. A.: The central nervous system in childhood leukemia. II. Subacute Leukoencephalopathy. Cancer *35,* 306–318 (1975)
33. Rider, W. D.: Radiation damage to the brain – a new syndrome. J. Canad. Assoc. Radiol. *14,* 76–79 (1963)
34. Rubin, P., Casarett, G. W.: A direction for clinical radiation pathology. The tolerance dose. Front. Radiat. Ther. Onc. *6,* 1–16 (1972)
35. Rubinstein, L. J., Herman, M. M., Long, T. F., Wilbur, J. R.: Disseminated necrotizing leukoencephalopathy: a complication of treated central nervous system leukemia and lymphoma. Cancer *35,* 291–305 (1975)
36. Salazar, O. M., Rubin, P., Feldstein, M. L., Pizzutiello, R.: High dose radiation therapy in the treatment of malignant gliomas: final report. Int. J. Radiat. Oncol. Biol. Phys. *5,* 1733–1740 (1979)
37. Schettler, T., Shealy, C. N.: Experimental selective alteration of blood-brain barrier by x-irradiation. J. Neurosurg. *32,* 89–93 (1970)
38. Schmitt, H. P.: Akute und intervalläre Strahlenschäden des Zentralnervensystems. Sitzungsber. d. Heidelberger Akad. d. Wiss. Math.-Naturwiss. Klasse, 1. Abhandlung. Berlin, Heideberg, New York: Springer 1979
39. Schuler, D., Gács, G., Révész, T., Koós, R., Keleti, J.: Hypophysenfunktion und Wachstum bei Kindern unter Leukämiebehandlung. Monatsschr. Kinderheilkd. *128,* 773–779 (1980)
40. Shalet, S. M., Price, D. A., Beardwell, C. G., Morris-Johnes, P. H., Pearson, D.: Normal growth despite abnormalities of growth hormone secretion in children treated for acute leukemia. J. Pediat. *94,* 719–722 (1979)
41. Shapiro, W. R., Chernick, N. L., Posner, J. B.: Necrotizing encephalopathy following intraventricular instillation of methotrexate. Arch. Neurol. *28,* 96–101 (1978)
42. Sheline, G. E., Wara, W. M., Smith, V.: Therapeutic irradiation and brain injury. Int. J. Radiat. Oncol. Biol. Phys. *6,*1215–1228 (1980)

43. Soni, S. S., Marten, G. W., Pitner, S. E., Duenas, D. A., Powazek, M.: Effects of central nervous system irradiation on neuropsychologic functioning of children with acute lymphocytic leukemia. N. Engl. J. Med. *293,* 113–118 (1975)
44. Spunberg, J. J., Chang, C. H., Goldman, M., Auricchio, E., Bell, J. J.: Quality of long-term survival following irradiation for intracranial tumours in children under the age of two. Int. J. Radiat. Oncol. Biol. Phys. *7,* 727–736 (1981)
45. Terry, R. D., Hyams, V. J., Davidoff, L. M.: Combined nonmetastasizing fibrosarcoma and chromophobe tumour of the pituitary. Cancer *12,* 791–798 (1959)
46. Trott, K.-R.: Strahlenbiologische Probleme bei der Strahlentherapie von Hirngeschwülsten. Röntgen-Bl. *31,* 282–288 (1978)
47. Verzosa, M. S., Aur, R. J. A., Simone, J. V., Hustu, H. O., Pinkel, D.: Five years after central nervous system irradiation of children with leukemia. Int. J. Radiat. Oncol. Biol. Phys. *1,* 209–215 (1976)
48. Wara, W. M., Phillips, T. L., Sheline, G. E., Schwade, J. G.: Radiation tolerance of the spinal cord. Cancer *35,* 1558–1562 (1975)
49. Whinger, H., Slanina, J., Jacobi, H., Musshoff, K., Dietz, V., Sauer, M., Dilger, M.: Prophylactic central nervous system therapy with cranial irradiation and intrathecal methotrexate in acute lymphoblastic leukemia of childhood. Strahlenther. *148,* 590–598 (1974)
50. White, A., Hornsey, S.: Radiation damage to the rat spinal cord: the effect of single and fractionated doses of x-rays. Brit. J. Radiol. *51,* 515–523 (1978)
51. Wilson, G. H., Byfield, J., Hanafee, W. N.: Atrophy following radiation therapy for central nervous system neoplasms. Acta Radiol. Ther. *11,* 361–368 (1972)
52. Zeman, W.: Pathogenesis of radiolesion in the nature central nervous system. In: 5th Intern. Congr. Neuropath. 1965. Luthy, F., Bischoff, A. (eds.) Amsterdam: Excerpta Medica Found. 1966
53. Zülch, K. J., Harder, W. A, Lechtarpe-Grüther, H.: Zur Pathogenese der Strahlenspätnekrose aufgrund experimenteller und humanpathologischer Beobachtungen. 52. Tagung Dtsch. Roentgengesellsch., Düsseldorf 1971

Radiation Technique and the Planning of Treatment in Brain Tumours in Children

J. KUTZNER

Next to operation radiation is the most effective treatment of brain tumours in children.

The addition of chemotherapy has improved the prognosis in some tumours. If at all possible a biopsy should be taken because the choice of radiation portals depends a great deal on the histology of the tumour. Tumour tissue can be obtained at the time of operation or by needle biopsy.

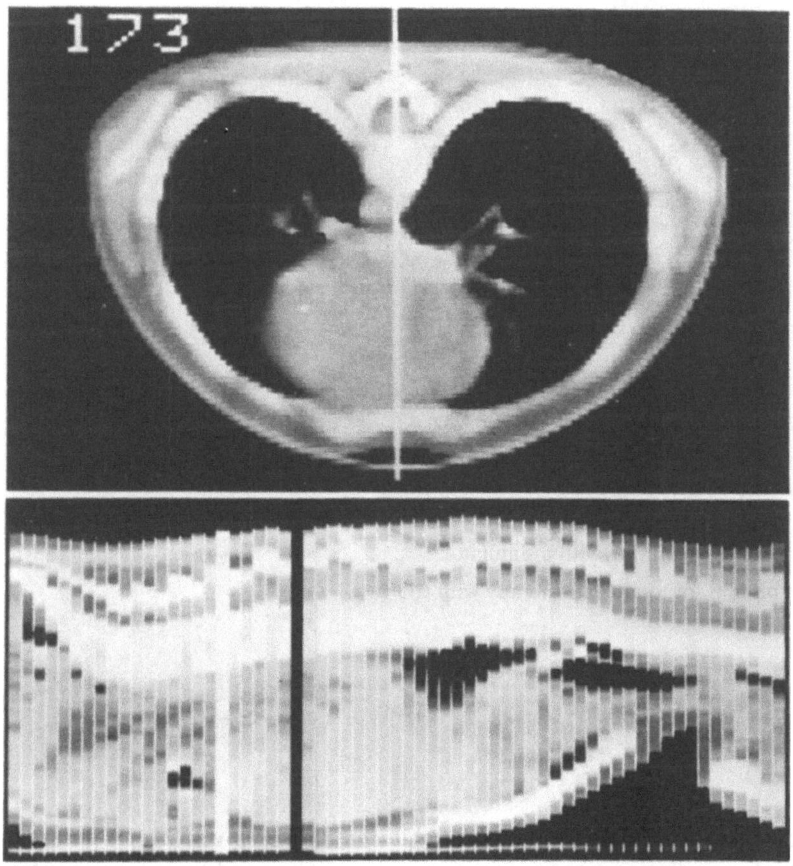

a

b

Fig. 1a, b. CT and topogram for dose calculation in the spinal axis

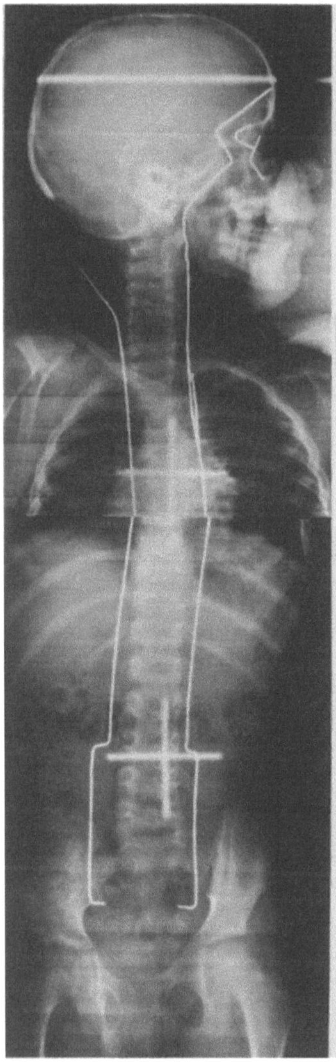

Fig. 2

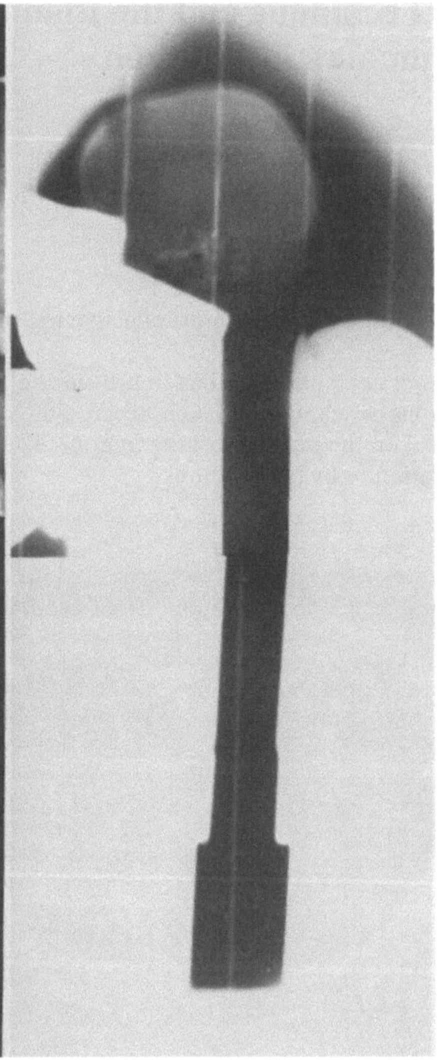

Fig. 3

Fig. 2. CNS – treatment-planning with a simulator

Fig. 3. Verification film for total CNS-therapy with CO^{60}

Policies of Treatment

Generally radiotherapy of brain tumours in children will be given with a curative intention. Palliative radiation treatment is rarely done. The conditions therefore for radiotherapy are either malignancy by histclogy or a highly suspected malignancy because of a synopsis of different examinations such as angiography or computerized tomography.

Biopsy should not be performed if it means an intolerably high risk for the patient. The policies of radiation therapy are:

1. Definitive radiotherapy with a curative intent,
2. Postoperative radiotherapy in case of
   a) a macroscopic complete tumour excision (so called prophylactic radiation therapy) or
   b) incomplete removal of the tumour.
3. Combined therapy with or without surgical treatment and chemotherapy.

Localized Disease

Localized tumours of the child are gliomas, gliomas of the optic nerve, astrocytomas or craniopharyngiomas as well as central brain stem tumours [11]. Postoperative radiation therapy is indicated in all cases of incomplete tumour removal. The same is true in severe degrees of malignancy because tumour recurrence is likely.

The target volume includes the volume of the original tumour site plus a safety zone of approximately 2 cm in which tumour can be assumed. Generally the size of the target volume is based upon examinations before operation, such as CT and angiography. Postoperative CT scans are required to take into account defects resulting from any resection.

Metastasizing Tumours

Pinealomas, ependymomas and medulloblastomas belong to the group of malignant brain tumours which do not remain confined to the site of origin.

Tumour recurrence is likely in all cases of glioblastoma grade IV even though the tumour has been completely excised macroscopically. Metastases or multicentric tumour growth has been blamed for the tumour recurrence. This is why radiotherapy should not only deal with the primary site but should be directed to the whole brain. Tumour spread via the cerebrospinal fluid is known to occur in medulloblastomas, high-grade ependymomas and also pinealomas.

Operation alone accounts for a five year survival rate of under 10%. Additional radiotherapy to the posterior fossa which has been done since 1925 has improved the results considerably. With radiation including the whole skull and spinal canal the five year survival rates increased to 70% [7, 9, 15, 16]. Collective data by McFarland report that metastases in medulloblastoma occur in one third of all cases [23].

In 430 patients there were 142 metastases to the central nervous system. 94% were found in the spinal canal and 6% in the cerebrum. In myelograms Deutsch saw unexpected spinal metastases in 7 of 16 children [13]. Even though some authors like Banner and Brutschin have reported cases of extra-cerebrospinal involvement mainly in bones and lymph nodes, this is a rare occurrence [2, 8, 12].

AV-shunt operations are sometimes done to decrease intracranial pressure in patients with medulloblastoma. This procedure contains the possibility of spreading tumour cells through the shunt system. Pichler found distant metastases in three children with AV-shunts [25].

Choice of Radiotherapy

External Beam Radiation

The most common form of radiotherapy is external beam therapy. The tumour site is irradiated with a source-skin distance (SSD) from 40 to 100 cm, by one or more portals.

Local Application

In some cases it will be possible to irradiate the tumour directly during surgical treatment. A radioactive source (^{182}Tantalum, ^{192}Iridium) can be positioned close to the tumour.

A high dose can be applied to the tumour with a low dose to the surrounding tissue.

The afterloading method is recommended in order to keep the radiation dose as low as possible for physicians and technicians.

Implantation Technique

For the interstitial technique a radioactive source is introduced directly into the tumour tissue. Depending on the isotope the source may remain implanted (e.g. ^{90}Yttrium seeds in the pituitary gland). The source has to be removed again if the nuclide has a long half-life.

The advantage of this treatment is the short range of beta and gamma rays. Fluid isotopes are only used in a few special cases. Injections of fluid radioactive preparations into the tumour or around it should not be performed, because the radiation dose delivered to the tumour is not homogeneous and the radioactive substance may vanish into the blood or cerebrospinal fluid. The administration of fluid isotopes is possible in tumours such as cystic craniopharyngiomas with cavities. Here mostly colloids of merely beta-emitting isotopes (e.g. ^{90}Y) or beta- and gamma-emitting isotopes (e.g. ^{198}Au) are used. Simultaneous gamma-ray emission has the advantage that the distribution and location of the isotope can be monitored by gamma-camera. X-rays, however, will raise the dose for patients and personnel.

D'Angio used intrathecal radiogold in patients with medulloblastoma. After cerebrospinal radiation therapy with 35 Gy in 3½ weeks, he injected 10 to 15 mCi ^{198}Au intrathecally in ten children. This treatment was repeated four times at intervals of six weeks. A cauda equina sydrome occurred in four patients, possibly as a result of arachnoiditis.

Therefore he decreased the dose to 10 mCi ^{198}Au and the radioactive material was only given twice to children under six years. Furthermore the patients were placed in a head down position after the injection and kept there for a several minutes. In two of six patients treated in this way a bilateral internal carotid occlusion occurred.

The arterial reaction is possibly due to hotspots shown on scintigram images days after the intrathecal therapy [10]. Six out of 16 children treated with radioactive gold died. A redistribution of the radioactivity must be considered after administration of fluid radioactive isotopes given as a fluid suspension. For instance the isotope can settle on the walls after an indefinite time. Lewis [17, 19] found less than 20% of radioactive gold in the cerebrospinal fluid 24 hours after administration. The effective radiation dose cannot easily be estimated and depends on the radionuclide, the energy of its beta- or gamma-rays, the half-life, the distribution and the absorption within the solution. Disappearance of radioactivity is also possible.

Radiation Quality

External beam radiation depends on the equipment used in a department. At first conventional x-ray therapy with 200 to 250 KV was used. The disadvantage of this radiation energy with its short range is a high dose delivered to the skin and bone. Lindgren [20] reported seven cases of aseptic skull necrosis associated with conventional radiotherapy of medulloblastoma with 170 KV. The estimated radiation dose absorbed by the skull was 110 Gy.

Cobalt-60-Therapy

The introduction of cobalt-60 machines made it possible to deliver higher doses to the tumour with no significant cutaneous reactions due to the build-up effect.

Accelerator

Electron accelerators either in form of circular or linear accelerators show a more efficient build-up effect due to the high energies of the photons. Accelerators are less likely to irritate the skin. There is also the possibility of using electrons with a defined range to the depth for irradiation of the spinal canal.

Management of Treatment

The individual treatment-planning takes into consideration the results of conventional x-ray examinations, computerized tomograms and operations to indicate the extent of the tumour.

Above all computerized tomograms are the basic information for a special treatment-planning computer regarding the set of portals and dose response curves. Depending on the extent of the tumour it is possible to use opposing portals from left and right.

A moving technique can be used in cases of a small target volume. It is necessary to protect the eyes and face by special lead blocks due to low radiation tolerance of the lens.

Lommatzsch [22] estimated a progressive cataract development in 50% of all patients who received a dose of 7.9 Gy and more [4].

In children under three years the dose of tolerance is even lower. Wedge-filter-technique can be used to compensate for the convexity of the skull or for irregularities caused by tissue-excision at operation. The critical point is to irradiate the whole cerebrospinal axis. Paterson and Farr [24] described in 1953 a technique of radiation of the whole skull and spinal column down to the second coccygeal vertebra using x-ray therapy with 250 KV and protecting the paravertebral region by lead blocks. Bottril [6] improved dose homogenity using a special compensator for the different depths of the tumour site.

As described by van Dyk [29] we irradiate the skull with bilateral fields and the spine simultaneously by 2–3 p.a. parts.

Scherer and Bamberg [26] have summarized the different radiation techniques for the central nervous system at the radiation Congress in Munich (1981).

By setting portals adjacent to each other, hot spots and low spots can occur up to 30%. Therefore this technique should be controlled by dose measurement in phantoms [1].

We found an irregularity in dose distribution of 10% in spinal fields as computed by the therapy-planning-system with cobalt 60 (field 6 cm × 10 cm).

Using a moving technique of 3 cm this irregular dose distribution was reduced below 5%. Griffin [14] thus recommends overlapping wedges at the borders of bilateral skull and spinal portals to equalize the isodoses.

Tokars [28] recommends radiating the whole cerebrospinal axis simultaneously in one field. The patient is placed in the prone position with the skull facing to one side. Other body regions are blocked out by satellites. Unwanted high doses are delivered to the eyes if the side of the skull is not correctly positioned in a horizontal plane. For a long source-skin distance of 160–170 cm cobalt units have a low output which makes long irradiation times necessary and this might reduce the biological effectiveness.

Landberg [18] points out that the subdural space also includes the nerve root recesses. In the thoracic spine, nerve root pockets reach beyond the width of the vertebra extending to the tip of the transverse process. Thus, the field width of the spinal portal has to be wide enough.

Dosage

The lethal dose for the tumour depends on histology, method of treatment and age of the child.

The delivered dose in external beam radiation varies between 30 Gy and 60 Gy considering time – dose – fraction. Local tumour relapse is found even after radiation with up to 60 or 70 Gy. To improve results chemotherapy is justified [3, 4, 5]. Interaction of radiotherapy and chemotherapy has to be considered and therefore dose reduction is indicated.

Table 1. Radiation doses in Gy for medulloblastoma

Author	Unit	Skull	Fossa post.	Spinal channel	Single dose	Pat.	Year
1) Wannenmacher and Knüfermann [30]	Cobalt-60 Linac	30 – 40	50 – 55	30 – 35	1.5		
2) Cumberlin et al. [9]		45	55 (38 – 57)	40 (26 – 46)	1.6 – 1.8	n = 20	1962 – 78
3) Tokars et al. [28]	Accelerator	40	50	40	1.0 – 2.0	n = 9	1966 – 76
4) Bamberg et al. [1]	Linac	30 – 36	45 – 50	30 – 36	2	n = 18	1974 – 77
5) Pichler et al. [25]	Cobalt-60 Linac	35 – 45	55	30 – 35		n = 15	1975 – 80

Littmann [21] reports two cases of radiation induced myelitis in adjuvant chemotherapy with actinomycin D in medulloblastoma. Total radiation dose for medulloblastoma with adjuvant chemotherapy should be reduced to 50–55 Gy at the tumour site, and in children under two year to 45 Gy. Brain oedema with increased intraventricular pressure can be expected in cases of primary radiotherapy without ventricular shunt operation or without tumour resection. Depending on the size of the target volume a gradually increasing dose is necessary. Radiotherapy begins with 0.5 Gy and increases to 1.5 Gy daily. Cortison is administered during this time.

Positions of Patients

Radiotherapy lasts for several weeks and may lead to problems in repositioning the patient exactly the same way as for treatment planning. Today generally a laser beam marker with either three points or line positioning is centred on the isocentre of the machine. Marking the laser beam position on the patient's skin allows a good reproduceable positioning of the patient. Children may need sedation and a plaster cast to keep them restricted in a prone position during the radiation of the spinal portals. A simple form of fixation is a vacuum cushion. More elaborate is the construction of individually fitted plastic moulds. Use of stereotactic equipment with the aid of computerized tomography has proven valuable in the administration of radioactive isotopes [27].

Forms of radiation therapy for treating CNS tumours in children:

1. Radiation therapy alone, as a curative measure
2. Postoperative radiation therapy
   a) with macroscopically complete tumour excision
   b) with incomplete removal of the tumour
3. Combined radiation therapy and chemotherapy

Factors affecting the radiation dose with the use of fluid isotopes

1. Nuclide used, with range of beta or gamma radiation depending upon energy (^{32}P, ^{90}Y, ^{198}Au)
2. Half life
3. Spatial distribution
4. Absorption by distribution medium
5. Possible disappearance

References

1. Bamberg, M., Schmitt, G., Quast, U., Bongartz, E. B., Nau, H. E., Bayindir, C., Reinhardt, V.: Therapie und Prognose des Medulloblastoms. Strahlentherapie *156*, 1–17 (1980)
2. Banna, M., Lassmann, L. P., Pearce, G. W.: Radiological study of skeletal metastases from cerebellar medulloblastoma. Brit. J. Radiol. *43*, 173–179 (1970)
3. Bloom, H. J. G., Wallace, E. N. K., Henk, I. M.: The treatment and prognosis of medulloblastoma in children. Am. J. Roentgenol. *105*, 43–62 (1969)
4. Bloom, H. J., G., Walsh, S.: Tumours of the central nervous system. In: Cancer in children. Berlin, Heidelberg, New York: Springer 1975
5. Bloom, H. Julian G.: Medulloblastoma: Prognosis and prospects. Int. J. Rad. Oncology Biol. Phys. *2*, 1031–1033 (1977)
6. Bottril, D. O., Rogers, R. T., Hope-Stone, H. F.: A composite filter technique and special patient jig for the treatment of the whole brain and spinal cord. Brit. J. Radiol. *38*,122–130 (1965)
7. Brown, R. C., Gunderson, L., Plenk, H. P.: Medulloblastoma. Cancer *40*, 56–60 (1977)
8. Brutschin, P., Culver, G. J.: Extracranial metastases from medulloblastoma. Radiology *107*, 359–362 (1973)
9. Cumberlin, R. L., Luk, K. H., Wara, W. M., Sheline, G. E., Wilson, Ch. B.: Medulloblastoma. Cancer *43*, 1014–1020 (1979)
10. D'Angio, G. L.: Intrathecal radiogold for medulloblastoma and ependymoblastoma. In: Hilaris B. S., (ed.) Afterloading: 20 years of experience 1955–1975 New York
11. Danoff, B. F., Kramer, S. Thompson, N.: The radiotherapeutic management of optic nerve gliomas in children. Int. J. Radiation Oncology Biol. Phys. *6*, 45–50 (1980)
12. Debnam, I. W., Staple, T. W.: Osseous metastases from cerebellar medulloblastoma. Radiology *107*, 363 (1973)
13. Deutsch, M., Reigel, D. H.: The value of myelography in the management of childhood medulloblastoma. Cancer *45*, 2194–2197 (1980)
14. Griffin, T. W., Schumacher, D., Berry, H. C.: A technique for cranial-spinal irradiation. Brit. J. Radiol. *49*, 887–888 (1976)
15. Gutjahr, P., Kutzner, J.: Kombinierte Radio-Chemotherapie des Zentralnervensystems bei malignen Neoplasien im Kindesalter. Dtsch. med. Wschr. *100*, 1651–1656 (1975)

16. Hirsch, J. F., Renier, D., Czernichow, P., Benveniste, L., Pierre-Kahn, A.: Medulloblastoma in childhood. Survival and functional results. Acta Neurochir. *48,* 1–15 (1979)
17. Kieffer, St. A., D'Angio, G. J., Nowak, T. J.: Laboratory studies of intrathecal radiogold with a new rationale for its use. Radiology *87,* 1120–1121 (1966)
18. Landberg, T. G., Lindgren, M. L., Cavallin-Stahl, E. K., Svahn-Tapper, G. O., Sundbärg, G., Garwicz, S., Lagergren, J. A., Gunnesson, V. L., Brun, A. E., Cronqvist, S. E.: Improvements in the radiotherapy of medulloblastoma 1946–1975. Cancer *45,* 670–678 (1980)
19. Lewis, C. L.: Treatment of meningeal system by means of radioactive gold and x-rays. Proc. Roy. Soc. Med. *46,* 653–655 (1953)
20. Lindgren, M.: Therapie der Tumoren des Gehirns und Rückenmarks bei Kindern. Sonderband *66,* Strahlentherapie, 180–189 (1967)
21. Littman, P., Rosenstock, J. G., Bailey, C.: Radiation myelitis following craniospinal irradiation with concurrent Actinomycin-D therapy. Med. Pediatr. Oncol. *5,* 145–151 (1978)
22. Lommatzsch, P.: Die therapeutische Anwendung von ionisierenden Strahlen in der Augenheilkunde. Leipzig: VEB Georg Thieme Verlag 1977
23. McFarland, D. R., Horwitz, H., Saenger, E. L., Bahr, G. K.: Medulloblastoma – a review of prognosis and survival. Br. J. Radiol. *42,* 198–214 (1969)
24. Paterson, E., Farr, R. F.: Cerebellar medulloblastoma: Treatment by irradiation of the whole central nervous system. Acta Radiol. *39,* 323–335 (1953)
25. Pichler, E., Kogelnik, H. D., Reinartz, G., Kärcher, K. H., Zaunbauer, F., Jürgenssen, O. A., Koos, W., Kundi, M.: Ergebnisse der Therapie des Medulloblastoms in den letzten 15 Jahren. Strahlentherapie *157,* 508–515 (1981)
26. Scherer, E., Bamberg, M.: Methoden und Ergebnisse der Strahlentherapie beim Medulloblastom. 62. Tg. Dtsch. Rö.-Gesellschaft April 1981
27. Schmidt, K., Potthoff, P. C.: Stereotaktische Hirnoperationen – heutiger Stand. Dtsch. Ärztebl. 1981, S. 387
28. Tokars, R. P., Sutton, H. G., Griem, M. L.: Cerebellar medulloblastoma. Cancer *43,* 129–136 (1979)
29. Van Dyk, J., Derek, R., Jenkin, T., Leung, Ph. M. K., Cunningham, J. R.: Medulloblastoma: Treatment technique and radiation dosimetry. Int. J. Radiation Oncology Biol. Phys. *2,* 993–1005 (1977)
30. Wannenmacher, M., Knüfermann, H.: Fortschritte in der Therapie des Medulloblastoms. Onkologie *1,* 92–96 (1978)

Experiences with the Treatment of Cystic Craniopharyngiomas by Stereotactically Injected Radioisotopes

V. STURM, P. GEORGI, H. NETZEBAND, K. E. SCHEER, L. STRAUSS, W. SCHLEGEL, H. SCHARFENBERG, H. SINN, H. GAHBAUER, and H. PENZHOLZ

Introduction

Although they are histologically benign, the treatment of craniopharyngiomas posses many serious problems, as the methods of treatment are still controversial. This is due to their extension into the hypothalamic region and their close adherence to the peritumoural cerebral tissue, optic nerves and blood vessels [4, 5]. In about 60% of the cases, the tumours consist of one or more cysts and a comparatively small solid part [2, 3]. In the development of clinical symptoms the solid part is most commonly of lesser importance than the more rapidly expanding cysts.

For treatment, some authors advocate an attempt at a radical microsurgical extirpation of the tumours at "first attack" [5, 12], but even in the hands of the most skilled neurosurgeons there is an operative mortality of about 11%. According to Shapiro et al. [12], radical removal of craniopharyngiomas exceeding 3 cm in diameter, is nearly impossible.

Because of the risks of radical extirpation other authors advocate a limited operation [9]. At present, there is nearly general agreement, that subtotal excisions should be accompanied by radiotherapy, which according to the review of the literature by Amacher [1] lowers the incidence of recurrences from 75% (after subtotal excisions without radiotherapy) to 30.4%.

The best results of percutaneous irradiation combined with a limited operation such as tapping of a cyst, have been reported by Kramer et al. [6], but even in their series of 26 patients there were three deaths due to tumour recurrence and one death due to irradiation necrosis.

In the late fifties, Leksell [7] introduced the method of contact-irradiation of craniopharyngioma cysts by stereotactically injected Yttrium-90. This method was standardized by Backlund and coworkers [2, 3]. It has been in routine use at the Karolinska Hospital, Stockholm, since 1965 and was taken over by our group three years ago. The aim is necrotizing irradiation of the cyst-wall and sparing of the surrounding tissue.

Material and Methods

Since May 1979, 25 consecutive cases of cystic craniopharyngiomas have been treated by intracavitary irradiation by Yttrium-90 (n=21), Rhenium-186 (n=2) and both Yttrium-90 and Rhenium-186 (n=1). In one case, Rhenium-186 was given after refilling of a cyst, treated six months earlier with Yttrium-90. In two cases with large solid components, intracavitary irradiation was combined with percutaneous irradiation according to Kramer et al. [6]. Fifty per cent of the patients were children (aged up to 15 years).

Choice of Radionuclides

As a routine, Yttrium-90 is used as therapeutic agent. It is a pure β-emitter and is available as stable colloidal silicate (mean β-energy 2.273 MeV, half layer in soft tissue 1.1 mm, half life 64 h). According to Leksell's and Backlund's experiences [7, 2, 3, and personal communication 1981], an accumulated radiation-dose of 200 Gy to the inner surface of the cyst-wall was aimed at.

For the last six months, we have used Rhenium-186, if the optic nerves were severely compromised by tumour pressure. This isotope has a lower β-energy than Yttrium-90 and a shorter range in tissue. Thus the danger of radiation-damage to the optic nerves is smaller than when using Yttrium-90 [13]. The drawbacks of this isotope are the γ-component and the less stable sulphide-form, in which it is available.

Operative Procedure

For operation we used the modified stereotactic apparatus of Riechert and Mundinger [10], which was provided by our group with a new carbon fibre fixation-system. It enables us to perform a CT-scan without artifacts, with the stereotactic frame fixed to the patient's skull, and to calculate the coordinates of any target point directly from transversal CT-sections (Fig. 1 a). This system will be described elsewhere.

For choosing the safest stereotactic approach, the tumour-outlines are reconstructed using a special computer-program from the transversal CT-sections, magnified to the stereotactic x-ray distortion and transferred to the operative x-ray films by superimposition [cf. 11]. The definitive route for the puncture is chosen according to the individual pattern of the intracranial vessels, which is assessed by intraoperative stereotactic serial-angiography (Fig. 1 b). Thus the risks of causing a haemorrhage or any injury to the optic nerves is minimized.

In order to avoid leakage of the cyst fluid, fine probes [2, 3] have to be used. Penetration of ventricles should be avoided. After puncturing the centre of the cyst, the exact volume is assessed by use of a radio-dilution method (mixing the cyst fluid with colloidal Technetium-99) and compared with the cyst-volume calculated from the CT-scan.

Thus, both leakage and communications with other cysts can be detected. The activity to be injected (200 Gy to the inner surface of the cyst) is calculated by use of the formula of Loevinger et al. [8].

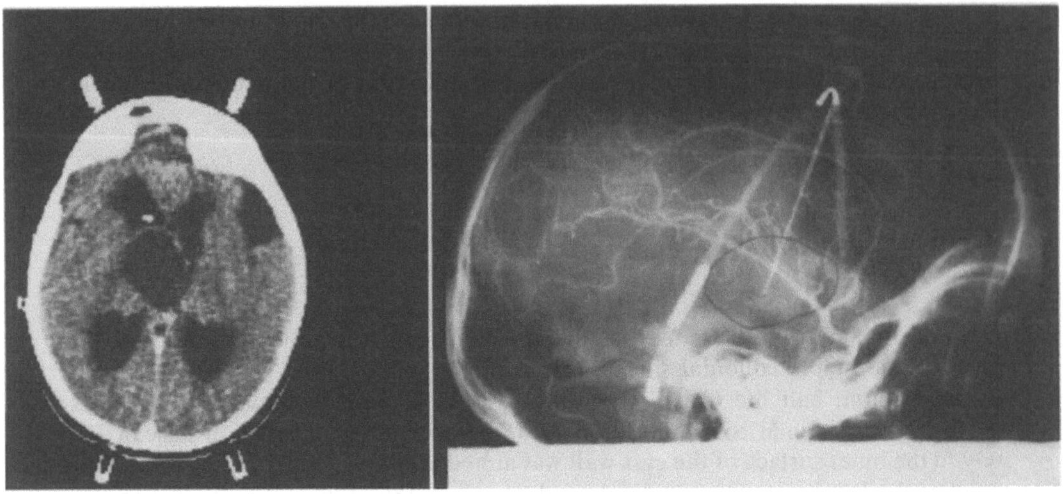

a b

Fig. 1. Localization of the target-point within a tumour from horizontal CT-scan (left panel). Note the white dots representing steel wires in plexiglas sheets. They are fixed to the stereotactic frame and give x, y and z coordinates of target-points. Stereotactic approach, chosen according to the intra-operative serial angiograms and the outlines of the tumour, which are transferred from computer-calculated longitudinal CT-sections to the stereotactic angiographic film (right panel). The stereotactic probe has reached the target-point within the cyst

In order to achieve proper irradiation of all parts of the cyst wall and to avoid dangerous rapid decompression, the volume of the cyst is not significantly reduced during operation and the first 12 days. i.e. 4–5 half life periods, after operation. If there is a hypersecretion during the period of irradiation, after 4–5 half life periods partial evacuation is performed by re-puncture.

The distribution of the radiocolloids within the cysts and possible leakage to CSF are assessed by intra- and postoperative gamma-camera investigations.

Results

In all cases the growth of the cysts could be stopped by the treatment. During the postoperative weeks or few months a gradual progressive shrinkage of the cysts up to complete disappearence could be observed in most cases, resulting sometimes in impressive clinical improvement. A typical example is given in Fig. 2.

There was no operative mortality. Four patients died during the first two years after operation, two of them from reasons not related to tumour growth or treatment, one patient died ten months after operation from thrombo-embolism, caused by a venous catheter, which was implanted because of a hyperosmolar state. One patient with an extremely large solid and polycystic lesion who was treated by both Yttrium instillation and percutaneous irradiation died nine months after irradiation from unknown causes, possibly from radiation necrosis.

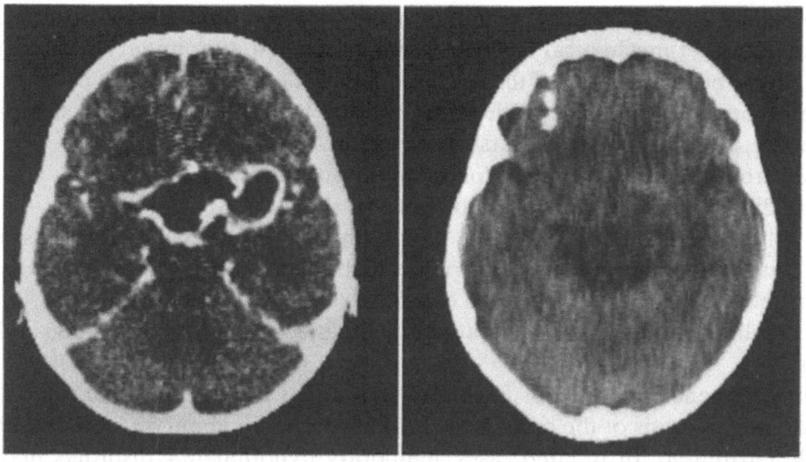

a b

Fig. 2. Typical course following intracavitary Yttrium-90 treatment. Horizontal CT-section through a craniopharyngioma, consisting of two communicating cysts before (left panel), and two years after, treatment (right panel). The contact irradiation has caused complete disappearance of the tumour

There was one refilling of the cyst six months after Yttrium instillation, which necessitated additional treatment with Rhenium-186. In this case with pre-existing severe atrophy of the optic nerves, the refilling of the cyst after initial shrinkage caused a further decrease in visual acuity and temporary hypothalamic symptoms.

In one case, nine months after Yttrium-90 treatment, which had led to considerable shrinkage of the cyst, the visual acuity which had been severely reduced preoperatively deteriorated completely. The remaining tumour was totally removed by a transfrontal operation. No living tumour tissue was found on histological examination.

Discussion

In our series of 25 patients the growth of the craniopharyngioma cysts stopped in all cases after treatment. In most cases a gradual shrinkage of the cysts could be observed during the following weeks or months, up to a total disappearance.

There was no operative mortality. Two patients died from disease and/or treatment (one of them ten months after the Yttrium treatment from thrombo-embolism which occurred during treatment of a hyperosmolar state), the other one nine months after combined intracavitary and percutaneous irradiation, possibly from radiation necrosis. Both patients were aged 50–60 years and were in a very poor clinical condition pre-operatively. The treatment produced considerable shrinkage of their tumours and impressive temporary clinical improvement.

There were two patients with permanent side effects, both from injury to the optic nerves, which had been severely compromised by pressure from the tumour before the operation. In one of them, radiation necrosis of the optic nerves occurred and in the other case a mechanical factor (refilling of the cyst after initial shrinkage) is thought to have been the cause of the further deterioration of visual acuity.

Because of the slow shrinkage of the cysts and the benign nature of the stereotactic procedure, the postoperative course was extremely mild.

It is clear, from the limited time of follow-up in our series, that no definite conclusions regarding the value of this procedure can be drawn.

On the other hand, our results agree well with the results of the Karolinska group [2, 3], who have had 16 years experience with more than 100 patients. They are also corroborated by Szikla (personal communication 1981) and Mori et al. [9], who report excellent results after cyst treatment with injections of Rhenium-186 and Phosphorus-31.

Our own experience and that of Backlund shows that the only specific side-effects are radiation necrosis of the optic nerves, which occurs in about 5% of the cases treated with Yttrium-90. In isolated cases, temporary hypothalamic disorders may occur. It might be expected, that the incidence of radiation damage to the optic nerves could be reduced, if Rhenium-186 is used in cases with pre-existing severe optic atrophy. From our limited data, the results of Backlund [2, 3] and the comparison with the results of conventional therapy (cf. Introduction) we conclude, that stereotactic intracavitary irradiation is a highly effective method with comparatively low risks, by which destruction of the cystic epithelium and sparing of the peritumoural tissue can be achieved.

References

1. Amacher, A. L.: Craniopharyngioma: The controversy regarding radiotherapy. Child's Brain *6,* 57–64 (1980)
2. Backlund, E. O., Johansson, L., Sarby, B.: Studies on craniopharyngiomas. II. Treatment by stereotaxis and radiosurgery. Acta Chir. Scand. *138,* 749–759 (1972)
3. Backlund, E. O.: Studies on craniopharyngiomas. III. Stereotaxis treatment with intracystic Yttrium-90. Acta Chir. Scand. *139,* 237–247 (1973)
4. Ghatak, N. R., Hirano, H., Zimmermann, M.: Ultrastructure of a craniopharyngioma. Cancer *27,* 1465 (1971)
5. Humphreys, R. P., Hoffmann, H. J., Hendrick, E. B.: A long-term postoperative follow-up in craniopharyngiomas. Child's Brain *5,* 530–539 (1979)
6. Kramer, S., Southard, M., Mansfield, C. M.: Radiotherapy in the management of craniopharyngiomas. Further experiences and late results. Amer. J. Roentgen. *103,* 44–52 (1968)
7. Leksell, L., Backlund, E. O., Johansson, L.: Treatment of craniopharyngiomas. Acta Chir. Scand. *133,* 345–350 (1967)
8. Loevringer, R., Japha, E. M., Brownell, G. L. In: Hine and Brownell (eds.), Radiation Dosimetry. New York: Academic Press 1956
9. Mori, K., Handa, H., Murata, T., Takeuchi, J., Miwa, S., Osaka, K.: Results of treatment for craniopharyngioma. Child's Brain *6,* 303–312 (1980)
10. Riechert, T., Mundinger, F.: Beschreibung und Anwendung eines Zielgerätes für stereotaktische Hirnoperationen (II. Modell). Acta Neurochir. Suppl. *3,* 308–337 (1955)
11. Schlegel, W., Scharfenberg, H., Sturm, V., Penzholz, H., Lorenz, W. J.: Direct visualization of intracranial tumours in stereotactic and angiographic films by computer calculation of longitudinal CT-sections: A new method for stereotactic localization of tumour outlines. Acta Neurochir. *58,* 27–35 (1981)
12. Shapiro, K., Till, K., Grant, D. N.: Craniopharyngiomas in childhood. A rational approach to treatment. J. Neurosurg. *50,* 617–623 (1979)

Radiosurgery in Intracranial Tumours and Arteriovenous Malformations in Children

L. STEINER

Radiosurgery in Leksell's definition is the focusing of a radiation energy on a limited intracranial target without opening the skull [17].

The concentration of a high necrotising single dose of radiation on the target, without damaging the surrounding brain tissue may be achieved by using stereotactic localisation and a field of radiation with steep dose gradients.

The new method was thought to replace the needle electrode of the open stereotactic technique and to make possible the treatment of functional diseases (e.g. Parkinsonism, intractable pain, psychiatric disorders) without the risk of haemorrhage or infection.

The first clinical application of radiosurgery was made with low-energy x-ray [20] and proton beams [15]. However, clinical and technical reasons led finally to the use of gamma beams and a Gamma Unit was built at the Karolinska Hospital. With this prototype small disc-shaped brain lesions could be produced, appropriate for thalamotomies [10, 21, 29]. Nevertheless, as soon as the work with the Gamma Unit started, the initial scope proved narrow and new fields had to be explored. Backlund started to irradiate tumours in the pineal region, pituitary tumours and craniopharyngiomas. Leksell started to treat acoustic neurinomas. Rähn treated Cushing's disease and Steiner started the use of radiosurgery in arteriovenous malformations (AVM) of the brain.

For the radiation of tumours and arteriovenous malformations the small disc-shaped lesions were not adequate. To obtain larger fields of radiation, spherical in shape, a new Gamma Unit (Unit II) with cylindrical apertures and wider distribution of the radioactive sources was built.

The Co-60 Gamma Unit

The Gamma Unit was devised by Leksell [18]. Sarby and Larsson [16] and Dahlin et al. [9] carried out the radiophysical measurements and computing.

In Fig. 1 a schematic drawing illustrating a section through the Gamma Unit is given. From 179 shielded ^{60}Co sources the narrow beams are radially directed by means of a collimator system towards the target point positioned in the centre of a collimator helmet. This is attached to the operating table. The table is moved in and out of the spherical body of the Unit by a remote controlled hydraulic system. The collimator helmets containing the diaphragms that define the geometric cross sec-

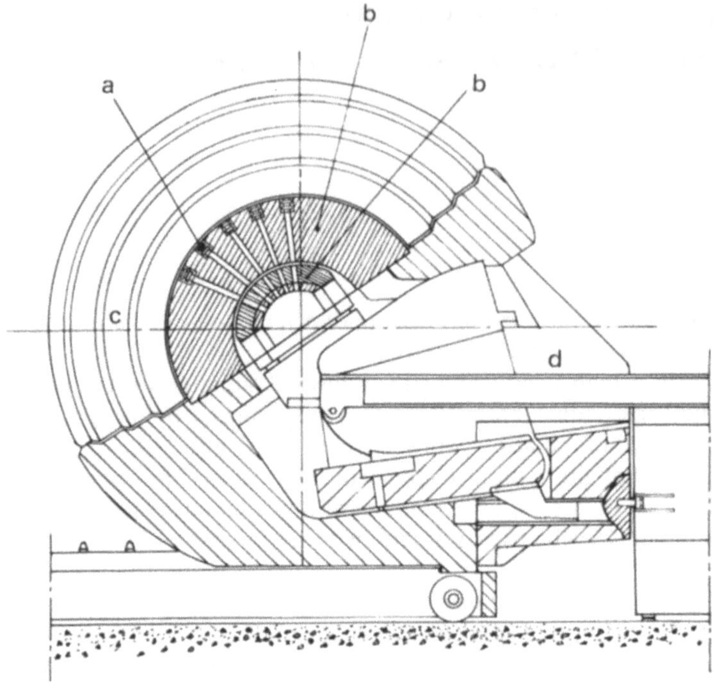

Fig. 1. Section of the Gamma unit: *a* Co-60 beam source, *b* collimator helmets, *c* shielded body, *d* operating table

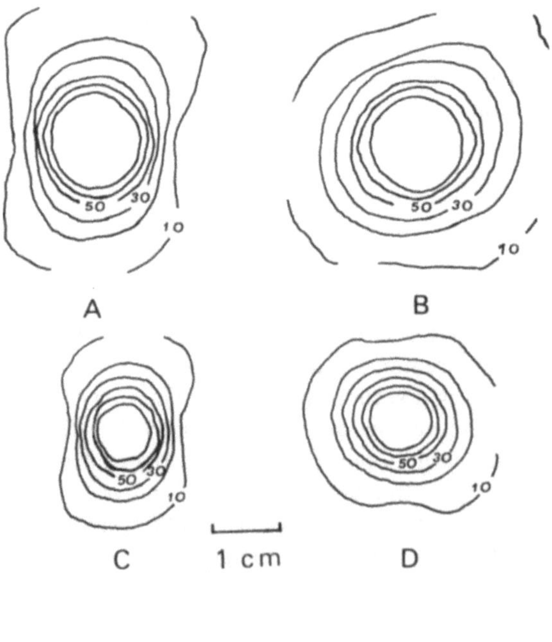

Fig. 2. Dose distribution. Lateral (*A, C*) and frontal (*B, D*) views obtained with the collimator 14 mm (*above*) and 8 mm (*below*)

tion of the beams are interchangeable. Thus with Unit I cross sections of the beams of 3 mm×5 mm or 3 mm×7 mm at the centre can be obtained, while the cross sections of the beams with Unit II are 4 mm, 8 mm or 14 mm in diameter. The available radiation fields range from a disc-shaped volume of 3×6×8 mm to roughly 10×16×18 mm corresponding to the 50 per cent isodose level. By plugging the collimator channel of any of the 179 sources, the shape of the summated dose distribution around the target area can be altered and in this way critical structures (i.e. optic pathways, oculomotor nerves, hypothalamus, brain stem) may be protected.

The radiation doses given in the text represent the dose at the stereotactic target point and the relative isodose levels are expressed as a percentage of this target dose.

The Radiosurgical Procedure

The procedure includes the following steps:

1) The stereotactic coordinate frame is fixed on a plastic shell moulded around the patient's head or a circular metal frame provided with coordinate scales is fixed directly to the skull.
2) The visualization of the target or of reference structures is obtained by stereotactic plain x-rays, stereotactic angiography or stereotactic computed tomography (CT) [6, 7, 11].
3) The determination of X, Y and Z coordinates [6].
4) The values obtained for the X and Y coordinates determine the place of two metal bearings for the axis rods of the collimator helmet. The bearings are secured to the plastic shell or to the scales of the metal frame.
5) The head of the patient is positioned in the collimator helmet according to the Z coordinate.
6) The table with the patient is moved into the apparatus and the radiation starts.

Results in Tumours and Arteriovenous Malformations

We report here the clinical experience gained in the treatment of intracranial tumours and AVM with special reference to paediatric material.

Tumours of the Pineal Region

This summary is based on Backlund's material [4].

If well delineated and of appropriate size, the tumours of the pineal region may be irradiated with good results. Stereotactic fine needle biopsy secures usually the histologic diagnosis and the tumour is treated according to the diagnosis: if benign

Table 1. Radiosurgery in tumours in the pineal region in children

Patient	Age	Sex	Histology	Tumour Diameter cm	Target Dose Gy	Follow-up (years)	Results
1	13	F	Pineocytoma	2	50	12	Good
2	7	M	Pineocytoma	1	40	11	Good
3	12	M	Pineocytoma	2.5	20	4	Good
4	7	M	Medulloblastoma	3	50	2	Died
5	9	F	Astrocytoma GR II	2	50	1	Good

by radiosurgery, if malignant by radiotherapy. Shunt insertion is often required before or after radiation.

Table 1 summarizes the results after radiosurgery in 13 cases, among them five children with tumours in the pineal region.

The average tumour diameter varied between one and three cm. Target doses of 20–50 Gy were given in children. The average observation time of these children is 6 years. One of the cases with an astrocytom Grade II had a one year follow-up. The tumour was no longer visible on CT at that time and the boy was in excellent condition. Unfortunately, he lived abroad and the follow-ups were not continued. One patient with medulloblastoma died two years after the treatment. The remaining three children were in good condition at the time of the last follow-up.

Craniopharyngiomas

Lately more and more neurosurgeons seem to adopt an eclectic approach in the management of craniopharyngiomas. Frequent unsatisfactory surgical results and the development of alternative therapeutic methods lead to a choice of radical microsurgical exstirpation, limited operation combined with additional radiotherapy [35, 37] or intracystic treatment with radiocolloid and radiosurgery [5].

Backlund [1] published the results in eleven patients where a solid part of the craniopharyngioma was treated by radiosurgery and his experience may be summarized as follows.

Intracystic treatment with radiocolloid solves most of the problems met with in cystic craniopharyngiomas. Nevertheless, the solid portion of the tumour cannot be neglected. It may grow in size and it represents a substrate for cyst development. Stereotactic radiosurgery appears as an appealing alternative to radiotherapy permitting precision irradiation of the tumour exclusively.

The eleven cases where solid tumour components required radiosurgery represented about 15 per cent of all craniopharyngiomas treated in ten years. Four of the irradiated patients were children.

The diagnosis was usually verified by biopsy either during previous open operation or most often by stereotactic technique. In the cases where a cystic component existed, radiosurgery was given to the solid portion only after the treatment and

Table 2. Radiosurgery in craniopharyngiomas in children

Patient	Age	Sex	Gross Anatomy	Dose Gy	Results
1	15	M	Cyst + solid part	20	Good
2	13	F	Cyst + solid part	30	Good except right sided amaurosis[a]
3	9	F	Solid part	50	Good
4	8	M	Solid part	30	Good

[a] The patient had a previous operation and her visual acuity on the right side at the time of the irradiation was 02 – 03

shrinkage of the cyst by intracystic radiocolloid Y-90. No part of the tumour received doses under 2–3 Gy. The average follow-up time was four years.

The details of the patients and of their treatment are given in Table 2.

Cushing's Disease

The material concerning radiosurgery in Cushing's disease is borrowed from the Ph. D. thesis of Rähn [25].

In patients with pituitary dependent Cushing's syndrome, a small adenoma of the anterior pituitary lobe is generally considered as the cause of the symptoms [37]. The results following conventional irradiation of the pituitary in Cushing's disease proved unsatisfactory in a significant number of patients [23]. Irradiation with proton beams [14, 16], pituitary implants [8] with steeper dose gradients, higher doses and better dose distributions led to an increased rate of success. The work of Backlund et al. [3], Thorén et al. [36] and Rähn et al. [24] proved that with the radiosurgical method selective destruction of small spatially well-defined volumes of tissue in the sella turcica is feasible. Thus the premises for a selective radiosurgical obliteration of microadenomas were created. Rähn treated 17 patients with Cushing's disease, among them five children. See Table 3.

Rähn found that the predilection site of the ACTH-producing adenoma seems to be the mid-anterior part of the adenohypophysis. He contends that complete clinical remission can be obtained after radiosurgery if the radiological examination permits a correct choice of the target area. A single dose dexamethasone suppression test usually showed that the previously moderate or failing suppressibility was more pronounced after treatment. When the suppression test was followed by ACTH-stimulation, a pre-operative increased cortisol secretion changed to a normal rise in plasma cortisol after the ACTH administration. The basal plasma cortisol levels used to be within normal range after treatment. In one case a subnormal level was found and replacement therapy with cortisol was used. A normal secretion of the other pituitary hormones was usually seen. No side effects from the treatment were encountered. The observation time ranged between two and three years.

Clinical remission occurred in all the five irradiated children and no one presented hormonal deficiencies after the treatment.

Table 3. Radiosurgery in Cushing's disease in children

Patient	Age at treatment (years)	Dose (Gy)	Results	Follow-up time	Complications
1	13	70	Remission 3 years		0
	16	60	Then new gamma lesion in adjacent area 6 months ago, not followed-up yet		
2	13	70	Remission	2 years	0
3	11	60	Remission	2 years	0
4	9	60	Remission	3½ years	GH-insuff. (substituted)
5	5½	50	Remission	2½years	0

Rähn assumes that a single radiation dose of 70 Gy in adults and 60 Gy in children is an optimal dose in patients with Cushing disease.

Arteriovenous Malformations (Fig. 3)

It is now generally agreed that vessels are sensitive to ionizing radiation. The alterations in vessel walls occur shortly after the radiation and continue for years as a reactive reparative process. Proliferation of the endothelial cells and of the subendothelial connective tissue is characteristic for the late periods. Even proliferation of medial elements and collagen deposition have been described. The changes are progressive and may lead to obliteration of the vascular lumen. There is enough evidence to contend that the often described difference between small and large vessels as regards obliteration is only apparent. It may be explained by the difference in lumen size, and in the long term the large vessels may also be occluded.

Radiotherapy in AVM has been used as a last resort since 1914 [22]. Since the details of treatment were usually lacking in the publications on this subject, it is meaningless to speculate on the reasons for the overwhelming failures which discredited the method. Johnson's material [12, 13] indicated, however, that radiotherapy in AVM should be reassessed.

Radiosurgery for the treatment of a cerebral AVM was used for the first time in March 1970. Results of the study in progress have been published [27, 28, 30, 31] or will appear in the near future [32, 33, 34].

Fig. 3. Vertebral angiography, frontal (**a**) and lateral (**d**) views. AVM located on the medial surface of the occipital lobe close to the tentorial notch fed by branches from the posterior cerebral artery and drained through the great vein of Galen to the straight sinus. The dose distribution completely covers the cluster of pathological vessels. The periphery of the AVM is included in the 30 per cent isodose curve (**b, e**). Vertebral angiography, frontal (**c**) and lateral (**f**) views one year after the treatment. No filling of the malformation

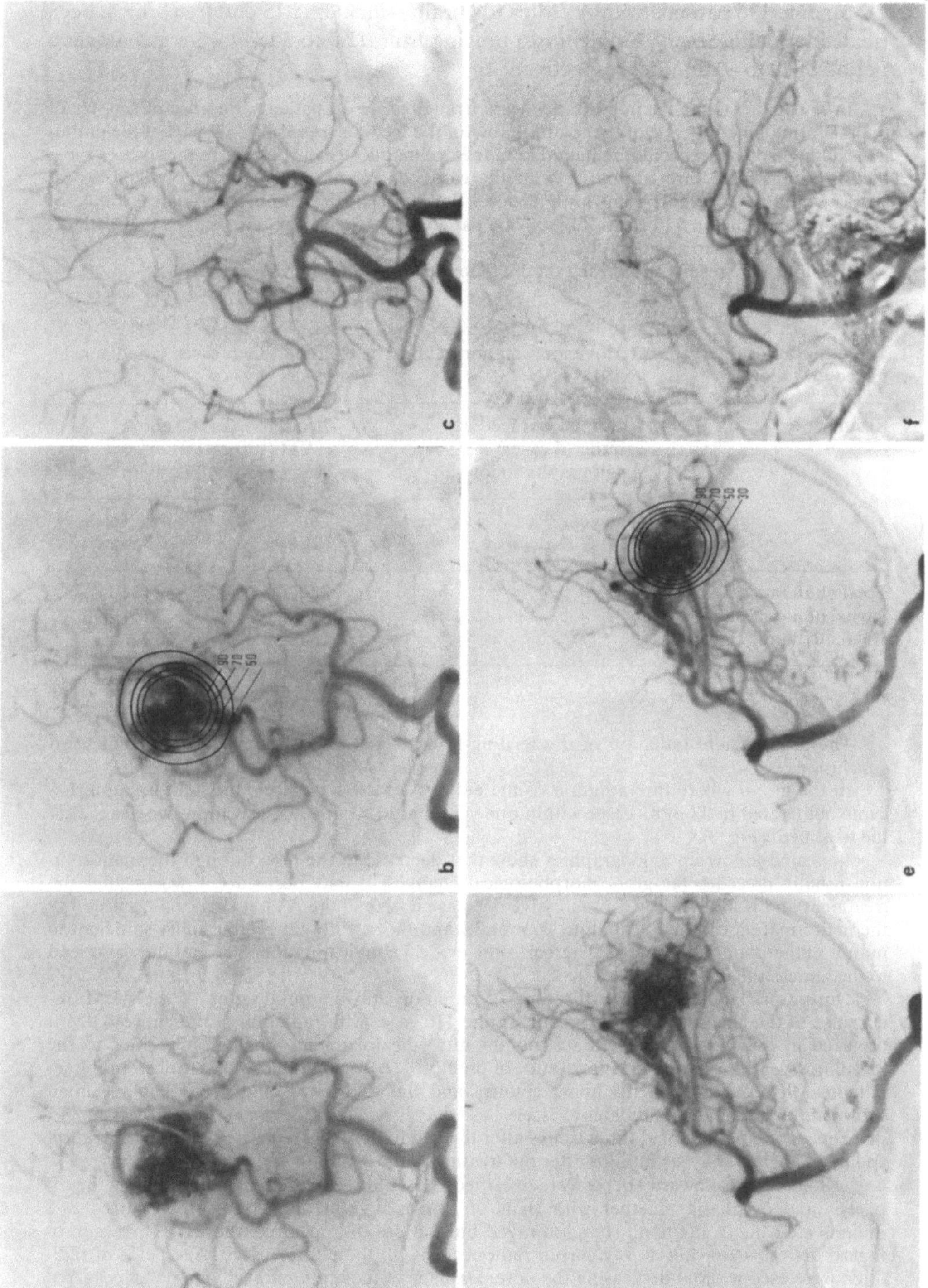
3a
b
90
70
50
c
d
e
90
70
50
30
f

To date 136 patients with AVM of the brain – including 15 children – have been treated by radiosurgery. Single doses ranging from 12.5 to 30 Gy were given over a period of 20 to 40 minutes respectively.

In four patients the feeding arteries were irradiated. In 20 patients, because of the size of the malformation, only one of the total number of the feeding vessels or only part of the pathological tangle of vessels could be included in the optimal dose distribution. In these cases satisfactory results were rare compared with the cases where the entire cluster of pathological vessels could be covered by an optimal dose. Radiation of the entire pathological tangle of vessels was possible in 110 cases. Eighty-one patients have had their one year and 63 patients their 2 years follow-up angiography.

In Table 4 the results as assessed on the follow-up angiographies are presented.

Table 4. Radiosurgery in arteriovenous malformations in children. Two cases could not be traced for follow-up

Results	Irradiation of feeding arteries (4 cases) Angiography follow-up		Irradiation of the entire AVM (110 cases) Angiography follow-up	
	One year	Two years	One year (81 cases)	Two years (63 cases)
Total obliteration		1	32 (39.5%)	53 (84.1%)
Partial obliteration			33 (40.7%)	7 (11.1%)
Haemodynamic changes	1		16 (19.7%)	3 (4.7%)

The group where radiation of the feeding arteries was carried out is too small for valid conclusions.

In the group where the radiation of the entire AVM was possible, the malformation became obliterated in 32 of 81 cases within one year and in 53 of 63 cases within two years after the treatment (Fig. 3).

Repeated follow-up angiographies show that decrease in the flow through the malformation usually precedes the gross morphological changes. It may occur a few weeks after the treatment and is followed by a progressive decrease in size of the AVM. The total occlusion of the malformation can take from 6 to 24 months and more. Fifty Gy were usually sufficient to induce obliteration of the AVM. There is some evidence indicating that 30 Krad may also lead to the same results.

During the latency between the time of radiation and the obliteration of the AVM, recurrence of the haemorrhage may occur. In the 110 cases with radiation of the entire AVM it occurred in two cases. One bled six months after the treatment. Angiography prior to the bleeding revealed a partial disappearance of the AVM. After the rebleed an intracerebral haematoma was evacuated in his home country and the AVM was extirpated. The specimen showed both obliterated and patent vessels.

The second patient bled three weeks after the irradiation. She recovered without operation and in an angiography six months after the treatment, the AVM no longer filled.

In four cases untoward effects were observed [31]. In three of them hemianaesthesia, hemiparesis and dysphasia together with signs of increased intracranial pressure occurred 3–8 months after the irradiation. They improved but did not disappear completely. These neurological deficits were caused by delayed radionecrosis. In these three cases large fields of radiation were used without decreasing the dose. Damage in the brain parenchyma never occurred when only one radiation field with collimators up to 14 mm in diameter, was used and single target doses of 30–50 Gy were given over 20–30 minutes.

In the fourth case no changes suggesting delayed radionecrosis could be seen on a computed tomography done when a hemianopia occurred after the radiation of an occipital AVM in a 52-year-old woman. On the follow-up angiography one year after the treatment the AVM was obliterated. Additionally, delayed and incomplete filling of peripheral branches supplying the medial portion of the occipital lobe could be seen and we assumed that this was the cause of the hemianopia.

Conclusion

Radiosurgery is used in the Department of Neurosurgery, Karolinska Hospital, for the treatment of e.g. AVM, craniopharyngiomas, pituitary tumours, pinealomas, acoustic neurinomas, meningiomas, retinoblastomas and glomus tumours. In the management of some of these diseases the method has already acquired an established place. Its value in the treatment of some of them still remains to be investigated.

References

1. Backlund, E. O.: Solid craniopharyngiomas treated by stereotactic radiosurgery, 271–281, in Stereotactic Cerebral Irradiation. Editor Szikla, G. Elsevier, North-Holland Biomedical Press 1979
2. Backlund, E. O.: Treatment of craniopharyngiomas, a 10 year material, 1966–1975. Proc. 6th Int. Congr. Neurol. Surg., Sao Paulo 1979
3. Backlund, E. O., Rähn, T., Sarby, B., de Schryver, A., Wennerstrand, J.: Closed stereotaxic hypophysectomy by means of ^{60}Co gamma radiation. Acta Radiol. (Ther. Phys. Biol.) *11,* 545–555 (1972)
4. Backlund, E. O., Rähn, T., Sarby, B.: Treatment of pinealomas by stereotaxic radiation surgery. Acta Radiol. (Ther. Phys. Biol.) *13,* 368–376 (1974)
5. Backlund, E. O.: Stereotaktisk Behandling av Kraniofaryngeom med intracystiskt Y-90 och Extern Co-60-Bestrålning. Thesis. Stockholm 1972
6. Bergström, M., Greitz, T., Steiner, L.: An approach to stereotaxic radiography. Acta Neurochirurgica *54,* 157–165 (1980)
7. Bergström, J., Greitz, T.: Stereotaxic computed tomography. Amer. J. Roentgenol. *127,* 167–170 (1976)
8. Burke, C. W., Fraser, R., Joplin, G. F., Doyle, F. H., Mac Erlaine, D. M.: Cushing's disease treated by pituitary implant. Clin. Sci. *44*: 5 P passion (1973)
9. Dahlin, H., Rossander, K., Svedberg, J.: On the selection of dose distribution in clinical cerebral radiosurgery. Proc. 9th Symposium Neuroradiologicum. Gothenburg 1970
10. Forster, D. M. C., Meyerson, B. A., Leksell, L., Steiner, L.: Stereotaxic radiosurgery in intractable pain. In: Pain, pp. 194–198 (Janzen, R., ed.). London: G. Thieme 1972
11. Greitz, T., Bergström, M., Boethius, J., Kingsley, D., Ribbe, T.: Head fixation system for integration of radiodiagnostic and therapeutic procedures. Neuroradiology *19,* 1–6 (1980)
12. Johnson, R. T.: Surgery of intracerebral haemorrhage. In Recent advances in neurology and neuropsychiatry, pp. 102–128. London: Churchill 1969
13. Johnson, R. T.: Radiotherapy of cerebral angiomas. With a note on some problems in diagnosis. Cerebral angiomas – advances in diagnosis and therapy. Springer Verlag, 256–258 (1975)
14. Kjellberg, R. N., Kliman, B.: A system for therapy of pituitary tumours. In: Diagnosis and treatment of pituitary tumours, pp. 234–252. Eds. Kohler, P. O., Ross, G. T., Amsterdam: Excerpta Medica 1973

15. Larsson, B., Leksell, L., Rexed, B., Sourander, P., Mair, W., Andersson, B.: The high-energy proton beam as a neurosurgical tool. Nature *182,* 1222 (1958)
16. Lawrence, J. H., Tobias, C. A., Linfoot, J. A., Born, J. L., Chong, C. Y.: Heavy particle therapy in acromegaly and Cushing's disease. J.A.M.A. *235,* 2307–2310 (1976)
17. Leksell, L.: The stereotaxic method and radiosurgery of the brain. Acta Chir. Scand. *102,* 316–319 (1951)
18. Leksell, L.: Stereotaxis and radiosurgery – an operative system. Springfield, Ill.: Ch. C. Thomas 1971
19. Leksell, L.: A note on the treatment of acoustic tumours. Acta Chir. Scand. *137,* 763–765 (1971)
20. Leksell, L., Herner, T., Lidén, K.: Stereotaxic radiosurgery of the brain. Report of a case. Kungl. Fysiogr. Sällsk. Lund Förhandl. *25,* 1–10 (1955)
21. Leksell, L., Cerebral radiosurgery, gamma thalamotomy in two cases of intractable pain. Acta Chir. Scand. *134,* 585–595 (1968)
22. Magnus, V.: Bidrag till hjernchirurgiens klinik og resultater. 138 pp. Kristiania: Merkur 1921
23. Orth, D. N., Liddle, G. W.: Results of treatment in 108 patients with Cushing's syndrome. N. Engl. J. Med., *285,* 243–247 (1971)
24. Rähn, T., Thoren, M., Hall, K., Backlund, E. O.: Stereotactic radiosurgery in Cushing's disease. Acute radiation effects. Surgical Neurology. in press (1980)
25. Rähn, T.: Stereotactic radiosurgery in Cushing's disease. Thesis. Sundt Offset, Stockholm 1980
26. Sarby, B., Larsson, B.: Fysikaliska experiment rörande förutsättningar för användning av smala gammastrålar vid cerebral strålkirurgi. Report from the Gustaf Werner Institute, Uppsala, Sweden 1965
27. Steiner, L., Leksell, L., Greitz, T., Forster, D. M. C., Backlund, E. O.: Stereotaxic radiosurgery for cerebral arteriovenous malformations. Report of a case. Acta Chir. Scand. *138,* 459–464 (1972)
28. Steiner, L., Leksell, L., Forster, D. M. C., Greitz, T., Backlund, E.-O.: Stereotactic radiosurgery in intracranial arteriovenous malformations. Acta Neurochir. (Wien) Suppl. *21,* 195–209 (1974)
29. Steiner, L., Forster, D., Leksell, L., Meyerson, B. A., Boethius, J.: Gammathalamotomy in Intractable Pain. Acta Neurochirurgica *52,* 173–184 (1980)
30. Steiner, L., Greitz, T., Leksell, L., Norén, G., Rähn, T., Backlund, E.-O.: Radiosurgery in intracranial arteriovenous malformations. II: A follow-up study. In Neurological Surgery, pp. 168–180. Eds. Carrea, R., Le Vay, D., Amsterdam-Oxford: Excerpta Medica 1977
31. Steiner, L., Greitz, T., Backlund, E.-O., Leksell, L., Norén, G., Rähn, T.: Radiosurgery in arteriovenous malformations of the brain. In Stereotactic Cerebral Irradiation pp. 257–269. Ed. Szikla, G., Elsevier, North-Holland Biomedical Press 1979
32. Steiner L.: Radiosurgery in arteriovenous malformations of the brain. In: Textbook of Cerebro-vascular Surgery. Eds. Flamm, E., Fein. New York, Berlin, Heidelberg: J. Springer. To appear 1982
33. Steiner, L.: The place of radiosurgery in the treatment of arteriovenous malformations of the brain. In: Symposium on arteriovenous malformations. Barcelona, Dec. 1980. Ed. Isamat, F. Acta Neurochirurgica. To appear 1982
34. Steiner, L.: Treatment of the intracranial arteriovenous malformations by radiosurgery. In "Intracranial Arteriovenous Malformations" in the Series Current Neurosurgical Practice. Eds. Wilson, Ch. B., Stein, B
35. Thompson, I. L. et al: Int. J. Radiation Oncology Biol. Phys. *4,* 1059–1063 (1978)
36. Thorén, M., Rähn, T., Hall, K., Backlund, E.-O.: Treatment of pituitary dependent Cushing's syndrome with closed stereotactic radiosurgery by means of ^{60}Co gamma radiation. Acta Endocrinol. *88,* 7–17 (1978)
37. Wilson, C. B., Tyrell, J. B., Fitzgerald, P.: Cushing's disease revisited. Am. J. Surg., *138,* 77–79 (1979)

Radiation Therapy in the Treatment of the Astrocytomas and Midline Tumours of Childhood

M. HERBST

Prior to the publication by WHO of the "Histological Typing of Tumours of the Central Nervous System" by Zülch in 1979 [17], both clinicians and pathologists were using a variety of different terminologies. Zülch listed five different readily differentiable astrocytomas (astrocytic tumours), together with a number of subtypes. Worthy of special mention is the pilocytic astrocytoma, which is also met with in the literature under the name juvenile astrocytoma. This tumour, which histologically resembles a spongioblastoma, is a slowly growing neoplasm, often located in the posterior cranial fossa. It can be completely removed surgically, and is considered to be not very sensitive to radiation [6, 10, 14]. However, Marsa et al. [13] report good long-term results from radiotherapy in such tumours located in the optic chiasm, the third ventricle, the hypothalamus and the cerebellum.

In Great Britain, the incidence of childhood tumours is 90.5 in one million children [14], of which 20% are gliomas. The incidence of astrocytomas and midbrain tumours is correspondingly low – Arendt quotes an incidence of childhood astrocytomas of 5% in 503 post-mortem and surgical speecimens [17]. If this low rate of incidence be correlated with the possibilities of histological classification, it proves difficult, when considering the various types of astrocytoma, to assess a particular treatment retrospectively, and even more so prospectively. Table 1 summarizes a

Table 1. Brain tumours: Reported cases of astrocytoma and midline tumours in childhood

	No.	Adult	Child	Astro-cytoma	Mid-line tumours
Fazekas [8]	68	41	27	27	
Camins et al. [6]	126	70	56		56
Hünig et al. [10]	63	–	63	10	
Bouchard [4]	119	–	119	16	14
Burr et al. [5]	72	–	72	38	47
Abramson et al. [1]	136	–	136	35	24
Lindgren [12]	53	–	53	6	
Salazar et al. [15]	148	124	24	24	
Sheline [16]	21	–	21	21	
Leibel et al. [11]	122	84	38	36	2
Marsa et al. [13]	37	37		16	6
Marsden and Steward [14]	318		318	124	112

number of publications which present data on childhood astrocytomas. Here, too, the numbers of cases with astrocytoma and midbrain tumours are small. Not all the reports list the midbrain tumours separately.

Pathology

Childhood astrocytomas behave in the same way as those seen in adults with respect to malignancy, growth and clinical picture, so that the latter can be included in any assessment of the results of treatment [4]. In the figures quoted by Fazekas et al., Camins et al., Salazar et al. and Leibel, childhood astrocytomas and midline tumours are reported separately from the astrocytomas in adults.

The majority of astrocytomas in adults are supratentorial, only 20% to 25% being infratentorial in position [1, 4]. In children this correlation varies, depending upon age. Arendt et al. [3] carried out a more detailed differentiation and, on the basis of their post-mortem material, state that up to the age of ten the infratentorial tumours predominate over the supratentorial growths while, thereafter the reverse is true.

Table 2. Sites of astrocytoma

Cerebellum
Midbrain
Cerebrum
Brain stem
Optic chiasm

In Table 2, the various sites of astrocytomas are indicated in decreasing order of incidence. Astrocytomas of the cerebral hemispheres are most frequently located in the frontal lobe and, according to Bouchard [4], diffusely growing astrocytomas in the temporal lobe. In this region, these infiltrating growths often extend beyond the midline – a fact that must be taken into account for postoperative radiotherapy. If the selected target volumes are too small, the whole of the tumour might not be irradiated. On the basis of his post-mortem material, Concannon [7] was able to show that in only two out of 21 cases had the entire tumour been included in the volume of tissue irradiated.

Cerebellar astrocytomas only rarely present as an infiltrating growth and they can usually be completely extirpated surgically. They have the best prognosis of all the astrocytomas as regards long-term survival [4, 6, 9, 11, 13, 14, 15].

Midbrain tumours, together with the tumours of the brain stem and the optic chiasma, form a special group. The distribution of brain tumours affecting this region in childhood, can be seen in Fig. 1. Here, a wide range of different types of tumour can be met with. Both Burr and Camins [5, 6] report a predominance of the astrocytomas (see Table 3).

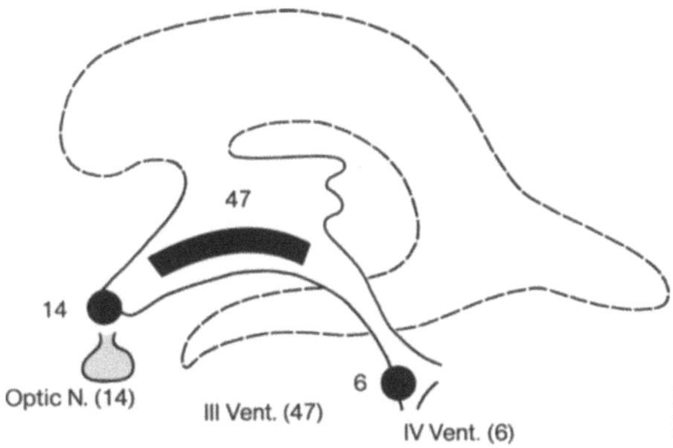

Fig. 1. Anatomical distribution of midline tumours. (After Burr et al. [5])

Tumours of the third ventricle have a special place, not so much on the basis of their histology, but rather on account of their growth and the resulting clinical symptoms.

Tumours in the posterior part of the third ventricle can block the flow of CSF, thus giving rise to an increase in intracranial pressure, nausea, papilloedema and atrophy of the optic nerve. In contrast, tumours of the anterior part of the ventricle rapidly lead to nystagmus and only later give rise to optic nerve atrophy and other ophthalmological symptoms.

A further reason for the special importance of tumours of the third ventricle is the fact that they are difficult to deal with surgically. In this region, numerous vital structures are found, so that total extirpation of a tumour is only rarely possible. In the majority of cases, the resection has to remain subtotal, or frequently serves

Table 3. The most important histological types of third ventricle tumour (Burr [7] and Camins [10])

Tumour	No. of patients	
	Burr	Camins
Astrocytoma	37	21
Astroblastoma	5	2
Mixed astrocytoma/oligodendroglioma	1	
Mixed astrocytoma/spongioblastoma	1	
Mixed astrocytoma/ganglioneuroma		1
Spongioblastoma	5	1
Ependymoma	2	5
Ganglioglioma/Ganglioneuroma	1	2
Pineal tumours		
Pinealoma		8
Teratoma		10
Ectopic pinealoma		3

merely as a decompression procedure involving the insertion of a drain. Improved microsurgical techniques will make more frequent tumour resection possible, but, in the last resort, will not entirely resolve the problem of treatment.

Indications for Radiotherapy

Before radiotherapy is started, the diagnosis must be clearly established unequivocally, either surgically or, at least, radiologically.

Astrocytomas of the cerebellum are readily accessible and, since they are only rarely infiltrating, can usually be completely extirpated. The radiotherapist, however, needs information from the surgeon and pathologist as to how radical was the operative intervention. If tumour extirpation has been complete, no further therapy is required. If, however, excision was only partial – which, fortunately, is not usually the case – post-operative irradiation is indicated. This also applies to astrocytomas of the cerebral hemispheres. In the cerebrum, however, astrocytoma growth is predominantly of an infiltrative nature, and this is often difficult to assess from the gross appearance. According to Bouchard and Fazekas, about one third of these tumours are completely resectable, while the remaining two-thirds permit only a subtotal operation. Tumours of the midbrain do not need to be differentiated to the same extent. Only rarely can they be completely removed [5]. Even a partial tumour resection leads to high complication rates. This is the reason why Bouchard and Camins recommend curative radiotherapy after an earlier exclusively shunting operation with the removal of biopsy material.

Radiotherapy Technique

For the radiotherapeutic treatment of brain tumours of childhood, two aspects should always be taken into account:

1) The higher the total dose, the greater is the probability of destroying the tumour.

2) The dose must be seen in relation to possible late injury of healthy tissue. In this respect, special consideration should be given to growth disturbances and interference with mental development, particularly since the child's brain appears to be more sensitive to radiation than the adults.

Astrocytomas of low-grade malignancy do not metastasize. Accordingly, irradiation of the whole brain or of the cerebrospinal axis is not necessary. Local irradiation of the tumour volume with an adequate treatment margin suffices. Pendulum therapy is least injurious to healthy tissue structures. The question as to whether the "pendulum volume" irradiated suffices to include the whole of the tumourous growth, or whether the target volume would be better included with the aid of a multi-field technique employing wedge filters, or by opposing lateral fields, must be decided from case to case. In the presence of extensive tumours of the cerebral hemispheres, a three-field technique with the additional use of wedge filters is recommended. The total dose should lie between 45 and 60 Gy. According to Leibel, of four children given doses of 3,500 rad none survived for five years. Furthermore, at doses of between 35 and 45 Gy, no differences in survival rates were observed compared with higher doses [11]. The total dose is fixed according to the age of the child. Below the age of two, children should receive a total dose of less than 50 Gy, while children above this age readily tolerate 55 Gy, or 1650 ret [16]. In exceptional cases, doses of up to 60 Gy might be necessary to achieve the destruction of the tumour. Under megavolt conditions, fractionation is 5×2 Gy per week.

The good tolerance of electron therapy by healthy brain structures may be mentioned. Hünig et al. [10] reported that doses of between 1,700 and 2,000 ret of electrons having an energy of 25 MeV and more, were tolerated without any clinically manifest brain damage.

Results of Treatment

Despite numerous publications to the contrary, the value of radiotherapy in the treatment of astrocytomas with a low degree of malignancy (I and II), has not yet been generally recognized. Two reasons might be mentioned for this:

1) Small numbers of cases do not permit large-scale comparisons.

2) Frequently, the patient material is not clearly defined with regard to extension, site and grading of the astrocytomas, the extent of the primary and secondary treatment and the correlation of survival rates among the various therapy groups.

Table 4 provides an summary of the results of treatment obtained by various investigators.

In a retrospective analysis, Fazekas makes a comparison between cases subjected to operation alone, and those who had operation and subsequent radiotherapy. Both groups contain both totally and subtotally removed tumours. The five and ten-year survival rates were 54% and 26% in the irradiated group, and 32% for both five-year and ten-year survival in the non-irradiated group. Similar survival rates are quoted by Marsa et al., and Salazar et al. These latter are somewhat more favourable than those quoted by Bouchard and Leibel.

If the completely resected tumours are examined separately, we find a five-year survival rate of 90% and, in a series reported by Leibel, 100% after 5, 10 and 20 years. In contrast, in the Manchester Group [14], after operation alone, 70%–80% survived for three years. Here, however, only juvenile astrocytomas were involved, while none of the 39 children with adult astrocytomas survived for three years. An additional piece of information was that 20 cases with juvenile astrocytoma were given subsequent radiotherapy; this did not lead to any therapeutic gain in this group.

In the case of midline tumours, the five-year survival rates lie between 40% and 57% [4, 6, 11]. In the report by the Manchester Group, only the three-year survival rate is indicated [14]. Most investigators are of the opinion that, on account of the

Table 4. Summary of survival rates reported by various investigations

		2 years			3 years		
		total Op	subtotal Op+Rt	subtotal Op	total Op	subtotal Op+Rt	subtotal Op
Fazekas [8][a]	Astrocyt.						
	Midbrain						
Camins et al. [6][a]	Astrocyt.						
	Midbrain						
Hünig et al. [10]	Astrocyt.						
	Midbrain						
Bouchard [4]	Astrocyt.						
	Midbrain						
Abramson et al. [1]	Astrocyt.		26 (42)				
	Midbrain		12 (24)				
Lindgren [12]	Astrocyt.						
	Midbrain						
Burr et al. [5]	Astrocyt.					28 (64)	
	Midbrain						
Sheline [16]	Astrocyt.						
	Midbrain						
Leibel et al. [11]	Astrocyt.						
	Midbrain						
Marsa et al. [13]	Astrocyt.						
	Midbrain		4 (6)			1 (6)	
Marsden and Steward [14]	Astrocyt.				88 (117)		
	Midbrain					15 (34)	
Salazar et al. [15][a]	Astrocyt.					20 (37)	
	Midbrain						

[a] Adults included

high rate of postoperative complications, midbrain tumours should be irradiated after preliminary biopsy, shunting or partial resection of the tumour has been performed [4, 5, 6].

Conclusions

Astrocytomas that have been completely removed with a good margin of healthy tissue, and the pilocytic astrocytomas, rarely require postoperative radiotherapy. If, however, a tumour is only partially resected, the five-year survival rate can be doubled by postoperative irradiation [8, 11, 13, 16]. In the case of midbrain tumours, on account of the high postoperative mortality rate, a cautious surgical approach involving shunting and tumour biopsy has now gained general acceptance. Postopera-

5 years			10 years			> 10 years		
total Op	subtotal Op+Rt	subtotal Op	total Op	subtotal Op+Rt	subtotal Op	total Op	subtotal Op+Rt	subtotal Op
20 (22)	13 (32)	2 (15)	5 (22)	9 (32)				
	55 (126)							
	6 (9)			5 (9)			5 (9)	
	1			1				
	12 (16)							
	8 (14)							
	5 (6)			4 (6)				
	18 (21)			16 (21)				
9 (9)	17 (21)	4 (8)	9 (9)	17 (21)	3 (8)	9 (9)	8 (21)	0 (8)
	9 (16)			8 (16)				
	1 (6)			1 (6)				

tively, the patients are then treated exclusively by radiotherapy. The aim of irradiation is the rapid elimination of the neurological symptoms and destruction of the tumour. For this purpose the modern megavolt therapy permitted by linear accelerators, adequate target volumes and doses of up to 60 Gy are to be recommended.

References

1. Abramson, N., Raben, M., Cavanaugh, P. J.: Brain tumours in children. Analysis of 136 cases. Radiology *112,* 669–672 (1974)
2. Arendt, A: Histologisch-diagnostischer Atlas der Geschwülste des Zentralnervensystems und seiner Anhangsgebilde. VEB Gustav-Fischer-Verlag: Jena, 1977
3. Arendt, A., Möller, B.: Hirngeschwülste im Kindesalter. Arch. Geschwulstforsch. *41,* 164–171 (1973)
4. Bouchard, J.: Radiation therapy in brain tumours in children. In: Fletcher, G. H. (ed.): Textbook of Radiotherapy. pp. 482–498. Lea & Febiger: Philadelphia 1980

5. Burr, J. I. M., Slonim, A. E., Danish, R. K., Gadoth, N., Butler, J.: Diencephalic syndrome revisted. J. Pediatr. *88,* 439–444 (1976)
6. Camins, M. B., Schlesinger E. B.: Treatment of tumours of the posterior part of the third ventricle and the pineal region: A long term follow-up. Acta Neurochir. *40,* 131–143 (1978)
7. Concannaon, J., Kramer, S., Berry, R.: The extent of intracranial gliomata at autopsy and its relationship to technique used in radiation therapy of brain tumours. Am. J. Roentgenol. *84,* 99–107 (1960)
8. Fazekas, J. T.: Treatment of grade I and II brain astrocytomas. The role of radiotherapy. Int. J. Rad. Onc. Biol. Phys. *2,* 661–666 (1977)
9. Hendrick, E. B., Hoffmann, H. J., Humphreys, R. P.: Treatment of infratentorial gliomas in childhood. In: Hekmatpanah, J.: Gliomas, Current concepts in biology, diagnosis and therapy. Recent results in cancer research. pp. 102–106. Springer-Verlag; Berlin, Heidelberg, New York: 1975
10. Hünig, R., Walther, E., Sauer, R.: Die Strahlentherapie von ZNS-Tumoren bei Kindern und Jugendlichen. Strahlentherapie *147,* 573–597 (1974)
11. Leibel, S. A., Sheline, G. E., Wara, W. M., Boldrey, E. D., Nielson, S. L.: The role of radiation therapy in the treatment of astrocytoma. Cancer *35,* 1551–1557 (1975)
12. Lindgren, M.: Therapie des Gehirns und Rückenmarks bei Kindern. Deutscher Röntgenkongreß 1967, Teil B, Strahlenbehandlung und Strahlenbiologie. Strahlentherapie Sdbde. *66,* 180–189 (1967)
13. Marsa, G. W., Probert, J. C., Rubinstein, L. G., Bagshaw, M. A.: Radiation therapy in the treatment of childhood astrocytic gliomas. Cancer *32,* 646–655 (1973)
14. Marsden, H. B., Steward, J. K.: Tumors in children. Recent results in cancer research. pp. 1–13, 137–193. Springer-Verlag; Berlin, Heidelberg, New York: 1976
15. Salazar, O. M., Rubin, P., McDonald, J. V., Feldstein, M. L.: Patterns of failure in intracranial astrocytomas after irradiation: analysis of dose and field factors. Am J. Roentgenol. *126,*279–292 (1976)
16. Sheline, G. E.: Radiation therapy of primary tumours. Seminars of Oncology *2,* 29–42 (1975)
17. Zülch, K. J.: Histological typing of tumours of the central nervous system. World Health Organization, Geneva, pp. 43–45 (1979)

Radiotherapeutic Principles in the Combined Treatment of CNS Tumours in Children

M. Bamberg and E. Scherer

For more than 50 years radiotherapy has played an important part in the treatment of CNS tumours in adults and children. As early as 1924 post-operative X-irradiation of the tumour region in medulloblastomas obtained better results as compared to those with operation alone. Due to the frequent occurrence of spinal metastases, irradiation was extended to include all the CSF pathways. By means of this systematic prophylactic irradiation a significant improvement of the cure rate was achieved in the following decades through the differential application of certain radiation properties and continually improved radiation techniques [1].

Based on these long term clinical experiences, successful radiotherapy for brain tumours nowadays especially in children, demands an exact knowledge of

1) the tolerance of the healthy surrounding brain tissue. Here it must be considered that these tolerance levels are not only subjected to individual variations but also differ in various regions of the brain. Because of the incomplete maturation process of the human brain, a phase of hypersensitivity towards radiotherapy exists even up to the third year of life.

2) the sensitivity of the various types of tumours to radiation. This is closely related to the growth aggressivity, and the scale stretches from the highly radiosensitive germinomas and medulloblastomas to the less radiosensitive glioblastomas. This differential behaviour towards radiotherapy requires that the dose is adapted to each individual case.

3) the complications, which can arise during treatment. These include those reversible side effects occurring during irradiation, as well as those arising after a period of latency which may lead to possible late effects [7].

In order to achieve favourable effects from the radiation and to avoid complications definite preconditions for successful radiotherapy must be established. These include a temporal dose distribution adapted to the various tumour types, whereby the total dose, the irradiation time and the number of fractions must be optimally adjusted to one another. By changing the fractionation pattern e.g. superfractionation, attempts are currently being made to establish a more effective treatment schedule in adult patients with gliomas, by using several single irradiations daily and therefore leading to a reduction in the total irradiation period [6].

The effectiveness of radiotherapy is also dependent on a homogeneous spatial dose distribution in the tumour volume to be irradiated. For these purposes one selects suitable irradiation properties with appropriate irradiation techniques, as well as irradiation planning procedures, with the aid of CT.

By means of this optimized radiotherapy the prognosis for cure with CNS tumours in children has been significantly enhanced in the last four years. Especially impressive is the improvement for medulloblastomas, where 5-year survival rates of up to 50% have been obtained (Table 1). The prerequisite is the exact carrying out of the sophisticated methods of total CNS irradiation, which should be left to departments of radiotherapy with the appropriate technical and personal equipment [5].

Even better results are seen with tumours of the pineal region. This group of tumours shows numerous different histological forms, of which about 70% are considered radiosensitive (Table 2). Because of the strong tendency to metastasize, whole-brain irradiation is given and has led to an improvement in prognosis compared to irradiation with smaller fields, as shown by the findings of Salazar et al. [9].

Table 1. Survival rates of patients with medulloblastoma after combined treatment by operation and irradiation

Author	Total no. patients	3-year	5-year
Paterson and Farr (1953)	31	54%	40%
Smith et al. (1961)	41	33%	33%
Bloom et al. (1969)	77	35%	32%
Probert et al. (1973)	17	–	27%
Marsa et al. (1975)	28	–	47%
Harisiadis and Chang (1977)	59	60%	40%
Sheline (1977)	8	–	63%
Quest et al. (1978)	16	–	41%
Bamberg et al. (1981)	22	55%	–

Table 2. Tumours of the pineal region

1) Tumours of germ cell origin (germinomas, teratomas)
2) Tumours of the pineal parenchyma (pineocytomas, pineoblastomas)
3) Gliomas (astrocytomas, oligodendrogliomas, ependymomas)
4) Other (lymphoma, metastases, meningiomas, angiomas, pineal cysts, epidermoids)

Table 3. Survival rates of patients with irradiated brain stem tumours

Author	Total no. patients	Dose (Gy.)	5-year rate
Bouchard (1966)	34	50 – 60	29%
Whyte et al. (1969)	61	10 – 60	38%
Urtasun (1972)	21	30 – 45	17%
Marsa et al. (1973)	15	50 – 71	20%
Sheline et al. (1975)	27	40 – 60	41%
Onoyama et al. (1975)	32 (< 15 y.)	50 – 60	13%
Salazar et al. (1977)	13	50 – 60	23%
Littmann et al. (1980)	62 (< 17 y.)	25 – 65	30%
Kim et al. (1980)	44	50 – 60	35%

However, a different pattern is seen with tumours of the brain stem where up to now the survival times, after primary radiotherapy in all age groups, are only slightly improved (Table 3). Because of a high percentage of malignant gliomas and tumours in unfavourable sites local recurrences arise continually and these limit the success of local long-term control after radiotherapy, as with all other brain tumours in children. Thus, interest has centred on the combination with other forms of therapy, which can increase the effectiveness of a particular form of treatment. At present these prerequisites appear to be fulfilled most effectively by radiosensitizing and cytotoxic substances. The increased radioresistance of hypoxic groups of cells in these brain tumours is considered responsible for the occurrence of local recurrences which limit survival. The use of radiosensitizers, which act selectively on hypoxic cells, has opened up new therapeutic possibilities. These are drugs belonging to the nitro-imidazole group of which Metronidazole and Misonidazole are of particular importance clinically [10]. Instead of oxygen these substances are able to sensitize hypoxic, radioresistant cells, thus making them more responsive to radiotherapy. Initial therapeutic success, achieved by Urtasun et al. [12] in the treatment of glioblastoma multiforme, appears to confirm these ideas. In this randomized study, the combination of Metronidazole and irradiation significantly increased the survival time in adult patients compared to radiotherapy alone. Whereas only minor gastrointestinal disorders were observed after administration of Metronidazole, the neurotoxic side-effects produced by Misonidazole limits the single and total doses which can be used. After crossing the blood-brain barrier, both substances are found in the CSF and tumour tissue, in concentrations paralleling those in plasma. The measured plasma levels are closely correlated to the observed sensitizing effect (Fig. 1) [2]. In randomized clinical studies, the efficacy of the more effective

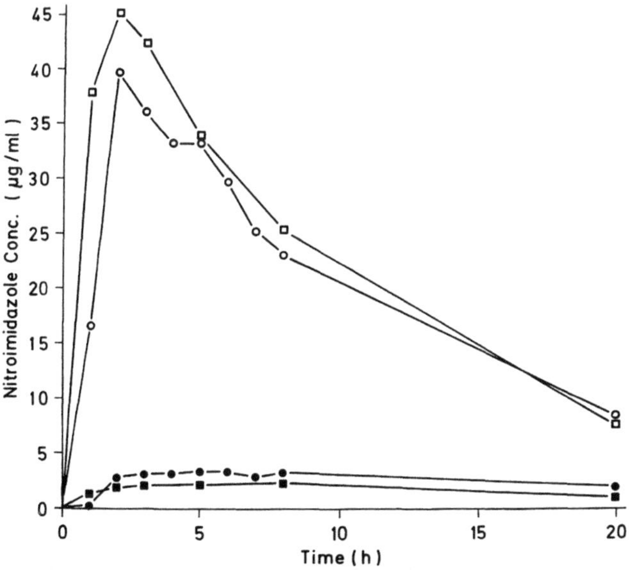

Fig. 1. Plasma misonidazole (○, □) and demethylmisonidazole, Ro-05-9963 (●, ■) in two glioma patients after oral administration of misonidazole at 1 g/m²

Misonidazole in combination with radiotherapy is being tested in adults with highly malignant gliomas. The present results of individual trials show no therapeutic gain either with large single doses of Misonidazole in combination with atypical irradiation fractionation or with the adminstration of numerous small amounts of Misonidazole with conventional fractionation schemes [3, 10]. The latest results of the trial initiated in the FRG in 1978 with malignant gliomas show us no therapeutic gain for the group using the combined techniques [2].

Derivatives of Misonidazole appear to promise more favourable prospects, since they are less toxic, and are stronger radiosensitizing agents. These substances are also of interest in combination with chemotherapy, because recent radiological investigations have shown them to possess strong cytostatic and cytogenetic properties. Misonidazole, given simultaneously or several hours previously, has shown an enhancement of the effect of certain cytotoxic agents e.g. nitroso-ureas [2].

In combining radiotherapy with CSF-penetrating substances, the choice and combination of suitable cytostatic agents as well as the sequence of both forms of therapy play an important role. It thus appears that the adjuvant chemotherapy has not only proved effective in randomized studies with medulloblastomas and ependymomas, but also avoids the enhancement of side-effects occurring during irradiation when given after radiotherapy [4].

Using these two types of tumour as example, an impressive interaction between the effects and side-effects of multimodality treatment is seen, whereby the extended radiation treatment considerably reduces the simultaneous administration of myelotoxic substances. Thus, severe toxic side-effects can result from the simultaneous administration of aggressive combinations of cytostatic drugs with ionizing radiation [11]. Whether or not chemotherapy given before radiotherapy can give new impulses towards improving the treatment of medulloblastomas remains to be evaluated from the current study of the German GPO [8].

In all attempts to achieve new forms of treatment one should remember the warning message from Bloom, one of the main initiators of the SIOP study, that the advances in treatment in the last few years for patients with medulloblastomas should not be jeopardized by the premature use of untried and possibly harmful methods [4]. Hence, one should be careful in reducing the single and total irradiation dose in favour of a chemotherapeutic treatment, since the established effect of a full dose of radiotherapy might be endangered thereby.

Through the use of combined methods there is an increased danger of additive effects on healthy tissues, which could give rise to lasting dangerous effects. It is important to detect these by means of carefully planned long-term investigations.

References

1. Bamberg, M., Schmitt, G., Quast, U., Bongartz, E. B., Nau, H.-E., Bayindir, C., Reinhard, V.: Therapie und Prognose des Medulloblastoms. Strahlentherapie *156,* 1–17 (1980)
2. Bamberg, M., Tamulevicius, P., Streffer, Chr., Scherer, E.: Klinische Erfahrungen mit dem Strahlensensibilisator. Misonidazol. Strahlentherapie *157,* 524–536 (1981)
3. Bleehen, N. M.: Pharmacokinetic and therapeutic studies with misonidazole and desmethylmisonidazole in man. International Conference on the "Chemistry, Pharmacology and Clinical application of nitroimidazole". Cesenatico, Italy, August 27–30, 1980

4. Bloom, H. J. G.: Recent concepts in the conservative treatment of intracranial tumours in children. Acta neurochir. *50,* 103–116 (1979)
5. Bongartz, E. B., Bamberg, M., Nau, H.-E., Schmitt, G., Bayindir, C.: Optimal therapy in medulloblastoma. Acta neurochir. *50,* 117–125 (1979)
6. Bourgeois, J.-P. Le., Schlienger, M., Constans, J.-P., Askienazy, S.: Irradiation concentrée des astrocytomes malins et des glioblastomes. Bulletin du Cancer *64,* 145–150 (1977)
7. Lindgren, M.: Therapie der Tumoren des Gehirns und Rückenmarks bei Kindern. Strahlentherapie Sdbd. *66,* 180–189 (1967)
8. Neidhardt, M. K.: Die Behandlung des Medulloblastoms aus pädiatrisch-onkologischer Sicht. Vortrag auf dem 62. Deutschen Röntgenkongreß, München, 10. April 1981. Strahlentherapie, – in press
9. Salazar, O. M., Castro-Vita, H., Bakos, R. S., Feldstein, M. L., Keller, B., Rubin, P.: Radiation therapy for tumors of the pineal region. Int. J. Radiat. Oncol. Biol. Phys. *5,* 491–499 (1979)
10. Tamulevicius, P., Bamberg, M., Scherer, E., Streffer, C: Misonidazole as a radiosensitizer in the radiotherapy of glioblastomas and oesophageal cancer. Pharmacokinetic and clinical studies. Brit. J. Radiol. *54,* 318–324 (1981)
11. Thomas, P. R. M., Duffner, P. K., Cohen, M. E. et al.: Multimodality therapy for medullobastoma. Cancer *45,* 666–671 (1980)
12. Urtasun, R. C., Band, P., Chapman, J. D., Feldstein, M. L., Mielke, B., Fryer, C.: Radiation and metronidazole for glioblastoma (Letter). New Engl. J. Med. *196,* 757–763 (1975)

Postoperative Chemotherapy Prior to Radiotherapy in the Combined Treatment of Medulloblastoma, Ependymoma and Tumours of the Pineal Region: Early Results

H. J. HABERMALZ, U. STEPHANI, H. RIEHM, and F. HANEFELD

Introduction

Medulloblastoma, ependymoma and tumours of the pineal region occur mainly in children and young adults and tend to spread through the subarachnoid space. If radiation therapy (RT) takes this tendency into account a major part of these tumours can be cured by meticulous technique. Recurrence within the primary tumour is responsible for failure to cure about half of these cases [2, 8, 9]. Therefore to improve the results intensification of treatment of the primary seems to be necessary. Cure rates well above 50% are reported for medulloblastomas in a few small series using diligent surgical technique and precise RT [3, 4, 11]. Comparable results are obtained with additional chemotherapy (ChT) [5, 12]. Besides improving survival rates the combination of operation, RT and ChT should also reduce the undesirable side-effects of RT [5, 7, 10] by reducing the radiation dose.

Our experience and the early results of combined treatment with postoperative ChT prior to RT in brain tumours are presented.

Patients

The study is based on 69 patients with medulloblastoma, ependymoma and tumours of the pineal region treated since 1951 in the departments of Radiology and Paediatrics of the Free University of Berlin. We have excluded three medulloblastomas who died from postoperative complications before adequate RT. The diagnosis of four of the eight tumours of the pineal region was made on clinical grounds and ventriculography. In all other cases histology was obtained from the surgical specimen. Most of the patients were operated in the department of Neurosurgery of the Free University of Berlin, in Charlottenburg.

Among the 69 patients were 35 with medulloblastoma, 26 with ependymoma and eight with tumours of the pineal region. Age and sex distribution are shown in Table 1.

Postoperative treatment was either small volume RT alone to the primary or, later on, a combination of large volume RT with adjuvant ChT.

The treatment of medulloblastoma varied at different times: RT of the primary alone was followed by neuroaxial RT with variable technique and RT with standardised technique (Fig. 1, Table 1). A similar technique was described by Tokars in 1979 [11]. The patient lies in the prone position, the head turned to the side. Brain and upper part of the spinal canal are treated together in a single individually shaped field. After half of the dose the head is turned to the opposite side each day. Another field directed to the rest of the spinal canal is added with changing separations every day. The technique is demonstrated in a case of plexus carcinoma (Fig. 1) using cobalt. As shown in Fig. 2 because of field irregularities different depths and fo-

Table 1. Distribution of age, sex and histology in brain tumours treated since 1951 at the Dept. of Radiology and Paediatrics at the Free University of Berlin

Histology	n	Male/fem.	Age (mean)	
1) Medulloblastoma	35	20/15	0.4 – 49 y	(11.7)
2) Ependymoma	26	16/10	0.5 – 60 y	(24)
3) Tumours of the pineal region	8	6/ 2	8 –36 y	(17.2)
Total	69	42/27	0.4 – 60 y	(16.9)

Table 2. Treatment of medulloblastoma

1) *Radiotherapy – technique*

Period	n	Region irradiated
1951 – 1970	14	posterior fossa
1971 – 1976	9	CNS – variable technique
1976 – 1980	12	CNS – standardised technique
	35	

2) *Radiotherapy – dose*

Region	Dose	Mean dose
Posterior fossa	30 – 55 Gy	46 Gy
Brain	20 – 36 Gy	30.8 Gy
Spinal canal	20 – 36 Gy	27.7 Gy

Fractionation: 5 times 1.5 Gy per week

3) *Adjuvant chemotherapy*

Period	n	
1972 – 1977	9	During and after RT: Dexamethasone, Cyt. – Arab., Ctx, Mtx i. t.
1978 – 1980	7	Prior to RT for 8 weeks: Dexamethasone, Procarb., Mtx i. v. (500 mg/m^2) with CF-Rescue, Mtx i. t. Ver.
	16	

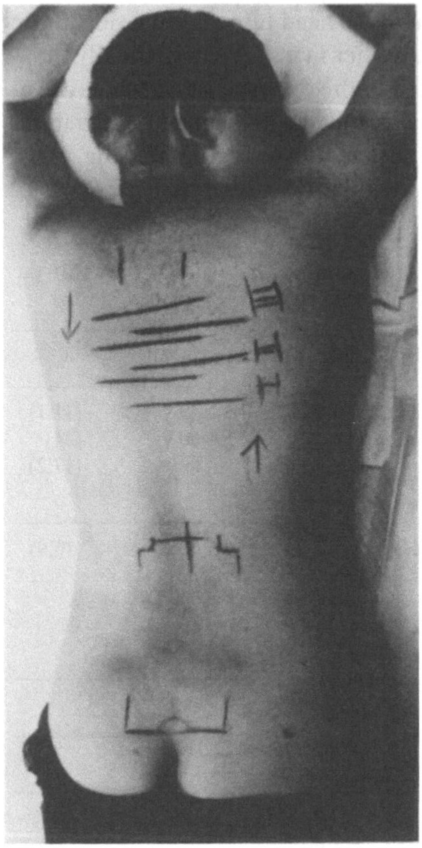

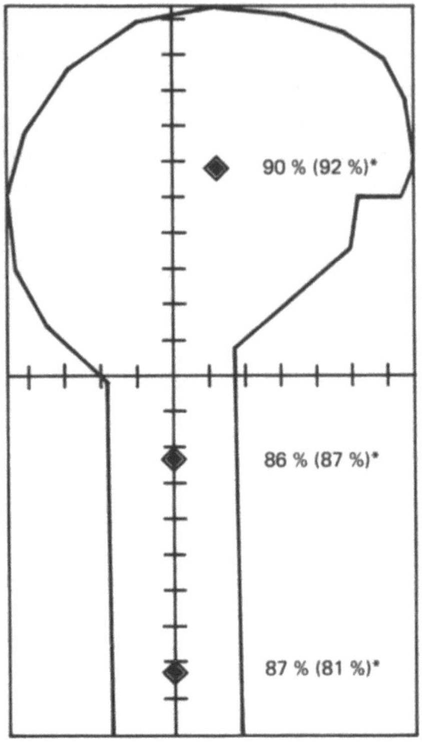

Fig. 2

Fig. 1

Fig. 1. Treatment of whole CNS by a standardized technique with cobalt using large focus-skin distance. Patient is in prone position, with the head turned to the side. Treatment volume and separation between upper and lower field is outlined

Fig. 2. Irradiation of CNS with standardized technique using cobalt. Distribution of depth dose corrected for (1) irregular shape of the field, (2) different depths, (3) different focus-skin distances. 100% = no correction of depth dose; corrected for irregularity of the field only

cus-skin distances, the dose distribution within the field becomes uneven and has to be corrected. The radiation dose given to the posterior fossa and the neuroaxis is shown in Table 2.

Adjuvant ChT in the beginning was administered during and after RT for 4 to 6 months. A combination of Vincristine, Cytoxine, Cytosine-Arabinoside and Methotrexate intrathecally was used, together with Dexamethasone. Cytoxine was omitted later on. Since 1978 ChT was given prior to RT. For a period of eight weeks ChT consisted of Procarbasine and Methotrexate systemically (500 mg/m²) with Citrovorum Factor rescue, Methotrexate intrathecally and oral CCNU (Table 2). Small changes in this combination were made later when it became part of a nation-

Table 3. Treatment of ependymomas

Period	n	Treatment
1953 – 1976	19	Small volume RT Dose 20 – 55 Gy No chemotherapy
1976 – 1981	7	Large volume RT Dose 50 – 60 Gy In 5 pat. ChT prior to RT
	26	

al study of the German Society of Paediatric Oncology. More details are published by Neidhardt et. al. [6].

The treatment of ependymomas is summarized on Table 3. Once again small volume RT alone and large volume RT combined with adjuvant ChT was employed.

Similarly treatment of pineal region tumours was small volume RT in six and combined therapy in two patients.

Results

Of 69 patients 23 are still alive – two with tumour – after five months to 25 years (median 29 month):

2 of 38 after small volume RT alone
21 of 31 after large volume RT combined with ChT
11 of 13 when ChT preceded RT.

Actuarial survival of patients treated for medulloblastoma is shown on Fig. 3. All patients who were radiated only locally died after a median survival time of 18 months. After four years 56% of those with neuroaxis RT are alive and 92% of the patients who received standardized RT technique – again usually combined with ChT.

Of 19 patients with ependymoma 18 died after small volume RT while six of seven patients with large volume RT and ChT are alive after a median observation time of 13 months.

Of six patients with tumours of the pineal region one is alive having received small volume RT. Two patients who were treated with large volume RT ara alive after 19 and 39 months.

ChT during and after RT was complicated by severe bone marrow toxicity. Three children with medulloblastoma died from complication of ChT, one with leuko-encephalopathy, another of cerebral oedema associated with interstitial pneu-

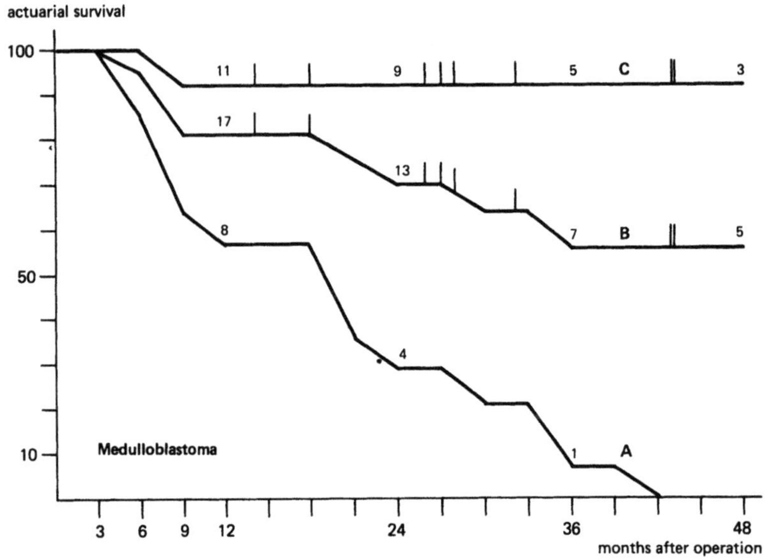

Fig. 3. *A* – Actuarial survival after local irradiation alone (n = 14). *B* – Actuarial survival after neuraxis irradiation, 16 of 21 in combination with chemotherapy (n = 21). *C* – Actuarial survival after standardized neuraxis irradiation, 9 of 12 in combination with chemotherapy (n = 12). The number of patients at risk for the interval is indicated. *Vertical bars* represent living patients at the particular interval after operation

monia and one of bone marrow insufficiency during treatment of recurrent tumour. In another child marginal misdirection of RT in the spinal canal resulted in recurrent tumour and death.

The 13 patients who received ChT prior to RT showed no major complications. Because of leucopenia and thrombocytopenia RT had been interrupted but not for more than a few days. Twice RT was interrupted for three weeks because of haemolytic anaemia and shunt sepsis.

Quality of life has been evaluated without detailed psychological testing (Table 4). Of 23 patients 16 live lifes comparable to that of their peers.

Table 4. Quality of life after combination therapy of medulloblastoma, ependymoma and tumours of the pineal region

1) Not or slightly disabled – quality of life comparable to their peers	16
2) Disabled – active life	5
3) Disabled – needs constant support	2
	23

Median interval since operation 29 months; 17 of 23 were treated with adjuvant Chemotherapy

Discussion

The combination of Methotrexate with high dose CNS – RT can be disastrous for the brain in producing leuko-encephalopathy. According to Bleyer [1] this can be avoided when Methotrexate is given prior to RT provided that CSF circulation is not disturbed. Our own observations support these assumptions.

It seems that by using ChT prior to RT the number of tumour cells can be reduced sufficiently to produce good results with relatively low doses of RT.

To evaluate the results in patients with ependymoma and tumours of the pineal region the number of cases is too small and the observation time too short. The results in medulloblastoma, however, are encouraging and they caused the national study of the German Society of Paediatric Oncology using postoperative combination ChT prior to RT. Early results have just been reported [6].

References

1. Bleyer, W. A., Griffin, T. W.: White matter necrosis, mineralizing microangiopathy and intellectual abilities in survivors of childhood leukemia: Associations with central nervous system irradiation and methotrexate therapy. In: Radiation Damage to the Nervous System edited by H. A. Gilbert, A. R. Kagan, pp. 175–180. New York: Raven Press 1980
2. Bloom, H. J. G.: Medulloblastoma: prognosis and prospects Int. J. Radiat. Oncol. Biol. Phys., *2,* 1031–1033 (1977)
3. Chin, H. W., Maruyama, Y.: Results of radiation treatment of cerebellar medulloblastoma Int. J. Radiat. Oncol. Biol. Phys. *7,* 737–742 (1981)
4. Hardy, D. G., Hope-Stone, H. F., Mc Kenzie, C. G., Scholtz, C. L.: Recurrence of medulloblastoma after homogeneous field radiotherapy J. Neurosurg *49,* 434–440 (1978)
5. Hirsch, J. F., Renier, D., Czernichow, P., Benveniste, L., Pierre-Kahn, A.: Medulloblastoma in childhood. Survival and functional results. Acta Neurochirurgica *48,* 1–15 (1979)
6. Neidhardt, M. K., Hanefeld, F., Henze, G., Langermann, H. J., Riehm, H.: Treatment of medulloblastoma with postoperative chemotherapy before neuroaxis irradiation: An interim progress report on the West Berlin pilot study and the West German cooperative trial (p. 349)
7. Raimondi, A. J., Tomita, T.: The disadvantages of prophylactic whole CNS postoperative radiation therapy of medulloblastoma. In: Multidisciplinary aspects of brain tumor therapy. Edited by Paoletti, P., Walker, M. D., Butti, G., Knetich, R., pp. 209–218, Elsevier/North Holland Biomedical Press, 1979
8. Salazar, O. M., Rubin, P., Bassano, D., Marcial, V. A.: Improved survival of patients with intracranial ependymomas by irradiation: Dose selection and field extension. Cancer *35,* 1563–1573 (1975)
9. Salazar, O. M., Castro-Vita, H., Bakos, R. S., Feldstein, M. L., Keller, B., Rubin, P.: Radiation therapy for tumors of the pineal region. Int. J. Radiat. Oncol. Biol. Phys. *5,* 491–499 (1979)
10. Spunberg, J. J., Chang, C. H., Goldman, M., Auricchio, E., Bell, J. J.: Quality of long-term survival following irradiation for intracranial tumors in children under the age of two. Int. J. Radiat. Oncol. Biol. Phys. *7,* 727–736 (1981)
11. Tokars, R. P., Sutton, H. G., Griem, M. L.: Cerebellar medulloblastoma. Results of a new method of radiation treatment. Cancer *43,* 129–136 (1979)
12. Venes, J. L., McIntosh, S., O'Brien, R. T., Schwartz, A. D.: Chemotherapy as an adjunct to the initial management of cerebral medulloblastomas. J. Neurosurg. *50,* 721–724 (1979)

Radiotherapy of Medulloblastoma: Radiation Technique, Results, and Complications

E. A. Bleher, P. G. Poretti, and P. C. Veraguth

Approximately 15%–20% of all brain tumours in children of less than 15 years of age are medulloblastomas. The tumour develops in close anatomical relation to the fourth ventricle and tends to metastasize early into the cerebrospinal fluid pathways, thereby leading the way for metastases in the entire subarachnoid space, including the skull and the spinal column. Age and sex influence its prognosis, but treatment plays the most important role [12].

Although salvage by surgery alone is only occasionally possible, Norris [9] recently showed an increased survival with more complete resection.

Surgical removal should be followed by radiotherapy. Introduced by Bailey in 1919, it has improved the results in the last 60 years from survival of only a few months to a 70% 5-year survival in selected series [3].

The reason for these improved results was the adaptation of the irradiated volume to the area of tumour spread, inclusion of the ventricular system, the entire skull and the entire spinal column, simultaneous rather than sequential irradiation of all volumes and a sufficiently high dose to the primary tumour as well as to possible subarachnoid metastases. Since the early 1970's further improvements in adjuvant systemic chemotherapy have been sought and achieved. For instance, the therapy-related improvement in survival of patients treated here in Berne correlates with the advances in methods of treatment in the last 20 years (see Fig. 1).

Twenty-one patients were treated between 1959 and 1979. Seven received chemotherapy, consisting in six cases of vincristine, procarbazine and prednisone, within the setting of a cooperative study of the Swiss Paediatric Oncology Group [11]. However, published survival rates differ considerably; 5-year survivals of between 35% and 86% have been noted. Thus, the 3-year survivals of the large cooperative studies of CCSG (Children's Cancer Study Group) and SIOP (Societé Internationale d'Oncology Pédiatrique), with and without chemotherapy, of ca. 63% and 46%, respectively [11], fall short of the 86% 5-year survival of selected patients mentioned by Cumberlin [5]. This may have any of several causes, differences in irradiation technique being primary among them, irrespective of operation, as previously referred to. In the SIOP study the rate of recurrence apparently increased in those radiotherapy departments which contributed fewer than 20 patients [11]. For some time it was assumed that the location of the first relapse was always the posterior fossa, but more refined diagnostic procedures have revealed their incidence in the entire subarachnoid space adjacent to the borders of the radiation volumes [4, 8]. Of interest in this context are such supratentorial recurrences at the cribriform plate caused by shielding of the eyes [6].

Thus, irradiation technique is the central problem in treatment. Its goal is a homogenous daily dose-distribution in the target-volume. The oval vault of the skull and the dose-loss at the borders of the radiation fields necessitate either very large fields which widely overlap the target-volume but which also expose the surrounding healthy tissue to a not inconsiderable dose of radiation, or special shielding which permits an optimal protection of the normal tissue, and, at the same time, a homogenous dose-distribution to the borders of the fields.

Another difficulty arises from extension of the target-volume which encompasses the entire subarachnoid space including S 3. Organs at risk at the borders are the lenses, in very young children the maxillary tooth primordium, the kidneys and the gonads.

In 1953 Paterson and Farr [10] reported a technique with orthovoltage whereby they achieved a 70% three-year survival rate. They irradiated a single posterior portal, including the skull and the entire spinal column and one frontal field of the forehead. We attempted to reproduce this technique with high-voltage equipment, using posterior electrons of 20–25 MeV, depending upon the depth on the spinal column, and sweeping with them horizontally over the total length of the field by moving the equipment table beneath the fixed radiation source. We added a split beam of ^{60}Co and 8 MeV x-rays with a linear accelerator to the forehead, shielding the face with Lipowitz's alloy (thickness 10 cm), thus defining the caudal border of

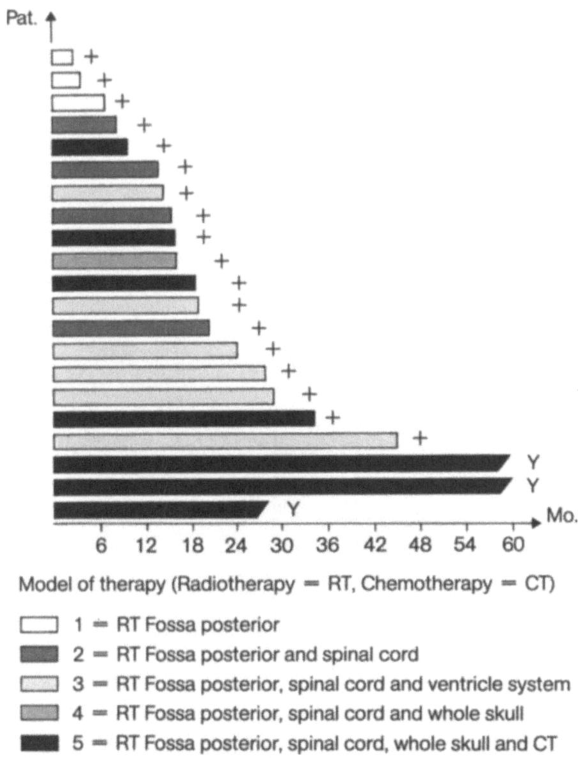

Fig. 1. Survival of 21 patients with medulloblastoma (Dept. of Radiotherapy, Univ. of Berne, 1959–1979)

the field by the centre of the beam. The results, however, were disappointing. Neither a wedge-filter in the splitbeam nor a different weighting enabled us to avoid more than 25% higher daily doses to the posterior fossa than to the rest of the volume. Jones and Innes described a second method in 1957, which today is the generally-approved technique: opposing side fields of the skull and/or more fields from the back to the spinal space. Figures 2a and b show the type of application used in Berne: horizontal translation with an electron beam, as discussed earlier, and at the side opposing fields with ^{60}Co to the skull. These are tilted by 7° toward the cranium corresponding to the 12 divergence angle of the field sizes, to get the matchline parallel to the posteriorly and caudally adjacent electron field. The portals to the skull enclose upper segments of the spinal cord. Blocks of Lipowitz's alloy shield the face and the anterior part of the neck. Critical in this technique is the dose-distribution at the base of the skull caused, for example, by the shielding of the eyes, as well as the tricky problem of junctional dosage. In order to reduce the number of posterior fields, Kuttig [7] recommended a horizontal translation to the spine. To avoid overdosage, the matchlines are moved daily by two vertebrae, alternately, or, as Bamberg [1] pointed out, in four steps, or after 10 Gy each. In practice, the added isodosis of the alternating cobalt-portals and the added isodosis of the alternating

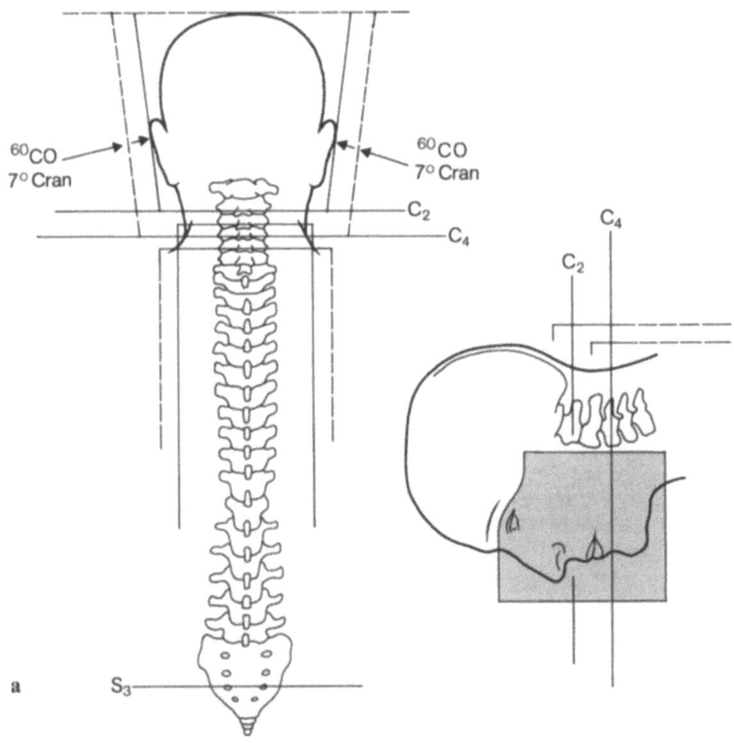

Fig. 2. a Model of supervoltage-radiotherapy according to Jones (1957). Overlapping changes individually in agreement with the optimal dose distribution. **b** Horizontal translation. **c** Isodoses in the junction between the radiation volume to the skull and the volume to the spine. Alternating field arrangement: --- day 1, —— day 2

electron-transversal fields are fitted together in order to get an optimal dose-distribution in the junction (Fig. 2c). Thus, the arrangement of the fields varies a little from patient to patient, which means that the best distribution must be arranged individually for each patient. The calculations have been confirmed by dosimetry with phantoms.

A preliminary requirement for this complicated irradiation is a reproducible fixation of the patient, for example in an individual bed of plaster of Paris.

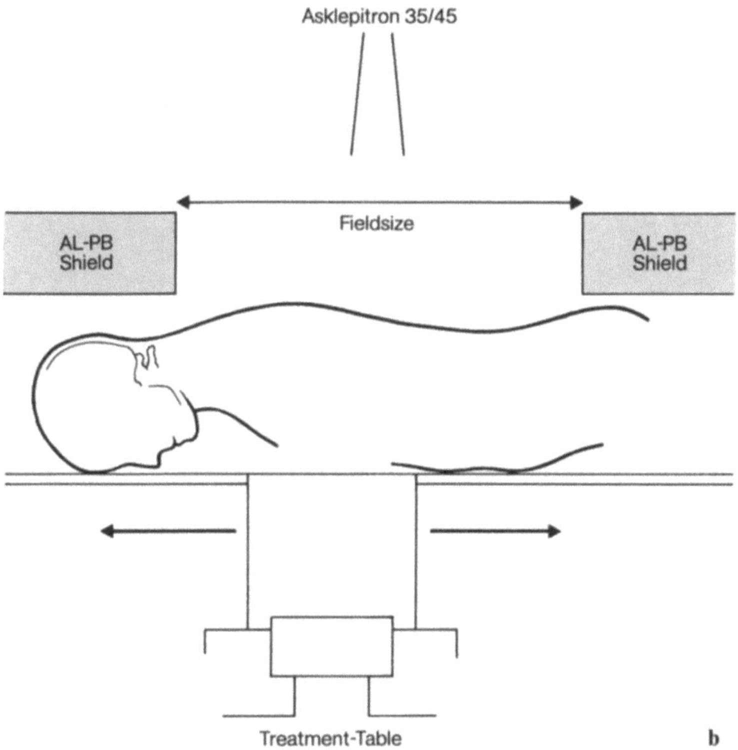

b

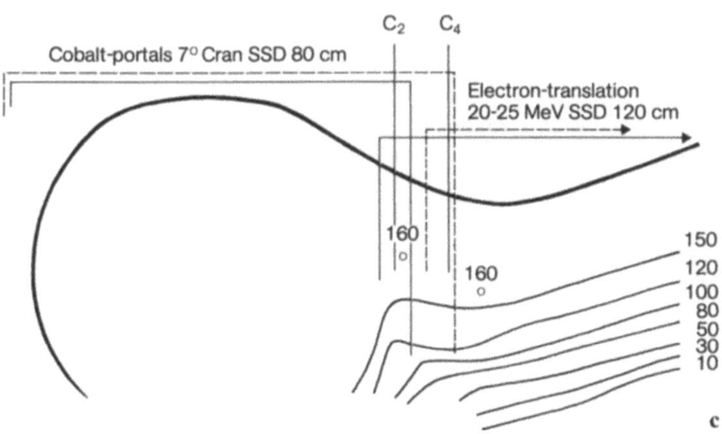

c

There is controversy in the literature as to the definition of a curative dose of radiotherapy. We give 35 Gy to the subdural space and 50–55 Gy to the posterior cranial fossa, and this is then followed by chemotherapy. The boost at the posterior cranial fossa is applied by way of small opposing fields at the two sides of the head. The dose to this area should be reduced by 10 Gy from 50–55 Gy in children of less than two years of age, with daily doses of 1.5 Gy, 5–6 times a week.

Sometimes a radiotherapy-related, long-lasting leucopenia or thrombocytopenia may be observed during treatment, which prevents delivery of the recommended dose within the planned time-span. Accounts of severe late changes, despite longer survival times, appear infrequently in the literature and when they do they usually concern children under two years of age [2]. Inasmuch as both the frequency and severity of the complications, e.g., lowered IQ scores, impairment of learning ability, etc., which follow combined administration of radiotherapy and chemotherapy, are increasing, we are becoming concerned as to the validity of the present concept of treatment.

References

1. Bamberg, M., Schmitt, G., Quast, U., Bongartz, E. B., Nau, H.-E., Bayindir, C., Reinhardt, U.: Therapie und Prognose des Medulloblastoms, Fortschritte durch neuartige Bestrahlungstechniken. Strahlentherapie. *156,* 1–17, (1980)
2. Broadbent, V. A., Barnes, N. D., Wheeler, T. K.: Medulloblastomas in childhood – long-term results of treatment. Cancer *48,* 26–30 (1981)
3. Brown, R. C., Gunderson, L., Plenk, H. P.: Medulloblastoma. A review of the LDS' Hospital experience. Cancer. *40,* 56–60 (1977)
4. Clark, E. E., Haffner, R. S.: Brain scintigraphy in recurrent medulloblastoma. Radiology. *119,* 633–636 (1976)
5. Cumberlin, R. L., Luk, K. H., Wara, W. M., Sheline, G. J., Wilson, Ch. B.: Medulloblastoma. Treatment results and effect on normal tissues. Cancer. *43,* 1014–1020 (1979)
6. Jereb, B., Sundaresan, N., Horten, B., Reid, A., Galicich, J. H.: Supratentorial recurrences in medulloblastoma. Cancer. *47,* 806–809 (1981)
7. Kuttig, H.: Strahlentherapie der Tumoren des Zentralnervensystems im Kindesalter. Strahlentherapie. *147,* 333–343 (1974)
8. Landberg, T. G., Lindgren, M. L., Cavallin-Ståhl, E. K., Svahn-Trapper, G. O., Sundbärg, G., Garwicz, S., Lagergehn, J. A., Gunneson, V. L., Brun, A. E., Cronquist, S. E.: Improvements in the radiotherapy of medulloblastoma 1946–1975. Cancer. *45,* 670–678 (1980)
9. Norris, D., Bruce, D., Byrd, R., Schut, L., Littmann, P., Bilaniuk, L., Zimmermann, R., Copp, R., Rorke, L.: Medulloblastoma (MBL): Improved relapse-free survival time (RST) with modern management. Proc. Am. Soc. Clin. Oncol. *21,* Abs. C-287 (1980)
10. Paterson, E., Farr, R. F.: Cerebellar medulloblastoma: treatment by irradiation of whole central nervous system. Acta Radiol. *39,* 323–336 (1953)
11. Seiler, R. W., Bernasconi, S., Berthold, W., Feldges, A., Imbach, P., Lüthi, A., Plüss, H. J., Vasella, F., Wyss, M., Wagner, H. P.: Adjuvant chemotherapy with procarbazine, vincristine and prednisone for medulloblastomas. Helv. paediat. Acta. *36,* 249–254 (1981)
12. Van Eys, J.: Malignant tumours of the central nervous system. In: Clinical Pediatric Oncology. Sutow, W. W. (ed.), pp. 487–505. St. Louis, Miss.: C. V. Mosby 1977

Report on the Medulloblastoma Study of the Society of Paediatric Oncology – Present Position

M. NEIDHARDT

On the basis of the favourable experiences with postoperative chemotherapy given before radiotherapy in medulloblastomas (cf. pp. 338–343), a committee of the Society for Paediatric Oncology worked out during 1979 a routine of treatment, in children with medulloblastomas, which involved the use of procarbazine and vincristine, and combined treatment with intrathecal and moderately high systemic doses of methotrexate, for a period of 10–12 weeks in the interval between operation and the time of starting radiotherapy.

Since Jan. 1st 1980 this protocol has been used in 40 patients. A further 14 patients with other types of brain tumour were also given the same treatment but they will not be considered here. Five patients were excluded from the study (two on account of later revision of the histological diagnosis and three on account of gross departures from the protocol). In ten patients the follow-up period is less than three months, that is to say they have not yet completed the initial treatment and according to the existing interim assessment they are also excluded. Thus there remain to be assessed 25 patients who were treated in 17 participating centres.

In 15 patients the primary tumour was macroscopically totally removed, in ten patients a residue of tumour, varying in size, but apparent through the microscope or by other magnification. In four patients examination of the CSF for tumour cells was positive.

Up to now two patients have suffered a recurrence (one in the posterior fossa and one in the spine) from which they have died. In a further patient there are urgent clinical symptoms suggesting a recurrence. Two further patients have died and this must be regarded as due to the treatment (one infection with thrush associated with an indwelling central catheter, and one encephalopathy presumably caused by the methotrexate). In the last-named patient there was, in addition, a disturbance of CSF drainage, which constituted a contraindication to methotrexate administration.

In the remaining patients the initial chemotherapy was, on the whole, well tolerated; in eleven patients there were reversible side-effects such as bone marrow depression, inflammation of mucous membranes, rashes, and also nausea and vomiting. In two patients it was necessary to reduce the dosage of the chemotherapy. It was possible in all cases to continue with the radiotherapy with no interruption worth mentioning.

In view of the relatively short follow-up period, it is still too early for an analysis of the survival times in the whole series. Furthermore the late results can only be accurately assessed at a later stage.

Considering it as a whole, we regard this new therapeutic approach as better suited to the embryonal nature of the tumour and, thus, theoretically more promising than radiation on its own. The treatment is in general easily controlled, but needs to be in experienced hands. The number of deaths produced by the treatment must definitely be further reduced. In addition, a randomized control trial with other tried and tested methods of treatment should be arranged.

Data on the Biology of Medulloblastomas

W. Müller, D. Afra, O. Wilcke, F. Slowik, R. Schröder, and M. Kordas

The introduction of the so-called "desmoplastic" phenotype of the medulloblastoma by Rubinstein and Northfield in 1964 [1] produced a lot of problems particularly concerning its biological behaviour. In the following report we attempt to make some contribution to the solution of these problems.

Altogether we have investigated the data from 260 patients. The specimens of the operated tumours where adequate have been reclassified before the analysis of the biological data.

Table 1 shows the tumour site and the distribution in two age groups, the first one comprises the young children and infants from 0 to 15 years and the other one the adults older than 15 years. In this table the well-known fact of the overwhelming localization of the medulloblastoma in the midline of the cerebellum is also confirmed. However, in the group of the adults the number of hemispheric tumours is evidently elevated.

In Table 2 the relationship between the histological type of the medulloblastoma and its location in both age groups is shown. For the sake of clarity only the numbers for the desmoplastic type are indicated. The completion of these numbers to 100% naturally corresponds to the classic type. In the adults we find twice as many of the desmoplastic medulloblastomas as in the childrens group. In the childrens group the distribution of the midline and hemisphere tumours is equal. In the adults a small, but not significant preponderance of the desmoplastic type in the lateral parts of the cerebellum is apparent. Therefore we can state that actually the frequency of the desmoplastic medulloblastoma increases with increased age of the patients. However, no preferential location is evident.

In Table 3 as a further factor the follow-up data are drawn into the analyses. The total number of the series is reduced, because some cases died two months after operation (i.e. operative mortality) and those which could not be observed for longer than two months after the operation have been eliminated. The figure shows a division of this series into four age groups and their average survival time in months. The average values are not indicated as arithmetic media. As usual in biological statistics we prefer the median. Evidently with increase of the patients age the median survival time continuously increases. So in general we can state, that in operated patients the life expectation is obviously closely related to the time of onset of the illness. The influence of the complicated postoperative treatment is not taken into consideration in this study.

The following question concerns the possible influence of the histological type of the medulloblastoma on the survival time in the children and adult groups (Table 4). The analysis in both groups demonstrates the same average survival time not only for the classic but also for the desmoplastic type of medulloblastoma. However, in contrast to the childrens group it is evident, that in the adults the striking prolongation of the survival time is likewise associated with both histological types. However, if the age distribution is ignored, then the desmoplastic type obviously seems to behave much better. Considering the widely different age composition of the both histologically defined series the total groups of all classic and all desmoplastic medulloblastomas are not homogeneous and are therefore not statistically comparable.

The relationship between average survival time and location of the tumour demonstrates in both age groups a nearly identical behaviour on follow-up (Table 5). In the group of the adults corresponding to the expectation the median survival time is two to three times longer than in the children.

Table 1. Localization (n=260)

	Medial	Lateral	
0 – 15 years	85%	15%	(n=204)
> 15 years	61%	39%	(n=56)

Table 2. Desmoplastic type

	All cases	Localization	
		Medial	Lateral
0 – 15 years	11%	12%	10%
> 15 years	22%	20%	27%
Total	14%	13%	18%

Table 3. Average follow-up (n=179)

0 – 5 years	11 months	n=45	n=131
6 – 10 years	15 months	n=64	
11 – 15 years	24 months	n=22	
> 15 years	39 months	n=48	

Table 4. Average follow-up related to histological type (n=179)

	Classic	Desmoplastic
≦ 15 years	13 months (n=114)	14 months (n=17)
> 15 years	39 months (n=37)	39 months (n=11)
All cases	15 months (n=151)	30 months (n=28)

Table 5. Average follow-up related to localization (n = 175)

	Medial	Lateral
≦ 15 years	13 months (n = 108)	15 months (n = 21)
> 15 years	39 months (n = 27)	39 months (n = 19)
All cases	18 months (n = 135)	22 months (n = 40)

In summarizing we come to the conclusion that the desmoplastic medulloblastoma has no preferred location and occurs with nearly the same frequency in the midline and in the hemispheres. In adults it appears approximately twice as often as in children. The significantly better prognosis of the medulloblastoma in adults is correlated neither to a higher frequency of the desmoplastic type nor to a preferred location in the hemispheres. The better prognosis for the adults is obviously dependent on the time of manifestation of the medulloblastoma.

This is finally demonstrated in the curves representing the probability of death (Fig. 1). In contrast to the presentation of the probability of survival the curves show ascending lines not starting at zero, i.e. at the time of operation, but in relation to the operative mortality at the two months mark. The three curves indicate the probability of death of the age groups 0 to 5, 6 to 10 and over 15 years. On account of the small number of cases the group 11 to 15 years is not taken into consideration. Not only the differences of the median probability of death but also the different prog-

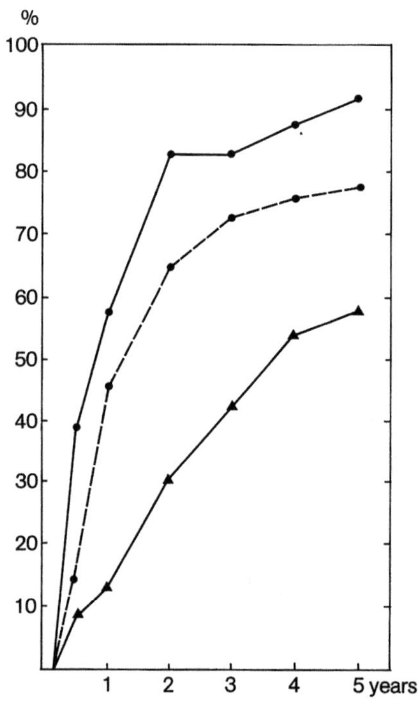

Fig. 1. Probability of death in dependence of time after operation in different age groups. ● 0 – 5 years, ●---● 6–10 years, ▲ > 15 years

ress of the three curves is striking. Thus, after 5 years in the two children groups 92% and 78% respectively and in the adults 58%, are dead.

On the basis of the results of our analysis we consider the desmoplastic type as a histological variant of the medulloblastoma occurring more frequently in adults. This variant does not seem to be connected with a better prognosis than the classic medulloblastoma.

Reference

1. Rubinstein, L. J., Northfield, D. W. C.: The medulloblastoma and the so-called "arachnoidal cerebellar sarcoma". A critical re-examination of a nosological problem. Brain *87*, 379–412 (1964)

Treatment of Meningeal Malignancy with Intrathecal ^{198}Au-Colloid and Methotrexate. The Example of Acute Lymphoblastic Leukaemia (ALL)

O. Metz

^{198}Au-colloid injected intrathecally ascends in the subarachnoid space as far as the cerebral hemispheres (scintigraphic control, Fig. 1) and a small amount of it is absorbed by the arachnoidal granulations. The bulk of the radiogold (90%) is adsorbed and phagocytized by the spinal and arachnoidal tissue (Fig. 2) [1–3, 6–8]. Thus the distribution sites of radiogold and of latent meningeal leukaemia are identical [11, 13]. Distribution, absorption, adhesion and phagocytosis of intrathecally injected radiogold take place only in the first 24 hours after injection. After that the distribution scintigram remains unchanged. One cannot measure the proportion of ^{198}Au-colloid phagocytized by the arachnoid and the proportion which is bound adhesively. Because of the minimal distance between them (capillary cleft) the radiogold radiation from the pia mater and that from the arachnoid membrane will interact. This fact makes an exact calculation impossible [2, 3, 7]. Because of the phagocytized radiogold, the actual arachnoidal dose is probably far above the calculations quoted [11].

In Jena [5], and later on also in other clinics of the GDR [9, 14], we have given colloidal gold-198 and methotrexate intrathecally to 249 children with acute lymphocytic leukaemia as a prophylaxis against meningeal involvement (4 different therapy protocols from 1972 to 1981). Altogether 21 children (8.4%) developed an isolated meningeal leukaemia, and five children (2%) a combined marrow and meningeal relapse. There are marked differences between the various protocols, because, on the one hand, cytostatic therapy has become more aggressive in the last few years, and, on the other hand, radio-gold was given in higher dosage. After an initial pilot study the doses were increased. An outline of the ^{198}Au-activity given for meningosis prophylaxis is given in Table 1. The four protocols show the following results: Table 2. Those are the latest results of a computer analysis extending up to March 31, 1981.

In less than 10% of all children radio-gold treatment caused mild post-punctural complaints. There were headaches (10%), nausea and vomiting (6%) and/or a rise of temperature (5–6%). The complaints did not last longer than 24 hours and did not differ from familiar postpunctural complaints. Apathy-syndromes or leukoencephalopathy did not occur. Computer-tomographic investigations showed that in all children the brain appeared normal after this prophylactic use of ^{198}Au [12]. In cases of bone-marrow and gonad relapses we gave a second prophylactic course of radio-gold with successful results. If the radionuclide was not distributed in the subarachnoidal space (in contrast with cytostatics, distribution of radio-gold can be scintigraphically controlled), we immediately irradiated the brain with telecobalt. It was, however, very rarely that we observed an insufficient distribution of the radio-

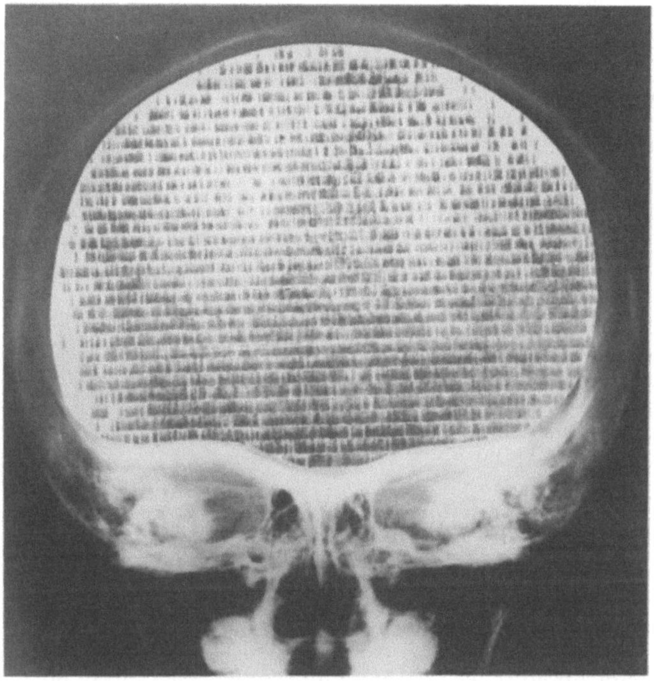

Fig. 1. Cranial scintigram (AP) two days after colloidal gold-198 injection (74.74 MBq = 2.02 mCi per lumbar puncture) and AP X-ray of skull (photo-montage)

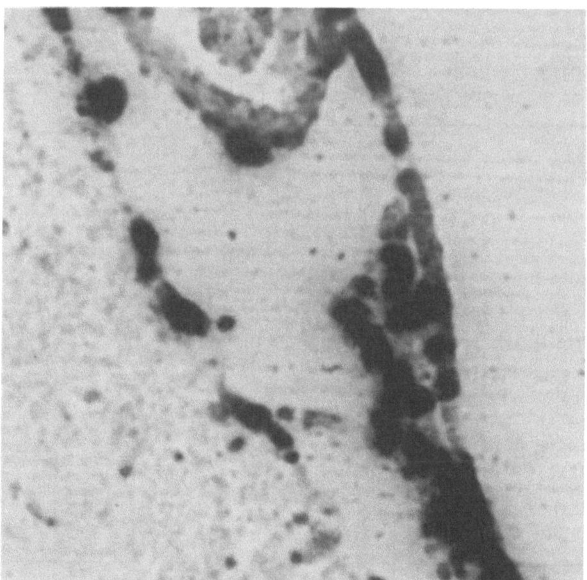

Fig. 2. Autoradiogram of rabbit brain (H. and E., ×600): Colloidal gold-198 (*black blots*) is phagocytized by arachnoidal tissue

Table 1. Activity of intrathecally injected colloidal gold-198. Development since 1972

Period I (1972 – 1975, June)
All patients: ca. 55.5 – 111 MBq[a]

Period II (1975 – 1978, June)

Patients:	2 years age =	37 MBq
	2 – 3 years age =	44.4 – 55.5 MBq
	4 – 12 years age =	74 MBq
	13 – 14 years age =	92.5 MBq
	14 years age =	111MBq

Period III (1978 – 1980, May)

Patients:	2 years age	= 60 MBq
	2 – 3 (4) years age	= 90 MBq
	4 (5) – 10 years age	= 120 MBq
	10 – 14 years age	= 130 MBq
	14 years age	= 150 MBq

Period IV (in Jena only) (since 1980, May)
Patients with ALL-high risk: activity as in period III twice (distance = 2 wks.)

[a] 37 MBq = 1 mCi

nuclide in the cerebral subarachnoid space (7% of all injections). There were no additional complications in the cases of children irradiated after radio-gold.

In several children we used radio-gold for treatment of florid meningeal leukaemia [10]. According to our experience a single injection was enough to clear the fluid of leukaemic involvement. Thus therapeutic CNS-irradiation can already begin after a few days. Unlike CSF clearance by intrathecal cytostatic drugs, radiogold reduces to a single one the number of lumbar punctures necessary and the CSF

Table 2. Results in all ALL therapeutic regimes (1972 – 1981) where intrathecal colloidal gold-198 and methotrexate were given as prophylaxis against meningeal involvement

Protocol (Patients) years	Risk	Bone-marrow relapses (%)	Isolated meningeal relapses (%)
L 3 (53) 1972 – 1976	Standard and high risk	13 + 9[a] (41.5)	5 + 3[a]
L 4 (40) 1976 – 1978	Standard risk	14 + 1[a] (37.5)	2 + 0[a] (5)
L 4 (40) 1976 – 1978	High risk	14 + 0[a] (35)	6 + 0[a] (15)
L 5 (73) 1978 – 1981	Standard risk	8 + 0[a] (11)	3 + 0[a] (4.1)
LSA2L2 (41) 1978 – 1981	High risk	5 + 0[a] (12.1)	2 + 0[a] (4.9)

[a] Sign indicates patients after cessation of ALL-therapy

pathways can be assessed scintigraphically. However, as the cerebral sulci or the perivascular space above the hemispheres are jammed by tumour cells (not at the time of meningosis prophylaxis!), cytostatics and radionuclids cannot act cytotoxically on all leukaemic cells. Colloidal gold-198 has a maximum range of 3.6 mm in tissue (beta rays). That is why a therapeutic irradiation with telecobalt must follow. Cases of meningeal leukaemia occurring after ^{198}Au-colloid can be irradiated with a curative dose. That is no longer possible after meningosis prophylaxis with telecobalt, unless one wishes to risk cerebral lesions.

We have not yet treated children with brain tumours (medulloblastoma, ependymoblastoma) with intrathecal colloidal gold-198 [4].

References

1. Döge, H., Henning, K., Woller, P.: Dosimetrie bei der intrathekalen Radiogoldtherapie. I. Verteilungskinetik. Radiobiol. Radiother. *19,* 219–228 (1978)
2. Döge, H., Henning, K.: Dosimetrie bei der intrathekalen Radiogoldtherapie. II. Quantitative Bestimmung des an der Oberfläche absorbierten 198Au-Kolloids. Radiol. Radiother. *19,* 229–233 (1978)
3. Döge, H., Hliscs, R., Henning, K.: Dosimetrie bei der intrathekalen Radiogoldtherapie. IV. Bestimmung der wirksamen Dosis. Radiobiol. Radioth. *20,* 111–120 (1979)
4. Fuller, L., Rogoff, E., Deck, M., Galicich, I., Ghavimi, F., Levitt, S., Smith, C., d'Angio, G.: Recent experience with intrathecal radiogold for medulloblastoma and ependymoblastoma: a progress report. Amer. J. Roentgenol. *122,* 75–79 (1974)
5. Metz, O., Stoll, W., Plenert, W., Unverricht, A.: Über die Anwendung von kolloidalem Radiogold (198Au) zur Meningosisprophylaxe bei der Leukosebehandlung des Kindesalters. Dtsch. Ges.wesen *28,* 2039–2043 (1973)
6. Metz, O., Stiller, K. I., Stoll, W., Reim, G., Plenert, W.: Verteilung von 198Au-Goldkolloid nach intraventrikulärer und intracisternaler Injektion bei Kaninchen. Radiobiol. Radiother. *16,* 117–123 (1976)
7. Metz, O., Unverricht, A., Walter, W., Stoll, W.: Zur Methodik der Meningosis-Prophylaxe bei Leukämien und Non-Hodgkin-Lymphomen im Kindesalter mit 198-Goldkolloid. Dtsch. Ges.wesen *32,* 67–70 (1977)
8. Metz, O., Stoll, W., Plenert, W.: Meningosis-Prophylaxe mit Radiogold (198Au) bei der Leukämie im Kindesalter. Dtsch. med. Wschr. *102,* 43–46 (1977)
9. Metz, O., Blau, H. J., Weinmann, G., Zastrow, I.: Zum gegenwärtigen Stand der ZNS-Prophylaxe mit 198-Goldkolloid und 60-Telekobalt bei akuten Leukämien und Non-Hodgkin-Lymphomen im Kindesalters. Dtsch. Ges.wesen *31,* 2472–2476 (1976)
10. Metz, O., Stoll, W.: Zur intrathekalen Anwendung von 198Au-Kolloid bei akuten Leukämien und Non-Hodgkin-Lymphomen im Kindesalter. 1. Mitteilung: Therapie der floriden Meningosis neoplastica. Dtsch. Ges.wesen *34,* 1621–1623 (1979)
11. Metz, O., Stoll, W.: Therapieabschluß bei akuter lymphatischer Leukämie im Kindesalter. Langzeitbeobachtungen nach Meningosisprophylaxe mit intrathekalem 198Au-Kolloid und Methotrexat. Dtsch. med. Wschr. *106,* 1026–1029 (1981)
12. Metz, O., Dietrich, I, Plenert, W.: in Vorbereitung.
13. Price, R., Johnson, W.: The central nervous system in childhood leukemia: I. The arachnoid. Cancer *31,* 520–534 (1973)
14. Zastrow, I., Schwartz, K. D., Reddemann, H., Schöneich, R., Griefhahn, B., Suhrbiert, P.: Intrathekale Gold-198-Kolloid-Applikation bei Leukämie und Non-Hodgkin-Lymphomen im Kindesalter. Dtsch. Ges.wesen *34,* 2133–2136 (1979)

Infratentorial Tumours – Treatment and Results in 109 Children

P. GUTJAHR, D. VOTH, J. HEIDFELD, B. WALTHER, J. KUTZNER,
and K. KRETZSCHMAR

Infratentorial neoplasms represent a group of tumours, if topographical aspects are primarily considered. These tumours are *heterogeneous,* however, as regards morphology, treatment and prognosis, as well as partly for aetiology. If clinical data are reported here in summarizing the group of different tumours, the clinical background for this is firstly to demonstrate the *different current methods of treatment,* their effect and importance, and secondly to give an actual standard for treatment and prognosis.

One hundred and nine children with primary infratentorial tumours represent 52% of a total of 213 primary CNS tumours, and these again are 23% of the total of 925 malignant neoplasms in children seen in our institution.

About one half of the children with infratentorial tumours were admitted within the past seven years, the other half were seen in the previous 20 years.

Eleven of the tumours were *pontine* lesions, 38 were *cerebellar astrocytomas,* and 45 were *medulloblastomas;* the remaining 15 were cerebellar ependymomas, haemangioblastomas of the Lindau type, arachnoid sarcomas and some other rare neoplasms. Only the main three types will be discussed here.

Intrapontine lesions were generally not operable, in part or totally. After the diagnosis had been established by ventriculography and/or angiography (during the past years only in part have these investigations been sufficiently replaced by computerized tomography), a shunting procedure was usually performed, mostly as a ventriculocisternal shunt.

After a postoperative interval of about two weeks, this was usually followed by *radiation therapy* (^{60}Co, 45–60 Gy within 5–8 weeks). To this treatment, *chemotherapy* was added following different regimen (Cyclophosphamide alone or in combination with Vincristine, CCNU alone or in combination with Vincristine).

The *disappointing results* of treatment are shown in Fig. 1: 37% of the children survived the first year, and *none the second.* The histology in four children, examined post mortem revealed, grade I astrocytomas and grade III and grade IV tumours as well.

Figure 2 shows the results of treatment of *cerebellar astrocytomas,* 1956–67 (n = 8) and 1968–80 (n = 30).

In general, treatment in both periods was almost exclusively by *operation. Local radiotherapy* (e.g. with 45–55 Gy) was given only in children with *gross residual* tumour after operation. In recent years, this was done in younger children only, when clinical and CT signs clearly proved a *progressive lesion.*

Survival rates after five and ten years, respectively, have *improved* remarkably (although these early results have been affected lately by one death due to a recurrence after 13 years; Fig. 2). Strictly speaking improvement in the results of treatment does not owe much to therapeutic oncologic progress: this improvement results more from *progress in the operation field* (improved techniques including microneurosurgery), and from *improved methods of postoperative paediatric intensive care.*

At present, *five-year and nine-year survival rates of 90%* are our current standard. However, one late death due to recurrent tumour and another due to a traffic accident cannot be left unmentioned.

Thus, the rate of *permanent cures is reduced to at least 77%.* Two of the children currently survive with demonstrable tumour on CT, without clinical signs of progression, however, after three and six years. Cytostatic chemotherapy was *not* instituted, of course, during the past ten years.

Thinking about the late outcome in medulloblastoma some years ago (number of our patients then 30, including early deaths and children not having come to radiation therapy), and comparing our results with comprehensive data from the literature [1], we noted that treatment results did not significantly differ from each other (25% survival versus 20%). We had assumed better results for our own patients, as our analysis referred to the period 20 years prior to 1977, and the survey of McFarland and others [1] summarized the results from an at least partly former and older period (with probably less favourable forms of treatment available). This gave us cause to *analyse our results of medulloblastoma treatment in more detail.*

In our patients, *treatment from 1961–67* was operative; postoperative treatment consisted of local radiotherapy to the posterior fossa; the majority of children then was treated with chemotherapy using a single agent namely cyclophosphamide.

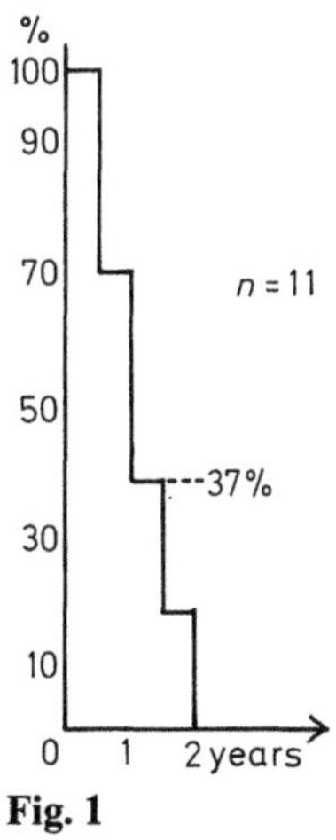

Fig. 1

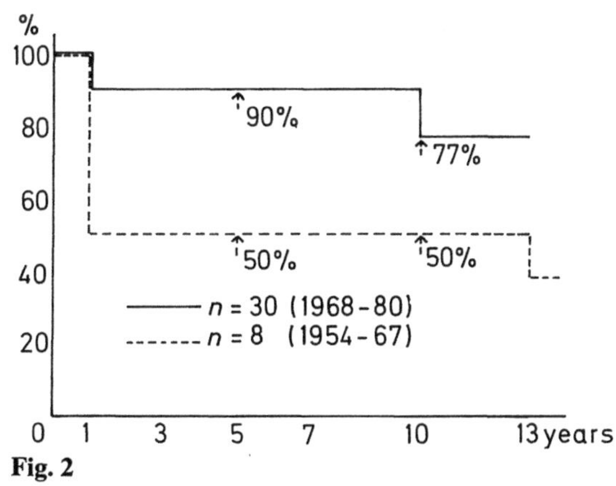

Fig. 2

Fig. 1. Treatment results in children with pontine tumours (n = 11); 1-year survival is 37%, and 2-year survival is 0%, respectively

Fig. 2. Treatment results in children with cerebellar astrocytomas (n = 38). 8 children treated between 1954 and 1967, 30 children treated between 1968 and 1980. 5- and 10-year survival in the first group is 50% and 5- and 9-year survival is 90% in the latter group. Deaths after more than 10 years did occur

During the *second period* (1968–74), *craniospinal irradiation* followed operation, and for chemotherapy we had the use of Cyclophosphamide or Cyclophosphamide plus Vincristine; in most of the cases intrathecal Methotrexate was used during the radiation phase.

In the *third period* (since 1975), operation was no longer ultraradical. Radiotherapy was still craniospinal, with the total doses reduced (35 Gy to whole CNS, 55 Gy to posterior fossa compared with 40 and 60 Gy, respectively, in the previous course of treatment). As for chemotherapy, *CCNU was added* to Vincristine, and Cyclophosphamide was no longer given. Intrathecal Methotrexate was given 6–8 times during the phase of radiation treatment.

The *results* are as follows (Fig. 3): None of the 11 children from the first period survived for more than one year. Concerning the other 34, there is a *5-year survival rate of 36%,* and a 10-year survival rate of 29%. This analysis includes *all* patients and therefore also those, who were early deaths postoperatively and others, who could not be irradiated for other reasons; one death which occurred before treatment is also included.

During the past five years, 1975–80, our chemotherapy followed the pattern of the International Society of Paediatric Oncology [2], which provided the use of Vincristine plus CCNU. We added intrathecal Methotrexate to the treatment (during the irradiation phase).

Analysing our results for *children who had had radiation therapy,* and excluding those who had died prior to irradiation, the survival curve for the period before 1967 remains unchanged. For the group of children diagnosed and treated after 1967, the *5-year survival rate is 43%,* and the *10-year survival rate is 36%* (Fig. 4).

These data now correspond with those of different authors from departments of radiology and radiotherapy, from which at the moment the most representative publications emerge [3, 4, 5, 6].

Finally, we have divided the children, seen since 1968, into two groups, and the major differences in the two are: the first group was the older one (1968–75), pos-

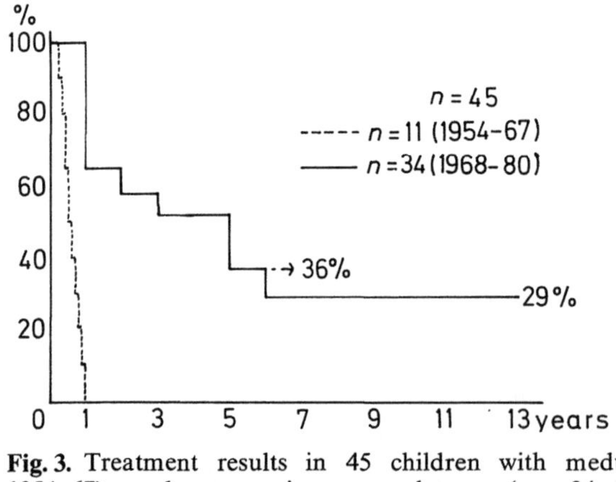

Fig. 3. Treatment results in 45 children with medulloblastomas. First group (n = 11; 1954–67): no 1-year survivor; second group (n = 34; 1968–80): 5-year survival rate is 36%, and 10-year survival is 29%. All children diagnosed are included (also postoperative and preradiotherapeutic death, and one pretreatment death)

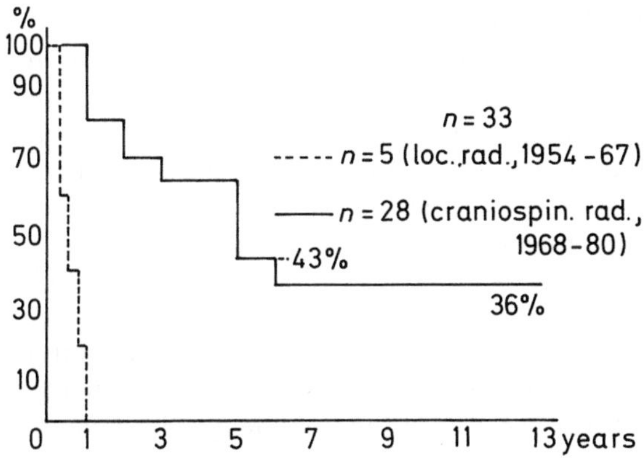

Fig. 4. Treatment results in children with medulloblastomas (irradiated patients only): --- = local radiotherapy posterior fossa only; — = craniospinal radiotherapy completed (n = 28): 5-year survival rate in the latter group is 43%, and the 10-year survival rate is 36%, respectively

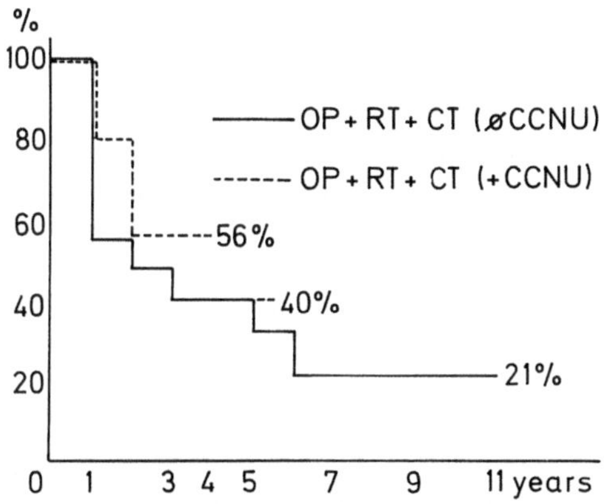

Fig. 5. Treatment results in medulloblastoma; —— = operation, craniospinal radiotherapy, chemotherapy without the use of CCNU; --- = operation, craniospinal radiotherapy, chemotherapy including CCNU. 5-year survival in the first group is 40%, 10-year survival 21%; 4-year survival in the latter group is 56%, and 2-year survival in this group is even 80%

sibly with less experience in medulloblastoma treatment at our institution (not only as regards neurosurgery, but also considering paediatric oncology care at that time and paediatric intensive care). Furthermore another difference is that the first group was treated with cyclophosphamide or cyclophosphamide plus vincristine, and intrathecal methotrexate was added in these patients, whereas the second group (1975–80) received CCNU plus vincristine and intrathecal methotrexate.

For the period 1968–75 (n = 21) there is a *5-year survival rate of 40%* and a 10-year survival rate of 21%; for the later period (1975–80) (n = 13) the *4-year survival rate is 56%* and the *2-year survival rate is even 80%* (Fig. 5)!

We draw the following *conclusions* from our results:

1) The *intrapontine* tumours have an *extremely poor prognosis,* which has remained *unchanged.* As radiotherapy and/or chemotherapy have proved to be ineffective in achieving cures or long-term remissions, other and more promising treatment techniques have to be looked for. One must again ask about the possibility of operative intervention at the pons, at least to achieve a biopsy is help with more reasonable additional postoperative treatment.

Radiation therapy giving the usual doses and modes of application seems to be superfluous in my opinion, regarding the *possibility of a permanent cure.* The same is certainly true for the *chemotherapeutic* agents in use up to the present; maybe future drugs will be more effective. Fundamentally however, new ways of tumour therapy have to be found, to realize a great break-through in the treatment of intrapontine tumours.

With the extremely poor prognosis in mind, it must not be overlooked that radiotherapy and/or chemotherapy in fact *often have a favourable effect,* namely regression of tumour symptoms and of the children's complaints for a relatively longer period of the remaining life-span. These latter aspects *justify the further use of the treatment described above,* which, although ineffective for permanent cures, is *often highly palliative,* at least for a certain time.

2) In children with *cerebellar astrocytomas* it was fortunately a rare event that local irradiation was given in these children. *We have never seen a proven positive antitumour effect from irradiation of cerebellar astrocytomas.* We therefore question reporting positive tumour responses in children with cerebellar astrocytomas. Especially in younger children with this type of tumour any consideration of a local radiotherapy should be postponed as long as possible, depending of course on signs of clinical progression and partly also on the results of CT examinations.

The occurrence of very *late deaths* in our series (n = 3 after more than ten years) requires a *long-term follow-up before judging the effects of treatment,* especially so-called innovative elements in therapy.

3) In *medulloblastomas,* improved operative techniques including microneurosurgery and improved postoperative paediatric intensive care have shown positive results. This is reflected in the reduced number of postoperative deaths and probably also by the reduced number and severity of late sequelae (which will be discussed in another part ot this volume).

For a number of years, we advocated the restricted operative procedure in medulloblastoma children and eschewed ultraradical surgical attempts. We *question this concept,* however, in view of modern microneurosurgical techniques and in view of the results of radiotherapy and chemotherapy, which even now have *not brought the great success that seemed possible five or seven years ago.*

Craniospinal radiotherapy holds its place, and it is certainly of great importance, although every modern statement on its value is based only on historical controls.

To *reduce radiation doses* to – for instance – 30 Gy (total CNS) and 40 Gy (posterior fossa) is desirable in order to reduce the number and severity of late adverse effects (which, however, must only partly be ascribed to the effect of radiation). I believe we should also *think about the possibility of totally renouncing supratentorial irradiation* in medulloblastomas. Nobody can clearly delineate the risk of supratentorial recurrences under modern treatment techniques without supratentorial radiation treatment; in our experience (four of the irradiated long-term survivors developed massive supratentorial lesions despite 35 or 40 Gy in 4–5 weeks and 55–60 Gy to the posterior fossa), it seems that without supratentorial irradiation *this incidence might be no higher than with it;* of course, this hypothesis presumes positive effects of modern operative procedures and of modern chemotherapy on medulloblastoma spread via the CSF pathways to the third and the lateral ventricles. Similar thoughts may be justified for *spinal irradiation in certain cases.* Now and then we should question our faith in established treatments and think again about the value of historical control groups.

Up to the present, it is *not clear, to what extent chemotherapy can contribute* to a reduction of radiation doses and fields. Chemotherapy can indeed have positive antitumour effects and we have seen regressions of medulloblastoma (partial responses) after chemotherapy alone (single agent treatment with a nitrosourea derivative) *at least in two children with recurrent inoperable disease,* who had previously been irradiated.

However, even today the importance of chemotherapy in medulloblastoma patients is by no means as great as it is in other childhood malignancies such as acute lymphocytic leukaemia, Wilms' tumours and others.

Clinical trials with a *combined regime of chemotherapy* before radiation appear to be a possible way of further improving the results of medulloblastoma treatment (see pp. 338–343 and 349).

4) The above mentioned results in our patients can be used to demonstrate how questionable the presentation of survival curves may be, depending on possible previous selection of cases.

Our *own data can be expressed* as:

- 29% 10-year survival for the total group 1968–80;
- 36% 5-year survival for the total group 1968–80;
- 36% 10-year survival for the craniospinally irradiated patients 1968–80;
- 43% 5-year survival rate for the craniospinally irradiated patients 1968–80;
- 56% 4-year survival for the craniospinally irradiated patients since 1975, who also received CCNU within a combined chemotherapy regime;
- 80% 2-year survival for the craniospinally irradiated patients since 1975, who also received CCNU within a combined chemotherapy regime.

It would be easy to attribute an improved survival rate as described above in these curves of survival to one of the new therapeutic elements introduced in our regime during the past years. Such a *"handling of survival curves"* must sometimes be assumed in one or the other modern reports of improved prognosis for medulloblastomas, especially when they deal with short-term results.

In our opinion, the *prognosis of medulloblastoma patients,* as regards 10-year or permanent cures, is *currently not above 30–35% in an unselected group of cases.*

Reports from radiological or radiotherapeutic institutions may – in this context – give a *too positive impression,* as only patients with initiated and completed radiotherapy are included in the analyses.

Therefore, careful reading of such reports is mandatory, including considerations of the institutional origin of the publications. *Scepticism* must be articulated, if we hear about dramatic improvements in medulloblastoma therapy during the past five to eight years.

Finally a remark dealing with the problem of *optimally organizing patients' treatment and long-term care.* In our institution we prefer to delegate the "total care" of the children to the *paediatric oncologist,* including the intensive long-term care, analysis of adverse late effects, problems of rehabilitation, care in questions of school and vocational guidance. Radiotherapy and operation are undertaken on an *outpatient basis* in the different institutions and clinics, while the *child remains in the care of the paediatrician.*

By this means, we believe we are better able to continue to answer questions about the *"total care"* in every phase of the treatment, which cannot be the task of a radiotherapist or neurosurgeon, and which has – in each of the above mentioned respects – to be organized from the very beginning of the treatment. We also suggest this kind of organizational care to other centres treating children with brain tumours, when they do not already practise it in this manner.

References

1. McFarland, D. F., Horwitz, H., Saenger, E. L., Bahr, G. K.: Medulloblastoma – a review of prognosis and survival. Brit. J. Radiol. *42,* 198–214 (1969)
2. Bloom, H. J. G., Walsh, L. S.: Tumours of the central nervous system; in: Bloom, H. J. G., et al. (eds.): Cancer in Children; Clinical Management; pp. 93–119; Berlin-Heidelberg-New York: Springer 1975
3. Jenkin, R. D. T.: The treatment of medulloblastoma; lecture at the Brain Tumour Symposium, Niagara Falls, New York, 1981
4. Mealey, J., Hall, P. V.: Medulloblastoma in children. J. Neurosurg. *46,* 56–64 (1977)
5. Landberg, T. G., Lindgren, M. L., Cavallin-Stahl, E. K., Svahn-Tapper, G. O., Sundbarg, G., Garwicz, S., Lagergren, J. A., Gunneson, V. L., Brun, A. E., Cronqvist, S. E.: Improvements in the radiotherapy of medulloblastoma, 1946–1975. Cancer *45,* 670–678 (1980)
6. Bloom, H. J. G.: Medulloblastoma: Prognosis and prospects. Int. J. Radiat. Oncol. Biol. Phys. *2,* 1031–1033 (1977)

Discussion

Habermalz (Berlin) considered again the question of radiation dosage and expressed the opinion that it was reasonable to make an effort to reduce the total dose still more. Together with the possibilities of chemotherapy this should not make the results of treatment noticeably worse.

B. Kornhuber (Frankfurt) asked *J. Kutzner (Mainz)* if there were differences between the Cobalt-60 source and the possibilities of the linear accelerator. The frequency of loss of hair is certainly different. However, there also exist possible differences in the sensitivity of the tumours, as well as in the possibility of damage to adjoining organs due to radiation scatter.

J. Kutzner (Mainz) pointed out that basically the radiation technique with a Cobalt-60 source did not differ in quality from an accelerator; what was normally understood by the latter was an electron accelerator. The possibility of radiation with neutrons or with heavy particles, or alpha particles is essentially still 'pie in the sky'. In children's brain tumours these procedures were, in practice, scarcely used at all. The difference between the cobalt source and accelerator is mainly that in the former the source has a diameter of 1.5–2.0 cm with a correspondingly larger penumbra, while the accelerator has a small focus, so that the field of radiation is more accurate and more sharply delimited, and correspondingly the volume dose is smaller with the accelerator and also the skin protection is better. The side effects can be influenced by the type of radiation technique.

M. Bamberg (Essen) does not consider interstitial treatment for dysgerminomas to be sensible, as these tumours are extremely radiosensitive and, furthermore, with conventional radiation technique there is a tendency to metastasize in the CSF pathways. Because of that a large field radiation with doses up to 50 Gy are sufficient and reasonable.

F. Mundinger (Freiburg) replied that he certainly held this objection to be justifiable, but the discussion on the matter is not yet concluded. He stated that in his material he had not seen a single instance of a local recurrence, even after percutaneous irradiation of the whole cerebrospinal axis 8–14 months after metastases.

H. J. Habermalz (Berlin) said that in his opinion local recurrence is still the most frequent. For this reason he was expecting good results from the combination of interstitial radiation and external radiation.

F. Mundinger (Freiburg) said that he was not able to answer this question as he had not observed a local recurrence in any of his cases.

B. Kornhuber (Frankfurt) reminded them of the possibility of tackling the dysgerminomas or the pineal tumours in general with cytostatic drugs; he then referred to cases in whom a recurrence after radiotherapy had been successfully treated with bleomycin and cysplatinum. He asked Dr. Mundinger to what extent an implanted radiation source could move around.

F. Mundinger (Freiburg) replied that the implant was very light and consequently it had no tendency to change its position in the tissues. However, it did happen occasionally when there was a cystic necrosis around the radiation source.

E. Halves (Würzburg) referred to the paper by *V. Sturm (Heidelberg)* and asked what was the rationale of the treatment with radionuclides. In general it seemed to be a treatment of the cyst and the immediate marginal structures, and less of the solid portion of the craniopharyngioma. That is to say, would the vessels lying on the outside be damaged by the radiation and, indeed, could damage possibly occur to the chiasm and optic nerves or the hypothalamus because of this.

V. Sturm (Heidelberg) replied that he regarded direct contact radiation of the cysts of a craniopharyngioma as the primary therapeutic measure, because there was comparatively low risk associated with it. From time to time, it also succeeds in getting rid of the cysts for many years, or even permanently. The solid portion of the tumour is apparently not adequately irradiated, but by the reduction in size of the cysts, any microsurgical operation on the solid part is facilitated. With very large craniopharyngiomas and those with a large solid component, external irradiation is definitely indicated. The main effect of the injected radionuclide is on the cyst epithelium, but the penetration into the tissue is really very slight. The peritumoural vessels may indeed be scarcely damaged.

D. Voth (Mainz) asked *L. Steiner (Stockholm)* for information about how he used stereotactic focussed gamma rays for inoperable angiomas of the brain stem and if he though that it was justifiable.

L. Steiner (Stockholm) replied that the difficulties of the treatment he was using lay in the fact that the effect only appeared after weeks or months. This was particularly the case with vascular malformations. If the patient had already had one or more haemorrhages, the rapidly acting operative excision would be preferable. If a patient has still not bled, this procedure seemed to him less risky that an operation. Also with angiomas of the brain stem, the possibilities of exactly locating the feeding vessels which are to radiated are now so good, that an optimum dose distribution is possible.

J. M. Schröder (Aachen) asked *M. Neidhardt (Augsburg)* if the causal connection between the administration of methotrexate and the development of leukoencephalopathy is adequately proved. From experimental work on monkeys it seemed to be evident that the radiation was the cause of the leukoencephalopathy and, much less, the treatment with the methotrexate.

M. Neidhardt (Augsburg) and also *J. Kutzner (Mainz)* both stated that the leukoencephalopathy was clearly associated with the administration of methotrexate and their figures for the combination of methotrexate and radiotherapy are definitely higher than those with radiation on its own.

M. Neidhardt (Augsburg) thought that disturbances of CSF circulation apparently played an important part in the development of this complication. Finally, it seems to be a convincing argument that methotrexate on its own can cause leukoencephalopathy, that in the present study by the German Society for Paediatric Oncology, in one case under treatment with methotrexate, a complication of this sort developed before any radiation was given.

In a subsequent discussion between *K. Kretzschmar (Mainz)* and *J. M. Schröder (Aachen)* it was stated that there are various forms of leukoencephalopathy. One form, predominantly vascular in origin is indeed well known as a sequal of radiation treatment. Apparently this has nothing to do with virus infections.

Frau *G. M. Zu Rhein (Madison, Wis.)* also pointed out that in her opinion methotrexate could definitely cause such demyelinating lesions, apparently however, only when there are disturbances of the CSF circulation.

It was further pointed out from the 'floor' that if such a favoured chemotherapy were started a relatively short time after the operation, one had to reckon with such disturbances of the CSF circulation and hence, also with the increased possibility of a leukoencephalopathy.

M. Neidhardt (Augsburg) considered that one should deliberately allow two to three weeks to elapse after the operation, before starting this treatment. In this way the CSF circulation would have had the opportunity to return to normal.

In a further discussion between *J. Kutzner (Mainz)* and *P. Gutjahr (Mainz)* consideration was given as to whether one could support a reduction in the amount of radiation, as well as to what extent this was possible. Kutzner pointed out the fact, that by omitting certain fields from the radiation, it was predominantly here that the recurrences or metastases developed and that gaps in the planning of the radiotherapy in medulloblastoma were shown as a rule by recurrences. He regarded the complete radiation of the neuro-axis as essential.

P. Gutjahr (Mainz) added that although the principle of cranio-spinal radiotherapy was started in 1953, the ultimate assessment of it effectiveness in the final analysis however, is based only on historical control groups, which originated from a long time before the era of craniospinal radiotherapy. Historical controls of this sort however, exhibit many uncertainties, if one thinks for example to what extent the mortality of neurosurgical operations has fallen from figures between 40% and 50% to practically nil.

Cytostatic Monotherapy of Tumours of the Central Nervous System in Children

B. KORNHUBER

Introduction

In this context side-effects of therapy will be discussed. The following statements should therefore not be considered as an evaluation of chemotherapy in view of the total policy for treatment, nor as a comparison between monotherapy and polychemotherapy. The rarity of CNS tumours in neurosurgical departments as well as the changes in the mode of treatment itself in the past few years, have resulted in information gained and published from a small number of case studies. Large multicentric studies, as far as their results have been published, concern polychemotherapy and will therefore not be referred to here. For this reason, the content of this paper has a more historical character and does not concern itself with present-day studies. Problems are also found in the evaluation of the success of the treatment. The hard data cannot be found in terms of years of survival, but only in rate of cure. It is often seen, in this context, that the quality of living for these patients is given little consideration.

Chemotherapy in CNS Tumours

The cytotoxic drugs are only effective in tumours of high malignancy. In children, these are mostly medulloblastomas, ependymomas and glioblastomas although rarely, one also sees intracranial germinomas (pinealomas).

The Blood Brain Barrier

The concentration of systemically administered drugs in the cerebrospinal fluid is dependent on the size and lipophilia of the molecule. The concentràtion of cytotoxic drugs in brain tissue is also less than in other body tissues. However, this fact is not true for CNS tumour cells. Hirano and Matsui, as well as Waggener and Beggs report on a damaged blood brain barrier in patients with CNS tumours with resulting higher concentrations in such tumour cells. There also seems to be a weakness in the blood brain barrier after irradiation of the central nervous system. This phenomenon can already be found with low doses of radiation, for example, the dosage ad-

Table 1. Chemotherapy in brain tumours

Cytotoxic agent	Single dose	Application repeated every	Effectivity as monotherapeutic agent
BCNU	60 – 120 $mg/m^2 \times 3$	6 – 8 week i. v.	+ + +
CCNU	100 – 200 mg/m^2	6 – 8 week p. o.	+ +
MeCCNU	200 – 220 mg/m^2	6 week p. o.	+ +
Procarbazine	150 $mg/m^2 \times 28$ (14)	8 week p. o.	+ +
Epipodophyllotoxine (VM-26)	100 – 130 mg/m^2	6 – 8 week i. v.	+
Vincristine	1 – 2 mg/m^2 (max. 2 – 3 mg)	week i. v.	+
Methotrexate (M) HD + CVR	15 – 900 mg/kg	1 – 2 week i. v. infus.	+ + +

ministered in the treatment of leukemia (18–24 gy) [17]. The possibility of encephalopathy due to cytostatic agents is enhanced by radiation therapy. This was especially found in treatment with methotrexate at high or medium dosage.

Effective Cytotoxic Drugs

Effective drugs have proved to be those substances which, on account of their molecular structure and lipophilia can pass the blood brain barrier. Foremost in efficiency are the nitroso-urea drugs which were already proved to be effective in the 1960's.

Nitroso-Urea Drugs

BCNU, CCNU and MeCCNU have been clinically tested. All three rapidly cross the blood brain barrier. The intact molecules can be found in plasma and cerebrospinal fluid; the concentration in CSF is approximately 15–30% of that in blood plasma. These substances are rapidly metabolized, but their effect can be seen for a long period of time. There is general agreement in the various therapy groups that nitrosourea drugs should not be readministered until six weeks have passed.

BCNU

The dosage generally given is between 60–125 $mg/m^2/day$ during three successive days. The drug is administered intravenously. This cycle is repeated after 6–8 weeks. The side effects necessitate this interval. BCNU has been tried in a series of phase II and III studies. BCNU is considered an effective drug for malignant tumours of the CNS. The clinical response is pronounced to be 45–62%. The success of this drug could only be partially proven by RN-scans. Long-term success is rare.

The largest number of patients is found in a study by Walker et al. [15]. Of 303 patients with anaplastic gliomas, 222 could be evaluated. Through randomization, the patients were divided into four subgroups. The median of survival of patients who had no chemotherapy or radiation therapy was 14 weeks, those given BCNU lived 18.5 weeks, those patients who only received radiation therapy lived 35 weeks and those with combination BCNU/radiation therapy survived 34.5 weeks [15].

Another randomized study was performed with 115 patients suffering from anaplastic gliomas (grade II and IV) treated with and without radiotherapy or with and without BCNU or MeCCNU. The chemotherapy alone showed no significant advantage in median length of survival, Radiotherapy, with or without chemotherapy did show hopeful results [2].

CCNU

CCNU is given orally for a period of six weeks. The dosage is 100–130 mg/m^2/day. The results of monotherapy with this drug are comparable to BCNU. The clinical rate of improvement is somewhat less (37% according to Rosenblum et al. [10]); the increase in median length of survival compared with operated patients suffering from malignant glioma was not significant. Also, CCNU in combination with radiotherapy was not superior to irradiation alone [6].

The median period of survival (not rate of cure) of patients with relapse is found to be longer in those patients treated with CCNU, then in those without therapy. CCNU is being used in combination with other cytotoxic agents in newer studies [6].

MeCCNU

MeCCNU is given orally in doses of 200–220 mg/m^2 once every 6–8 weeks. The clinical use of the drug has not shown uniform results. This is due to the small number of cases treated with MeCCNU as well as differing methods of evaluating the success of such therapy. Tranum [13] found that 8 of 29 patients suffering from recurrent malignant glioma responded to therapy with MeCCNU. This response was assessed by RN scan and/or neurological examination. The improvement lasted a mean of 44 weeks. Walker et al. [15] performed a randomized study with four groups: MeCCNU, radiotherapy, MeCCNU plus radiotherapy and BCNU plus radiotherapy. The data on 253 patients showed a median rate of survival of three weeks for the first group, 34.6 weeks in the group with MeCCNU and radiotherapy and 50.3 weeks in the group with BCNU plus radiotherapy.

Chin et al. compared radiation therapy with and without MeCCNU or BCNU. Nitroso-urea agents alone did not lead to a significant increase in length of survival. However, radiation therapy with or without nitroso-urea drugs did show better results. Four of 25 patients suffering from malignant glioma given radiation therapy were still alive after two years of therapy. Of those receiving BCNU as well as radiotherapy, seven of 26 patients were still alive after two years. Three of ten patients who also received MeCCNU survived this two year period as well. A combination with other cytotoxic drugs is also possible.

Procarbazine

Procarbazine is given orally for a period of 2–4 weeks. The daily dosage is 150 mg/m^2. The pause between courses is usually four weeks. The effectiveness of this drug has been proved. The best response was seen in the treatment of medulloblastoma. Kumar et al. report that three of four patients respond to procarbazine. This response was documented by RN scan, clinical examination and the amount of steroids needed. The use of polychemotherapy is, as with other agents, more effective than monochemotherapy. Cross resistance between procarbazine and nitroso-urea substances is suspected.

Methotrexate

MTX has been used to treat CNS tumours in low dosage without CVR (Citrovorum factor rescue), in median dosage (500 mg/m^2) with CVR and concurrent intrathecal instillation and in high dosage (200 mg/kg MTX-HD) with CVR but without intrathecal instillation as well as solely by intrathecal instillation using lumbar puncture or an Ommaya reservoir.

Djerassi et al. found effective concentrations (between 0.7 and 2.25 μg/ml) in cerebrospinal fluid 12–24 hours after intravenous infusion of 15–100 mg/kg MTX. Upon examination, the neurological state had improved in six of seven children with medulloblastoma. Rosen showed similar results. Two of four patients with glioma of the brain stem and five of seven children with medulloblastoma improved with MTX therapy. Most information gained on MTX-HD (high-dosed MTX) refer to MTX-HD combined with radiotherapy and other cytostatic drugs, especially vincristine and BCNU. For this reason it is difficult to evaluate the effectiveness of MTX-monotherapy. There is no doubt that MTX-MHD or MTX-HD is the most efficient treatment for medulloblastoma next to radiotherapy. The danger of a leukoencephalopathy due to MTX is enhanced by previous irradiation of the central nervous system. In a new study, one is trying to minimize the toxicity of treatment by administering the six MTX infusions postoperatively and before radiotherapy (see pp. 338–343).

Vincristine (VCR)

In 1969 Braham et al. [1] reported on four patients with relapse of glioma after operative measures and radiotherapy. These patients were then given vincristine on its own. They received 0.5–0.1 mg/kg weekly for a period of three months. All of the patients responded to vincristine. The improvement lasted 5–18 months. Rosenstock and colleagues treated 16 children with recurrent CNS tumours by giving them weekly injections of vincristine (1.5 mg/m^2, maximum dose 2 mg/m^2) for a period of 12 weeks, followed by an injection every two weeks. Eight of these 16 patients responded to treatment. The cases which had not improved but remained stable were viewed as a positive response.

Epipodophyllotoxin (VM-26)

VM-26 is given intravenously in a dose of 100–130 mg/m². The injections are given every week for a period of 6–8 weeks. Skylansky et al. repeat this course after a two week recuperation period. With this treatment, they found that five of 13 patients showed objective improvement which lasted 3–14 months. Clinical improvement using VM-26 alone was found in 38% of tumour patients. However, the effectiveness of VM-26 on CNS tumours is less than that of the nitroso-urea compounds.

Discussion

The effectiveness of chemotherapy on intracranial tumours is well documented. However there is still dissatisfaction with the results of cytostatic therapy. As in the treatment of other tumours, chemotherapy is indicated in the treatment of malignant CNS tumours in children.

The criteria for the evaluation of chemotherapy must be clearly defined. The term "remission" is used differently with respect to CNS tumours than with leukemia. In leukemia, "remission" means that the tumour is no longer detectable. In CNS tumours remission describes a clinical improvement. For this reason, the term "in remission" is not as suitable for a multicentric study as the term "stable disease". The comparison of publications becomes more difficult with these subjective data.

Besides gaining information on the post-therapy observation period and the number of survivors, data should also be published on the quality of life after treatment. Information is valuable on the patients ability to attend school, to continue working in his profession or on any change of profession.

The number of patients examined in the studies to date are too few. For this reason the data gained cannot be used as statistically-based evidence. They may only be considered in pilot studies to examine new treatments. The studies must be planned more prospectively. Monotherapy shows a poorer response than polychemotherapy. Therefore, monotherapy was used almost solely to treat relapsed patients. An exception could be MTX-HD and MTX-MHD plus intrathecal with CVR.

Because of the rarity of central nervous system tumours, multicentric studies are necessary. In West Germany 220 new cases between 0–15 years of age are expected. These will include varying diagnoses. This means that no centre can make relevant statements on treatment based on their results alone.

The drugs discussed here show varying therapeutic effectiveness on CNS tumours. The side-effects are manifold and considerable. The most effective drugs appear to be the nitroso-urea compounds, MTX-HD and procarbazine. Radiotherapy cannot be replaced nor reduced by chemotherapy. Chemotherapy administered postoperatively and before radiotherapy in the treatment of medulloblastomas, promises to minimize the toxic side-effects.

Summary

Cytostatic therapy is becoming increasingly more significant in paediatric oncology. However, in the chemotherapy of malignant tumours of the central nervous system, the blood brain barrier presents an obstacle to the selection of cytotoxic agents. In these cases the cytotoxic agent must be chosen in terms of its ability not only to destroy the tumour cells, but primarily to reach the site of the tumour. Of crucial importance are the molecular size and lipophilia of the molecule. The rarity of the various CNS tumours in children and the problems described above explain the small numbers of patients in the series of studies on treatment published to date.

Previous irradiation of the tumour influences the blood brain barrier in a beneficial therapeutic manner. It is also possible that the blood brain barrier is less well maintained within a CNS tumour. The clinical efficacy of some cytotoxic drugs on CNS malignant tumours has been proved. This is true for the nitroso-urea compounds (BCNU, CCNU, MeCCNU), Procarbazine and Methotrexate in high and medium dosage with leucovorin-rescue as well as, to a certain extent, Vincristine and Epipodophyllotoxin (VM 26).

Studies of treatment in which one sole cytotoxic drug was used are important for the evaluation of chemotherapy. However, because of the superiority of combination chemotherapy, monotherapy can no longer be justified today. This makes the evaluation of new drugs more difficult. Prospective multicentric studies with a sufficient number of cases will yield new insights regarding the effect of new drugs.

References

1. Braham, J., Sarova-Pinhas, I., Goldhammer, Y.: Glioma of the brain treated by intravenous vincristine sulfate. Neurochirurgia (Stuttg.), *12,* 195 (1969)
2. Chin, H. W., Young, A. B., Maruyama, Y.: Survival response of malignant gliomas to radiotherapy with or without BCNU or Methyl-CCNU chemotherapy at the University of Kentucky Medical Center. Cancer Treat. Rep. *65,* 45 (1981)
3. Djerassi, I., Abir, E., Royer, G. L. et. al.: Long-term remissions in childhood acute leukemia: use of infrequent infusions of methotrexate. Clin. Pediatr. (Phila) *5,* 502 (1966)
4. Djerassi, I., Kim, J. S., Shulman, K.: High-dose methotrexate-citrovorum factor rescue in the management of brain tumours. Cancer Treat. Rep. *61,* 691 (1977)
5. Edwards, M. S., Levin, V. A., Wilson, C. B.: Brain tumour chemotherapy: an evaluation of agents in current use for phase II and III trials. Cancer Treat. Rep. *64,* 1179 (1980)
6. EORTC Brain Tumour Group: Effect of CCNU on survival rate and objective remission and duration of free interval in patients with malignant brain glioma – final evaluation. Europ. J. Cancer *14,* 851 (1978)
7. Hirano, A., Matsui, T.: Vascular structure in brain tumours. Hum. Pathol. *6,* 611 (1975)
8. Kumar, A. R. V., Renaudin, J., Wilson, C. B. et al.: Procarbazine hydrochloride in the treatment of brain tumours: phase 2 study. J. Neurosurg. *40,* 365 (1974)
9. Rosen, G., Gharimi, F., Nirenberg, A. et al.: High-dose methotrexate with citrovorum factor rescue for the treatment of central nervous system tumours in children. Cancer Treat. Rep. *61,* 681 (1977)
10. Rosenblum, M. L., Reynolds, A. F., Smith, K. A., Rumack, B. H., Walker, M. D.: Chloroethyl-cyclo-hexyl-nitrosourea (CCNU) in the treatment of malignant brain tumours. J. Neurosurg. *39,* 306–314 (1973)

11. Rosenstock, J. G., Evans, A. E., Schut, L.: Response to vincristine of recurrent brain tumours in children. J. Neurosurg. *45,* 135 (1976)
12. Skylansky, B. D., Mann-Kaplan, R. S., Reynolds, A. F. et. al.: 4′-dimethyl-epipodophyllotoxin-β-D-ethylidene-glucoside (PTG) in the treatment of malignant intracranial neoplasms. Cancer *33,* 460 (1974)
13. Tranum, B. L., Haut, A., Rivkin, S. et al.: A phase II study of methyl-CCNU in the treatment of solid tumours and lymphomas, a Southwest Oncology Group study. Cancer *31,* 1148 (1975)
14. Waggener, J. D., Beggs, J. L.: Vasculature of neural neoplasms. Adv. Neurol. *15,* 27 (1976)
15. Walker, M. D., Alexander, E., Hunt, W. E. et. al.: Evaluation of BCNU and/or radiotherapy in the treatment of anaplastic gliomas. A cooperative clinical trial. J. Neurosurg. *49,* 333 (1978)
16. Walker, M. D., Hurwitz, B. S.: BCNU (1,3-bis (bis (2-chloroethyl)1-nitrosourea); in the treatment of malignant brain tumour – a preliminary report. Cancer Chemother. Rep. *54,* 263 (1970)
17. Welte, K., Engert, A., Siegert, M., Gadner, H.: Verhalten von Gerinnungsproteinen im Liquor cerebrospinalis bei Kindern mit Akuter Lymphoblastischer Leukämie (ALL) während der kombinierten Induktionstherapie. Monatsschrf. Kinderheilk. *127,* 262 (1979)
18. Wilson, C. B., Boldrey, E. B., Enot, K. J.: 1,3-bis (2-Chlorethyl)-1-nitrosourea (NSC-409962) in the treatment of brain tumours. Cancer Chemother. Rep. *54,* 273 (1970)

Rationale of Combined Chemotherapy of Brain Tumours

J. HILDEBRAND and D. ZEGERS DE BEYL

In this review dealing with the rationale for combination chemotherapy of brain tumours, two main issues will be considered: (a) what are the characteristics of brain tumours most likely to determine the choice of chemotherapeutic drugs, and (b) is there any clinical evidence supporting the view that combination chemotherapy is superior to single-drug therapy in human brain neoplasms.

Characteristics of Malignant Brain Tumours

The most peculiar feature of human malignant brain tumours is that they are confined to the central nervous system (metastases are exceptional), and are therefore protected, at least partially, by the *blood-brain barrier.* This blood-brain barrier is no longer present in the centre of the tumour in which capillary endothelium displays open intracellular junctions, whereas at the periphery of the tumour where malignant cells infiltrate normal brain parenchyma, the barrier is preserved [8]. The fact that small neoplastic nodules are protected by the blood-brain barrier has also been shown in experimental tumours of the central nervous system [1]. Thus, to reach the peripheral part of brain tumours where the rate of proliferating cells is the highest, one should use lipid soluble non-ionized drugs which cross the blood-brain barrier. The use of drugs which rapidly cross the blood-brain barrier is particularly important for intracarotid administration, since the advantage of this technique exists only for the first passage of the drug. The blood-brain barrier, however, may be temporarily suppressed by intracarotid perfusion of hypertonic solutions such as mannitol. Clinical trials are currently assessing this approach [9]. This technique, however, leaves the normal brain tissues unprotected and it is therefore not suitable for neurotoxic agents.

The second characteristic of most human brain tumours, which probably determines their relative resistance to chemotherapeutic agents, is their *small growth fraction.* Limited data are available on this subject, and most authors usually refer to the work of Hoshino et al. [6] who found a mean growth fraction of 8.6 to 17.8 per cent in glioblastoma and only 1.1 to 2.1 per cent in astrocytoma. As mentioned previously, the largest growth fraction is found in the peripheral part of the tumour. These figures indicate that the majority of brain tumours cells would be sensitive only to phase non-specific agents which are active on non-dividing cells. In children, astrocytomas which are very slowly growing tumours, have probably a very low growth fraction whereas medulloblastoma, which grow rapidly, are theoretically more sensitive to chemotherapy as they also are to irradiation.

A third very important characteristic of brain tumours is their *heterogeneity.* Both experimental and human tumours are formed by clones which differ from each other not only by karyotypes but also by their sensitivity, at least *in vitro*, to various chemotherapeutic agents [12]. If these data are confirmed, then tumour heterogeneity is probably one of the strongest arguments for the use of drug combinations in the treatment of brain neoplasms.

A fourth factor, emphasized by Victor Levin [7], is the importance of *intercapillary distance* since the amounts of drug delivered to a given cell decrease with the distance separating that cell from the nearest capillary. This distance is of about 100 μ in the brain and this places, according to Levin, some strong theoretical limitations on the efficacy of the current chemotherapeutic agents including nitrosoureas.

Another particularity of brain tumour chemotherapy is that it can be administered *intrathecally.* However, this route of drug administration is of restricted value in the treatment of solid tumours because (a) drug diffusion is limited, (b) several drugs are neurotoxic and (c) even agents like methotrexate which are reasonably well tolerated may become extremely toxic and cause severe encephalopathy when CSF flow is impaired [10, 11]. Today intrathecal administration is currently used in the treatment of meningeal carcinomatosis but has been abandoned in the treatment of solid tumours, even medulloblastomas.

Thus drugs chosen for brain tumour chemotherapy should fulfil, at least theoretically, the following criteria:

- have some antitumour activity when used *alone*,
- be able to cross the *blood-brain barrier,*
- have *different mechanisms* of action,
- include at least one *phase non-specific* agent,
- have *non-cumulative toxicities.*

The sequence in which the various agents should be administered remains largely empirical despite an impressive number of studies devoted to the problem. For example, the role of cell synchronisation remains controversial. In human tumours, unlike in some experimental work, cell divisions occur in a random fashion. Therefore, it seems that synchronisation of cell divisions by agents such as vincristine or podophyllotoxine derivatives, which temporarily block cell mitoses could increase the cytotoxicity of phase-specific agents administered subsequently. This very attractive approach has served as a rationale for many drug combinations but there is no firm evidence that this recruitment mechanism is actually involved in the efficacy of combined chemotherapies of human neoplasms [13].

Clinical Data

The number of controlled studies evaluating single-agent chemotherapy in brain tumours is rather small and trials testing adequately combination treatments are even more scarce.

At least three factors may be measured in such studies:

(1) the rate and length of objective remission,
(2) the total survival time,
(3) the free interval, i.e. the time interval between operation and relapse.

Because the activity of presently used chemotherapy in human brain tumours is low, various agents may affect these factors differently so they should therefore be considered separately.

Objective remission, usually defined as an improvement or stabilization of the neurological status, has been achieved with the three nitrosoureas currently used: CCNU, BCNU and methyl-CCNU [14]. These drugs are lipid soluble, cross the blood-brain barrier and act, at least partially, as alkylating agents. They are considered today as the most active single chemotherapeutic agents in the treatment of malignant brain gliomas, although their overall effect is modest. The addition of a "syndromizing" drug such as vincristine to BCNU [4] or VM_{26} to CCNU [3] did not increase the length and rate of objective remission in adults with malignant hemispheric gliomas. Next to nitroso-ureas, procarbazine appeared as an active agent in several studies [14]. However, there is no firm evidence that the combination of procarbazine, vincristine and CCNU (PVC) is superior to nitrosoureas used alone in supratentorial gliomas, whereas this combination appears at present as the best treatment in previously irradiated recurrent medulloblastomas [15].

There is less agreement concerning the effects of chemotherapy on the *total survival* time. Several studies indicate that nitroso-ureas prolong the survival time in adults operated and irradiated for brain gliomas but there is no indication that any other single-agent chemotherapy or combination treatment could do better.

Finally, in two consecutive randomized trials, the EORTC brain tumour group failed to demonstrate any benefit of CCNU or VM_{26} plus CCNU in prolonging the *free interval* in adults operated on for supratentorial gliomas [2, 3].

Thus, it does appear today that we are lacking active adjuvant chemotherapy in malignant gliomas of the adult. The situation could be different, however, in child medulloblastomas where CCNU plus vincristine could delay and, in certain age groups, even decrease the rate of recurrence.

References

1. Blasberg, R., Patlack, C., Shapiro, W., Fenstermacher, J.: Metastatic brain tumours: local blood flow and capillary permeability. Neurology *29,* 547, 1979
2. EORTC brain tumour group: Effect of CCNU on survival, rate of objective remission and duration of free interval in patients with malignant brain glioma: final evaluation. Europ. J. Cancer *14,* 851–856, 1978
3. EORTC brain tumour group: Evaluation of the CCNU, VM_{26} plus CCNU and procarbazine in supratentorial brain gliomas. Final evaluation of a randomized study. J. Neurosurg. *55,* 27–31, 1981
4. Fewer, D., Wilson, C. B., Boldrey, E. B., Enot, K. J., Powell, M. R.: The chemotherapy of brain tumours: clinical experience in the carmustine (BCNU) and vincristine. JAMA *222,* 544–559, 1972
5. Hildebrand, J., Nouwynck, C.: Malignant gliomas. In: Randomized trials in cancer, a critical review by sites. M. J. Staquet (ed.), pp. 377–388. New York: Raven Press 1978

6. Hoshino, T., Barker, M., Wilson, C. B.: The kinetics of cultured human glioma cells. Acta Neuropathol. *32,* 235–244, 1975
7. Levin, V. A., Patlack, C. S., Landahl, H. D.: Heuristic modelling of drug delivery to malignant brain tumour. J. Pharmacokinet. Biopharm. *8,* 257–296 (1980)
8. Long, J. M.: Capillary ultrastructure and blood-brain barrier in human brain tumours. J. Neurosurg. *32,* 127–144, 1970
9. Neuwelt, E. A., Diehl, J. T., Long, H. W., Hill, R. N., Michael, A. J., Frenkel, E. P.: Monitoring of methotrexate delivery in patients with malignant brain tumours after osmotic blood-brain barrier disruption. Ann. Intern. Med. *94,* 449–454, 1981
10. Norell, H., Wilson, C. B., Slagel, D. E., Clark, D. B.: Leukoencephalopathy following the administration of methotrexate in the cerebrospinal fluid in treatment of primary brain tumours. Cancer *33,* 923–932, 1974
11. Shapiro, W. R., Chernik, N. L., Posner, J. B.: Necrotizing encephalopathy following intraventricular instillation of methotrexate. Arch. Neurol. *28,* 96–102, 1973
12. Shapiro, J. R., Yung, A., Wei-Kwan, Shapiro, W. R.: Isolation, karyotype and clonal growth of heterogeneous subpopulation of human malignant gliomas. Cancer Res. *41,* 2349–2359, 1981
13. van Putten, L. M., Keizer, H. J., Mulder, J. H.: Syndromization in tumour chemotherapy. Europ. J. Cancer *12,* 79–85, 1976
14. Wilson, C. B., Gutin, P., Boldrey, E. B., Crafts, D., Levin, V. A., Enot, J.: Single agent chemotherapy of brain tumours. Arch. Neurol. *33,* 739–744, 1976
15. Wilson, C. B., Yorke, C. H. Jr., Levin, V. A.: Intracranial malignant growth, primary and metastatic. In: Current problems in cancer. R. C. Hickey (ed.), Year Book Medical Publishers, Vol. I, Nr. 8, 1977

Acute Toxicity of Chemotherapy of Tumours of the Central Nervous System in Children

W. Havers

Many investigations reported a variety of chemotherapeutic agents tested in children suffering from tumours of the central nervous system. The following substances (Table 1), whether used on their own or in combination, have numerous side effects. The toxicity of chemotherapy will be directly discussed, but it should never be forgotten that the toxicity should be seen as a part of the total plan of treatment and never alone.

Table 1. Acute side effects of drugs used in chemotherapy of brain tumours in children

Drug	*Mean side effects*
Nitroso-ureas (BCNU, CCNU, mCCNU)	Myelosuppression Nausea, vomiting Local irritation (BCNU)
Procarbazine	Myelosuppression Nausea, vomiting Hyperexcitability Somnolence
Vincristine	Loss of deep tendon reflexes Paraesthesia Paretic gait Seizures Inappropriate ADH-secretion Constipation, abdominal pain Alopecia
Methotrexate	Myelosuppression Gastrointestinal mucositis Hepatitis Chemical arachnoiditis Motor dysfunction Renal dysfunction Acute desquamative dermatitis
Epipodophyllotoxin (VM 26)	Myelosuppression Vomiting Alopecia

Nitroso-Ureas

BCNU (1,3-bis(2-chloroethyl)-1-nitroso-urea, CCNU (1-(2-chloroethyl)-3-cyclohexyl-1-nitroso-urea) and methyl-CCNU have been successfully used in brain tumours in children. BCNU is given intravenously, CCNU and methyl-CCNU is given orally.

The nitroso-ureas are highly toxic for the bone marrow, therefore there has to be a waiting period of six weeks between courses of treatment. Depending on the dose leucopenia and thrombocytopenia have been observed, but anaemia is seldom seen. The lowest levels are seen around the thirtieth day after administration. Then the bone marrow recovers spontaneously. If given for one year or more there is a definite danger of irreversible damage to the bone marrow [1]. There have been reports on the frequency of this acute myelosuppression: Of the 51 patients reported by Walker, 30% developed thrombocytopenia below 50 000 mm^3 and 18% leucopenia below 2 000 mm^3 after administration of BCNU [2]. In this group of patients no sepsis or bleeding was seen. On the other hand deaths from sepsis and/or bleeding after nitroso-ureas have been reported [3], but today serious toxicity can be controlled by scrupulous patient supervision and supportive care.

Nausea and vomiting are harmless side-effects seen regularly several hours after giving nitroso-ureas. BCNU can also cause a local thrombophlebitis. Liver damage shown by elevation of SGOT and alkaline phosphatase is unusual and is reversible.

Recently intra-arterial BCNU was tried for metastatic brain tumours [4]. All the patients had periorbital and/or occipital pain with more than 10% suffering from focal seizures and confusion. No toxicity was seen in the liver, kidneys, lungs, or gastro-intestinal tract. All side-effects were reversible.

Procarbazine

Procarbazine is an inhibitor of monoamine oxidase and therefore should never be used with tricyclic antidepressants because of possible central nervous system complications. Hyperexcitability and somnolence are seen but are unusual. Procarbazine is given orally. Some patients suffer from nausea and vomiting but do adjust to the medication.

The main side-effect is myelosuppression which affects all three cell types. In monotherapy the myelosuppression is easy to control and should never cause a dangerous situation. When giving more than one drug side-effects are to be expected especially in connection with nitroso-ureas and radiotherapy. The combination could lead to bone marrow depression and death [5].

Vincristine

Vincristine is commonly given with other agents. It is administered weekly in doses of 1 to 2 mg/m^2 intravenously. One should be extremely careful with the intravenous injections as it can cause irritation at the site of injection or even necrosis.

Its toxicity is primarily neurological, and myelosuppression is very uncommon. Neurological side-effects start with a loss of deep tendon reflexes. This if often reversible and should not cause a discontinuation of the treatment. If severe neurological symptoms such as disturbances of movement through pain in the extremities and/or paraesthesias occur, then one should consider stopping the treatment. Paralysis and central nervous system symptoms demand an end to the use of vincristine in the treatment. In severe cases a replacement has to be found. We have the impression that neurotoxicity is more frequent in older children than in younger ones.

Abdominal pain and constipation are not dangerous but can lead to serious impairment of the patients health. That is why it is necessary to provide for regular bowel movements during vincristine therapy. A paralytic ileus is an extreme example and is rarely seen.

All children get a reversible alopecia from this therapy. Central nervous complications including inappropriate ADH-secretion with weight gain, hypertonia, and hyponatraemia are unusual.

Methotrexate

There are many ways of giving methotrexate. The substance can be given orally, on a daily or weekly basis. In the conventional intravenous method the patients receive between 20 and 80 mg/m² every seven to fourteen days. A higher dosage would be 500 mg/m² intravenously over a period of 24 hours. With the highest dosage of 20 g/m² a citrovorum factor rescue and forced diuresis must follow. In some cases methotrexate is given intrathecally or into the ventricle. Even intra-arterial infusion has been tried.

The three main side effects, independent of dosage are myelosuppression, gastro-intestinal irritation, and liver damage [6]. The toxicity increases with frequency and amount of dosage. Myelosuppression affects all cell types. Mucositis can be followed by fungus infection, bleeding, and weight loss. Gastrointestinal tract lesions are often the site for bacterial infections. Liver damage in most cases is completely reversible. Hepatocellular changes were portal inflammation and fibrosis. Double nucleated hepatic cells were often seen as well as mitochondrial swelling [7].

The common form of toxicity of intrathecal or intraventricular methotrexate is chemical arachnoiditis. This is characterized by headache, stiff neck, vomiting, fever, and a cerebrospinal-fluid pleocytosis. Subacute forms of neurotoxicity of methotrexate are motor dysfunctions and seizures [6]. Previous damage to the spinal cord through radiotherapy or other neurotoxic substances increases the frequency of neurotoxicity, but serious complications may be expected even without previous damage and may occur from a few hours to a few days. The cause of chemical arachnoiditis may be the pH of the solution, the high osmolarity, an acute sensitivity or a local citrovorum factor deficiency. The frequency of such side-effects is not known. Of 50 patients with regular intrathecal methotrexate over a period of two years we observed two cases of acute pareses that disappeared spontaneously, although several cases of residual pareses were reported [8]. Cerebrospinal fluid problems of every type increase the incidence of chemical arachnoiditis and necrotizing demyelinating leukoencephalopathy, which may occur months or years after treatment [9, 10, 11].

In addition to the general side effects seen with higher doses of methotrexate, central nervous system complications such as apathy and seizures have been reported [12]. Experience with high-dose methotrexate with citrovorum factor rescue in the treatment of brain tumours in children is minimal [13, 14]. Acute side-effects of this treatment are seizures, rashes, desquamative dermatitis and impaired kidney function. It is worth mentioning that the mortality rate of treatment with the highest doses is about 5% [15].

Lung fibrosis is a rare complication, seen mostly after long-term therapy but may also be seen when using a low dosage.

Epipodophyllotoxin

There is less experience in the treatment of central nervous tumours in children with epipodophyllotoxin (VM 26). During treatment vomiting and alopecia are observed and myelosuppression is the most serious complication. In polychemotherapy including epipodophyllotoxin bone marrow toxicity has often been seen: Half of the 22 patients treated with CCNU and VM 26 had a leucopaenia below 2000/mm^3 [16]. In this group of patients lethal complications following myelosuppression were not observed.

Polychemotherapy

All of the preceding substances with the exception of vincristine are myelotoxic and increase the danger of leucopenia and thrombocytopenia. Therefore polychemotherapy can lead to serious complications such as sepsis and/or bleeding. In the development of polychemotherapy it is important to remember that each substance has a different length of time before myelosuppression is produced. For all children receiving polychemotherapy during radiotherapy there is a special danger of bone marrow toxicity [5, 17]. Radiotherapy also increases the neurotoxicity of certain drugs.

Therefore chemotherapy should not be seen in isolation but rather as an integral part of the total plan of treatment. In connection with this one must remember the immunosuppressive effects of steroids.

References

1. Shapiro, W. R.: Chemotherapy of primary malignant brain tumours in children. Cancer *35*, 965–972 (1975)
2. Walker, M. D., Alexander, Jr., E., Hunt, W. E., MacCarty, C. S., Mahaley, Jr., M. S., Mealy, Jr., J., Norrell, H. A., Owens, G., Ransohoff, J., Wilson, C. B., Gehan, E. A., Strike, T. A.: Evaluation of BCNU and/or radiotherapy in the treatment of anaplastic gliomas. A cooperative clinical trial. J. Neurosurg. *49*, 333–343 (1978)

3. Fewer, D., Wilson, C. B., Boldrey, E. B., Enot, K. J., Powell, M. R.: The chemotherapy of brain tumours. Clinical experience with carmustine (BCNU) and vincristine. JAMA *222,* 549–552 (1972)
4. Madajewicz, S., West, C. R., Park, H. C., Ghoorah, J., Avellanosa, A. M., Takita, H., Karakousis, C., Vincent, R., Caracandas, J., Jennings, E.: Phase II study – Intra-arterial BCNU therapy for metastatic brain tumours. Cancer *47,* 653–657 (1981)
5. Crafts, D. C., Levin, V. A., Edwards, M. S., Pischer, T. L., Wilson, C. B.: Chemotherapy of recurrent medulloblastoma with combined procarbazine, CCNU, and vincristine. J. Neurosurg. *49,* 589–592 (1978)
6. Bleyer, W. A.: The clinical pharmacology of methotrexate – new applications of an old drug. Cancer *41,* 36–51 (1978)
7. Sharp, H., Nesbit, M., White, J., Krivit, W.: Methotrexate liver toxicity. J. Pediat. *74,* 818–819 (1969)
8. Luddy, R. E., Gilman, P. A.: Paraplegia following intrathecal methotrexate. J. Pediat. *83,* 988–992 (1973)
9. Price, R. A., Jamieson, P. A.: The central nervous system in childhood leukemia. II. Subacute leukoencephalopathy. Cancer *35,* 306–318 (1975)
10. Rubinstein, L. J., Herman, M. M., Long, T. F., Wilbur, J. R.: Disseminated necrotizing leukoencephalopathy: A complication of treated central nervous system leukemia and lymphoma. Cancer *35,* 291–305 (1975)
11. Shapiro, W. R., Chernik, N. L., Posner, J. B.: Necrotizing encephalopathy following intraventricular instillation of methotrexate. Arch. Neurol. *28,* 96–102 (1973)
12. Rechnitzer, C., Scheibel, E., Hendel, J.: Methotrexate in the plasma and cerebrospinal fluid of children treated with intermediate dose methotrexate. Acta Paediatr. Scand. *70,* 615–618 (1981)
13. Rosen, G., Ghavimi, F., Nirenberg, A., Mosende, C., Metha, B. M.: High-dose methotrexate with citrovorum factor rescue for the treatment of central nervous system tumours in children. Cancer Treat. Rep. *61,* 681–690 (1977)
14. Shapiro, W. R.: High-dose methotrexate in malignant gliomas. Cancer Treat. Rep. *61,* 753–756 (1977)
15. Djerassi, I., Kim, J. S., Najak, N. P., Ohanissian, H., Adler, S.: High dose methotrexate with citrovorum factor rescue. A new approach to cancer chemotherapy. In Recent Advances in Cancer Treatment, Vol. 3, H. J. Tagnon and M. J. Stakuet Eds. New York: Raven Press 1977
16. Gutin, P. H., Walker, M. D.: I.v.methyl-CCNU, VM-26, and cranial irradiation in therapy for malignant brain tumours. Cancer Treat. Rep. *61,* 1715–1717 (1977)
17. Thomas, P. R. M., Duffner, P. K., Cohen, M. E., Sinks, L. F., Tebbi, C., Freeman, A. I.: Multimodal therapy for medulloblastoma. Cancer *45,* 666–669 (1980)

Late Effects After Treatment of Brain Tumours in Childhood

P. GUTJAHR and B. WALTHER

A cautious therapeutic optimism is justified with regard to the treatment and prognosis of the primary brain tumours of childhood although progress in treatment is far behind the results obtained in other childhood malignancies such as acute lymphoblastic leukaemia and Wilms' tumours.

In the permanent and frequent *long-term care* of children with cancer in our paediatric-oncologic outpatient service we noticed early [3, 4] that a great number of children with primary CNS tumours evidently suffered from *severe late sequelae* after the tumour and its treatment.

One author has reported [10] that some patients, having survived cancer in childhood, even see *positive aspects* in their disease, which they had overcome (e.g. with regard to the development of their personality), an interesting fact, which has also been pointed out by some of our own patients with different malignancies outside the CNS. However, this usually does not apply to children after primary CNS tumours. In these, the late adverse effects often cause great problems, in different respects.

In 1975, we started intensive work in the field of late effects. Several publications have emerged from this work [1, 2, 5, 7–9, 11, 12, 14, 15] and a comprehensive survey was published in 1979 [6].

The *following problems* have to be considered in an analysis of the late effects after brain tumours of childhood:

- the *clinical* status, *neurological* status, alterations of *sense – organ* functions and physical *development;*
- changes of structure and/or function of the *skeleton; soft-tissue* defects (e.g. after irradiation of the spinal column);
- a possibly increased risk of infections with the *hepatitis B virus;*
- *endocrine* changes;
- *EEG – changes* or *epilepsies*;
- alterations in the *peripheral nerves* (mostly due to Vincristine medication);
- *second malignancies* as a possible consequence of treatment;
- *psychological and psychosocial late consequences* as well as delayed intellectual damage.

Some of our results will be presented here incidentally. Others such as the late sequelae after inadequate (paravenous) injection of cytostatics (e.g. Vincristine), paralysis after intraspinal tumours, or the wide field of CT – demonstrable changes of brain structure are referred to in other publications [7–9, 11, 13].

Table 1. Neurological findings in children treated for medulloblastomas and cerebellar astrocytomas (Dept. of Paediatrics, Univ. of Mainz)

	Medullo-blastomas	Cerebellar astrocytoma
	$n=16$	$n=24$
Sensorimotor system, arms and legs		
normal	5	10
slightly disturbed	6	5
medium changes	5	7
severe changes	0	2
Gross motor function, coordination lower limbs		
normal	0	0
slightly disturbed	5	13
medium changes	5	8
severe changes	6	3
Fine motor function, coordination upper limbs		
normal	0	0
slightly disturbed	4	12
medium changes	6	6
severe changes	6	6
Balance of trunk		
normal	0	5
slightly disturbed	2	7
medium changes	4	10
severe changes	10	2
Quality of performance of movement dynamics		
normal	0	10
slightly disturbed	5	5
medium changes	5	8
severe changes	6	1

The different items of the neurological performance were evaluated according to the principle of the best possible. The scores were obtained by the assessment of the following functional aspects:
Sensorimotor system: resistance against passive movements, muscle power, deep tendon reflexes, plantar response (signs of lesions of pyramidal tract), lateralization of symptoms;
Gross motor function, coordination lower limbs: heel-knee-test. standing on one leg, jumping (hopping) on one leg, lateralization of symptoms;
Fine motor function, coordination upper limbs: diadochokinesis, pronation and supination, finger opposition test, finger-nose test, fingertip-touching test, posture with arms extended, lateralization of symptoms;
Balance of trunk: Romberg's test, walking along a straight line, eyes opened and eyes closed, walking on heels, walking on tiptoe;
Quality of performance of movement: Dynamics, speed, goal-direction, extent of movement, involuntary and associated movements, lateralization of movements

Table 2. Results of ophthalmological fundoscopy in children after acute lymphoblastic leukaemia (treatment had included cranial irradiation) and several types of primary CNS tumours

	n	Fundus right side	Fundus left side
Acute lymphoblastic leukaemia	38	Normal in 38	Normal in 38
Primary CNS tumours	73	Normal in 44	Normal in 46
		Partial optic nerve atrophy in 25	Partial optic nerve atrophy in 22
		Total optic nerve atrophy in 4	Total optic nerve atrophy in 5 children

After *infratentorial* tumours we have never found a child totally normal as regards *neurological performance.* There were indeed several children who appeared normal in their sensorimotor system but totally normal findings as regards gross and fine motor function as well as coordination were never found (Table 1).

Changes of medium and severe degree occurred more often than slight ones. Children after *medulloblastomas* had a *worse performance* than children after cerebellar astrocytomas.

It seems that improved neurophysiological diagnostic methods will reveal more and more important neurological late sequelae, which some investigators for a long time have denied or underestimated.

Table 2 shows the results of *fundoscopy* in a former investigation in our patients (the actual detailed analysis is given in another part of this book with regard to the ophthalmological aspects). The table compares the results in children after irradiation of the skull in acute lymphoblastic leukaemia with those in children after primary CNS tumours. Different types of brain tumour were investigated.

Two of the long-term survivors of cerebellar astrocytomas are blind, as a result of longstanding raised intracranial pressure before treatment owing to a long history of delayed diagnosis.

In general, *visual disturbances* predominantly affect children with craniopharyngiomas and optic nerve gliomas. Others may be affected, however, as described above.

Growth disturbances occur for instance as vertebral arrests or retardations after *radiotherapy* for medulloblastoma, but also as *endocrine* short stature associated with Craniopharyngiomas and HGH – deficiency. *Spontaneous regrowth* (and so-called catch-up growth) may happen, but often *HGH-substitution* is necessary. We also identified two children with HGH-deficiency after medulloblastomas.

From the group of 21 *craniopharyngioma* patients six had negative results on stimulation of HGH by two tests (L-arginine and L-Dopa/Carbidopa).

About 35% of the craniopharyngioma patients need long-term treatment with DDAVP (Minirin). We prefer the intranasal preparation to the intramuscular drugs, even in younger children.

In two medulloblastoma children stimulation of TSH by TRH gave clearly elevated values after 30 minutes, which is compatible with the assumption of a *latent hypothyroidism*. As *thyroid carcinoma* seems to be a possible event after medulloblastoma (and craniospinal irradiation), careful *long-term evaluation* of this organ seems mandatory.

We further investigated *motor and sensory nerve conduction velocities* in long-term survivors of childhood cancer. Motor nerve conduction velocities were normal in the groups of children after different types of brain tumour (treated with or without Vincristine); however, by determination of sensory nerve conduction velocities we found that these were *prolonged* in children after brain tumours who also had had Vincristine treatment, whereas sensory nerve conduction velocities in brain tumour children without Vincristine treatment remained normal.

The field of late *EEG-findings* has been investigated by Dieterich et al. (pp. 95–98). In summary, EEG-findings are *not directly correlated with clinical findings* (EEG in infratentorial tumour survivors are often normal, whereas the clinical status may reveal severe handicaps, and *cerebral convulsions* must be considered especially in children after supratentorial tumours, although their clinical states may be perfectly normal).

It is impossible to give a detailed analysis of *long-term psychosocial problems* in this survey. However, it has to be mentioned that also in this regard most of the severe sequelae apply to the children with medulloblastomas, and we consider these to be rather a result of the tumour itself than of the treatment.

About one half of the children had to be *put back* a stage from their former levels at school, and a considerable number of them have to attend a *school for backward children* (see also: Walther et al.: pp. 389–398). Unfortunately at the moment, most of the efforts to improve the situation of these children and to promote *rehabilitation* measures, are based on private initiatives.

One other important late adverse effect is the risk of a *second neoplasm*. Based on the current knowledge, acute leukaemia (especially the acute nonlymphoblastic variety), thyroid carcinoma, osteogenic sarcoma and possibly glioblastoma multiforme have to be considered after irradiation of the brain and skull and after chemotherapy.

Furthermore, some of the children with brain tumours have a risk of a second neoplasm, which is apparently *unrelated to radiation and/or chemotherapy*. Within a cooperative group of Germain paediatric oncologists, we have identified 41 second malignancies and neoplasms after irradiation and/or chemotherapy for non-malignant primaries in different centres of paediatric oncology during 1981.

Among these children were *four CNS tumours as second neoplasms* (Table 3): one glioblastoma after irradiation for craniopharyngioma, one glioblastoma after chemotherapy for acute lymphoblastic leukaemia and irradiation of the skull with 24 Gy[1]; two other CNS tumours occurred after operations for tumours in other sites: one medulloblastoma after an operation on an adrenocortical carcinoma[1] (the brother of this patient had developed unilateral retinoblastoma), and one pilocytic astrocytoma[1] after operation on a gangliocytoneuroma in a patient with von

1 One patient of the Dept. of Paediatrics, Mainz; two patients of Prof. Kornhuber, Dept. of Paediatrics, Frankfurt/M.; one patient of Priv.-Doz. Dr. Brandeis, Heidelberg

Table 3. CNS tumours as second neoplasms in children with cancer; results from a German cooperative group (1981)

First neoplasm	Treatment of first neoplasm	Second neoplasm
Craniopharyngioma	Radiotherapy 60 Gy, Cyclophos.	Glioblastoma within irradiation field
Acute lymphoblastic leukaemia	Radiotherapy 24 Gy, combination chemotherapy	Glioblastoma multiforme
Adrenocortical carcinoma	Operation alone	Medulloblastoma (brother of patient had retinoblastoma)
Gangliocytoneuroma (retroperitoneal)	Operation alone	Pilocytic astrocytoma (patient suffers from von Recklinghausen's neurofibromatosis)

Recklinghausen's disease. The two latter cases may provide evidence for a *genetic susceptibility* for tumours.

In summarizing the possible late effects described above, we stress the fact that *intensive long-term care* and *detailed analysis of late adverse effects* in the survivors of childhood brain tumours is needed. It is needed for early recognition and possibly *early treatment of late sequelae;* late effects – at least in part – should *influence future concepts of treatment* regimen. However a great misunderstanding after the above survey (for a complete review see (6)) would be to develop a pessimistic attitude towards combined treatment of childhood brain tumours in view of the many and varied possible late effects.

References

1. Baumann, W., Gutjahr, P., Arnold, W., Meyer zum Büschenfelde, K. H.: Spätfolgen nach Tumortherapie im Kindesalter: HB_sAg – Persistenz und Lebererkrankungen. Mschr. Kinderheilk. *125,* 574–575 (1977)
2. Dieterich, E., Göbel, B., Gutjahr, P.: EEG-Befunde nach Vincristin-Behandlung. Mschr. Kinderheilk. *126,* 709–710 (1978)
3. Gutjahr, P., Kutzner, J.: Kombinierte Radio- und Chemotherapie des Zentralnervensystems bei malignen Neoplasien im Kindesalter. Dtsch. med. Wschr. *100,* 1651–1656 (1976)
4. Gutjahr, P., Wallenfang, T., Meinig, G., Einsiedel, E., Nakayama, N., Voth, D.: New Problems in the Therapy of Medulloblastomas. In: Modern Problems in Paediatrics, Vol. *18,* pp. 75–79; Karger, Basel, 1977
5. Gutjahr, P., Kretzschmar, K.: Akute lymphoblastische Leukämien und maligne Non-Hodgkin-Lymphome im Kindesalter. Computertomographische Befunde nach prophylaktischer Schädelbestrahlung und Chemotherapie. Dtsch. med. Wschr. *104,* 1068–1071 (1979)
6. Gutjahr, P.: Das Schicksal tumor- und leukämiekranker Kinder – Untersuchung Langzeitüberlebender nach Realisierung moderner Konzepte der pädiatrischen Onkotherapie. Habilit.schr., Mainz 1979
7. Gutjahr, P.: Untersuchungen zum Spätstatus Langzeit-Überlebender und Geheilter nach bösartigen Neubildungen im Kindesalter. Fortschr. Med. *98,* 289–292 (1980)

8. Gutjahr, P., Kretzschmar, K.: Akute lymphoblastische Leukämien und maligne Non-Hodgkin-Lymphome im Kindesalter. Computertomographische Befunde *vor* Behandlung des Zentralnervensystems und ihre Beziehung zu klinischen Parametern. Dtsch. med. Wschr. *105,* 1389–1392 (1980)
9. Gutjahr, P., Walther, B.: Bösartige Neubildungen als chronische Erkrankungen in der Pädiatrie. Sozialpädiat. *2,* 224–231 (1980)
10. Holmes, H. A., Holmes, F. F.: After ten years, what are the handicaps and life styles of children treated for cancer? Clin. Pediat. *14,* 819–823 (1975)
11. Kretzschmar, K., Gutjahr, P., Kutzner, J.: CT studies before and after CNS treatment for acute lymphoblastic leukemia and malignant non-Hodgkin's lymphomas in childhood. Neuroradiol. *20,* 173–180 (1980)
12. Lowitzsch, K., Gutjahr, P., Ottes, H.: Clinical and neurophysiological findings in 47 long-term survivors of childhood malignancies treated with various doses of Vincristine. In: Canal, N., Pozza G. (eds.): Peripheral neuropathies; Elsevier/ North-Holland Biomedical Press, pp. 459–465, 1978
13. Price, R. A., Jamieson, P. A.: The central nervous system in childhood leukemia. II. Subacute Leukoencephalopathy. Cancer *35,* 306–318 (1975)
14. Walther, B., Gutjahr, P., Beron, G.: Therapiebegleitende und -überdauernde neurologische und neuropsychologische Diagnostik bei akuter lymphoblastischer Leukämie im Kindesalter. Klin. Pädiat. *193,* 177–183 (1981)
15. Ziegler, R., Schönberger, W., Gutjahr, P., Grimm, W.: Ergebnisse der Schilddrüsendiagnostik nach Radiotherapie maligner Tumoren im Halsbereich. Mschr. Kinderheilk. *124,* 484–485 (1976)

Development After Treatment of Cerebellar Medulloblastoma in Childhood

B. WALTHER and P. GUTJAHR

Introduction

Among paediatric oncological patients in general and especially those with central nervous system tumours, the group with cerebellar medulloblastoma is characterized by numerous additional problems: tumour therapy, comprising operation, radiation and polychemotherapy is increasingly aggressive, thus adding to the neurological symptoms of the tumour itself [1]; the survival rates are still rather low, the risk of recurrence persists up to 5–10 years after diagnosis [24]; the long-lasting effects of tumour treatment as well as the underlying disease involve somatic as well as neurological and psychological functions.

Thus, the long-term medical care of medulloblastoma patients has to extend to the initiation of rehabilitation programmes for preventive and curative therapy of chronic disabilities.

In the literature of the last 20 years there exist contradictory reports respecting the quality of life and the frequency and amount of handicap in survivors of medulloblastoma in childhood. Therefore, in addition to a first preliminary assessment which suggested multiple disabilities in the majority of patients [10, 11, 12], the children and adolescents treated for medulloblastoma at the Department of Paediatric Oncology of the Children's University Hospital at Mainz underwent an extensive diagnostic procedure aimed at a comprehensive evaluation of neurological and neuropsychological function of the survivors.

Patients of the Study Group

Between the years 1954 and 1980 there were 885 children treated for malignant lesions at the Department of Paediatric Oncology of our clinic, including 211 patients with tumour of the central nervous system: the diagnosis of cerebellar medulloblastoma was verified in 43 cases, representing 20% of the brain tumours and 4.9% of all patients.

None of the 12 patients with onset of disease before 1967 survived, whereas five out 20 who were admitted to the department between 1967 and 1974 were still alive at the beginning of the follow-up study; treatment consisted of operation, craniospinal irradiation and chemotherapy with cyclophosphamide partly combined with vincristine and/or intrathecal methotrexate; three of them participated in the study, the fate of one patient is unknown and another patient could not be contacted. In the following years – from 1975 to 1980 – there were 14 children with cerebellar medulloblastoma, of whom eight began their treatment within the last 12 months before the re-evaluation. All of them underwent operation, craniospinal radiation and polychemotherapy with intrathecal methotrexate, vincristine and – for the majority – CCNU; 12 survived up to the date of the investigation and could thus be included in the study.

According to the time elapsed since diagnosis, the 15 patients were divided into two groups: group I comprises the seven patients with onset of disease between 1969 and 1977; group II refers to the eight children with less than 12 months since diagnosis. The psychosocial factors of the study group are summarized in Table 1: there were eight boys and seven girls with onset of disease at the age of 2 to 14 years with a median at 8, 10 years. The length of survival was 51 months in the median for group I and 5 months for group II. Patients in group II were younger at the follow-up investigation (median of 9.6 years) than the group I patients (median of 13.5 years). School achievement was normal prior to the diagnosis of the tumour in all

Table 1. Psychosocial characteristics of the patients. Group I: long-term Survivors. Group II: survival less than one year

Characteristics		All subjects n=15	Group I n=7	Group II n=8
Year of onset of disease		1969 – 1980	1969 – 1977	1979 – 1980
Sex	Boys	8	4	4
	Girls	7	3	4
Age at onset of the disease	Variation	2 – 14 years	2 – 14 years	3 – 12 years
	Median	8, 10 years	8, 10 years	8, 10 years
Length of survival in years	<1	8	0	8
	1 – 5	4	4	0
	>5	3	3	0
	Median	6 months	51 months	5 months
Age at follow-up assessment in years	<6	2	0	2
	6 – 10	4	1	3
	>10	9	6	3
	Median	11, 1 years	13, 5 years	9, 6 years
School achievement at onset of the disease	Not yet at school-age	5	2	3
	Primary school	6	4	2
	Secondary school	1	1	0
	High school	3	0	3
	Special school	0	0	0
Socio-economic class	Upper/middle	8	2	6
	Lower	7	5	2

Table 2. Symptoms of history and clinical assessment before treatment

Characteristics		All subjects $n=15$	Group I $n=7$	Group II $n=8$
Symptoms of cerebellar disease	in history	9	5	4
	on admission	13	5	8
Cranial nerve symptoms	in history	9	5	4
	on admission	9	5	4
Symptoms of increased intracranial pressure	in history	14	6	8
	on admission	12	6	6
Neuroradiological diagnosis	Internal hydroceph.	14	7	7

cases, in group II with higher rate of upper social class membership, 3 children attended high schools.

The history of early development was uncomplicated in 12 children, disease of the nervous system existed in no case prior to the tumour diagnosis. The duration of tumour history varied from 2 weeks to 6 months; nausea and vomiting were the first symptoms in six patients; in five children the early symptoms were interpreted as manifestations of a cerebral concussion after acute head injury [15]; the first diagnosis was different from suspicion of an intracranial space-occupying lesion in nine cases.

Disorder of gait was observed by the parents in nine children, on admission 13 patients presented with clear symptoms of a cerebellar lesion (Table 2); cranial nerve dysfunction was evident in nine patients, symptoms of increased intracranial pressure were found in 12 patients; papilloedema existed in 13 cases and amounted to at least 2 dioptres in seven. The X-ray of the skull was abnormal in 12 out of 13 cases, in 10 out of 11 electroencephalograms there was slow wave activity with a maximum in the parieto-occipital leads. Angiography was suspicious of a space-occupying lesions in all of the eight patients were it was done and ventriculography showed dilatation of the ventricular system in all patients. Thus, in 14 out of the 15 cases, there was a diagnosis of internal hydrocephalus with symptoms of complete occlusion in eight patients.

The therapeutic procedures are summarized in Table 3: the resection of the tumour was subtotal in eight cases and infiltration of the rhombencephalon was verified in six children. Internal shunts were implanted five times, ventriculoperitoneal shunts in three patients. Complications in the early postoperative period occurred in eight children with symptoms of unconsciousness and peaks of intracranial pressure; attacks of cerebral convulsions occurred in two patients.

The stay at the hospital for the initial treatment varied from 8 to 24 weeks; on discharge, all children were ataxic, speech disorder was manifest in five patients,

Table 3. Neurosurgical procedure, and characteristics of radiation and cytostatic therapy. Symptoms in the early phase of disease after starting treatment. *CP* Cyclophosphamide; *MTX* Methotrexate; *VCR* Vincristine

Characteristics			All subjects $n=15$	Group I $n=7$	Group II $n=8$
Local situation at operation: infiltrat. of rhombencephal.			6	1	5
Extent of tumour extirpation		Total	7	3	4
		Subtotal	8	4	4
Implantation of shunt		Internal	5	0	5
		External	3	1	2
Full dose radiation in rad		Post. fossa	5500 – 6000	5500 – 6000	5000 – 6000
		Spinal canal	3000 – 4500	3500 – 4500	3000 – 3500
Chemotherapy with cytostatic agents		CP	6	6	0
		MTX, i.th.	14	6 (1 on recurrence)	8
		VCR	13	5 (1 on recurrence)	8
		CCNU	8	1 (1 on recurrence)	7
Postoperative complications			8	3	5
State at the time of discharge	Ataxia	All	15	7	8
		Severe	5	2	3
		Hemi-ataxia	9	2	7
	Speech dysfunction		5	4	1
	Cranial nerve symptoms		11	7	4
	Reduction of vision		6	4	2
	Psychological changes		6	2	4

behavioural problems in six children. The full extent of handicap often became apparent only in the ensuing months. Physiotherapy was prescribed for the majority of the patients.

Realization and Design of the Study

The diagnostic sessions – up to six for each patient – were coordinated in most cases with dates for therapy control at the oncological clinic and they comprised 15 to 20 hours for the older patients. Family members often attended the investigation. In the majority, the children and adolescents enjoyed the examination, though often this constituted the first experience of complete failure in formerly well – controlled functions: but the diagnostic procedures revealed disabilities underlying the general or very specific learning difficulties and thus could point to remedial measures and functional training supporting the child's efforts for reintegration.

The neuropsychological investigation included the following functions:

1) sensorimotor system, postural abilities and coordination of movement, including motoscopic and motometric test measures,
2) level of general and cognitive development with distinction of speed and power in the conditions of testing,
3) mode of problem solving and cognitive style, individual psychomotor speed,
4) visual and graphomotoric coordination, auditory and visual perception,
5) concentrative capacity, short-term memory, speed and duration of attentive behavior,
6) developmental level of cultural techniques – reading, spelling, mathematics,
7) psychodiagnostic evaluation and history taking with patients and parents.

Results of the Study

Parental Reports

Impairment of movement was attested by all; physical tiredness existed in all group II patients, but only in half of the long-term survivors. Reduction of mental abilities exclusively affected group I. Instability of mood and exaggerated irritability were observed by nearly all parents.

For the majority of the long-term survivors, the parents confirmed symptoms of disability in learning and defective concentration, frequent aggressive outbursts and loss of extrafamiliar contacts in combination with serious problems within the family; these changes were lacking in group II.

In summary, according to the parents' reports, there exist lasting neurological handicap and mood disorder, whereas physical strength seems to improve with the ending of treatment. Changes in psychosocial behavior and socialization become obvious only later in the course of the disease. The time sequence in the emerging and persistence of symptoms and problems underlines the necessity for long-term care and observation.

School Attainment

For group II patients the time elapsed since the onset of the disease is too short for conclusive assessment, but so far two of the five surviving patients have experienced severe school problems. In the long-term survivors the consequences of the tumour disease for the educational development are obvious: the youngest child has twice been prevented from starting school, thus being retarded for two years in educational achievement; the oldest girl left the ordinary school without receiving a final certificate, she had no professional training and until now is without any occupation. Four children attend special schools for physically handicapped pupils in classes for teaching retarded children. Only one child living in a rural community, remained in the ordinary local school. Thus, school attainment was normal in one out of seven patients.

Individual Activities and Contacts

According to the reports of the patients themselves and their parents, the friendships of the time prior to the disease rapidly decrease in number and intensity after the patient returns home from the hospital. This is caused and enhanced by at least two facts: first, the patient can no longer participate in the usual play activities and secondly, the patients are extremely vulnerable by experience of failure even in game activities; they demonstrate intense motivation to compete with the others and to win, thus appearing egocentric and unfair. This isolation is aggravated if removal from the former school becomes necessary.

None of the patients was member of a club, only a few were engaged with a hobby; often individual interests and occupations had to be abandoned because of impairment of vision or manual skills.

In the short-term survivors there existed a deep motivation to compensate for the handicaps and social isolation by educational success, whereas in the long-term survivors resignation and lack of creativity and spontaneity were dominating. These tendencies were affirmed by the results of the psychodiagnostic tests; self-concerned reaction tendencies in social interaction, neurotic attitude especially in the short-term survivors, strong motivation for social contacts, denying of the restricted ability and opportunity of engagement in age-specific activities.

Neurological Assessment

All 15 patients were able to walk at least a few steps without being supported. Disturbance of cranial nerve function existed in all cases (Fig. 1): nystagmus (n = 15), phonetic problems (n = 12), loss of visual accuracy (n = 8), motility disorder of the tongue (n = 5), impairment of hearing (n = 3).

Symptoms of cerebellar affection were present in all patients: ataxia of the trunk was combined with significant lateralization of neurological handicap in 13 cases. Tasks of postural stability and motor coordination – as walking on a straight line, standing on one leg, standing and walking on tiptoe, walking backwards – if at all, could not be performed without balancing movements of the trunk and the upper limbs. Directional movements and diadochokinesia of the upper limbs were impaired in all group II cases and in five out of seven patients in group I. Sensorimotor functions were more affected in the patients still under therapy because of the additional adverse effects especially of vincristine on the peripheral nerves. The psychomotor speed was slowed in all but one child with pre-existing developmental retardation and hyperkinetic behaviour disorder.

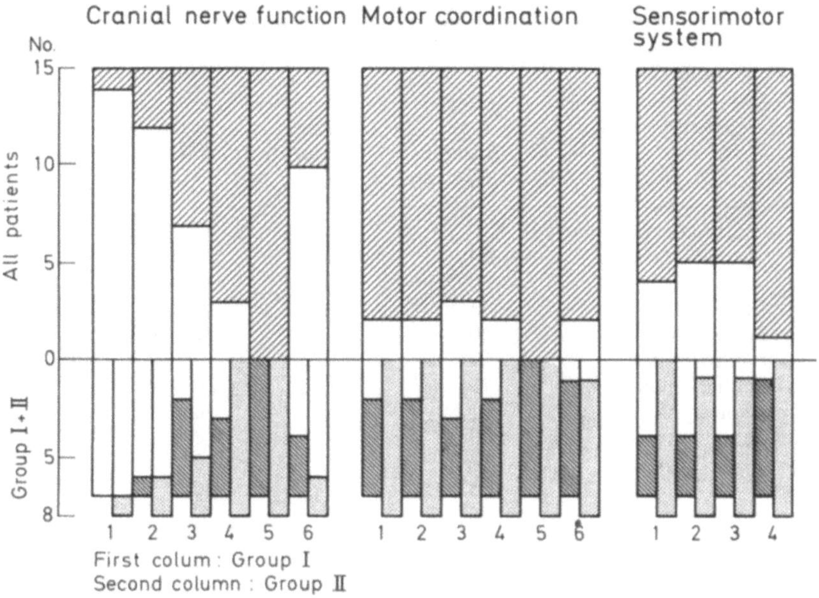

Fig. 1. Frequencies of dysfunction of the neuromotor system. White: Unaffected; Black: disturbed. Cranial nerve function: facial innervation (*1*), auditory system (*2*), visual system (*3*), speech (*4*), vestibular system (*5*), tongue motility (*6*). Motor coordination: metria (*1*) and diadochokinesia (*2*) of upper limbs, praxia of upper limbs (*3*), bimanual coordination (*4*), balance and posture of trunk (*5*), lateralization of symptoms (*6*). Sensorimotor system: resistance to passive movements (*1*), muscle power (*2*), threshold and intensity of tendon reflexes (*3*), amount of movement (*4*).

In accordance with the high degree of neurological disorder, the test results of the motometric scale (coordination test for children) all ranged below 3 standard deviations from the mean; in a second standardized procedure including skills of upper and lower limbs, there were only two patients who performed at least 10 of the 18 items, three out of 12 patients ranged within 3 standard deviations below the mean. Kinaesthetic function and body scheme were intact in half of the cases. When performing the "Draw a Man" test, the majority portrayed asymmetrical bodies, accentuating the side affected in the patient himself.

Neuropsychological Functions

The assessment aimed at the recognition of functional disorders resulting in impairment and difficulties of learning. In contrast the well-known syndrome of minimal cerebral dysfunction, visual perception was affected in only one third of the patients; whereas visuomotoric coordination and graphomotoric performance involving manual skills as well as perceptual-motor integration were impaired in half of the patients. Visual short-term memory was less frequently reduced than auditory memory. Severe handicap was observed in speed of reaction to stimuli and capacity

Table 4. Pattern and frequency of disorders (in per cent of the sample) at follow up. For test-measures, the following cut-off-points are chosen: No disability: beyond the 25th percentile; slight disability: beyond the 3rd percentile

Medulloblastoma – Groups I and II -function		No disabil. (%)	Slight disabil. (%)	Severe disabil. (%)	No. of pat.
Sensorimotor system, motor coordination		0	13	87	15
Kinaesthesia		54	15	31	13
Body scheme		60	30	10	10
Visual motor	Coordination	53	33	14	15
Graphomotor	Performance	40	33	27	15
Visual	Figure ground	67	33	0	15
Perception	Spatial orientation	70	10	20	10
Visual short-term memory		71	29	0	14
Auditory short-term memory		58	34	8	12
Power of concentration		15	0	85	13
Speed of reaction		38	16	46	13
Verbal fluency		40	40	20	15
Cognitive ability (IQ)		60	27	13	15
School achievement test		22	56	22	9
Cognitive style		23	62	15	13
Culture	Reading	13	37	50	8
Technique	Spelling	0	11	89	9
	Mathematics	33	25	42	12

to concentrate under time-limited test conditions. Verbal fluency, even for common words such as colour names, was abnormal in the majority.

Cognitive ability in a test procedure without time-limited administration order was below the age level in 40%; only two adolescents ranged within the level of mental retardation. However, the results in school achievement clearly contrasted with this approximately normal level of intelligence: only a quarter of the patients reached the age-specific standard. Strategies of problem solving and cognitive style were impaired in most cases: in relation to the attained level of solved problems, the reaction time was too long, often the cue of the test items had to be repeatedly demonstrated until it was understood (Table 4).

Thus, the prerequisites for learning and educational progress – memory, concentration, speedness, ease in problem solving, graphomotoric skills – are manifold impaired especially in the long-term survivors. The low level of abilities in the cultural techniques – reading, spelling, mathematics – can be explained by these handicaps. The effects of poor motivation together with the lack of encouragement and individual assistance following failure in the normal school may add to these results. Apart from other handicaps, the underachievement in the cultural techniques means restricted chances for further professional education and occupation. In summarizing the patients' and parents' reports and the results of the investigation, the quality of life appears affected by the disease in all patients, though with different degrees of disability. In adopting the grouping proposed by Bouchard [6], to which several authors refer, there was no one patient in our study leading an active life without being disabled. 14% in group I and 13% in group II were slightly impaired, 57% (74% in group II) were affected by partial but severe dysfunction, 29% (13% in group II) had to be considered as being incapable of looking after themselves.

Discussion

In the literature there exists a seemingly convincing accord in the evaluation of the frequency and degree of handicap in survivors of brain tumours of childhood in general and of medulloblastoma in particular [2, 5, 6, 7, 8, 9, 14, 16, 21]; Lasson [18] in reviewing the literature, reports on 80% of childhood brain tumour patients leading a normal life. This high degree of unaffected development holds true irrespective of the method of treatment and the year of onset of the disease. In an early paper, McFarland [19] suggested in contrast to the published data 'that brain damage suffered in the period prior to the treatment, which may be increased by some degree of central nervous system damage as a direct result of heavy irradiation' should be expected in these patients. There exist a few papers with less encouraging results, two of them base their evaluation on actual follow-up assessment and closely correspond to our results: Berthold [4] on the basis of interviews and historical data rated 58% of the survivors four years after diagnosis as leading a normal life; Raimondi [20] classified only 38% after two years survival as lacking any handicap; Ullmo [22] published results on intelligence testing, one third ranged as learning disabled. Bamford [3] retrospectively investigated 30 long-term survivors of intracranial space-occupying lesions and demonstrated physical and neurological handicap in the majority – 40% with cranial nerve palsies, 27% with severe neurological disorder, 57% with lower educational attainment, 42% with emotional problems. The best agreement with our study is provided by the detailed investigation of Hirsch [13] comparing the functional disorders after treatment of medulloblastoma and astrocytoma. In survivors of medulloblastoma in childhood he confirmed specific learning disorders in 82% (our study: 84%), behaviour disorder in 93% (our study: 93%) and falling off in school achievement in 75% (group I in our study: 86%).

Whereas Hirsch suggested a relation of the degree of mental impairment with infiltration of the brain stem, this association could not be confirmed by our study; however, our data indicate a correlation of the later cognitive development with the degree and persistence of increased intracranial pressure, a fact which is also emphasized by other authors [3].

Though survivors of malignant lesions in childhood other than brain tumours also suffer neurological and neuropsychological handicap [23], the high frequency and degree of disorder appear to be disease-specific. The number of patients is too small to allow for general conclusions; nevertheless, the results underline the need of detailed follow-up investigations including neurological, neuropsychological and educational aspects as well as early introduction of rehabilitation programs. Efforts of a multicentred study should be encouraged also in this aspect of patient care [17] to identify the factors of disease and therapy which, at comparable levels of survival rate, minimize the adverse effects and improve the functional prognosis of the long-term survivors.

References

1. Allen, J. C.: The effects of cancer therapy on the nervous system. J. Pediat. *93*, 903 (1978)
2. Bamberg, M., Schmitt, G., Quast, U., Bongartz, E. B., Nau, H.-E., Bayindir, C., Reinhardt, V.: Therapie und Prognose des Medulloblastoms. Fortschritte durch neuartige Bestrahlungstechniken. Strahlentherapie *156*, 1–17 (1980)
3. Bamford, F. N., Jones, P. M., Pearson, D., Ribeiro, G. G., Shalet, S. M., Beardwell, C. G.: Residual disabilities in children treated for intracranial space-occupying lesions. Cancer *37*, 1149–1151 (1976)
4. Berthold, R., Janka, G., Lampert, F.: Kleinhirnmedulloblastom-retrospektive Untersuchung der Wertigkeit von Diagnostik und Therapie. Klin. Pädiat. *193*, 189–197 (1981)
5. Bloom, H. J. C., Wallace, E. N. K., Henk, J. W.: The treatment and prognosis of medulloblastoma in children: a study of 82 verified cases. Am. J. Roentgenol. *105*, 43–62 (1969)
6. Bouchard, J., Peirce, C. B.: Radiation therapy in the management of neoplasms of the central nervous system, with a special note in regard to children. Twenty years of experience, 1939–1958. Am. J. Roentgenol. *84*, 610–628 (1960)
7. Bouchard, J.: Radiation therapy of tumours and diseases of the nervous system. London: J. Kimpton 1966
8. Duffner, P. K., Cohen, M. E., Thomas, P. R. M., Sinks, L. F., Freeman, A. I.: Combination therapy in recurrent medulloblastoma. Cancer *43*, 41–45 (1979)
9. Gjerris, F.: Clinical aspects and long-term prognosis of intracranial tumours in infancy and childhood. Dev. Med. Child Neurol. *18*, 145–159 (1976)
10. Gutjahr, P.: Das Schicksal tumor- und leukämiekranker Kinder. Habil.schrift. Mainz 1979
11. Gutjahr, P., Walther, B.: Bösartige Neubildungen als chronische Erkrankungen in der Pädiatrie. Sozialpädiatrie *2*, 224–231 (1980)
12. Gutjahr, P., Dieterich, E., Walther, B.: Spätstatus Langzeitüberlebender nach infratentoriellen Tumoren im Kindesalter. Aktuelle Neuropädiatrie *2*, 94–104 (1981)
13. Hirsch, J. F., Renier, D., Czernichow, P., Benveniste, L., Pierre-Kahn, A.: Medulloblastoma in childhood. Survival and functional results. Acta Neurochirurgica *48*, 1–15 (1979)
14. Holmes, H. A., Holmes, F. F.: After ten years, what are the handicaps and life styles of children treated for cancer? Clinical Pediatrics *14*, 819–823 (1975)
15. Jacobi, G.: Klinik und Diagnostik kindlicher Hirntumoren. Aktuelle Neuropädiatrie *2*, 54–69 (1981)
16. Jenkin, R. D. T.: Medulloblastoma in childhood: radiation therapy. Canad. Med. Ass. J. *100*, 51–53 (1969)
17. Landbeck, G.: Konservative Therapie der Geschwülste des kindlichen Zentralnervensystems. Mschr. Kinderheilk. *126*,639–641 (1978)
18. Lasson, U., Nohl, M.: Neurologische Kontrolle des Krankheitsverlaufes. Mschr. Kinderheilk. *126*, 655–658 (1978)
19. McFarland, D. R., Horwitz, H., Saenger, E. L., Bahr, G. K.: Medulloblastoma – a review of prognosis and survival. Br. J. Radiol. *42*, 198–214 (1969)
20. Raimondi, A. J., Tomita, T.: Medulloblastoma in childhood. Comparative results of partial and total resection. Child's Brain *5*, 310–328 (1979)
21. Tokars, R. P., Sutton, H. G., Griem, M. L.: Cerebellar medulloblastoma-Results of a new method of radiation treatment. Cancer *43*, 129–136 (1979)
22. Ullmo, D., Lemerle, J., Schweisguth, O.: Traumatisme cerebrale, traumatisme psychique. Étude de 47 enfants atteints de medulloblastome et de leur devenir. Arch. Franc. Ped. *35*, 559–570 (1978)
23. Walther, B., Gutjahr, P., Beron, G.: Therapiebegleitende und -überdauernde neurologische und neuropsychologische Diagnostik bei akuter lymphoblastischer Leukämie im Kindesalter. Klin. Pädiat. *193*, 177–183 (1981)
24. Wilcke, O.: Therapie und Prognose der Medulloblastome im Kindesalter. Aktuelle Neuropädiatrie *2*, 86–93 (1981)

Spongioblastoma in Childhood. Remarks on Problems in Diagnosis and Treatment

W. ENTZIAN, L. DIAZ, and H. W. SCHUMACHER

The spongioblastoma (=piloid astrocytoma WHO) is a slowly-growing brain tumour of childhood, that generally shows a circumscribed expansion in the cerebellum and, with exceptions, a diffuse pattern of growth in the brain stem. They may also occur in the paraventricular regions of the lateral and third ventricles. The circumscribed lesions are generally completely excisable, without recurrence.

We presented the clinical data from consecutively treated patients with spongioblastoma (SP) in order to underline the difficulties in making an early diagnosis. In approximately half of our patients the period of pre-operative observation was noted to range between six months and six years.

Further, we will point out how the diagnostic advantages of CT and the use of the dissecting microscope have helped in the treatment of particular cases.

Material

Between 1966 and 1980, 66 paediatric patients up to the age of 16 years were operated on. In all cases the pathological specimen showed all the signs of SP; five patients are included with the signs of a mixed glioma (ependymospongioblastoma). Spongioblastomata of the chiasm and optic nerve were not included, because these tumours represent a separate entity. Brain stem tumours were not included unless a biopsy was taken. The age distribution (Fig. 1) confirms the known predominance in the first decade [1]. Among our patients, however, no SP was detected below the age of 24 months.

History

In 49% of our patients the clinical history was shorter than six months, but in 51% the clinical history was between six months and 6 years. Among the initial complaints were non-specific symptoms, specific localizing symptoms as well as those symptoms indicative of raised intracranial pressure. These occurred with more or less equal frequency (Table 1). A wry neck or stiff neck was reported by six patients. Complaints such as those found in "migraine" were reported by seven children, ad-

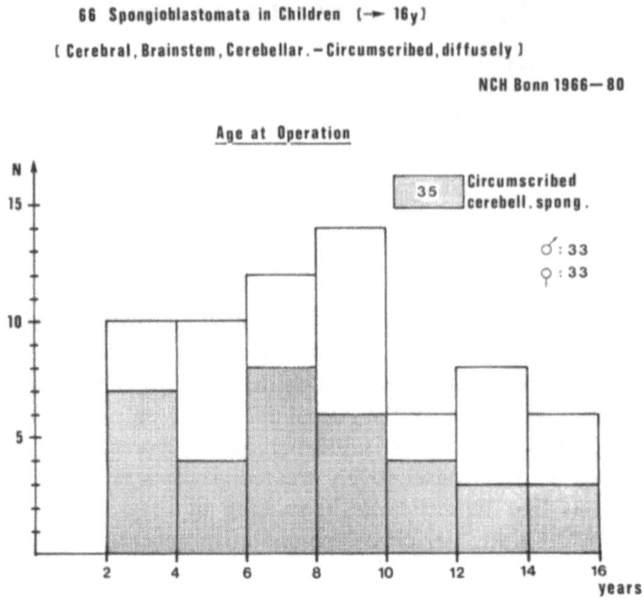

Fig. 1. Circumscribed SP in the cerebellum predominate over SP in the cerebral hemispheres and over those with a diffuse growth pattern

mitted in the last six years. One patient with a tumour of vermis and right cerebellar hemisphere, extending deeply through the floor of the fourth ventricle demonstrated all the symptomatic criteria of a "migraine accompagneé".

The *neurological findings* during the preoperative period are unknown, however up to the time of admission obvious neurological symptoms had developed in all cases: 60 patients presented with severe or at least clear neurological local disorders, but, six patients however (approx. 10%) had no or minimal findings. Forty-one patients (62%) had papilloedema; and there was no child, that did not have either papilloedema or evident neurological disturbances. The EEG was abnormal at least in those cases with raised intracranial pressure.

Table 1. Presenting symptoms in patients with SP in the brain stem and/or cerebellum may be unspecific or caused by raised ICP

Unspecific:	Headache (moderate)	19
	Deficits in school	3
	Behavioural disturbances	3
Cerebellar:	Unsteady (walking, manual)	15
Brain stem:	Pyramidal, CN deficits	6
ICP:	Severe headache, vomiting	15
	visual disturbances	11
Other:	Wry neck	6
	"Child's migraine"	7

Table 2. Circumscribed SP are in general completely removable

	Circumscribed		Diffuse	
	Dead	Living (follow-up)	Dead	Living (follow-up)
Subtotal excision Re-Op.	0 1	1 (5 y.) 1 (9 y.)	13 (1 d – 4 y)	4 (1 – 4 y.) 1 (2 y.)
Radical excision	6 (Intraop. infect., subdur. haemat., shunt sepsis, brain stem def., rebleeding)	26 (2 – 10 y.) (CT-control) 12 (no CT-control)		
Autopsy diagn.			1	
Total	7	40	14	5

Table 3. SP develop mostly in the cerebellum, less often they are paraventricular (lateral or third ventricle). Pontine tumours are included only when a biopsy was taken. With some exceptions, they grow diffusely

	Circum-scribed	Diffusely	Circum-scribed + diff.	Uncertain
Cerebral	4	–	–	–
Cerebral and brain stem	–	1	1	–
Oral brain stem	1	1	1	1
Ponto-mesencephalic	2	"3"	–	–
Medulla oblong. (+cervical)	1	2	–	–
Cerebellar	35	2	3	–
Cerebellar + pons	–	–	7	1
Total	43	9	12	2

In a few cases some misdirected measures delayed correct treatment. A "torticollis" was treated orthopaedically, a drop in mental abilities was treated psychotherapeutically and a cerebellar dysmetria was misinterpreted as nervousness.

Operative results (Table 2) depended upon the growth pattern: In three cases the surgeon avoided a complete removal because of the extension of the tumour near the brain stem. In all other cases no recurrence has yet been observed. However, tumours with a diffuse growth pattern cannot be totally removed. In addition, several cases of cerebellar spongioblastomata were encountered which presented intraoperatively as both a circumscribed lesion of the cerebellar hemisphere and a diffusely growing lesion of the pons.

Six patients died from reasons, related to the general risk of a posterior fossa craniotomy.

Case Reports

SP in the depths of a cerebral hemisphere may be detected very late because of its slow growth and the plasticity of infantile cerebral tissue. Nevertheless, the operative result may be satisfactory.

Case 1. The 14-year-old right-handed girl (file 102/78) had shown a slight drop of her abilities in school during the last six months. Findings: Mild hemiparesis and slightly impaired coordination on the right side. Large, poorly vascularized hemisphere tumour shown in the left carotid angiogram. CT confirmed the size and furthermore revealed a good demarcation. Excision by temporal approach. For some weeks after operation she had a global aphasia, a complete homonymous hemianopia and a paralysis of the right extremities. These defects improved to a state where she was able to continue her English and French studies with moderate results. The paralysis recovered to the preoperative stage. Because of an intention dyskinesia of athetotic character of her right hand, she learned to write with her left hand. There is no evidence of tumour recurrence in the CT-controls three years after the operation.

CT in this case supported the indication for the operation because of the sharp demarcation indicative of a SP or astrocytoma grade I, that seemed excisable in spite of its large size.

Case 2 (Intrapontine-mesencephalic location of spongioblastoma). This 13-year-old girl (614/77) showed very mild brain stem signs on her first admission: right-sided hemiparesis, facial paresis and cerebellar dysdiadochokinesia. Neuroradiology indicated the presence of a lesion within the pons. On exploration of the posterior fossa, a small biopsy was taken from an intrapontine tumour, that had elevated the floor of the fourth ventricle far laterally. The specimen showed a spongioblastoma. In the following year, lateral pyramidal defects, cerebellar symptoms and dysfunction of the fifth, sixth and seventh cranial nerves on the right and the sixth cranial nerve on the left developed to a serious degree so that the child was unable to stand. CT demonstrated a large oval lesion with a hyperdense margin and hypodense contents. A second operation was performed. When exposed the surface of the tumour was clearly demarcated and could be separated from the normal appearing brain stem tissue. Postoperatively her neurological deficits improved partially and approximately to the pre-operative stage. Though handicapped, she finished "Hauptschule" and seems able to continue commercial school. CT control four years postoperatively is questionable abnormal.

Conclusions

1. Attention is drawn to the fact, that the interval between the onset of initial clinical symptoms and operative treatment was surprisingly long in approximately one half of these patients with spongioblastoma. This can be explained by the slow growth of the tumours. Nevertheless efforts should continue for earlier diagnosis.

2. Spongioblastomas, if they develop as circumscribed lesions have a very good prognosis after operation, as is known. Nowadays, even very large and deep seated SP of the cerebral hemispheres and SP of the brain stem seem to be approachable under special circumstances.

References

1. Zülch, K. H.: Biologie und Pathologie der Hirngeschwülste. In Handbuch der Neurochirurgie Bd III. Berlin-Göttingen-Heidelberg: Springer 1956
2. Entzian, W.: On the extended Indication for Operation of Deep Seated Brain Tumours. Adv. Neurosurg. *10*, 64–72 (1982)
3. Entzian, W.: Tumours of the brain stem: Removal of intraponto-mesencephalic spongioblastoma. Intern. Microneurosurgery Symposium, Frankfurt/M., 1981

Medulloblastoma. Relationship of Histologic Type to Survival

H. Arnold, H. D. Franke, G. Langendorf, R. Olotu, and J. Grosch-Wörner

It is commonly held that the prognosis of medulloblastoma depends mainly on the histologic characteristics [6, 15] and on the age of the patient at the time of operation [10, 13]. According to Gullotta [5], in infancy and early childhood tumours preponderate, which display predominantly neuroectodermal structures. Beyond the fifteenth year of age almost no medulloblastomas other than desmoplastic ones [6] are found. These are also called arachnoidal sarcoma [14]. At the age of ten, when the tumour frequency is highest, mixed tumours consisting of mesenchymal and neuroectodermal parts are most common. Only rarely are desmoplastic medulloblastomas found in young children, or mixed tumours in adults. Usually, neuroectodermal and mixed tumours originate in the vermis, diffusely infiltrating the cerebellar hemispheres. In contrast, desmoplastic medulloblastomas often grow primarily in the cerebellar hemispheres or even in the cerebello-pontine angle. Generally, they are solid and well circumscribed. From the report of Gullotta and Neumann [6], covering the period from 1950 to 1976, about 150 cases of medulloblastoma, the conclusion might be drawn, that the age of the patient and the morphological structure of the tumour exclusively determine prognosis. This statement is not unequivocal. It stimulated us to correlate histologic data, with treatment and survival rates in our medulloblastoma patients.

Out of 88 patients treated for medulloblastoma in the period 1951 to 1977, 58 met the requirements of this study, which were adequately documented history, investigations, treatment, and follow-up data as well as tumour sections, which were qualitatively and quantitatively adequate to allow re-evaluation of the histological diagnosis.[1] Another 15 cases did not fulfil these conditions. The remaining 15 had died within two months of the operation, which means a total operation mortality of 19.3%. The late results of the group excluded from the study are somewhat more favourable than those of the group re-evaluated. Seven out of 15 patients are alive 15 to 25 years after operation.

Possibly, the diagnosis of desmoplastic medulloblastoma was established more frequently than in the average of comparable series because of the peculiarities of the operative procedure in which the tumour was never extirpated as a whole. Generally, soft tumour tissue was removed by suction, and the remaining solid portions of tumour were sent for microscopic investigation.

Desmoplastic medulloblastomas predominate in the older patients (Figs. 1 and 4). Long survivals, however, occur not only in patients with desmoplastic medul-

---

1 We wish to thank Prof. Dr. F. Gullotta, Department of Neuropathology, University of Bonn, for re-evaluating the tumour sections

loblastomas, but also in those with mixed tumours, and are found in adults as well as in children aged 2 to 15 years. Survival rates correlated positively with how circumscribed the tumour was and negatively with tumour size. Until the tenth postoperative year the survival rate in desmoplastic medulloblastoma was somewhat higher than that in the other tumour subgroup (Fig. 2). Beyond the tenth postoperative year there was no significant difference between the two histological tumour groups.

Patients were divided into two groups according to age (Figs. 3 and 4). The first group comprises all infants and children up to 15 years of age, the second one the older children and adults. A comparison between these groups demonstrates, as is expected, that the older patients have a better chance of surviving for a long time; but the difference is not as dramatic as was reported by others [6]. Survival times of five or even ten years can also be attained in children, who had to be operated on before the age of ten (Figs. 1 and 3).

From a neurosurgical point of view the material is not uniform. In the period from 1951 to 1970 the operative mortality amounted to 21.2%, whereas from 1971 to 1977 it was 4.8%. Microsurgical techniques and intensive care facilities are considered to be responsible for the improvement. Operative removal of the tumour was rare in those patients who died within two years after operation. Changes of survival improved if total removal of the tumour had been performed. After complete tumour removal 12 out of 31 patients were alive after five years; in comparison only three of 22 patients survived the fifth year after incomplete tumour removal.

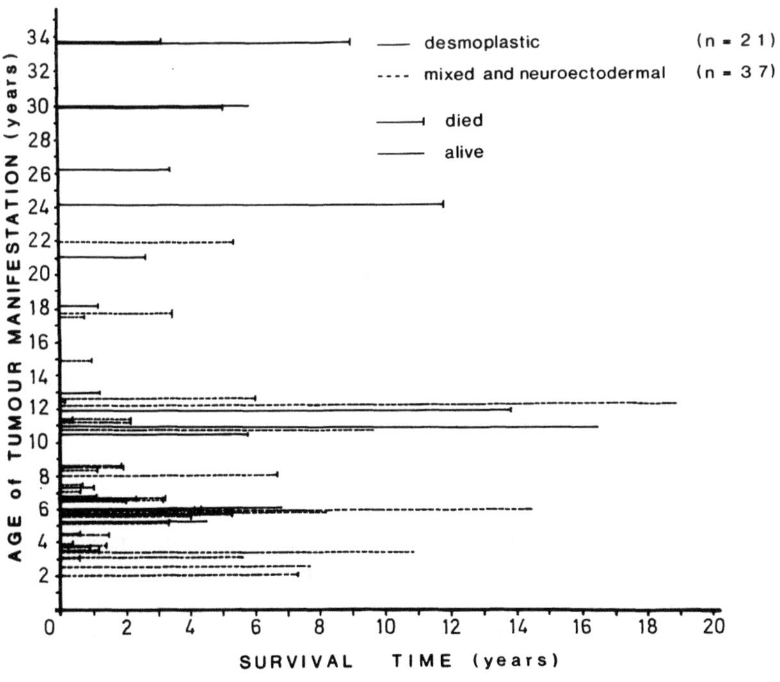

Fig. 1. Medulloblastoma. Type and survival time in relation to age

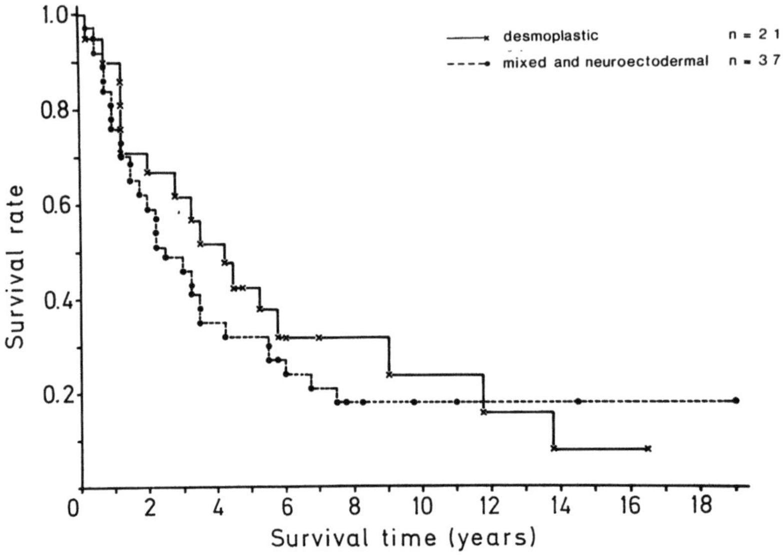

Fig. 2. Medulloblastoma (n = 58)

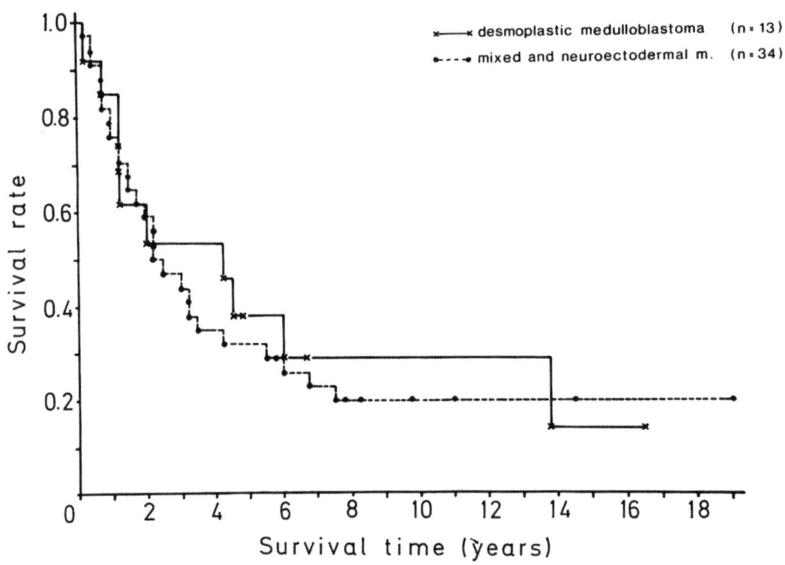

Fig. 3. Age of tumour manifestation < 15 years

With the introduction of microsurgery the percentage of radical tumour removals increased from 40% in the sixties to about 65% in the seventies.

The method of radiation has changed from the fifties to the seventies. During the period covered by this report three different radiotherapeutic regimens have been applied:

1) radiation of the primary tumour only,

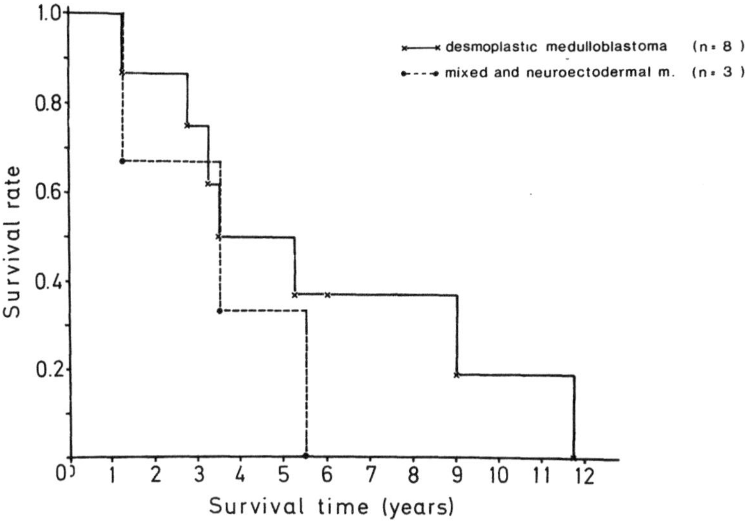

Fig. 4. Age of tumour manifestation > 15 years

2) radiation of the tumour and the spinal cord,
3) radiation of the whole neuraxis including tumour site, entire brain, spinal cord, and lumbar sac down to S3.

Posterior fossa irradiation dose was 40–60 Gy/4–6 weeks (Telecobalt), in the spinal cord 30 Gy/3 weeks (Telecobalt or fast electrons). Results improved nearly corresponding to the completeness of neuraxial radiation. Out of 44 patients, which received radiation of the entire neuraxis 18 survived more than 5 years. Among the remaining 14 patients, that were treated by irradiation of the posterior fossa and spinal canal or the posterior fossa only, three were alive after five years. Desmoplastic medulloblastomas slightly prevailed among the survivors. Metastatic seeding could not be prevented even in spite of irradiation.

During the last few years chemotherapy has been used. Methotrexate, cyclophosphamide, and vincristine have been given to 14 of our patients. The chemotherapeutic regime varied. Since surgical techniques, anaesthesia, intensive care and radiotherapy have changed during the same period, it is impossible to establish whether patients benefited from chemotherapy or not.

Discussion

Unquestionably, desmoplastic medulloblastomas occur more frequently in adults than in children, and their nodular growth facilitates the identification of tumour boundaries and usually permits surgical eradication of the tumour. Thus, the age of appearance and the morphological structure of medulloblastomas were thought to be the main determinants of prognosis although the location of the tumour and the type of growth (nodular or diffuse) were also important prognostic features. This view received support from the report of Gullotta and Neumann [6], whose series did not include a single patient younger than 15 years who had survived the second postoperative year. Today, however, things have changed, and the opinion reported above cannot be confirmed without reservation. Owing to improvements in pre-operative management, anaesthesia and intensive care, overative mortality has dropped to percentages lower than 5%. Generally, postoperative neurological deficit was less pronounced, and recovery was less eventful and more complete in the seventies than in former years. The effects of radical microsurgical tumour removal and adequate radiotherapy of the entire CNS should not be underestimated [1, 4, 8, 9, 11, 12]. The survival rate of children up to 15 years of age has considerably improved. It is a widespread view that children younger than five years have the worst chance of surviving for a longer period [10]. Since the evaluation of our series does not give support to this opinion (Fig. 1), we wonder whether such reports about discouraging results in young children may reflect difficulties in intensive care and anaesthesia rather than an above-average tumour malignancy.

Chemotherapy has been used only in a small group of children. Proof of its effectiveness is lacking, because operative procedures, intensive care, and radiotherapy improved simultaneously. Similar difficulties in judging treatment are known from other series, too [12]. According to Bloom [2, 3] chemotherapy appears promising. A randomised study will provide the information required for definite rating.

In former years, prognosis of patients with medulloblastoma was mainly determined by the age, and the histological type of the tumour. Seemingly, the development of several therapeutic measures is going to equalize those differences in survival rate which were due to tumour biology. Looking at the good prognosis associated with complete tumour removal [1, 7], early diagnosis deserves emphasis. Prognosis depends on time of diagnosis, extent of tumour removal, intensive care facilities, and completeness of neuraxial irradiation, as much as on the patient's age and tumour type. Nowadays the difference in survival chances between desmoplastic medulloblastoma on the one hand and mixed and neuroectodermal medulloblastoma on the other hand, although not insignificant, is not as striking as was stated formerly.

References

1. Berry, M. P., Jenkin, R. D. T., Keen, C. W. et al.: Radiation treatment for medulloblastoma. J. Neurosurg. *55,* 43–51 (1981)
2. Bloom, H. J. G.: Medulloblastoma: Prognosis and prospects. Int. J. Radiation Oncology Biol. Phys. *2,* 1031–1033, Pergamon Press 1977
3. Bloom, H. J. G.: SIOP Brain Tumour Trial, Sept. 1980 (unpublished)
4. Chatty, E. M., Earle, K. M.: Medulloblastoma. A report of 201 cases with emphasis on the relationship of histologic variants to survival. Cancer *28,* 977–983 (1971)
5. Gullotta, F.: Das sogenannte Medulloblastoma. Berlin-Heidelberg-New York: Springer 1967
6. Gullotta, F., Neumann, J.: Medulloblastome und zerebelläre Sarkome. Eine histologisch-katamnestische Untersuchung. Neurochirurgia *23,* 35–40 (1980)

7. Harisiadis, L., Chang, C. H.: Medulloblastoma in children: A correlation between staging and results of treatment. Int. J. Radiation Oncology Biol. Phys. *2,* 833–841, Pergamon-Press 1977
8. Lins, E.: Das Medulloblastom des Erwachsenen. Acta Neurochir. *31,* 67–72 (1974)
9. McIntosh, N.: Medulloblastoma – a changing prognosis? Arch. Dis. Child. *54,* 200–203 (1979)
10. Müller, W., Afra, D., Wilcke, O. et al.: Data on the biology of medulloblastomas. This volume, pp. 350–353
11. Nüchel, B., Andersen, A. P.: Medulloblastoma. Treatment results. Acta Radiol. Oncol. *17,* 305–311 (1978)
12. Pichler, E., Kogelnik, H. D., Reinartz, G., et al.: Ergebnisse der Therapie des Medulloblastoms in den letzten 15 Jahren. Strahlentherapie *157,* 508–515 (1981)
13. Quest, D. O., Brisman, R., Antunes, J. L., et al.: Period of risk for recurrence in medulloblastoma. J. Neurosurg. *48,* 159–163 (1978)
14. Rubinstein, L. J.: Tumours of the central nervous system. Fasc. 6. AFIP, Washington/D.C., 1972
15. Zülch, K. J.: Classification of brain tumours in childhood. This volume, pp. 1–16

Ophthalmological Findings in Long-Term Survivors After Primary Brain Tumours in Childhood

R. ROCHELS and Th. NEUHANN

Introduction

The primary ophthalmological signs of brain tumours in children are basically related to size, site and rate of growth of the tumour [1, 4]. Choked discs, acute strabismus, nystagmus, eye muscle palsies and visual field defects are frequently encountered [3].

Conversely, the late clinical pattern is mainly determined by the duration of raised intracranial pressure and by the position and extent of those brain structures, that had to be removed during operation.

While the primary signs and symptoms are well documented in the literature [1, 2], because of their value for making an accurate diagnosis, follow-up studies of late visual disturbances after brain tumours are lacking.

Clinical Studies

We had the opportunity to follow up 120 children (60 boys and 60 girls) between the ages of one and 14 years for an average period of three years postoperatively at intervals of at least six months. A survey of location and histological nature of the tumours encountered in our patients is given in Table 1.

Table 1. Primary brain tumours in 120 children

A. Infratentorial tumours	78	B. Supratentorial tumours	42
1. Cerebellum and fourth ventricle	68	1. Chiasma and Sella	24
1.1. Medulloblastoma	31	1.1. Craniopharyngioma	16
1.2. Astrocytoma	32	1.2. Glioma of the optic nerve	8
1.3. Ependymoma	2	2. Cerebral hemisphere tumours	18
1.4. Haemangioblastoma	1	2.1. Astrocytoma	10
1.5. Rhabdomyosarcoma of base of skull	1	2.2. Glioblastoma	1
1.6. Plexus papilloma	1	2.3. Ependymoma	5
2. Tumours of the brain stem	10	2.4. Oligodendroglioma	1
		2.5. Arachnoidal sarcoma	1

We evaluated visual acuity, visual fields, discs and ocular alignment and motility, including nystagmus. We present here the late findings in contrast to those at the time of diagnosis.

Results

Brain Tumours

Patients with Cerebellar Medulloblastomas

The rapid growth of cerebellar medulloblastomas, their proximity to the ventricular system and the limited infratentorial space explain the high rate (70%) of choked discs in this group. Sixth nerve palsies and visual field defects were present in only a few cases and visual acuity was not noticeably reduced.

Despite this high rate of choked discs, follow-up examinations revealed consecutive optic atrophy in only 20%, usually with no noteworthy reduction of visual acuity or field defect. Sixth nerve palsies, strabismus and nystagmus occurred in one fifth of the children.

Patients with Cerebellar Astrocytomas

The slow growth of these tumours in reflected in the fact, that when they first present only 40% of the children had papilloedema, but 16% already showed unilateral or bilateral optic atrophy in response to longstanding raised intracranial pressure. The occurrence of disorders of motility and visual field defects is also very high in this group.

Consequently, the pattern of late signs in cerebellar astrocytomas is characterized by a high proportion of optic atrophies with considerable visual loss and field defects.

Patients with Rare Cerebellar Tumours

The primary and late ophthalmological signs in this group (ependymoma, haemangioblastoma, one rhabdomyosarcoma and choroid plexus papilloma) are closely similar to those in cerebellar astrocytomas. Here, too, considerable loss of all visual functions was encountered.

Patients with Brain Stem and Pontine Tumours

In these tumours, the primary ophthalmic signs are an important guide to the location of the lesion. Acute abducens palsies and horizontal and vertical nystagmus, indicating an involvement of the gaze centres, were observed in one out of three children. Low grade papilloedema was of equal frequency.

Surgical intervention in these cases is hardly ever possible; thus, 60% of the children exhibit unilateral or bilateral sixth and seventh nerve palsies within a few months after the establishment of the diagnosis.

Patients with Craniopharyngioma

The anatomical site and the direction of growth of craniopharyngiomas cause optic nerve involvement as a primary sign in the majority of the cases. In our patients, optic atrophy was seen in 25%, papilloedema in over 30%.

Late findings consisted in optic atrophy in over 60% of the children. Visual field defects, mainly bitemporal hemianopsia, could be verified in 50%.

Patients with Optic Nerve Glioma

Optic nerve gliomas were seen in eight children. Six of these tumours were located intracranially, two intraorbitally; in the latter ones the exophthalmos had dominated the initial clinical picture. In the intracranial gliomas, ipsilateral optic atrophy was observed in 40%.

Late sequelae are characterized mainly by gross visual field defects with impaired vision.

Patients with Cerebral Hemispheric Tumours

In general, spongioblastomas and rare cerebral tumours (ependymoma, glioblastoma, oligodendroglioma and arachnoid sarcoma) constitute only a small fraction of all brain tumours in childhood. This proves to be true also in our series. At the time of first presentation, we saw choked discs in 50% and poor vision was of equally frequent occurrence. Follow-up examinations revealed a high incidence of optic atrophy (50%), accompanied by visual field defects (40%) and substantially reduced visual acuity.

Ocular Signs

Patients Without Pathological Ophthalmic Findings

At the time of the first eye examination, only 19 children (16%) were ophthalmologically normal; ten of them had cerebral tumours. After an average of three years, this figure had increased to 35 (29%). An analysis of the individual cases shows, that low grade papilloedema can resolve without demonstrable loss of visual functions.

Visual Loss and Optic Discs

As an initial sign, 43% of all children presented with reduced visual acuity, 20% already having complete optic atrophy at the time of their first examination. Craniopharyngiomas, optic nerve gliomas and cerebral tumours caused the most pronounced visual loss. In these tumour groups optic atrophy, mostly bilateral occurred in almost 40% of the cases. The mechanisms responsible were either direct compression injury of the optic pathways or long-standing and pronounced disc congestion.

Visual Field Loss

A minimum age and ability to cooperate are indispensable prerequisites for perimetry in children. Thus, in 44% of our patients, no evaluable visual fields could be recorded. In the remaining 67 children, normal field limits were found in 57%. Pathological findings always corresponded to the location of the tumour within the optic pathways: Homonymous hemianopia was found in five children; in all of them the lesion was behind the optic chiasm on the opposite side. There was one choroid plexus papilloma of the posterior fossa, one glioblastoma, one eccentrically growing craniopharyngioma and two spongioblastomas. Bitemporal hemianopia was present in six cases, all of them craniopharyngiomas. In advanced and asymmetrically growing tumours there was unilateral amaurosis and contralateral hemianopia, as was shown in two children with craniopharyngioma and one girl with an intracranial optic nerve glioma.

An enlarged blind spot, caused by papilloedema, was encountered mainly in medulloblastomas. In two intraorbital optic nerve gliomas there was unilateral amaurosis with a normal contralateral field.

Strabismus

In the cases of non-paretic permanent squint, a compression injury of the hypothetical centres for binocular single vision by the elevated intracranial pressure must be held responsible. In our patients, a divergent squint is twice as frequent as a convergent one. This is true at the first examinations as well as in the long-term controls. Cerebellar and brain stem tumours are responsible for most of these cases. Only in cerebral astrocytomas secondary squint is rare.

Another cause of secondary strabismus is unilateral amaurosis, mainly caused by optic nerve gliomas.

Nystagmus

Horizontal and vertical nystagmus generally indicate that the lesion is situated in the cerebellum or the brain stem: seven out of ten patients with brain stem tumours and 48% of those with cerebellar tumours, but only 10% of the children with a cerebral tumour exhibited nystagmus. As one would expect from their position, craniopharyngiomas were never associated with nystagmus, nor were optic nerve gliomas.

Cranial Nerve Involvement

Abducens palsies occurred in 33% of cerebellar and in 40% of all brain stem tumours. Oculomotor and trochlear impairment were not encountered in this series. Facial nerve palsies occurred mainly in brain stem tumours and in medulloblastoma.

Other Ocular Disturbances

We did not observe any damage of the lens or the retina induced by therapeutic X-rays in our 120 children. One girl with extensive rhabdomyosarcoma of the middle and posterior fossa presented with ipsilateral corneal anaesthesia and a dry eye, one year after treatment.

Discussion

The importance of appropriate ophthalmological care of children with brain tumours is twofold:

1. Within the diagnostic evaluation of a general clinical pattern, which could point to the existence of a brain tumour, the ophthalmologist has a prime responsibility in judging the appearance of the optic disc. Moreover, a meticulous neuro-ophthalmological examination can make important contributions to the diagnosis and localization of a lesion. While computerized tomography has rendered perimetry somewhat secondary in this respect, impairments of the cranial nerves 3, 4, 6 and 7 and their higher centres, especially the gaze centres and pathways, are still of paramount importance. They often allow a very exact localization of brain stem tumours which is difficult to obtain by other methods.

2. In the postoperative period, the ophthalmologist plays an even more important role. In this context it should be pointed out, that immediate postoperative control examinations are generally of only very limited value, because at this time the children are hardly ever able to cooperate to the extent that is necessary for a useful eye examination. However, as soon as the general physical state permits good cooperation again, an exact functional and anatomical ophthalmological evaluation is indispensable as a basis for future follow-up examinations, because the progression or development of functional disorders or disc changes may be the first sign of a recurrence before it can be anatomically verified.

Moreover, the ophthalmologist must be given the chance to take care of the ocular sequelae of the brain tumour and its treatment. This consists not only of ophthalmological treatment in a restricted sense, as, e.g. in muscle surgery for secondary squint, but also includes the introduction and continuation of rehabilitation measures. It is, last not least, that we have today in this field a variety of sophisticated possibilities, that are still not always made fully available to our patients.

References

1. Huber, A.: Augensymptome bei Hirntumoren. Bern: Huber 1956
2. Tönnis, W.: Augensymptome bei 3033 Hirngeschwülsten. Ber. Dtsch. Ophthalm. Ges. *59*, 6–27 (1956)
3. Walsh, F. B., Hoyt, W. F.: Clinical neuro-ophthalmology. 3rd Ed. Vol. III, 2075–2330. Baltimore: Williams & Wilkins 1969
4. Weinstein, P.: Ophthalmologische Differentialdiagnose bei Gehirntumoren. Stuttgart: Enke 1972

Endocrinological Investigations in 68 Children with Brain Tumours

W. Andler, K. Roosen, and H.-E. Clar

Endocrinological investigations were performed in 68 children with intracranial tumours. In 33 children the tumour involved the hypothalamic area, whereas in the other 35 it did not. While there was no significant pituitary dysfunction in all 35 patients with tumours not involving the hypothalamic region, endocrinological problems played a role in about 50% of patients with suprasellar tumours. According to the site of the lesion, pituitary dysfunction could be identified as suprahypophyseal in origin [1].

Results

Growth hormone deficiency (GHD), assessed by both insulin induced hypoglycaemia and the propranolol-glucagon stimulation test, was present in 15 patients with suprasellar tumours (Table 1). In 14 of them GHD was proven prior to surgical or radiological treatment. In only one child was GHD related to surgical treatment. On the other hand defective GH-secretion was not improved in any patient where the tumour therapy was otherwise successful.

Hypothyroidism due to hypothalamic thyrotropin releasing hormone deficiency was present in 12 of 33 children (Table 3). In five children thyroid dysfunction was documented before any treatment. In four children thyroid function was not sufficiently investigated prior to operation. In three children hypothyroidism was excluded before and documented after therapy. In one of these, however, hypothyroidism developed during unsuccessful radiotherapy. In this child the dysfunction may be due to further tumour growth rather than to the irradiation treatment. Furthermore none showed any improvement with therapy as regards thyroid dysfunction.

Table 1. Clinical data of 15 children with suprasellar tumours before treatment

Symptoms	n
Short stature (< 3 rd Pc.)	7
Precocious puberty	6
Emaciation syndrome	1
Diabetes insipidus	1

Table 2. Growth hormone deficiency 15 of 33 patients with suprasellar tumours

Growth hormone deficiency	n
Documented before treatment	14
Documented after treatment	1
Improved by tumour treatment	0

Table 3. Hypothalamic hypothyroidism in 12 of 33 patients with suprasellar tumours

Hypothyroidism	n
Documented before treatment	5
Not investigated before and documented after treatment	4
Excluded before and documented after treatment	3
Improved by tumour treatment	0

Table 4. Elevated basal prolactin levels (>20 ng/ml) in 6 of 33 patients with suprasellar tumours

Patient (No)	Therapy	Prl (ng/ml)
1	–	42
2	–	25
3	before surgery	75
	after surgery	83
4	before surgery	13
	after surgery	32
5	before surgery	17
	after surgery	50
6	before radiotherapy	10
	after radiotherapy	82

Table 5. Secondary adrenocortical insufficiency in 8 of 33 patients with suprasellar tumours

Adrenocortical insufficiency	n
Documented before treatment	5
Documented after treatment	3
Improved by treatment	0

Basal *prolactin* levels (Table 4) were elevated in three patients before any treatment and in two additional patients only after surgical treatment. In one patient the prolactin level increased during unsuccessful radiotherapy, secondary to further tumour growth rather than to the irradiation.

Secondary *adrenocortical insufficiency* (Table 5) has been documented even before treatment in five and in an additional three patients after surgical treatment. Clinical features such as hypoglycaemia and salt loss were present in four of eight patients, after a period of four to 36 months after biochemical documentation of cortisol deficiency.

Secondary *gonadal insufficiency* (Table 6) with decreased gonadotropin secretion was present in seven patients before and in another three patients after, neurosurgical treatment. No patient showed any improvement after therapy.

Six children presented with isosexual *precocious puberty*. Three of them suffered from gliomas of the optic chiasm, two from suprasellar tumours of unknown histology and one from a hormone-producing hamartoma of the tuber cinereum. Three of these patients with sexual precocity showed neurofibromatosis. Sexual precocity was the only endocrinological symptom in all six children whereas all patients with secondary hypogonadism showed at least one other hypothalamic dysfunction.

Diabetes insipidus, a rare pre-operative complication in suprasellar tumours but often manifest after operative treatment was present in 12 of 33 patients. Three additional patients showed hyperosmolarity which could not be corrected by ADH-substitution alone.

Discussion

Although symptoms of endocrine dysfunction such as retarded growth and delayed sexual development are common at the first presentation (Table 6) they are rarely the presenting complaint [2]. In most cases a suprasellar tumour is only suspected after clinical signs of increased intracranial pressure or ophthalmological disturbances, which often indicate a late stage of the disease. Polyuria and polydipsia could be alarming features of a suprasellar tumour but in contrast to their high postoperative frequency they are rare complaints before treatment. However, pre-

Table 6. Hypogonadism and precocious puberty in patients with suprasellar tumours

	n
Hypogonadism	10
Documented before treatment	7
Documented after treatment	3
Improved by treatment	0
Precocious puberty	6
Before treatment	6

cocious puberty or the diencephalic emaciation in infancy [3] could be important symptoms for early diagnosis of tumours involving the hypothalamic area.

What role does hypothalamic hypothyroidism play in patients with suprasellar tumours? The typical clinical signs of hypothyroidism are only moderate or may even be absent. However, hypothalamic hypothyroidism is clearly manifested by retardation of skeletal development and decreased longitudinal growth.

Growth hormone deficiency and hypothalamic thyroid dysfunction are often combined in patients with suprasellar lesions. In the individual case it is not clear whether GHD or hypothyroidism play a major role in growth retardation. However, at least after surgical treatment thyroid dysfunction seems to be of more importance and some patients show normal growth velocity after thyroxin replacement alone, despite biochemically documented GHD.

"Growth hormone independent" growth after successful surgical treatment is still an unresolved problem. Either hyperprolactinaemia [4, 5] or hyperinsulinaemia [6] are presumed to be the cause for normal somatomedin level and normal growth. But neither elevated prolactin levels nor hyperinsulinaemia are constant features in these patients. Possibly a partial instead of complete GHD is responsible for further longitudinal growth.

Hypothalamic lesions may produce disturbances of water and electrolyte balance which cannot be explained by defective ADH-secretion alone [7], but by additional hypothalamic osmoreceptor dysfunction. Clinical features in these patients are hypodipsia and episodical or permanent hypernatraemia, infrequently in the absence of clinical evidence of extracellular depletion. In some cases serum sodium level does not decrease in response to water loading, so that the pathophysiology appears to be related to an elevated osmotic threshold for ADH-release [8]. Prognosis is poor in such cases [9]: Osmoreceptor dysfunction indicates extensive involvement of the hypothalamus and death is frequently due to severe hyperosmolarity.

In conclusion only few patients with suprasellar tumours sought medical attention because of symptoms suggesting hormone deficiency, although about half of these patients show pituitary dysfunction secondary to hypothalamic insufficiency before any therapy. Surgical treatment may produce additional disorders in some cases. On the other hand clinical and experimental investigations [10] show that endocrine hypothalamic disorders in patients with suprasellar space-occupying lesions are definitely irreversible independent of the treatment which is given.

References

1. Andler, W., Stolecke, H., Kohns, U.: Thyroid function in children with growth hormone deficiency either idiopathic or caused by diseases of the central nervous system. Eur. J. Pediatr. *128*, 273–281 (1978)
2. Thomsett, M. J., Conte, F. A., Kaplan, S. L., Grumbach, M. M.: Endocrine and neurologic outcome in childhood craniopharyngioma. Review of effect of treatment in 42 patients. J. Pediatr. *97*, 728–735 (1980)
3. Burr, I. M., Slorim, A. E., Danish, R. H., Gadoth, N., Butler, I. J.: Diencephalic syndrome revisited. J. Pediatr. *88*, 439–443 (1976)
4. Gluckman, P. D., Holdaway, I. U.: Prolactin and somatomedin studies in the syndrome of growth hormone independent growth. Clin. Endocrinol. *5*, 545–549 (1976)

5. Kenny, E. M., Hutzaelta, N. F., Mintz, D., Drash, A., Garies, L. Y., Susen, A., Ascary, H. A.: Iatrogenic hypopituitarism in craniopharyngioma, unexplained catch-up growth in three children. J. Pediatr. *72,* 766–775 (1968)
6. Costin, G., Kogut, M. D., Phillips, L. S., Daughaday, W. H.: Craniopharyngioma: The role of insulin in promoting postoperative growth. J. Clin. Endocrinol. Metab. *42,* 370–379 (1976)
7. De Rubertis, F. R., Michaelis, M. F., Davis, B. B.: Essential hypernatriemia. Arch. Intern. Med. *134,* 889–895 (1974)
8. Khomami-Asadi, F., Norman, M. E., Parks, J. S., Schwartz, M. W.: Hypernatriemia associated with pineal tumour. J. Pediatr. *90,* 605–606 (1977)
9. Katz, E. L.: Late results of radical excision of craniopharyngiomas in children. J. Neurosurg. *42,* 86–93 (1975)
10. Andler, W., Clar, E., Stockmann, N.: Secondary hypothyroidism due to suprasellar lesions in dogs. Eur. J. Pediatr. *130,* 228 (1979)

Supratentorial Tumours in Infants and Children

S. TIYAWORABUN, S. KAZKAZ, N. NICOLA, and M. SCHIRMER

The first report on the results of treatment of brain tumours in infants and children was published by Starr in 1889 (257 cases) [8, 10, 12, 17]. In contrast to adults, brain tumours in the paediatric age group tend to occur along the central neural axis and the embryonic closure line in the midline, which complicated the effects of treatment [6, 8, 10, 12, 13, 15, 17].

In recent years there is no doubt that the results of treatment have improved considerably. This can be explained by quite a number of factors which include improvements in neuroradiological techniques in diagnosis, more efficient control of brain oedema, shunting of hydrocephalus, refinements in surgical equipment, progress in postoperative intensive care, supplementary postoperative irradiation and the use of promising methods of neuro-endocrine replacement therapy and cytostatic treatment.

In this short communication, we wish to report on the results of treatment in 174 supratentorial tumours in children, during the last 16 years.

Material

During the last 16 years, i.e. from 1965 to 1980, 174 supratentorial tumours in infants and children under the age of 16 years have been seen and treated in the neurosurgical department of the university hospital, Düsseldorf. Of these, 120 children were male and 54 female. The ratio of male to female was 2.2 to 1. Their age distribution on admission is shown in Fig. 1. The youngest patient was one month old and the oldest 16 years, the mean age being 9 years 10 months.

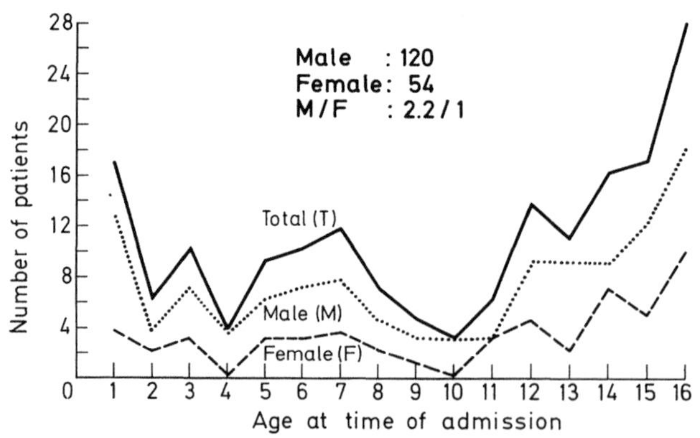

Fig. 1. Age distribution of 174 children on admission

The location of tumours in this series is shown in Fig. 2. There were 101 (57.9%) tumours located in the cerebral hemispheres and 73 (42.1%) tumours were in the diencephalon and midbrain.

The duration of clinical symptoms and signs prior to admission ranged from one day to 20 months, with an average of five months. From 1965 to 1976, nearly all children were investigated by EEG, skull X-ray, cerebral angiography, scintigraphy with ^{99m}Tc-pertechnetate, and air ventriculography prior to surgical treatment. Cranial computerized tomography (CT) has been used since 1977.

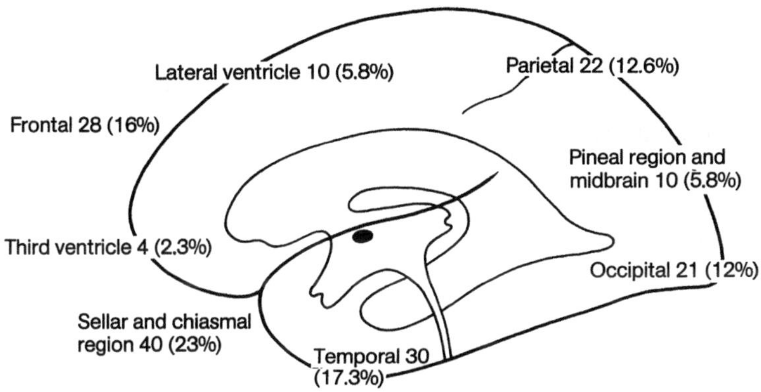

Fig. 2. The location of 174 supratentorial tumours. 101 (57.9%) tumours in cerebral hemisphere and 73 (42.1%) tumours in diencephalon and midbrain

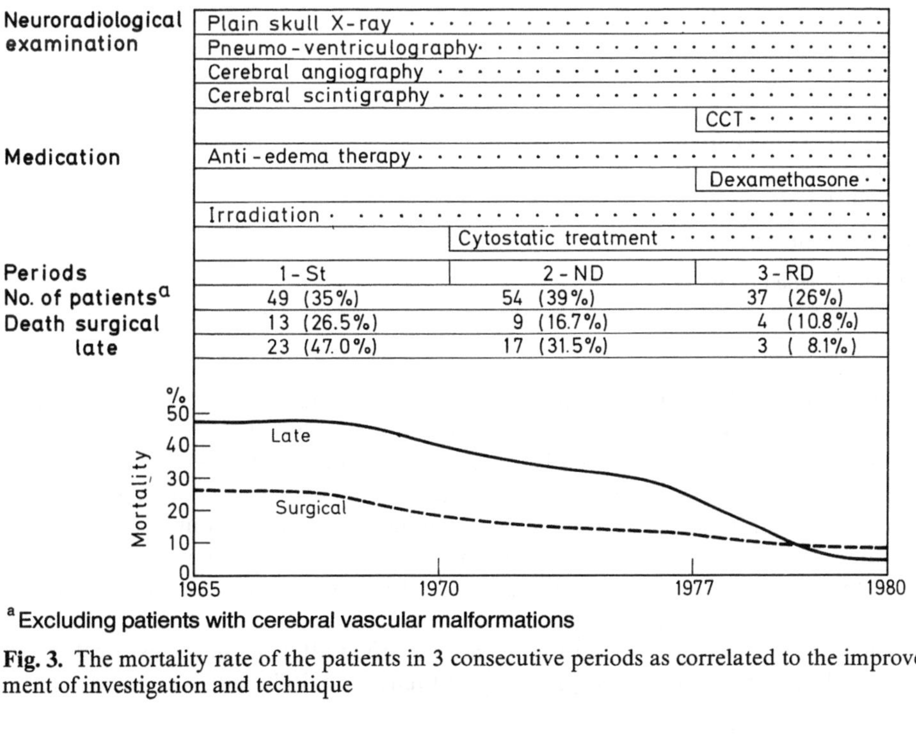

[a] Excluding patients with cerebral vascular malformations

Fig. 3. The mortality rate of the patients in 3 consecutive periods as correlated to the improvement of investigation and technique

Table 1. Incidence of 174 supratentorial tumours in infants and children (age 0–16), neurosurgical clinic Düsseldorf. Histological classification. (After world health organisation 1979)

Type of tumours	No. of patients		%	
I. Tumours of neuroepithelial tissue	70		40.2	
Astrocytic tumours		34		19.5
Ependymal tumours		16		9.2
Choroid plexus tumours		8		4.6
Oligodendroglial tumours		4		2.3
Pineal cell tumours		4		2.3
Glioblastomas		3		1.7
Gangliocytoma		1		0.6
II. Tumours of nerve sheath cells	0		0	
III. Tumours of meningeal and related tissues	9		5.2	
Meningiomas		4		2.3
Meningeal sarcomas		5		2.9
IV. Primary malignant lymphomas	1		0.6	
V. Tumours of blood vessel origin	2		1.2	
Monstrocellular sarcomas		2		1.2
VI. Germ cell tumours	3		1.7	
Teratoma		3		1.7
VII. Malformative tumours and tumour-like lesions	34		19.6	
Craniopharyngiomas		8		10.4
Epidermoid cyst		2		1.2
Other benign cysts		14		8.0
VIII. Vascular malformations	34		19.6	
IX. Tumours of anterior pituitary	0		0	
X. Local extension from regional tumours	2		1.2	
Chondroma		1		0.6
Other		1		0.6
XI. Metastatic tumours	7		4.0	
XII. Unclassified tumours	12		6.9	

Our policy in the surgical treatment of tumours is the most radical macroscopic removal possible. Among the tumours in the cerebral hemisphere removal was radical in 80 (79.2%) and only partial in 21 (20.8%). Of those in the region of the diencephalon and midbrain, 44 (60.3%) were partially and 29 (39.7%) radically excised. Pre-operative drainage of obstructive hydrocephalus was carried out in 63 cases; 48 had tumours in the midline and 15 had tumours of the cerebral hemisphere extending to the midline. Shunting of obstructive hydrocephalus in inoperable recurrent tumours was done in eight cases.

The histological types of the tumours are classified after the new classification of the World Health Organisation proposed at Geneva in 1979 [20]. The incidence of

Table 2. The correlation of location, grade of malignancy, irradiation and cytostatic treatment to the outcome of patients

Location	Grade of malignancy		Irradiation	Cytostatic therapy	Result	
					Death	Alive
Cerebral hemisphere 60 (52.6%)	Gr. I – II	43 (71.7%)	–	–	6	37 (86.1%)
	Gr. III – IV	17 (28.3%)	12	4	12	5 (29.4%)
Diencephalon and midbrain 54 (47.4%)	Gr. I – II	45 (83.3%)	1	–	18	27 (60.0%)
	Gr. III – IV	9 (16.7%)	7	3	7	2 (22.2%)

types of tumour in our series is shown in Table 1. Among the 34 children harbouring astrocytic tumours there were four astrocytomas, 20 pilocytic astrocytomas, six subependymal giant cell astrocytomas, and two each of astroblastomas and anaplastic astrocytomas. Seven metastatic tumours were one each of rhabdomyosarcoma, salivary gland carcinoma, seminoma, lymphoma, Wilms' tumour and two neuroblastomas.

We divided our patients in three consecutive periods, i.e. from 1965–69, 1970–76, and 1977–1980. Their surgical and late mortality rates are compared and shown in Fig. 3. Postoperative survival for up to one month or longer but while still in hospital was classified as a surgical death. Excluding those with cerebral vascular malformations (CVM) [18], 114 children who survived surgical treatment, were followed up for periods ranging from ten months to 16 years (Table 2, Fig. 3).

Results and Discussion

Intracranial tumours represent one of the most common neoplasms in childhood and just next to leukaemia [8, 10, 12, 13, 15]. In the major statistics, about 30–45% of brain tumours in the paediatric age group occur supratentorially [6, 8, 10, 12, 13, 15]. The incidence was 41.5% was in our series.

The sex distribution seen in our series shows a clear preponderance of male over female at all ages (Fig. 1) [8, 10, 12, 13, 15]. The incidence in relation to age was as follows: 9.8% in infants, 16.7% in the preschool age (2–5 years), 32.1% in school age (6–12 years), and 41.4% in older children (13–16 years). The age distribution in other series is different; this is probably due to the different incidence of tumour types and the different methods of neuroradiological examination. Recently, with the aid of CT, many tumours in infants and young children can be promptly diagnosed, especially when evaluating children with "congenital hydrocephalus" (Fig. 1).

Tumours of the cerebral hemispheres are slightly more numerous than those in the midline (Fig. 2) [8, 10, 12, 13, 15]. These latter were mostly found in the sellar and chiasmal region and were followed by those in temporal, frontal and other parts of hemisphere and midline.

The clinical manifestation of brain tumours in older children and adults are mainly identical and easy to evaluate. However, those in infants and young children are sometimes difficult to evaluate because of the immature functional development of the brain, and are thus easy to overlook or misinterpret. The most common symptoms and signs found in our collection were increased intracranial pressure (72%), focal or lateralizing signs (36%), and cerebral convulsion (29%). This clinical picture is mainly the result of the preponderance of midline tumours.

Since 1977, ventriculography and cerebral scintigraphy have been almost abandoned being replaced by CT. Cerebral angiography, without question, still plays an important role in the evaluation of morphologic and haemodynamic changes, except in cases with "cryptic" angiomas [19], in CVM. However, its role in the diagnosis of brain tumours is now only supplementary to CT and it be omitted in many cases in young children or in high risk cases. Prior to CT, pre-operative external drainage of the ventricles, both for diagnosis and treatment also had a favourable effect.

Although total removal of tumours is favoured, in many cases of malignant tumours or benign tumours in vital anatomical regions, subtotal resection is advisable. Conservation of tissue in some areas is occasionally beneficial and important, especially in those children with diminished life expectancy.

The histological characteristics of tumour alone do not usually foretell the outcome of treatment. Factors, such as age at onset, intrinsic growth property, site and size of tumour, focal and generalized raised intracranial pressure, changes in the ventricular system, neuroendocrine function, and vascular circulation, must also be considered. Many of the histologically benign tumours, are clinically malignant on account of these unfavourable factors.

One hundred and three of 140 tumours (73.5%), excluding CVM (18), were histologically benign. Their surgical mortality was 14.6%. Of these 62.1% are still alive (range: 10 months to 16 years and 8 months mean: 7 years and 3 months). Thirty-seven of 140 tumours (26.5%) were histologically malignant. The surgical mortality was 29.7%. Among the survivors, 12 of them received only postoperative irradiation and only one patient (8.3%) was still alive after seven years (range: 5 months to 2 years and 3 months. Mean: 1 year and 4 months). Seven patients received both irradiation and cytostatic drugs; six of them (85.7%) are still alive (range: 10 months to 2 years and 1 month. Mean: 1 year and 5 months). Owing to the diverse selection of tumour types, the relatively small number of patients with irradiation and the use of different forms of cytostatic treatment, the assessment of results is difficult. An absolute conclusion may not be possible, but comparisons could be made in the light of other reports [1–17]. Without doubt, the combination of postoperative irradiation and polychemotherapy appears promising and encouraging.

Second and third explorations were performed respectively in 30 and in two cases. They were eight astrocytomas, seven craniopharyngiomas, six ependymomas, four spongioblastomas, two each of sarcoma, carcinoma metastasis and choroid plexus papilloma and one chondroma. Among these we observed ten cases with malignant transformation: two choroid plexus papillomas, four astrocytomas and four ependymomas. The prognosis of any further operation depends mainly on the infiltrative character and malignant transformation of the tumours.

It can be seen that the surgical mortality is significantly decreased as a result of the tremendous advances in investigation and technique (Fig. 3). However, it is sad to realize that these improvements produced no satisfactory and certain effect on the late mortality. The mortality rate in the third period needs further evaluation because of the short postoperative period and the increasing number of "inoperable" tumours found by CT screening.

In conclusion, the general outlook for brain tumours in children is still not very satisfactory. Just a minority of patients are fortunate enough to survive. Further investigations and a fresh approach are still required.

References

1. Afra, D., Müller, W., Benoist, Gy., Schröder, R.: Supratentorial recurrences of gliomas. Results of reoperations on astrocytomas and oligodendrogliomas. Acta. Neurochir. *43,* 217–227 (1978)
2. Dohrmann, G. J., Farwell, J. R., Flannery, J. T.: Ependymomas and ependymoblastomas in children. J. Neurosurg. *45,* 273–283 (1976)
3. Guidetti, B., Gagliardi, F. M.: Epidermoid and dermoid cysts. Clinical evaluation and late surgical results. J. Neurosurg. *47,* 12–18 (1977)
4. Hase, U., Hock, H., Schindler, E., Schürmann, K.: Tumoren der Pinealregion. Teil II: Behandlungsergebnisse bei 23 Patienten. Neurochirurgia. *22,* 118–129 (1979)
5. Heikanen, O., Raitta, C., Torsti, R.: The management and prognosis of gliomas of the optic pathways in children. Acta. Neurochir. *43,* 193–199 (1978)
6. Hooper, R.: Intracranial tumours in children. Child's Brain. *1,* 136–140 (1975)
7. Jellinger, K., Kothbauer, P., Volc, D., Vollmer, R., Weiß, R.: Combination chemotherapy (COMP protocol) and radiotherapy of anaplastic supratentorial gliomas. Acta Neurochir. *51,* 1–13 (1979)
8. Koos, W. T., Miller, M. H.: Intracranial tumours of infants and children. Stuttgart: Thieme 1971
9. Lorenz, R.: Zur Frage der Rezidivoperation bei Gliomen. Zbl. Neurochir. *28,* 27–34 (1967)
10. Matson, D. D.: Neurosurgery of infancy and childhood. Springfield: Thomas 1969
11. Mercuri, S., Russo, A., Palma, L.: Hemispheric supratentorial astrocytomas in children. J. Neurosurg. *55,* 170–173 (1981)
12. Milhorat, T. H.: Pediatric neurosurgery. Philadelphia: Davis 1978
13. Paraicz, E., Szenàsy, J.: Brain tumours in infancy and childhood: A report of 843 treated cases. Acta. Paediat. Acad. Sci. Hung. *22,* 251–258 (1981)
14. Raimondi, A. J., Gutierrez, F. A.: Diagnosis and surgical treatment of choroid plexus papillomas. Child's Brain. *1,* 81–115 (1975)
15. Russel, D. S., Rubinstein, K. J.: Pathology of tumours of the nervous system London: 4th ed. E. Arnold 1976
16. Seiler, R. W.: Late results of multimodality therapy of high grade supratentorial astrocytomas. Surg. Neurol. *15,* 88–91 (1981)
17. Starr, M. A.: Tumours of the brain in childhood. Med. News. *54,* 29 (1889)
18. Tiyaworabun, S., Kramer, H. H., Lim, D. P., Bock, W. J.: Cerebral arteriovenous malformations in children: Clinical analysis and follow-up results. Child's Brain. *8,* 232 (1981)
19. Tiyaworabun, S., Nicola, N., Schirmer, M., Seibert, H., Parsch, U.: Detection of angiographically "cryptic" cerebral vascular malformations by computerized tomography. Presented at the 32th Annual meeting of German Society of Neurosurgery in Tübingen, 1981. Adv. Neurosurg. *10,* 117–123 (1982)
20. Zülch, K. J.: Historical development of the classification of brain tumours and the new proposal of the world health organisation (WHO). Neurosurg. Rev. *4,* 123–127 (1981)

Discussion

To start with *P. Gutjahr (Mainz)* and the audience discussed how one should regard such treatment regimes, if randomisation offered any advantages and where they should be encouraged and where not. Furthermore, on account of the small morbidity figures it was quite clear that nation-wide studies were necessary.

D. Schreiber (Erfurt) in discussing the problem of second tumours, pointed out that the accidental coincidence still had to be paid for. *P. Gutjahr (Mainz)* in answer to the particular question said that the interval between radiation and the appearance of a second tumour was between seven and ten years. If the intervals are short one should probably not accuse the treatment entirely for the appearance of the second tumour.

Habermalz (Berlin) stressed how very much his findings after lengthy treatment differed from those which had been collected by B. Walther and P. Gutjahr. He had never seen such extensive damage; he had performed thorough neurological examinations in the course of which he had carefully scrutinized fine motor function as well as co-ordination. It was pointed out in the discussion which followed that these different findings in the late results possibly were the results of differences in the technique of testing.

B. Walther (Mainz) stated that, for her part, she was extremely concerned by the extent of the damage to these children. The children were continually conscious in their everyday life of the disability produced by this damage. These findings are therefore most important and relevant to the life-style of thė child and are not 'created' by particularly subtle methods of investigation. She said in addition, that the condition of the child before the radiotherapy is important; children who are already in poor condition before any treatment, generally show definitely more marked injury both during and after treatment.

The findings of *W. Andler (Essen)* led to a series of comments in the course of the discussion. *J. Kutzner (Mainz)* asked to what extent retarded growth is considered the result of an overt hypothyroidism or possibly is the result of a growth hormone deficiency. *W. Andler (Essen)* replied that hypothyroidism was only apparent in 12 out of 33 patients, to the extent that there was an impairment of growth in height, that is to say a retardation of the skeletal bone age. The clinical symptoms in all patients had been very scanty. In every case, however, there had been a slowing of growth. He pointed out further, that naturally the diagnosis had been confirmed by laboratory studies.

H. Gerlach (Halle) noted that endocrine disturbances should be expected in lesions near the sella, whereas they are generally absent in lesions remote from the sella. There is, however, and exception to these findings; he mentioned a patient with a gangliocytoma of the posterior fossa with definite endocrine disturbances.

In reply to the paper from *S. Tiyaworabun (Düsseldorf) H. Gerlach* said that the reports about sex distribution are often extremely misleading. Thus, it had been stated that with material from childhood tumours medulloblastomas undoubtedly predominated in girls, while in adults it is predominantly the males who are affected. Choroid plexus papillomas show an equal sex distribution in children, in contrast to the findings in adults.

Final Comment and Summing-Up

P. GUTJAHR and D. VOTH

Among the neoplasms which occur in the paediatric age group, tumours of the CNS can be regarded as posing the most complex problems. This, however, is only a partial and very general explanation for the evident uncertainties in the clinical management of these tumours.

In general there are no uniform and standardized ideas as to the timing of any operation and what is to be achieved in treating these children. This is particularly true in deciding how aggressive one should be in the operative procedure. Similar problems also apply to radiation treatment. What is the precise value of irradiation as part of a concept of treatment by a variety of means? The role of chemotherapy remains largely undetermined, although various drugs have come into use during recent years, mostly after preliminary reports which were initially promising.

Uncertainties and contradictions even exist with regard to the problems of late sequelae in long-term survivors of brain tumours in childhood, although at first sight these results appear to have been analysed quite objectively.

All these facts, which at the moment suggest that the clinical aspects of tumours of the CNS in children represent – with certain exceptions – the most backward branch of paediatric oncology, have justified the holding of this symposium in Mainz during the three days, Oct. 22nd–24th, 1981.

The objective of this symposium was not to hope for the presentation of dramatic innovations in brain tumour research or treatment, but we intended firstly to put forward a summary of the present situation and secondly to improve the exchange of information among clinicians in different disciplines, such as neurosurgeons, paediatric oncologists, radiotherapists, neuroradiologists and neuropathologists. In this way, the mutual understanding of the problems could be encouraged, and further activities could perhaps be promoted in the future, possibly on a multicentre basis.

We also acknowledge with gratitude that several investigators of high repute from the fields of basic research and pathology have enriched the sessions by their valuable contributions.

Within the past three days, we have heard 65 papers and reports. It became evident at a very early stage of this symposium that much more time should have been available for the presentations and especially for the discussions from which so often many more important points emerged. However, within the limitations available, we believe that comprehensive, up-to-date views on the problems have been presented. These should serve in many ways as the possible starting point for future projects.

We learned that the WHO histopathological classification of brain tumours is not accepted everywhere in its entirety. However, to help the children who are affected, clear and unambiguous language is needed among pathologists, and the uniform classification system required should not only be used uniformly but should in addition incorporate relevant clinical information.

If we assume that a total of 400 new cases of brain tumour in children is seen every year in the Federal Republic of Germany, and hence, each treatment centre has a limited experience even of the more frequent tumour types, it is not acceptable that more than one classification system should be in general use, particularly when there are perhaps 80 or more histopathological subtypes in each of the classifications.

There were very interesting reports on chemical and viral carcinogenesis, referring in part to the question of defective DNA-repair mechanisms. Indeed, most of the participants in the symposium had the impression that cancer research has stepped forward during recent years. However, it is not yet enough to have a great number of potential chemical carcinogens identified. Data of molecular biological importance have to be further sought for, and one day a solid bridge must be built, which may then connect basic research projects intensively with basic clinical problems in favour of the affected children.

During one of the discussions clinicians justly stressed the fact that important knowledge concerning epidemiological research and chemical carcinogenesis has arisen from clinical observations and not from research laboratories; as an example of this the Diethylstilbestrol – consequences on unborn children were cited.

By clinical observation, a number of patients can be identified, who have a genetically determined risk for tumours of the CNS. The phakomatoses may possibly be a model for early detection and prevention of tumours in this regard.

The interferon problem was shown to have a fascinating theoretical background. Its clinical use, however, especially in brain tumours, is far from being indicated in humans. The same must be supposed concerning any other kind of immunotherapy of human brain tumours, at this time.

We heard of the different composition of tumour types in different child age groups, and of rarer neoplasms in infancy and childhood. These differences again suggest that various influences may lead to brain tumours in childhood, that their clinical expression evidently changes during life, and that there is not a single causative releasing factor; on the other hand, the rare tumour types make all the more necessary the need for regional, national or international clinical studies on brain tumours. Thus in certain regards, neonatal and infantile tumours need to be investigated in this manner.

The need for a careful neurological examination was examplified and underlined in one paper. This aspect needs to be be emphasized especially at a time, which – in our opinion – perhaps rather runs the risk of become too trusting in the CT and its present abilities. CT should be – in general – a means for the confirmation of a diagnosis and it does not in any way replace the neurological examination. In any case this should precede the planned CT examination; one must recognize early changes in the clinical states, and must suspect a lesion.

CT confirms a suspected diagnosis, but it is important in the primary diagnostic measures, as sometimes it may determine the tumour type with a high degree of certainty. Further experience, however, with follow-up examinations by CT and its clinical significance will have to be gained in the near future. Until now, there may be diagnostic and prognostic CT-problems in judging clearly e.g. meningeal seeding of tumour cells, recurrences in the former operation field and other treatment fields such as those exposed to radiation treatment. They often have to be cautiously interpreted and in most cases need detailed clinical information, and not merely the picture of a CT-investigation. It is not always possible with CT alone to decide that a mass is a tumour recurrence.

Other new diagnostic procedures from the field of neurophysiology were presented (acoustic and visual evoked potentials), with emphasis on their importance also in clinical follow-up investigations. CSF cytology may also have an important role especially in malignant disease; work in this field should be intensified. As the results of such investigations clearly depend on the long-term experience of the investigator and his laboratory personnel, this can be taken as another argument in favour of the centralization of treatment and long-term follow-up of children with brain tumours.

The current advances in the study of epilepsy made it necessary to have a report on this problem presented at our meeting. It is not advisable to put every child after brain tumour treatment on routine anticonvulsant drugs, the more so, as this procedure may even provoke adverse effects in some patients.

There was a controversy during the meeting concerning the need and also the frequency of so-called "conventional" x-ray diagnostic measures, such as ventriculography and cerebral angiography. It was quite clearly stated that there are certain indications for these investigations. Of course, the number of conventional neuroradiological examinations has been – and must continue to be – reduced in some institutions. However the decisions concerning the need for ventriculography and/or angiography must be made by the clinician responsible for the treatment. Close and continuing interdisciplinary discussion between neurosurgeons and neuroradiologists should of course, be encouraged.

The second day of the meeting dealt with operative and radiation treatment. Impressive contributions were made regarding the present day standards and abilities of neurosurgeons including microneurosurgical procedures. It became evident that the neurosurgical treatment of tumours has improved remarkably throughout the past decade.

Shunting procedures are frequently necessary in brain tumours in children. The question, which type of shunt system should be used, must consider other clinical data than merely the obstruction, e.g. the later radiation field and/or concomitant chemotherapy planned.

This again requires an early and close cooperation between neurosurgeons, radiotherapists, and paediatric oncologists. Similar problems have to be discussed with regard to implanting artificial devices, needed possibly, for intraventricular or other tumour therapy, e.g. with cytostatics.

Stereotactic biopsy and tumour treatment by implantation of radioactive seeds were presented as an often useful procedure. As for diagnosis however, there remains some uncertainty about this method, as shown by the number of specimens that do not allow one to establish an exact diagnosis. Accordingly this procedure should – in our opinion – be performed only in selected cases. As for the therapeutic importance of stereotactic treatment, this cannot yet be finally judged. Selected cases, however, may be suitable to be permanently and successfully treatment by this method. Evaluation of the results as a whole was difficult, as the results of treatment were presented as a whole, and were not specified according to tumour types and age of patients.

The possibilities and limitations of radiotherapy were detailed in another session of the meeting. We had the impression that the indications for irradiation are regarded differently at different institutions; occasionally radiotherapy may have to be performed in tumours without histological confirmation (brainstem).

To judge the results of radiotherapy, often quite old groups of patients have to serve as controls. Therefore, the real value of present-day radiotherapy (under circumstances of modern neurosurgery) often remains questionable.

In general, there is a need to try to reduce radiation doses. The side-effects of radiotherapy are well known. By this, one can understand that alternative methods of treatment such as internal radiotherapy (implantation of radioactive seeds and others) must be carefully followed with regard to their true effects. This also concerns the effects of long-term therapy. In this regard, there is one special aspect in children: it is not a goal in the treatment of perhaps a two-year-old child to prolong his life for a couple of months or one year; the situation – independant of the time which the patients remains in hospital – is quite different in a 70-year-old adult. Treatment in children aims at first at a permanent cure, not at palliation and prolonging life for a short span in infants and young children. It is only secondly that palliative procedures should be considered (e.g. palliative shunts, anti-oedematous treatment for pain relief etc.).

In another lecture it was pointed out that the quality of radiotherapeutic treatment is highly important as a prognostic factor. Adequate standards of radiotherapy have probably not yet been realized everywhere.

Other papers, concerning e.g. multiagent chemotherapy prior to radiotherapy, seem to present an alternate way of treatment in medulloblastoma patients; however, they cannot yet be judged definitely.

There were possibly some reservations concerning chemotherapy. In our opinion these are not justified. The use of chemotherapy does not originate from the wishes of chemotherapists. It has developed rather, from a need to offer a more promising outlook in brain tumour treatment in children, in whom operation and radiotherapy alone do not promise cure.

We further learned in our sessions that the results of treatment have to be carefully analysed. Some statistical analyses exclude a number of patients (e.g. medulloblastoma patients who have not come to radiotherapy); the selection criteria have to be read and interpreted carefully, in order not to have a misleading impression of treatment results reported from some centres.

The third day of the symposium was devoted to chemotherapy and the late sequelae.

Several single agents used in chemotherapy have shown some effects in the treatment of brain tumours of childhood. However, results do not yet suggest that chemotherapy alone – or in combination with radiotherapy – will be a substitute for a successful operation. Whenever the latter seems possible, or in cases where operation cannot result in cure (because of the site of the tumour or its special biological features) these chemotherapeutic agents should be used in the majority of cases.

Single agent chemotherapy has certainly proved effective in some patients. The more promising conceptions include combination chemotherapy; the rationale of the latter was presented in one lecture.

Various acute side-effects of combination chemotherapy have to be considered. Before starting such treatment, one should try to calculate the balance of risks and benefits. The possible side-effects – tumour-related or therapy-dependent – cover a large field. Doctors caring for survivors, and long-term survivors especially, should be aware of the wide range of these side-effects, and they must be able to maintain a permanent and close contact with other paediatric subspecialities in order to overcome the late adverse effects as far as possible. There was evidence of controversy in the diagnosis of late neurophysiological sequelae. Also in this regard we have to standardize the diagnostic routine and we must not rely on the pressures of wished-for and of desirable therapeutic success. The patients' fate and destiny are the factors which have priority in any consideration of treatment. This includes the quality of survival.

This first interdisciplinary cooperative symposium in our country on the subject of brain tumours in childhood made clear that several firm data can be accepted as a basis for the current diagnostic and therapeutic standards in managing children with primary brain tumours. Many questions remain open, however.

There is no doubt that benign CNS tumours, radically operated on, have a good prognosis. In other cases, there persists a great variability in deciding on treatment. A certain agreement about treatment policy has been reached in medulloblastomas, without, however, having dramatically changed and improved the results. The number and severity of late effects makes further thought about the treatment of medulloblastoma all the more necessary.

Radiotherapy and chemotherapy do not seem to offer any great break-through in treating brain tumours within the next few years as has been possible in other childhood malignancies.

During this meeting there were often huge numbers of patients and treatments reported in some of the lectures. They often reflected the great merits of an individual therapist or scientist. However, they sometimes did not give very much information about the actual outlook for certain tumours, e.g. based on prospective studies, or the statements we heard lacked clarity and any definite guidance to others!

One of the main aims of this symposium was to bring all the participating scientists and clinicians together, and to have the present day position of brain tumours in childhood defined. This has been reached, not without imposing some physical load on all of us. We hope that at the end of the symposium, everyone understands a little better the special and general problems of his colleagues in related medical disciplines concerned with diagnosis and treatment of brain tumours in childhood.

The formidable problems (for instance composition of combination chemotherapies and combination therapies in those tumours, where operation alone does not lead to cures) have to be worked on by intense collaboration among all of us. The value of additional types of treatment can – in our opinion – only be judged satisfactorily by regional or multicentre experience. It cannot be managed by one centre alone because of the lack of adequate numbers of patients with a single tumour type likely to be seen within a reasonable time span.

If this symposium has helped to promote further or to initiate interdisciplinary, interinstitutional and multicentre cooperation, it will have fulfilled its original purpose.

Subject Index

Page references of major topics discussed are given in *italics*

Abdominal pain, chemotherapy 380
Acoustic evoked potentials 429
ADH 418
ADH-secretion, inappropriate 380
Adiuretic hormone 418
Adrenocortical carcinoma and medullo-
 blastoma 387
Adrenocortical insufficiency 417
Age groups 1
Age preference 4
Ala cinerea 209
Alkylation 376
Anaplasia 18
Anaplastic astrocytoma 423
Angioblastoma 4
Angiography 107
Anorexia 75
Apathy-syndrome see somnolence
 Aquaeduct 4, 6
Arachnoidal sarcoma 404
Arachnoiditis, methotrexate 380
Area postrema 209
Arteriovenous malformations, radio-
 therapy 366
Astroblastoma 206, 423
Astrocytoma 2, 3, 5, 6, 9, 45, 54, 55, 56, 59, 63, 66, 81, *117*, 131, 249, 326, 359
 clinical history 399
 CT *117*
 giant cell 118
 late effects 384
 localization 401
 metastases of *165*
 neurology 400
 piloid 206, 208, 399
 radionuclide imaging 125
 radiotherapy 325, 358
 in v. Recklinghausen's disease 386
 sites 326
 treatment results 401
Au-Colloid 354

Backward children 386
Balance of trunk 384
BCNU 368
 side effects 378
Behaviour, changes in 80
Benefit of therapy 431
Bleomycin 365
Blind spot 413
Blood-brain-barrier
 alterations 292
 chemotherapy 374
Biopsy, CT-stereotactic 234, 247
Brain oedema
 peritumoural *229*
 therapy *223*, *229*
Brain stem 78, 100, *190*
 astrocytoma *147*
  prognosis 147
 organisation 190
 tumours 211
  chemotherapy 358
  radiotherapy 358
  results 334
Brain spatula 203
Broca's area 199

Calamus scriptorius 209
Carcinogens 11, *19*, 28
Catch-up growth 385
CBF 199
CCNU 340, 360, 361, 368, 376
 in medulloblastoma 390
 side effects 378
Cerebellar affection, long-term survivors 394
Cerebellar artery
 anterior inferior 209
 posterior inferior 209
Cerebellar astrocytomas see astrocytoma
 eye in 411
 radiotherapy 358
Cerebellar peduncle, infiltration of 209
Cerebral dysfunction 395
Cerebrospinal fluid, cytology *85*
Chemotherapy *338*, 360, *367*, 430
 acute side effects 378
 blood brain barrier 367

choice of drugs 375
combination 374
concentration in tumour cells 367
concentration of drugs in CSF 367
criteria remission 371, 376
impaired CSF-flow 375
intracarotid perfusion 374, 379
intrathecal 375
medulloblastoma 392
meningeal carcinomatosis 375
monotherapy 367
preradiotherapeutic 349
role of 427
side effects 341
Chiasm 6
Children, goal of treatment 430
Choked discs 410, 412
Chondroma 422
Choroid plexus papilloma 2, 6, 9, 44, 45, 54, 55, 59, 63, 66, 118, 206, 249
CT 118
Choroid plexus tumours 422
Choroidal arteries 202
Cis-Platinum 365
Citrovorum factor rescue 370
Classification of brain tumours 1, 3, 428
Clinical observation and basic research 428
Clinical presentation 75
CNS-toxicity, chemotherapy 378
Cognitive ability 396
Cognitive development, medullo-blastoma 393
Cognitive style 396
Collaboration 431
Combination chemotherapy 374
results 376
Conclusions *427*
Congenital hydrocephalus 423
Conventional investigations *105*
Convulsions, long-term survivors 386
Cooperation 431
Coordination 395
astrocytomas 384
medulloblastomas 384
Cortisol deficiency 417
Cranial nerve
palsies 411
symptoms *77*
Craniectomy, posterior fossa 200, *201*
Craniopharyngioma 2, 6, 44, 55, 59, 121, 131
CT 121
radionuclide imaging 125
radionuclides 365
transsphenoidal approach *270*, 276
Craniospinal
irradiation 390
radiotherapy 345, 361, 362
CSF
cytology *85*
circulation, disturbance 366
CT 106, *111*, *115*, *130*, 142
midline tumours *186*
role of 428
Cure, permanent 430
Cushing's disease 319
Cyclophosphamide 360
in medullobastoma 389
Cytocentrifugation 87
Cytosin-Arabinoside 340
Cytostatics see chemotherapy
Cytotoxics see chemotherapy
Cytoxan 340

Dandy-Walker Syndrome, postoperative 180
Dedifferentiation 9
Deep tendon reflexes, loss 379
Dermoids 64
Desmoplastic medulloblastoma 350
age 405
prognosis 406
Development after medulloblastoma 389
Devices for intraventricular therapy 429
Dexamethasone 222, *229*
Diabetes insipidus 75, 385, 415, 417
Diencephalic syndroms see Russell's syn-drome
Diktyoma see medulloepithelioma
Disorders, medulloblastoma survivors 396
Distance, intercapillary 375
DNA 39

EAEP, early auditory evoked potentials 99
EEG *90*, *95*, 99, 386
in long-term survivors 386
Electrolyte balance 418
Electrophysiological diagnosis *90*
Ellis formula 295
Emaciation 415
Endocrine disorders 385
Endocrine dysfunction 417
Endocrinology 415
Ependymoblastoma *50*
Ependymoma 1, 2, 4, 5, 6, 9, 45, 54, 59, 63, 66, 81, 88, 117, 131, 206, 208, 209, 249
CT 117
radionuclide imaging 125
treatment 339
Ependymospongioblastoma 399
Epidermoids 64
Epilepsy 97, 386
after brain tumours 429
Epipodophyllotoxin 371
side effects 381

Evoked potentials 429
early auditory *99*
visual *90*
Exophthalmos 412
Eye *410*
disturbance 385

Facial nerve 209
Final comment *427*
Fine motor function 384
Follow-up studies *130*
Fundoscopy 385
Furosemide 229

Gangliocytoma 5, 9
Ganglioglioma 45, 66
Ganglioneuroma 4
Genetic mechanisms 37
Genetics *32*
Germ cell tumours 422
Germinoma 4, 6, 10, 45, 80, 121, 249
CT 120
radiotherapy 365
GFAP *58*
Glial fibrillary acidic protein see GFAP
Glioblastoma 17, 45, 47, 54, 59, 63, 81, 87, 131, 249
and acute leukaemia 386
and craniopharyngioma 386
giant cell 3
radionuclide imaging 125
Glioma 44, 47
Gonadal insufficiency 417
Gonadotropin secretion 417
Grading 6, 7, 18
Gross motor function 384
Growth disturbance 385
Growth fraction, glioblastoma 374
Growth hormone deficiency 415

Haemangioblastoma 45, 59
Haemangiopericytoma 45
Handicaps
long-term survivors 394
survivors 397
Headache 75
Hemianopia
bilateral 412
homonymous 413
Hemisphere tumours 423
HGH 385
Hormones *415*
Human growth hormone 385
Hyperinsulinaemia 418
Hypernatraemia 418
Hyperprolactinaemia 418
Hyperventilation 223, 224

Hypodipsia 418
Hypoglycaemia 417
Hypogonadism, secondary 417
Hypoplasia of the genitals 75
Hypothalamus 6
emaciation syndrome 418
Hypothyroidism 75, 386, 415
hypothalamic 418

ICP see intracranial pressure
Immunoblastoma 46
Immunodefense 39
Immunotherapy 428
Infancy, tumour-signs 424
Infratentorial tumours 358
removal *199*
Inoperable midline tumours, follow-up finding *186*
Instruments, microsurgical 205
Intensive care *222*
Interferon *42*, 428
Interstitial radiotherapy 304
Interventriculostomy see Leksell drainage
Intracranial pressure (ICP) *218*, 222, 278, 286
epidural recording 219
measurement 226
Intraventricular tumours 205
Isolated fourth ventricle *180*

Kinaesthesia 396

Labetalol *278*
Late effects *383*, 431
Late sequelae 383, 427
Late side effects, treatment *383*
Leksell drainage 211, *214*
results *283*
Leukaemia 354
Leukencephalopathy 295, 366, 380
subacute 292
Lipoma 64
Lobectomy 201
Long-term care 383
Long-term suvivors *383*
visual disturbances 385
Lymphoma 422
primary malignant 45

Malformations *19*
vascular 422
MeCCNU 369, 376
side effects 378
Medulloblastoma 2, 3, 6, 44, 45, 54, 59, 63, 66, 81, 82, 87, 88, 131, 208, 209, 249
adults 351
biology *350*
chemotherapy 339, 349, 360, 362, 407

Medulloblastoma
combination therapy 342
cranial nerve symptoms 391
CT 115
desmoplastic 5
eye in 411
histology 404
hydrocephalus 391
intracranial pressure 391
localization 351
long-term survivors 389
neurological late effects *389*
neurological state 391, 392
prognosis 351, 405
psychosocial state 390
radionuclide imaging 125
radiotherapy 344, 360, 407
results of treatment 334, 345
staging system 82
survival *360,* 361
in survivors 384
treatment 339, *358,* 389, 392, 405
treatment study 349
Medulloepithelioma 45, 49
of the eye *169*
prognosis 172
treatment 173
Meningioma 9, 45, 59, 63
Meningiosis 354
Mesencephalon, organisation 190
Metastases, extracranial *165*
Metastatic tumours 423
Methotrexate 296, 340, 354, 360
high dose 370, 380
liver toxicity 380
neurotoxicity 380
in medulloblastoma 389
side effects 378, 380
Methyl-CCNU see MeCCNU
Metronidazole 335
Microangiopathy, mineralising 296
Microneurosurgery *199*
historical retrospect 204
infratentorial lesions *207*
supratentorial tumours *205*
Microscope 204
Midbrain tumours 326
radiotherapy 325
Midline shift 229
Midline tumours 423
inoperable *186*
Misonidazole 335
Monstrocellular sarcoma 422
Morbidity of brain tumours 428
Mortality, operative 366
Motility disorders, medulloblastoma 394
Motor dysfunction, medulloblastoma 396
Motor function 384
Movement dynamics 384
Multicentre experience 431
Myelography 114
Myelosuppression, chemotherapy 378

Nerve conduction velocities 386
Neurinoma 4, 45, 59
Neurofibromatosis 33
Neurological signs *76*
Neuromotor dysfunction, medulloblastoma survivors 395
Neuro-oncogenesis, experimental *19*
Neurophysiology 429
Neuropsychological investigation 393
Nitroso-urea 368
side effects 378
Nominal standard dose 295
Nystagmus 410, 413

Obex 209
Ocular findings *77*
Oligodendroglioma 4, 45, 59, 63, 66, 81, 249, 422
Ommaya-Reservoir *265*
Operation, timing of 427
Operative mortality 211
Ophthalmology 385, 410
late findings *410*
Optic fascicle 6
Optic glioma 66, 90
Optic nerve atrophy 412
after treatment 385
Osmoreceptor dysfunction 418

Palliation 430
Papilloedema 411, 412
Paralysis, Vincristine 380
Performance 384
neurological 385
Pineal tumours 6, 9, 10, 334
treatment 339
Pinealoma 2, 4, 119
Pituitary adenoma 4, 45
Pituitary dysfunction 415
Polychemotherapy, acute side effects 381
Polydipsia 417
Polyuria 417
Pons 4
glioma of 117
Pontine tumours 359
prognosis 359
radiotherapy 362
Posterior fossa operations *207*
Post-irradiation syndrome 295
Procarbazine 344, 370, 376, 379
side effects 378

Prognosis, brain stem astrocytoma *147*
Prolactin 416, 417
Psychosocial, long-term state 386
Psychosocial state, medulloblastoma 390
Puberty, precocious 415, 417

Radiation dose, medulloblastoma 365
Radiation
  myelitis 307
  oedema 292
  quality 305
  technique *301*
Radiocolloids 312
Radiogold 354
Radionecrosis 292
Radionuclids 106, *122*, 311
  dosis 123
  indication for 128
  radiation dose 127
Radioreaction, acute 291
Radiosensitivity *291*
Radiosensitizers 335
Radiosurgery *315*
  arteriovenous malformations 320
  craniopharyngiomas 319
  gamma unit 315
  pineal tumours 318
Radiotherapy 8
  accelerator 365
  combined treatment *333*
  dosage 307
  dose-time diagram 297
  intentions 303
  medulloblastoma 358, 392
  midline tumours *186*
  neuroaxis 338
  subacute reactions 292
  technique 346
  tolerance doses 291
  treatment planning 306
Radiotoxicity 293
Remission, chemotherapy 376
Resection of a lobe 201
Resignation, long-term survivors 394
Results
  of operation 211
  selection of cases 430
Retinoblastoma 172
Rhombencephalon
  infiltration of 209
  organisation *190*
Risk of therapy 431
Rosenthal fibres 6
Russell's syndrome 65

Salt loss 417
Sarcoma *50*, 59
  cerebellar arachnoidal 5
  meningeal 422
  monstrocellular 3
School achievement 396
School attainment, medulloblastoma 393
Second malignancies 426
Second neoplasms 386, 387, 426
Sedimentation technique 87
Seizures *79*
Sellar region, tumours of *276*
Sensorimotor system, long-term
  survivors 385
Sex preferences 4
Sexual development 417
Short stature 415
Shunt
  complications 215
  systems *214*
  ventriculo-atrial 214
  ventriculo-peritoneal 214
Side effects
  long-term 384
  acute 431
Skull X-ray *105*
Somatomedin 418
Somnolence syndrome 295
Spinal cord 4, 114
  tumours of 5
Spongioblastoma see astrocytoma
  circumscribed 401
Squint 413
Stenosis of the aquaeduct 180
Stereotactic biopsy *234*
Stereotaxy *310*, 429
Strabismus 410, 413
Studies, clinical 428
Supratentorial radiotherapy, medullo-
  blastoma 362
Supratentorial tumours *420*
  chemotherapy 425
  histologic classification 422
  investigations 421
  localization 421
  mortality 421
  radiotherapy 425
  removal *199*
  shunt 422
  surgical death 423
Survival
  quality of 431
  curves 363
  times 7
Symptoms
  first 67
  of tumours 74
Synchronisation
  tumour cells 375

Tanycyte 18
Teratogenesis 28
Teratoma 3, 4, 45, 50, 54, 55, 63, 66, *69,* 174
  CT 174
Thalamus 4
Therapy, long-term sequelae *383*
Third ventricle, tumours 327
Thyrotropin releasing hormone 415
Thyroxin treatment 418
Tomography 106
Torkildsen drainage *214,* 223
Total care 364
Toxicity, chemotherapy *378*
Transventricular approach 206
Treatment, late, side effects 383
Trigonum hypoglossi 209
TRH see thyrotropin releasing hormone
Tuberous sclerosis 33
Tumours
  brain stem 211
  clinical presentation *75*
  CNS *62*
  dysontogenetic 64
  epidemiology 9
  experimental radiation 11
  extraventricular 5, 6
  familial aggregations 32
  familial occurrence 10
  genetic disorders 32
  heterogeneity 375
  identification, cell *85*
  induction 23
  meningeal *50*
  microsurgery *199*
  midline 145
  morbidity 428
  neuroepithelial 44, 45
  optic chiasm *90*
  pathogenesis 9
  radiation-induced 293
  removal of *199*
  sex incidence 44
  shunting procedures 429
  spinal *53,* 56
  supratentorial *420*
  trauma 11

Vascular malformation 127
Ventricle, isolated fourth *180*
Ventricular drainage 214
Ventricular fluid drainage *257*
Ventriculocisternal drainage see Torkildsen
  drainage
Ventriculocisternal shunt in pontine
  tumours 358
Ventriculocisternostomy see Leksell
  drainage *283*
Ventriculography *142, 145,* 199, 209, 223
  indications *140, 145*
  midline tumours *186*
Vertigo 75
Visual evoked potentials 429
Visual field 385, 410
  loss 412, 413
Vincristine 340, 344, 360, 370, 379, 389
  side effects 378
Virus 11
VM-26 371
  side effects 378
Vomiting 75

Wernicke's area 199

Computer Reformations of the Brain and Skull Base

By R. Unsöld, C. B. Ostertag, J. DeGroot, T. H. Newton

1982. 237 figures including 76 colored plates.
Approx. 245 pages
ISBN 3-540-11544-7

Contents: General Considerations. - Orbit and Paranasal Sinuses. - Anterior Cranial Fossa. - Temporal Lobe and Insula. - Sella, Pituitary Gland, Suprasellar Cistern, and Parasellar Area. - Supratentorial Circumventricular Structures. - Quadrigeminal Cistern. - Occipital Lobe. - Prepontine and Cerebellopontine Cisterns. - Cerebellum and Fourth Ventricle. - Lower Brain Stem, Cisterna Magna, Posterior Skull Base. - Index.

The first guide to the optimal use of computer reformation in almost every conceivable plane of the brain and skull base regions is provided in this book. It contains detailed descriptions of normal anatomy in the clinically most important section and reformation planes and compares them with normal CT anatomy. Diagnostic techniques and approaches are then described and illustrated on the basis of case histories.

Functional and pathologic anatomy of the cranial compartments is covered with a view toward localizing the symptoms most often encountered in clinical practice. The optimal choice of section and reformation plane prior to radiologic examination itself is facilitated by an index of clinical signs indicating the location of the suspected lesion or pathologic process. A brief description of common surgical approaches is also provided to allow radiologists to correctly interpret lesions resulting from earlier operations.

With its wealth of information, concise presentation and handy format, this book will prove an indispensable manual for work at the light box and at the CT console.

Springer-Verlag
Berlin
Heidelberg
New York

MIX
Papier aus verantwortungsvollen Quellen
Paper from responsible sources
FSC® C105338

If you have any concerns about our products,
you can contact us on
ProductSafety@springernature.com

In case Publisher is established outside the EU,
the EU authorized representative is:
Springer Nature Customer Service Center GmbH
Europaplatz 3, 69115 Heidelberg, Germany

Printed by Libri Plureos GmbH
in Hamburg, Germany